A Guide to Genetic Counseling

A Guide to Genetic Counseling

Second Edition

Edited by

Wendy R. Uhlmann
Division of Molecular Medicine and Genetics
University of Michigan

Jane L. Schuette
Division of Pediatric Genetics
University of Michigan

Beverly M. Yashar
Department of Human Genetics
University of Michigan

WILEY-BLACKWELL
A JOHN WILEY & SONS, INC., PUBLICATION

Wiley-Blackwell is an imprint of John Wiley & Sons, formed by the merger of Wiley's global Scientific, Technical, and Medical business with Blackwell Publishing.

Published by John Wiley & Sons, Inc., Hoboken, New Jersey
Published simultaneously in Canada

For general information on our other products and services or for technical support, please contact our Customer Care Department within the United States at (800) 762-2974, outside the United States at (317) 572-3993 or fax (317) 572-4002.

Wiley also publishes its books in a variety of electronic formats. Some content that appears in print may not be available in electronic formats. For more information about Wiley products, visit our web site at www.wiley.com.

Library of Congress Cataloging-in-Publication Data:

A guide to genetic counseling / [edited by] Wendy R. Uhlmann, Jane L. Schuette, Beverly M. Yashar. – 2nd ed.
        p. ; cm.
    Includes bibliographical references and index.
    ISBN 978-0-470-17965-9 (pbk.)
    1. Genetic counseling. I. Uhlmann, Wendy R., 1961- II. Schuette, Jane L., 1956- III. Yashar, Beverly M., 1957
    [DNLM: 1. Genetic Counseling. QZ 50 G946 2009]
    RB155.7.G85 2009
    616′.042–dc22
                                                    2009004199

Printed in the United States of America

10 9 8 7 6 5 4 3 2

*To our patients and their families, from whom we receive the
inspiration to pursue our work
and
to our students, who provide the
opportunity for us to look at our work in new ways.*

Contents

3   Interviewing: Beginning to See Each Other   71

Kathryn Spitzer Kim

4   Thinking It All Through: Case Preparation and Management   93

Wendy R. Uhlmann

5   Psychosocial Counseling   133

Luba Djurdjinovic

6 Patient Education   177

Ann C.M. Smith and Toni I. Pollin

7 Risk Communication and Decision-Making   207

Bonnie Jeanne Baty

Foreword

Genetic counseling is often thought of as a young profession. But that perception may be misguided. Genetic counseling as a clinical service was defined more than 60 years ago, the first genetic counseling class graduated nearly 40 years ago, the National Society of Genetic Counselors is 30 years old, and genetic counseling training programs span the globe. And now this book—the first comprehensive genetic counseling text—is in its second edition. We are not the new kids on the block anymore.

The appearance of youth is perhaps due to a widespread lack of awareness of the profession. Why would most people need to know about genetic services when such a narrow segment of the population initially needed our services?

Over the last four decades, the portion of the patient population that needs genetic counseling services has steadily expanded. When advances in genetic knowledge, theory, and technology inevitably found their way into the medical care and lives of families, a wider swath of the general public discovered anew the need for genetic counseling by properly trained professionals. In the early years, genetic counselors met mostly with parents of children with genetic diseases or adults who had relatively uncommon disorders like Neurofibromatosis, Marfan syndrome and Ehlers–Danlos syndrome. Then came pregnant women, at first, only those over 35, and eventually pregnancies with abnormal serum or sonographic findings and carriers of recessive diseases as carrier testing expanded to a wider range of conditions. This was followed by the 10% of breast/ovarian/colon cancer patients who have a hereditary basis to their disease. Now we are counseling patients and families who are at risk for cardiovascular, neurological, and other common diseases, as well as anyone with a computer who wants to utilize online genetic testing. We seem like a new profession to each segment of the population who suddenly need genetic services.

Genetic counseling is not primarily about diagnosing genetic diseases, although genetic counselors often play a key role in that process. Rather, genetic counseling is more about the steps leading up to deciding about a genetic test or what happens once a diagnosis is made or a test result is positive. This is where the human meets the genome, the stage on which the human drama—or comedy, as Balzac or Saroyan would broadly describe it—plays itself out as families learn to cope with and adapt to the medical, social, and psychological impact of hereditary diseases.

How do you tell a couple who have been trying to get pregnant for 10 years that their unborn baby—their one and only pregnancy—has a lethal condition? How do you break the news to immigrant parents, who barely speak English and are so proud of their first child born in a new country, that their son will be cognitively and physically challenged, without losing focus on the child's humanity and dignity and the family's cultural values? How do you discuss limiting physical activity with a 15-year-old star player of her school basketball team after a "'fainting spell" leads to a diagnosis of long QT syndrome? How do you tell a newly married 30-year-old woman that she faces a high risk of developing ovarian cancer, the same disease her mother and sister died of by the time they were 40, while maintaining hope and guiding her to take control of her risk before her risk controls her? How do you explain to a 70-year-old man that his Parkinson-like symptoms are related to his grandson's fragile X syndrome? What ethical principles guide you through these experiences? What counseling and educational skills do you need to help patients understand and act on their risks and diagnoses? How do you set up your clinic to make sure that your services are properly delivered and patients are appropriately evaluated and followed? How do you keep yourself educated in the rapidly expanding universe of genetic information? How do you maintain your sanity, health, commitment, and passion? How do you train the next generation of genetic counselors so they can use what we already know and adapt genetic counseling to discoveries about what we do not yet know?

Turn the page and find out.

Swedish Medical Center   ROBERT G. RESTA, M.A., M.S., C.G.C.
Seattle, WA

Preface

The first edition of this book was a landmark achievement—the first book written by genetic counselors on the principles and practice of genetic counseling. Since its publication in 1998, much has changed—the Human Genome Project has been completed, over 1700 genetic tests are available, and the profession has seen substantial growth, nationally and internationally. The goals of the second edition remain the same—to provide a comprehensive overview of genetic counseling, focusing on the components, theoretical framework, and unique approach to patient care that are the basis of this profession. The book covers the genetic counseling process, from case initiation to completion, and uses a broad lens that makes this information generally applicable to all areas of clinical genetic counseling.

Genetic counselors have created roles for themselves in an expanding array of medical specialties and assumed important roles in settings that extend beyond the clinic, including research, industry, commercial laboratories, Internet companies, public policy, education, and public health. In recognition of genetic counselors' role expansion, new chapters in this edition include "Genetic Counseling Research: Understanding the Basics," "Evolving Roles, Expanding Opportunities," and "Genetic Counselors as Educators." In addition, there is a new chapter on "Risk Communication and Decision-Making."

As in the first edition, the chapters are organized in a manner to facilitate academic instruction and skill attainment. Chapter 1 provides an overview of the history and field of genetic counseling. Chapters 2–11 describe the components of genetic counseling, including content on how to obtain family and medical history information, conduct a genetics medical evaluation, case preparation and management, genetic testing, medical documentation, patient interviewing, psychosocial considerations, multicultural counseling, patient education, risk communication and facilitation of decision-making. Chapter 12 focuses on some of the ethical and legal issues that arise in cases and in our professional interactions with patients and other healthcare professionals. Chapters 13–17 address professional issues, which include providing and receiving clinical supervision, writing research proposals and conducting research, giving presentations, continuing education, professional development, and expansion of genetic counselors' positions in clinical and non-clinical settings. The final chapter helps the reader see how it all fits together, using specific genetic counseling case examples.

All chapters in the second edition have been updated. Case vignettes are included in several chapters, and there are several tables that can be used as checklists for case preparation and management, presentations, clinical supervision, writing research proposals, and conducting research. Several chapters are lengthy, packed with content and details, and will be best approached by reading in more than one sitting. You will find some topics addressed in more than one chapter, covered from different perspectives and for varied applications. Some topics are not covered in great depth because it would take an entire book to appropriately cover the topic. Given how rapidly web addresses change, we have kept website citations to a minimum, mainly those that cannot be accessed from a name search. Since the focus of this book is the practice of genetic counseling and not genetic conditions, we recommend that you access GeneReviews, Online Mendelian Inheritance in Man, and the literature for specific information about cited conditions.

The field of genetic counseling began in the United States and has spread internationally, with genetic counseling programs in many countries. We wish to acknowledge that our book is written from an American perspective; it is beyond the book's scope to address genetic counseling in other countries. The principles of genetic counseling are universal, even though the practice of genetic counseling varies nationally and internationally. Whether you are a student, teacher, supervisor, healthcare professional or just interested in learning about genetic counseling, this book will serve as a comprehensive introduction and reference.

We wish to acknowledge Diane L. Baker, M.S., C.G.C. for her leadership, vision, and dedication to the first edition of this book. We wish to express our appreciation to John Wiley & Sons—Blackwell Publishing for their commitment to publishing this and other books about genetic counseling, particularly Thomas Moore (Senior Editor, Medicine), Kristen Parrish (Production Editor), and Sanchari Sil (Senior Project Manager, Thomson Digital).

Ann Arbor, Michigan   Wendy R. Uhlmann, M.S., C.G.C.
January 2009   Jane L. Schuette, M.S., C.G.C.
                                      Beverly M. Yashar, M.S., Ph.D., C.G.C.

Contributors

Evolving Roles, Expanding Opportunities

ELIZABETH A. BALKITE M.S., C.G.C., President/CEO, ABQ Associates, Inc., Durham, NC

Risk Communication and Decision-Making

BONNIE JEANNE BATY, M.S., C.G.C., L.G.C., Professor, Pediatrics; Program Director, Graduate Program in Genetic Counseling, Division of Medical Genetics, University of Utah Health Sciences Center, Salt Lake City, UT

The Ultimate Genetic Tool: The Family History

ROBIN L. BENNETT, M.S., C.G.C., D.Sc. Hon., Clinical Associate Professor, Senior Genetic Counselor and Co-Director, Division of Medical Genetics, Medical Genetics Clinic, University of Washington Medical Center, Seattle, WA

Putting It All Together: Three Case Examples

DONNA F. BLUMENTHAL, M.S., C.G.C., Senior Genetic Counselor, Division of Medical Genetics, Schneider Children's Hospital, New Hyde Park, NY

Genetic Counselors as Educators

DEBRA L. COLLINS, M.S., C.G.C., Genetic Counselor, Associate Clinical Professor, Department of Internal Medicine, University of Kansas Medical Center, Kansas City, KS

Medical Documentation

DEBRA LOCHNER DOYLE, M.S., C.G.C.,   State Genetics Coordinator, Washington State Department of Health, Manager, Genetic Services Section, Kent, WA

Psychosocial Counseling

LUBA DJURDJINOVIC, M.S.,   Executive Director, Genetic Counselor, Ferre Institute – Genetics Programs, Binghamton, NY

Understanding Genetic Testing

W. ANDREW FAUCETT, M.S., C.G.C.,   Assistant Professor, Department of Human Genetics, Emory University School of Medicine, Atlanta, GA

Professional Identity and Development

ELIZABETH A. GETTIG, M.S., C.G.C.,   Associate Professor, Human Genetics; Co-Director Genetic Counseling Program, Department of Human Genetics, Graduate School of Public Health, University of Pittsburgh, Pittsburgh, PA

Professional Identity and Development

KAREN GREENDALE, M.A., C.G.C.,   Director, Cancer Support and Survivorship Initiatives, Bureau of Chronic Disease Services, New York State Department of Health, Albany, NY

Student Supervision: Strategies for Providing Direction, Guidance, and Support

BONNIE S. LEROY, M.S., C.G.C.,   Associate Professor, Genetics, Cell Biology and Development; Director, Graduate Program of Study in Genetic Counseling, Institute of Human Genetics, University of Minnesota, Minneapolis, MN

Putting It All Together: Three Case Examples

MONICA L. MARVIN M.S., C.G.C.,   Clinical Instructor, Department of Human Genetics and Genetic Counselor, Department of Internal Medicine, University of Michigan, Ann Arbor, MI

Genetic Counselors as Educators

JOSEPH D. MCINERNEY, M.S., M.A.,   Director Emeritus, National Coalition for Health Professional Education in Genetics (NCHPEG), Lutherville, Maryland

Multicultural Counseling

GOTTFRIED OOSTERWAL, Ph.D., Lit. D,   Director, Center for Intercultural Relations, Professor of Medical Anthropology, Berrien Springs, MI

The Medical Genetics Evaluation

ELIZABETH M. PETTY, M.D., FACMG,   Professor, Departments of Internal Medicine and Human Genetics; Associate Dean, Office of Student Programs, University of Michigan Medical School, Ann Arbor, Michigan

Patient Education

TONI I. POLLIN, M.S., Ph.D., C.G.C., Assistant Professor, Division of Endocrinology, Diabetes and Nutrition, Department of Medicine, Program in Genetics and Genomic Medicine, Co-Track Leader, Human Genetics and Genomic Medicine Track, Graduate Program in Epidemiology and Human Genetics, University of Maryland School of Medicine, Baltimore, MD

Ethical and Legal Issues

SUSAN SCHMERLER, M.S., C.G.C., J.D., Supervisor, Genetics Division, St. Joseph's Children's Hospital, Paterson, NJ

The Ultimate Genetic Tool: The Family History
and
Putting It All Together: Three Case Examples

JANE L. SCHUETTE, M.S., C.G.C., Clinical Instructor, Department of Human Genetics; Genetic Counselor, Pediatric Genetics Clinic, University of Michigan Health System, Division of Pediatric Genetics, Ann Arbor, MI

Putting It All Together: Three Case Examples

CHERYL SHUMAN, M.S., C.G.C., Director, Genetic Counselling, Hospital for Sick Children; Associate Professor, Department of Molecular Genetics, Program Director, MSc Program in Genetic Counseling, University of Toronto, Toronto, Ontario, Canada

Patient Education

ANN C.M. SMITH, M.A., D.SC. (HON), C.G.C., Senior Genetic Counselor/ Contractor, Office of the Clinical Director, National Human Genome Research Institute, National Institutes of Health, Bethesda, MD

Evolving Roles, Expanding Opportunities

MAUREEN E. SMITH, M.S., C.G.C., Clinical Director, the NUgene Project, Center for Genetic Medicine, and Instructor, Clinical and Translational Sciences Institute, Northwestern University, Chicago, IL

Interviewing: Beginning to See Each Other

KATHRYN SPITZER KIM, M.S., C.G.C., Coordinator of Counseling Education, Genetic Counseling Program, Arcadia University, Glenside, PA

Thinking It All Through: Case Preparation and Management

WENDY R. UHLMANN, M.S., C.G.C., Clinical Assistant Professor of Internal Medicine and Human Genetics; Genetic Counselor/Clinic Coordinator, Medical Genetics Clinic, Division of Molecular Medicine and Genetics, University of Michigan Health System, Ann Arbor, MI

Student Supervision: Strategies for Providing Direction, Guidance, and Support

PATRICIA MCCARTHY VEACH, PhD., L.P., Professor, Educational Psychology and Distinguished Teaching Professor, Department of Educational Psychology, University of Minnesota, Minneapolis, MN

The Practice of Genetic Counseling

ANN P. WALKER, M.A., C.G.C., Adjunct Professor, Pediatrics and Obstetrics and Gynecology (Retired), Division of Clinical and Metabolic Genetics, Department of Pediatrics, University of California, Irvine, La Jolla, CA

Understanding Genetic Testing

PATRICIA A. WARD, M.S., C.G.C., Director, Genetic Counseling Services and Education, Medical Genetics Laboratories; Instructor, Department of Molecular and Human Genetics, Baylor College of Medicine, Houston, TX

Genetic Counseling Research: Understanding the Basics

BEVERLY M. YASHAR, M.S., C.G.C., Ph.D., Clinical Associate Professor, Human Genetics and Ophthalmology and Visual Sciences; Director, Genetic Counseling Graduate Training Program, Department of Human Genetics, University of Michigan Medical School, Ann Arbor, MI

1

The Practice of Genetic Counseling

Ann P. Walker, M.A., C.G.C.

THE PRACTICE OF GENETIC COUNSELING

Historical Overview

Until the beginning of the last century there existed little scientifically based information for those concerned about the chances of an apparently familial disorder or birth defect occurring (or recurring) in themselves or their offspring. Observations of such conditions had sometimes led to correct interpretations of their pattern of inheritance, as in the understanding of hemophilia evidenced by the Talmudic proscription against circumcising brothers of bleeders, in Broca's report of a seemingly dominant breast cancer predisposition in five generations of his wife's family (Broca, 1866), or in societal taboos against marriages between close relatives. Often, however, birth defects and familial disorders were attributed to exogenous causes—punishment (or perhaps, favor) by a deity, a misdeed on the part of the parents (usually the mother), a fright, a curse, or some natural phenomenon such as an eclipse. Indeed, similar beliefs are still widespread in many cultures and may even figure subliminally in irrational fears of people who are otherwise quite scientifically and medically sophisticated.

Throughout the late 1700s and the 1800s, investigators wrestled with how traits might be transmitted. Lamarck's theories regarding the inheritance of *acquired*

A Guide to Genetic Counseling, Second Edition, Edited by Wendy Uhlmann, Jane Schuette, and Beverly Yashar
Copyright © 2009 by John Wiley & Sons, Inc.

characteristics persisted into the twentieth century. Darwin recognized that characteristics that were advantageous in particular circumstances might increase the likelihood of survival and reproduction—eventually generating a population sufficiently different from its ancestors as to constitute a new species. Darwin's cousin Galton, by studying families and twin pairs, attempted to develop mathematical models to tease out the relative contributions of environment and heredity. By the start of the twentieth century, Bateson and Garrod had each recognized that the familial occurrence of alcaptonuria (described by Garrod in 1899) and other recessive "inborn errors of metabolism" could be explained by the neglected and recently rediscovered laws of Mendel (Garrod, 1902). Thus began a new era in which the pattern of inheritance of certain genetic conditions—and hence their risks of recurrence—could be deduced, providing a more scientific basis for genetic counseling.

During the last century, understanding of genetic disorders, variability, mechanisms, and contributions to common diseases grew exponentially. Medical technology exploded, leading to a host of new genetic testing capabilities, including prenatal and ultimately preimplantation genetic diagnosis. Less dramatic but equally important advances occurred in the study of human behavior, in public health policy, in ethics, and in counseling theory. Concomitantly, people began to assume greater responsibility for their own health care decisions. The *activity* of genetic counseling developed and changed accordingly over this period. It is only since the 1970s, however, that a *profession* specifically devoted to genetic counseling has arisen. The education and practice of these professionals encompasses all of the above elements, enabling them, as members of genetics health care teams, to bridge such diverse disciplines as research scientist, clinical geneticist, primary health care provider, social worker, and hospital administrator. More importantly, today's genetic counselor provides a service that is unique—distinct from the contributions of these other individuals—for patients and families who seek to understand and cope with both the genetic and the psychosocial aspects of disorders they confront.

Less than 40 years after the first master's degrees were awarded in genetic counseling, these new professionals have achieved a prominent place in genetic health care delivery, education, and public policy development. They have formed professional organizations in several countries, been involved in starting training programs, developed mechanisms for accrediting over 30 North American genetic counseling graduate programs, and become board certified, credentialed, registered, and/or licensed as distinct health professionals. This chapter gives an overview of these developments—and perhaps also a glimpse of the challenges and excitement to come.

Models of Genetic Counseling

Eugenic Model   Sheldon Reed is credited with introducing the term "genetic counseling" in 1947 (Reed, 1955). However, the practice of advising people about inherited traits had actually begun about 1906, shortly after Bateson suggested that the new medical and biological study of heredity be called "genetics." By then the public (and many scientists) had been intrigued by the thought that this new science might be able to identify hereditary factors contributing not only to medical diseases, including mental retardation, but also to social and behavioral diseases such as poverty, crime, and mental illness. Galton himself had suggested in 1885 that "eugenics" (a word he coined from the Greek ευγενηζ, meaning "well-born") become the study of "agencies under social control that may improve or impair racial qualities of future generations, either physically or mentally" (Carr-Saunders, 1929).

Enthusiasm over the possibility that genetics might be used to improve the human condition gave rise, for example, to the Eugenics Records Office at Cold Springs Harbor (a section of the Carnegie Institution of Washington's Department of Genetics) and establishment of a chair of eugenics (by bequest of Galton himself) at University College London. Not only did scientists in these institutions collect data on human traits, they also sometimes provided information to affected families— usually with the intention of persuading them not to reproduce. Unfortunately, at least at the Eugenics Records Office, data collection was often scientifically unsound, or was biased and tainted by social or political agendas. The eugenics movement, initially well-intentioned, ultimately had disastrous consequences. By 1926, 23 of the 48 United States had laws mandating sterilization of the "mentally defective" and over 6000 people had been sterilized (most involuntarily) (Carr-Saunders, 1929). Astoundingly, this practice persisted up into the 1960s and 1970s in some countries (Wooldridge, 1997). In 1924 the U.S. passed the Immigration Restriction Act, instituting quotas to limit immigration by various "inferior" ethnic groups. In Germany, euthanasia for the "genetically defective" was legalized in 1939—leading to the deaths of over 70,000 people with hereditary disorders in addition to Jews, Romanies (gypsies) and others killed in the holocaust (Neel, 1994). Revulsion at the specter of these past abuses in the name of mandatory eugenics is at the heart of the "nondirective" approach to genetic counseling that prevails today.[1]

Medical/Preventive Model   Distress at the outcomes of what had started out as legitimate scientific inquiry caused most geneticists to retreat from advising families about potentially hereditary conditions for at least a decade. However, by the mid-1940s, heredity clinics had been started at the Universities of Michigan and Minnesota and at the Hospital for Sick Children in London (Harper, 2004). A decade later, during a time when prevention had become a new focus of medicine, several additional genetics clinics were established. Information about risks was offered—based almost entirely on empirical observations—so that families could avoid recurrences of disorders that had already occurred. However in 1956, few diagnostic tests were available. Knowledge of the physical structure of DNA was only three years old; there was no way to prospectively identify unaffected *carriers* of genetic conditions; and given that it was still thought that there were 48 chromosomes in the human genome and that our mechanism of sex determination was the same as in *Drosophila* (Therman, 1993; Miller and Therman, 2001), the basis for chromosomal

---

[1] Robert G. Resta has written an excellent essay reviewing the complex issues around eugenics and nondirectiveness for the *Journal of Genetic Counseling* (1997, 6:255–258).

syndromes was completely unknown. Even with the goal of preventing genetic disorders, there was little for genetic counseling to offer families but information, sympathy, and the option to avoid childbearing. Many geneticists assumed that "rational" families would want to do so (Resta, 1997).

Decision-Making Model   The capabilities of genetics changed dramatically over the next 10 years as the correct human diploid complement of 46 was reported by Tjio and Levan (1956) and the cytogenetics of Down (Lejeune et al., 1959), Klinefelter (Jacobs and Strong, 1959), and Turner (Ford et al., 1959) syndromes and trisomies 13 (Patau et al., 1960) and 18 (Edwards et al., 1960; Patau et al., 1960; Smith et al., 1960) were elucidated. Over this decade it also became possible to identify carriers for α- or β-thalassemia (Kunkel et al., 1957; Weatherall, 1963), a host of abnormal hemoglobins, and metabolic diseases such as galactosemia (Hsia, 1958), Tay–Sachs disease (Volk et al., 1964), and G6PD deficiency (Childs, 1958), among others. Amniocentesis was first utilized for prenatal diagnosis—initially for sex determination by Barr body analysis (Serr et al., 1955)—and then for karyotyping (Steele and Breg, 1966). In 1967, the first diagnosis of a fetal chromosome anomaly was reported (Jacobson and Barter, 1967).

These advances in genetics meant that families had some new options to better assess their risks and possibly avoid a genetic disorder. However, the choices were by no means straightforward. Tests were not always informative. Prenatal diagnosis was novel, and its potential pitfalls were incompletely understood. Explaining the technologies and the choices was time-consuming. However, clinical genetics' tenet of nondirective counseling was beginning to be echoed elsewhere as medicine began to shift from its traditional, paternalistic approach toward promoting patient autonomy in decision-making. The emphasis in genetic counseling shifted too, from simply providing information that families would presumably use to make "rational" decisions (thereby preventing genetic disorders) toward a more interactive process in which individuals were not only *educated* about risks but also helped with the difficult tasks of exploring issues related to the disorder in question, and of making decisions about reproduction, testing, or management that were consistent with their own needs and values.

Psychotherapeutic Model   Although families often come to genetic counseling seeking information, they cannot really process or act on it effectively without dealing with the powerful reactions this information can evoke. For this reason, exploring with clients their experiences, emotional responses, goals, cultural and religious beliefs, financial and social resources, family and interpersonal dynamics, and coping styles has become an integral part of the genetic counseling process. Genetic disorders and birth defects often catch individuals completely off-guard—raising anxiety about the unfamiliar, assaulting the self-image, provoking fears for one's own future and that of other family members, and generating guilt. Even a client who brings a lifetime of experience with a disorder, or who has known about his or her own or reproductive risk for some time, will have cognitive or emotional "baggage" that may need to be addressed for counseling to succeed. A skilled genetic counselor must be able to elicit and recognize these factors, distinguish appropriate from pathological responses, reassure clients (when appropriate) that their reactions are normal, prepare them for new issues and emotions that may loom ahead, and help them marshal intrinsic and extrinsic resources to promote coping and adjustment. A few genetic counselors have chosen to develop these skills to a higher degree by obtaining additional training so that they can provide longer-term therapy for dysfunctional families or for individuals whose underlying psychopathology complicates genetic counseling.

DEFINITION AND GOALS OF GENETIC COUNSELING

1975 ASHG Definition of Genetic Counseling

In the early 1970s a committee of the American Society of Human Genetics (ASHG) proposed a definition of genetic counseling that was adopted by the Society in 1975. Though oft cited, no textbook of genetic counseling would be complete without it:

> Genetic counseling is a communication process which deals with the human problems associated with the occurrence or risk of occurrence of a genetic disorder in a family. This process involves an attempt by one or more appropriately trained persons to help the individual or family to: (1) comprehend the medical facts including the diagnosis, probable course of the disorder, and the available management, (2) appreciate the way heredity contributes to the disorder and the risk of recurrence in specified relatives, (3) understand the alternatives for dealing with the risk of recurrence, (4) choose a course of action which seems to them appropriate in their view of their risk, their family goals, and their ethical and religious standards and act in accordance with that decision, and (5) to make the best possible adjustment to the disorder in an affected family member and/or to the risk of recurrence of that disorder.
> —American Society of Human Genetics, 1975

This definition held up quite well for a time, articulating as it does several central features of genetic counseling. The first is the two-way nature of the interaction— quite different from the "advice-giving" of the eugenics period or the primarily information-based counseling characteristic of the mid-twentieth century. The second is that genetic counseling is a *process,* ideally taking place over a period of time so the client can gradually assimilate complex or distressing information regarding diagnosis, prognosis, and risk and formulate decisions or strategies. The third is the emphasis on the client's autonomy in decision-making related to reproduction, testing, or treatment, and the recognition that such decisions will *appropriately* be different depending on the personal, family, and cultural contexts in which they are made. The fourth acknowledges that the occurrence or risk for a genetic disorder can have a family-wide impact different from that in other kinds of diseases and indicates that there should be a psychotherapeutic component of genetic counseling to help people explore and cope with the reproductive implications and other burdens of a rare disorder. Implicit in the words "appropriately trained persons" is the admonition that, because of these particular features, genetic counseling requires special knowledge and skills distinct from those needed in other medical and counseling interactions.

Genetic Counseling Has Changed Since 1975!

More Indications for Genetics Services and Counseling The ASHG definition relates primarily to genetic counseling in the context of *reproductive* risk assessment and decision-making. In the three-plus decades since this definition was proposed, genetic counseling's purview has expanded considerably beyond the prenatal and pediatric realm, with many genetic counselors now focusing entirely on diagnosis and risk assessment for diseases that affect individuals as adults— frequently *after* they have completed their reproductive years. Moreover, genetic counseling often addresses conditions that are not solely, and sometimes not at all, genetic. Genetic counselors now provide information about potentially teratogenic or mutagenic exposures; about birth defects that may have little if any genetic basis; and about common diseases of adulthood that have complex and heterogeneous causes. Increasingly, counselors work in settings where they are involved in discussions about possible interventions like chemoprevention, prophylactic surgery, or other strategies, enabling patients to make choices that may reduce future disease risk. It is likely that in the future, as our understanding of the genome enables us to personalize medicine to individual genotypes, genetic counselors will have a role in discussing genetic polymorphisms that could affect a patient's response to therapeutic drugs or environmental pollutants or perhaps even in providing information about genetic variations that contribute to common behavioral and physical traits.

Changes in Clients and Health Care Delivery As individuals seeking genetic counseling have become more diverse and the technology ever more powerful and complex, new elements have gained prominence in the genetic counseling process. In 1975 one could not have predicted that access to genetic evaluation or appropriate treatment would be limited by lack of insurance or by constraints imposed by managed care, with the result that advocating for funding would become a new (and usually unwelcome) part of the genetic counseling process. Or that the counselor would need to inform clients not only about the nature of the disorder, risks, testing, and reproductive options, but also about ethical dilemmas that might arise as a result of testing, or about the possibility of resultant discrimination in employment or insurance. Or that the genetic counseling "process" might have to be accomplished in just half an hour. Or that counseling a recently arrived immigrant might be severely compromised by passage through two translations or the client's unfamiliarity with even rudimentary concepts of biology. The basic tenets and goals remain as they were in 1975, but the face of genetic counseling will continue to change.

2006 NSGC Definition of Genetic Counseling and 2007 Scope of Practice

Because genetic counseling has continued to evolve, in 2003 the National Society of Genetic Counselors (NSGC) appointed a task force to revisit the definition of genetic counseling. Recognizing that many types of professionals provide genetic counseling, the group's charge was to define *genetic counseling*, rather than to describe various *professional roles* of genetic counselors (Resta et al., 2006). In reviewing the literature, the task force found 20 previous definitions of genetic counseling, which are provided as an appendix to their article. They also considered the purposes for which a genetic counseling definition might be used. Among these are marketing the profession, not only to potential clients but also to insurance companies, hospital administrators, and health maintenance organizations; increasing public, professional, and media awareness; developing practice guidelines and legislation for licensure; and providing a basis for research in genetic counseling. They settled on crafting a succinct definition that would be readily understandable, broad enough to apply to the variety of settings in which genetic counseling might occur, and acknowledging the increasing importance of genetic counseling for common and complex diseases. Drafts were presented to the NSGC membership and an advisory expert panel, as well as to representatives of other professional genetics organizations, advocacy groups, legal counsel, and marketing consultants for comments, and revised repeatedly to reflect this input. As approved by the NSGC Board of Directors, the definition reads:

> Genetic counseling is the process of helping people understand and adapt to the medical, psychological and familial implications of genetic contributions to disease. This process integrates the following:
>
> - Interpretation of family and medical histories to assess the chance of disease occurrence or recurrence.
> - Education about inheritance, testing, management, prevention, resources and research.
> - Counseling to promote informed choices and adaptation to the risk or condition.

Note that the definition does not indicate who is qualified to *provide* genetic counseling. Nor does it address the scope of practice of genetic counselors. A second NSGC task force developed a complementary document to define genetic counselors' scope of practice and to capture the broad range of activities involved in genetic counseling.

"Scope of practice" is a term frequently used in the context of licensing non-physician medical professionals—particularly those with advanced practice degrees such as physician assistants, nurse practitioners, audiologists, etc. A scope of practice describes activities that an appropriately trained and qualified person in that profession should be able (and allowed) to do. It is usually developed by one or more organizations representing the profession as a means of educating others about their training, skills, and unique place in service delivery, and for encoding in regulatory language the tasks a licensed professional should be entitled to perform. Sometimes the scopes of practice of different professional groups overlap—occasionally causing tension if a newer professional group begins to provide services that historically have been the sole province of another. Since clinical geneticists and genetic counselors have practiced as a team since the beginning, this has been less of an issue in the provision of genetics services.

Describing a scope of practice is often viewed as an important step in a profession's development. While this was part of the reason the NSGC undertook the task, a more urgent reason was to provide a document that could be used in efforts to educate legislators about the need for genetic counselor licensure and to assist states in developing licensure regulations that would be as uniform as possible. The NSGC Scope of Practice describes elements of the genetic counselor's role as they relate to clinical genetics, to counseling and communication, and to professional ethics and values. The 2007 Scope of Practice is reproduced in the Appendix to this chapter, after the ABGC competencies. Because of the changing face of genetic counseling and its many potential future directions, it is anticipated that the Scope of Practice will be revised periodically to reflect how the profession is changing. The NSGC website should be accessed for the most up-to-date version.

Philosophy and Ethos of Genetics Services and Counseling

Voluntary Utilization of Services Genetic counseling operates on a number of assumptions or principles. Among these are that the decision to utilize genetics services should be entirely voluntary. Society at large and other entities such as insurance companies clearly have economic and eugenic interests in promoting prevention of genetic disease. However, at least in most developed nations, the prevailing philosophy is that information should be made available and tests offered when appropriate, but that patients and families should have the right to make their own decisions—particularly about genetic testing and reproduction—unencumbered by pressure or by the implication that they are being fiscally or socially irresponsible if they choose *not* to try and prevent a hereditary disease.

In reality, of course, patients sometimes get referred for genetics services not at their own request, but by virtue of a care provider's fear of litigation, or because they have been identified through a screening program about which they were not adequately educated. Furthermore, decisions about testing or reproduction are often influenced by financial considerations. Genetic disorders usually come with additional health care costs, which may or may not be covered by health insurance or public medical assistance programs. In some cases, insurers consider newer genetic tests to be "experimental" or see genetic counseling as unnecessary outside of the context of pregnancy. To assume that families can always make voluntary decisions about utilizing genetic services or about reproduction based solely on their preferences, personal goals, and moral views is, unhappily, somewhat naive. To maximize the ability of families to benefit from advances in genetics, it is incumbent on genetic counselors to educate insurers about the value of genetics services and testing, to advocate for access to these services, and also to be involved in developing public policies that promote responsible use of genetics, ensure that patients will be able to *make* choices, and also protect them from misuse of genetic information.

Equal Access Ideally, genetics services, including counseling, diagnosis, and treatment should be equally and readily available to all who need and choose to use them. Compared with other medical specialties, however, *genetics* services are more likely to be accessed by people living in heavily populated areas who have some sort of health coverage, enough education or medical sophistication to know that such services exist, and the ability to advocate for themselves in the health care system. Even patients lucky enough to have these attributes may find particular genetic technologies (e.g., preimplantation diagnosis) out of reach, just because of their cost, novelty, or limited availability. As capabilities continue to expand it will be important to assess expensive genetic services not only in terms of how likely they are to be available to *all* those who might benefit, but also by considering their costs relative to other public health care needs.

Client Education   A central feature of genetic counseling is a firm belief in the importance of client education. Expanding on the NSGC definition, this education typically includes information about (1) the features, natural history, and range of variability of the condition in question, (2) its genetic (or nongenetic) basis, (3) how it can be diagnosed and managed, (4) the chances it will occur or recur in various family members, (5) the economic, social, and psychological impact—positive as well as negative—that it may have, (6) resources available to help families deal with the challenges it presents, (7) strategies that can ameliorate or prevent it if the family so wishes, and (8) relevant research that may contribute to understanding the disorder or better treatment.

Complete Disclosure of Information   In providing education about diagnosis and related issues, most geneticists and genetic counselors subscribe to the belief that all relevant information should be disclosed. Being selective in what one tells a client is viewed as paternalistic—and disrespectful of the person's autonomy and competence. There is wide disagreement, however, both in philosophy and in practice, on what geneticists or counselors view as "relevant". Most would probably concur that a competent patient should be given the facts about his or her own diagnosis—even in a challenging scenario such as informing a phenotypic female with androgen insensitivity syndrome about her XY karyotype. But there is less consensus about what should be done with other dilemmas, like disclosing nonpaternity revealed through DNA testing when it does not affect risk. With genetic testing now widely available for a host of carrier states, there also has been considerable debate about whether all possible tests (e.g., for diseases more prevalent in specific populations but still quite uncommon) need to be discussed or offered. Nor is it clear whether a counselor should be obligated to address issues of potential genetic significance that are not related to the reason for referral (e.g., a familial cancer history uncovered in the context of prenatal diagnosis counseling).

At the same time as testing capabilities and understanding of genetic mechanisms have become more extensive and complex, clients have become more diverse in their cultural backgrounds, education, and health literacy. Concomitantly, the time available for counseling has often decreased. In the 1980s and early 1990s, when a typical session might last an hour and a half and the majority of clients were college educated, middle class, and English speaking, a "genetics lesson" was a prominent feature of genetic counseling. We believed that clients needed a basic understanding of genes, chromosomes, and how the test would be done in order to make informed decisions. Now, however, with burgeoning genetic knowledge and technology, the pressure to see more clients more quickly, and a more frequent need to work through interpreters, achieving this level of client education is often impractical. Moreover, full disclosure of all "relevant information" could paralyze even the most sophisticated patient. Despite these pressures, however, it will always be critical for the counselor to disclose any information *relevant to decision-making* in ways that the client can interpret and act on.

Nondirective Counseling   Although the counselor can use clinical judgment in choosing what information is most likely to be important and helpful in a client's adjustment to a diagnosis or for decision-making, it should be presented fairly and even-handedly—not with the purpose of encouraging a particular course of action. Adherence to a nonprescriptive (often less appropriately referred to as "nondirective") approach is perhaps the most defining feature of genetic counseling. The philosophy stems from a firm belief that genetic counseling should, insofar as is possible, be devoid of eugenic motivation. Although this is a time-honored tradition, it can be counter-productive for the counselor to avoid expressing *any* opinions. This is especially true when genetics evaluation reveals *personal* health risks, such as an increased liability to specific diseases that could be reduced by particular interventions (e.g., aggressive screening, chemoprevention, or prophylactic surgery to reduce breast or ovarian cancer risk in a *BRCA* mutation carrier; monitoring serum iron, dietary modifications, or therapeutic phlebotomy in a person with hemochromatosis). It is even true in certain situations involving reproductive decision-making—an area where genetic counselors have historically shied away from expressing opinions or offering advice. If a pregnancy risk could be reduced by various actions (e.g., avoiding exposure to a teratogenic drug, taking folate, or achieving good diabetic control before to pregnancy), few counselors would hesitate to advise the client accordingly. A client should expect a genetics professional to be able to provide guidance when the genetic and medical issues are complex, if there are limited data or medical opinions conflict, and even when choices raise problematic moral or psychosocial issues. Failing to share our knowledge and experience out of fear that we will be perceived as directive may leave the client to flounder.[2]

Attention to Psychosocial and Affective Dimensions in Counseling   Just giving information does not necessarily promote client autonomy. To succeed in empowering individuals to cope with a genetic condition or risk, and to make difficult decisions with which they are comfortable, the counselor needs to

---

[2] Seymour Kessler has explored nondirectiveness in genetic counseling—particularly in the context of reproductive genetics—in numerous publications, but the following is especially provocative: Kessler (1997) Psychological aspects of genetic counseling. XI. Nondirectiveness revisited. *American Journal of Medical Genetics* 72:164–171. Some more recent discussions of this challenging issue can be found in Elwyn, Gray, Clarke (2000) Shared decision making and non-directiveness in genetic counselling. *Journal of Medical Genetics* 37:135–138; in Oduncu (2002) The role of non-directiveness in genetic counseling. *Medicine, Health Care, and Philosophy* 5:53–63; and in Koch, Svendsen (2005) Providing solutions—defining problems: the imperative of disease prevention in genetic counselling. *Social Science & Medicine* 60:823–832.

encourage clients to see themselves as competent and to help them project how various events or courses of action could affect them and their family. This cannot be done without knowing something of their social, cultural, educational, economic, emotional, and experiential circumstances. The client's ability to hear, understand, interpret and utilize information will be influenced by all of these factors. An effective counselor will be attuned and responsive to affective responses and able to explore not only clients understanding of information, but also what it means to them, and what impact they feel it will have within their social and psychological framework.

Confidentiality and Protection of Privacy Respecting confidentiality and protecting personal health information has always been an essential part of any medical interaction, but it has become even more critical since passage of The Health Insurance Privacy and Accountability Act (HIPAA) in 1996. However, genetic counseling raises additional issues with regard to confidentiality and privacy protection. Information about an individual's genetic disease, family history, carrier status, reproductive risk, or related medical decisions is extremely sensitive and potentially stigmatizing. Very rarely, information about risk leads to discrimination in employment or difficulties in obtaining or retaining insurance. For these reasons it is especially critical that genetic information be kept confidential. On the other hand, knowing a person's diagnosis or genotype sometimes provides information not only about his *own* risk, but also that of family members who may be only remotely related. This can create a conflict between the client's right to privacy and the benefit to relatives of knowing about their potential risk. If the risk is substantial or serious, and when options are available to prevent harm, the client—and sometimes the counselor—may have an ethical duty to warn relatives. There are only a few other situations in medicine (e.g., a serious infectious disease or threat to another's safety disclosed in the course of psychotherapy) where breaching confidentiality may be warranted if the client refuses to share information with those at risk (please see Chapter 12 by Schmerler in this book for additional discussion).

With the advent of computerized databanks and of samples containing DNA being stored for many reasons, concerns have been raised about the *privacy* of genetic information. Genetic material obtained for one purpose (for instance, genetic linkage studies, newborn screening, or military identification) can also reveal information about unrelated features of the genotype (e.g., risk for late-onset disease, nonpaternity) that may be both unwanted and damaging. The privacy of genetic information increasingly will become a cause for both litigation and legislation.

COMPONENTS OF THE GENETIC COUNSELING INTERACTION

Information Gathering

An integral part of genetic evaluation is, of course, the family history. This usually is recorded in the form of a pedigree so as to clarify relationships and note phenotypic features that may be relevant to the diagnosis. Additional family history of potential genetic significance (ethnicity, consanguinity, infertility, birth defects, late-onset diseases, mental disability) should also be obtained as a matter of course. Adherence to conventions for symbols notating gender, biological relationships, pregnancy outcomes, and genotypic information, when known (Bennett et al., 1995) will ensure that any pedigree can be readily and accurately interpreted.

Medical history is routinely obtained, as is information about previous and current pregnancies, including complications and possible teratogenic or other exposures (such as smoking, radiation, or previous chemotherapy) that might have bearing on the outcome. Often, clinical features or history potentially relevant to a diagnosis must be confirmed—even before the visit—by obtaining medical records not only on the patient, but also on family members previously evaluated or treated for symptoms that may be relevant. In the context of cancer genetic counseling, it may be important to obtain not only records (such as pathology reports or test results) but actual tumor samples or slides from affected individuals.

Of equal importance to counseling success is learning about the client's or family's understanding about the reason for referral and their expectations about what will be gained through the consultation. Determining the family's beliefs about causation and assessing emotional, experiential, social, educational, and cultural issues that may affect their perception of information is a process that should be ongoing throughout the course of the evaluation.

Establishing or Verifying Diagnosis

Although a genetic diagnosis can sometimes be established or ruled out solely by reviewing medical records, evaluation usually involves at least one clinic visit. This might be for a diagnostic procedure, as in the case of prenatal testing, or for a physical examination by the clinical geneticist or another specialist experienced with the condition. Confirming a clinically suspected diagnosis often requires additional assessments, such as imaging studies, evaluations by other specialists, or examinations of particular family members. Increasingly, however, cytogenetic or molecular genetic testing alone may be sufficient not only to diagnose an affected individual or carrier, but also to provide important information about prognosis or severity. With so many of these tests commercially available, many genetic diagnoses can now be made or confirmed by the primary care physician or a specialist in a field other than genetics. The NSGC's Scope of Practice even indicates that genetic counselors may "order tests and perform clinical assessments in accordance with local, state and federal regulations." This is more likely to be appropriate in the context of prenatal diagnosis counseling or cancer risk assessment than in the general genetics clinic. Some commercial genetics laboratories have aggressively marketed genetic tests to nongeneticists and even directly to consumers—sometimes via the Internet, so testing increasingly is occurring outside of the context of genetics evaluation. This sometimes creates difficult situations in which genetic counseling must be provided post hoc to a client who was inadequately educated about testing or its implications.

Risk Assessment

In many cases, the client's concerns center not on diagnosis of an affected individual but on assessing future reproductive or personal health risk. The counselor can sometimes make such an assessment by analyzing the pedigree—taking into account the pattern of inheritance and the client's relationship to individuals with the condition. Mathematical calculations may be needed to incorporate additional information (e.g., carrier frequencies, test sensitivity and specificity, numbers of affected and unaffected individuals, the client's age) to modify the risk. Questions about carrier status may be resolved with appropriate laboratory tests. When a condition has a multifactorial basis or is genetically heterogeneous, the best risk estimates may come from epidemiologic data on other families with affected individuals. Answering concerns about potentially mutagenic or teratogenic exposures also usually relies on empirical data about the agent in question, and on evaluating the timing, duration, and dose of the exposure. In some areas of genetic counseling, such as cancer risk assessment, factors such as reproductive history, hormone use, and lifestyle issues such as smoking, obesity, or alcohol use are also important variables in risk assessment.

Information Giving

Once a diagnosis or risk is determined, the client and/or family needs to understand how it was arrived at and what the implications are for the affected person and other family members. This includes describing the condition, its variability, and its natural history—making sure that the family's prior perception of the disorder (if any) is still appropriate in light of current understanding of the genetics and treatment. It is important to make sure that, depending on the situation, the client, parents, or family are told about medical, surgical, social, and educational interventions that can correct, prevent, or alleviate symptoms. Discussions should also include available financial and social resources (e.g., support groups) to help treat and cope with the condition. When appropriate, it may be important to describe reproductive options (e.g., prenatal or preimplantation diagnosis) that could reduce risk or provide information during pregnancy. Clearly this depth of discussion would neither be warranted nor feasible in the time available for a routine prenatal session, but once a specific fetal diagnosis is made or suspected, the prospective parents should have access to as much information as they need to make a truly informed decision about their course of action.

Psychological Counseling and Support

Being given a diagnosis or learning about a personal or reproductive risk is likely to generate powerful emotional responses that must be acknowledged and dealt with if the information is to be assimilated. Part of counseling is preparing clients for these responses and helping them cope with them, often over a period of months or years. Sometimes, as in a fetal or neonatal diagnosis, critical decisions must be made rapidly on the basis of new and distressing data. In other situations, carrier or presymptomatic testing may reveal that a person is *not* at increased risk to develop a disease or have affected children. If this new knowledge overturns long-held beliefs, it can be quite disorienting. Clients often need help in trying possible scenarios "on for size" to help them imagine how various courses of action—including just the decision to *undergo* diagnosis—may affect them and their family. The counselor must be knowledgeable about resources that can help families adjust to the reality of a condition or risk, be alert to pathological reactions that are beyond his or her skills to treat, and be able to make an effective referral when necessary.

COUNSELING CONTEXTS AND SITUATIONS

Genetic Counseling for Reproductive Issues

As genetics becomes increasingly relevant to all areas of medicine, the contexts in which genetic counseling occurs also are expanding. Genetic counselors once worked mostly in pediatrics, prenatal diagnosis, and a few specialty clinics. Today, however, people may seek counseling *before* they conceive, because of concerns about the reproductive implications of their own or their partner's family history, or to discuss carrier screening for conditions that occur more frequently in people of their ethnic background. Others may come as part of an evaluation for infertility or fetal loss, or for donor screening if they are considering using assisted reproductive techniques. With the growing use of preimplantation genetic diagnosis—not only for known genetic disorders, but also to enhance the likelihood of a successful pregnancy after in vitro fertilization—"prenatal" counseling may actually occur before conception. Also, screening pregnancies for chromosome abnormalities has shifted from the second to the first trimester and is now becoming a standard part of prenatal care for women of *any* age (Breathnach et al., 2007; Sharma et al., 2007). Indeed, discussing the host of screening options for chromosomal aneuploidy and neural tube defects has become so complicated that it is daunting for both the counselor and the pregnant couple. Despite this complexity, blood for first trimester screening is often drawn in the primary care setting in the context of "routine prenatal blood work," sometimes without the patient fully understanding the implications of screening. As a consequence, many couples who embarked on a pregnancy with no known risk factors unexpectedly find themselves in the genetic counselor's office in the first trimester discussing multiple testing options after fetal ultrasound and serum markers suggest increased risk for Down syndrome or other aneuploidies. These testing options include combining first- and second-trimester serum screening (using several possible algorithms), CVS, amniocentesis, second-trimester detailed ultrasound, and various combinations of these. Genetic counseling for prenatal diagnosis of birth defects and genetic disorders not only has become more complicated as techniques have proliferated and improved, but increasingly has shifted from large university genetics units into HMOs, private obstetricians' offices, commercial laboratories, and private hospitals.

Genetic Counseling in Pediatrics

Most genetic conditions and birth defects appear without warning. Genetic counselors have an important role to play after the birth or stillbirth of an abnormal baby or when an infant with a genetic condition dies. The counselor can help the family understand the cause of the problem (if it is known) and also help them grieve for the baby's death or the "loss" of the normal child they had anticipated. At a time when families may feel abandoned by previously trusted professionals and friends who are un-comfortable dealing with a baby's death or a birth defect, the counselor can provide not only information but also ongoing emotional support that can even continue through subsequent, usually successful, pregnancies.

Many genetic conditions are not suspected until later in childhood or even in adolescence or adulthood. In some situations, as with delayed physical or cognitive development, problems may have become evident over time. In others, a newly recognized health problem or feature of a disorder may prompt concerns about a particular diagnosis. Genetic counseling in these circumstances includes gathering information relevant to establishing the diagnosis, anticipating its impact on the patient or family, addressing their fears and distress, educating them about the condition and its implications, and ensuring that they access necessary medical and social services. Because genetic counselors understand the unique genetic, psycho-social, and medical issues that attend many chronic conditions, they are often part of teams of professionals who provide ongoing management for diseases such as cystic fibrosis, craniofacial or bleeding disorders, muscular dystrophies, inherited metabolic conditions, and hemoglobinopathies.

Genetic Counseling for Adult-Onset Diseases

A newer arena for genetic counseling is in genetic testing for conditions that develop later in life. As molecular tests have become available for disorders such as Huntington disease, familial amyotrophic lateral sclerosis, and numerous hereditary cancer predispositions, healthy individuals who are at risk may consider learning about their genotype so as to diminish anxiety, remove uncertainty, or make personal and medical decisions. Numerous complex genetic and psychosocial issues arise in helping families consider testing and cope with the results. Many physicians who traditionally have cared for affected individuals in these families feel ill equipped to provide the necessary education and counseling that should surround testing. Consequently, genetic counselors now find themselves working in settings such as cancer centers, dialysis units, and adult neurology, cardiology, or dermatology clinics that historically may not have had close relationships with genetics. Many clinics are now hiring genetic counselors directly, rather than "borrowing" them from genetics units, with the result that some counselors now work more closely with an oncologist, neurologist, or cardiologist than they do with a clinical geneticist.

These new work settings are interesting in that genetic counselors are removed from the traditional "genetics team" and may be looked to for diagnostic expertise that formerly was provided by clinical geneticists. Up until recently, diagnosing most genetic conditions required the skill in physical diagnosis and acumen in synthesizing complex historical and laboratory information that physicians have. For many genetic conditions, this undoubtedly will always be the case. While genetic counselors are trained to understand genetic test results, their training does not develop these other diagnostic skills. However, with diagnosis of some disease predispositions, carrier states, and adult-onset genetic disorders able to be established solely through molecular or other types of genetic tests, genetic counselors in certain clinical settings are able to function more autonomously. The NSGC has indicated that ordering diagnostic tests and other clinical assessments, "in accordance with local, state and federal regulations," is within the genetic counselor's scope of practice.

PROVIDERS OF GENETIC COUNSELING

Geneticists

Elements of genetic counseling—risk assessment, information about genetic disorders and reproductive options, treatment for psychological distress related to these issues—are provided by many types of health care workers in diverse settings. However, with genetics now recognized as a distinct medical specialty, people with a genetic condition or birth defect ideally should be seen at some point by one or more professionals with specialized training in genetic diagnosis and counseling. In many centers, a genetics *team* that includes many of the geneticists described below, each with distinct disciplinary backgrounds, roles, and areas of expertise, provides these services. The NSGC Code of Ethics has a section relating to our obligations in regard to relationships with these colleagues. Specifically mentioned is the importance of respecting and valuing their knowledge, perspectives, contributions, and areas of competence and collaborating with them to provide the highest quality of service.

Genetic Counselors The first graduate program to educate master's-level professionals in human genetics and genetic counseling was started at Sarah Lawrence College in 1969 (Marks and Richter, 1976). There are now over 50 such programs in the United States, Canada, Cuba, the United Kingdom, the Netherlands, Norway, Sweden, France, Spain, Israel, Saudi Arabia, South Africa, Australia, Japan, China, and Taiwan. Most programs outside of North America have started since the beginning of the millennium, and several more countries are now actively planning to train counselors.

According to the NSGC Professional Status Survey (2006), to which about two-thirds of members responded, 79% of genetic counselors provide direct clinical services. Most work in an academic medical center (38%), but collectively even more work in a private (20%) or public (11%) hospital/medical facility, a diagnostic laboratory (8%), a private physician's office (5%), or an HMO (3%). About 55% are responsible for teaching or providing clinical supervision, and roughly one in five (usually those associated with an academic medical center) has some type of faculty appointment. Over a quarter coordinate clinics and/or research studies. Other primary roles include healthcare administration, public policy, management, and client services or marketing for a commercial laboratory. Some counselors see patients in just one specialty area, while others cover several areas. The most frequently reported was prenatal diagnosis (54%), followed by cancer genetics (39%), pediatrics (34%), adult genetics (24%), and specialty clinics (13%). Less frequent activities (reported in each case by less than 10% of counselors) were public health and screening programs and counseling related to infertility, neurogenetics, cardiology, psychiatric genetics, or possible teratogenic exposures.

Clinical Geneticists   Physicians who have completed accredited residency and/ or fellowship programs in North America may become eligible for certification in clinical genetics by the American Board of Medical Genetics (ABMG) or the Canadian College of Medical Genetics (CCMG). In the past, many of these physicians first trained in pediatrics, internal medicine, obstetrics, or another specialty before entering genetics. Recognition of the ABMG by the American Board of Medical Specialties in the early 1990s meant that residencies could have clinical genetics as the *primary* specialty. Some institutions also offer one or more combined residencies with both genetics and another specialty as the focus. There are several such programs in the U.S. and also in Canada (where clinical genetics training is under the aegis of the CCMG and the Royal College of Physicians).

Board certification in clinical genetics requires the physician to have knowledge and experience in diagnosing and treating genetic conditions and birth defects, as well as a thorough understanding of the underlying genetics principles. Genetic counseling is assumed to be part of their fellowship training. Clinical geneticists often have particular areas of interest, such as dysmorphology, neurogenetics, metabolic or adult disorders, or prenatal diagnosis, but should also be able to provide expertise on diagnosis and management of a wide range of genetic conditions.

Other Genetics Subspecialists   In addition to clinical geneticists (who must be physicians), the ABMG certifies several other categories of genetics professionals. These include cytogeneticists, molecular geneticists, and biochemical geneticists— many of whom direct genetics diagnostic laboratories. People usually seek ABMG certification if they intend to be involved in clinical activities—either seeing patients or doing diagnostic testing—so even laboratory-oriented certification examinations assess knowledge of genetic counseling in addition to expertise in the appropriate subspecialty(ies). Historically, the ABMG has been unusual among medical specialty boards in certifying Ph.D.s as well as M.D.s and in having been at one time (1982 to 1990) the certifying board for genetic counselors. Some geneticists who are certified in laboratory subspecialties also counsel and treat patients with diseases they diagnose. By the same token, clinical geneticists who perform and interpret diagnostic tests or who specialize in diagnosing and treating metabolic or chromosomal disorders may have additional certification(s) in these subspecialties, even if they are not directly involved in a diagnostic laboratory. Some laboratories doing genetic testing may be directed or staffed by clinical pathologists who have acquired knowledge and skills in molecular genetics or cytogenetics.

Genetics Nurses   There are enough nurses working in genetics to have their own professional society (The International Society of Nurses in Genetics, or ISONG), although relatively few are certified in *genetic counseling*. This is because eligibility for both the ABMG and the American Board of Genetic Counseling (ABGC) has required master's-level training in genetics, usually from an accredited genetic counseling program. However, advanced practice and other specialty nurses often work in clinics and programs where genetic disorders and birth defects are diagnosed and treated. Many have acquired their knowledge of genetics through years of clinical experience, and a few actually hold a graduate degree in genetics nursing from one of the handful of programs that have provided such training. Nurses' additional skills in physical and psychosocial assessment, case management, patient education, clinic administration, and community health are highly valued in specialty and outreach clinics, and in genetics screening programs. Those with specialization in areas such as infant special care, oncology, or midwifery may be astute "case-finders" of patients in need of genetics services and helpful allies in their care.

The Genetics Nursing Credentialing Commission uses a portfolio-based mechanism for appropriately prepared nurses to become credentialed in genetic nursing. Those with a graduate degree from an accredited program and 300 hours of training in a practice at least half devoted to genetics can qualify for a credential as an Advanced Practice Nurse in Genetics (APNG) by providing a logbook of 50 genetics cases and an in-depth written description of four cases, and by documenting sufficient recent genetics coursework or continuing education. Nurses with only a bachelor of nursing degree can qualify as a Genetics Clinical Nurse (GCN) through a similar process. This portfolio-based approach to credentialing is similar to what is used for genetic counselors in the UK and some other countries that do not have examination-based certification.

NonGeneticists

Many patients receive "genetic counseling" in the context of primary or specialty care from health providers who are not geneticists. Examples of such "genetics services" would include molecular or cytogenetic diagnostic testing, screening for potential genetic risks via a family history questionnaire, interview or blood test (e.g., to look for hemoglobinopathies or to measure maternal serum markers during pregnancy), or advising patients about reproductive risks and screening or testing options (as is now done in many prenatal care settings). Commercial availability of a host of tests for genetic diseases or predispositions and their use by nongeneticists means that people more frequently will be asked to consider these tests or will be given results by health providers who have had relatively little training in medical genetics. Many of these providers have not been exposed to the idea of nondirective counseling, and they frequently work under pressures that limit the time that can be spent in discussion. Economic constraints of managed care, fear of litigation, and patient demand are factors that may encourage providers to try to provide genetic tests themselves. For these reasons, geneticists and genetic counselors have an obligation to help educate other health care providers in (1) recognizing potential genetic risks; (2) being aware of phenomena such as variability, heterogeneity, and penetrance that can complicate genetic counseling; (3) understanding the complexities and limitations as well as the benefits of genetic testing; (4) appreciating the philosophy of nondirective counseling; (5) being sensitive to inherent ethical dilemmas; and (6) knowing when they should refer a client to a geneticist or genetic counselor.

The NSGC Code of Ethics specifically refers to genetic counselors' duty to share their knowledge of genetics with other health care providers and to provide mentorship and guidance with regard to genetics health care. The National Coalition for Health Professional Education in Genetics (NCHPEG) has developed useful resources that provide guidance for developing the genetics content of curricula and continuing education programs for *all* health care providers ("Core Competencies in Genetics Essential for All Health Care Professionals" and "Core Principles of Genetics for Health Professionals"). The NCHPEG website is a very useful source of materials that genetic counselors can access to help them educate nongeneticist colleagues.

PROFESSIONAL AND EDUCATIONAL LANDMARKS IN GENETIC COUNSELING

Development of Training Programs and Curricula for Genetic Counseling

In 1971, the year in which the first 10 "genetic associates" graduated from Sarah Lawrence, a report of the National Institute of General Medical Services predicted that by 1988, 68% more geneticists would be needed to provide appropriate services. By 1973, four more genetic counseling programs had been started. The next year, a meeting of various faculty, students, and graduates from four of the five existing programs was held at the California state conference grounds at Asilomar to discuss training goals and expectations for this new profession. Representatives from state and federal health care agencies, genetics centers, volunteer health organizations and legislators, as well as counseling program directors and graduates attended a second Asilomar meeting, sponsored by the March of Dimes in 1976. Both these meetings emphasized the importance of planning and program evaluation for genetic counseling training.

In the spring of 1979, the Office of Maternal and Child Health (MCH) sponsored a much more comprehensive meeting, involving about 50 people, in Williamsburg, Virginia. Participants represented constituencies similar to those in 1976, but also included planners from health maintenance organizations and the health insurance industry, nurses and social workers who provided genetics services, and representatives of the NSGC, which had been formed just the year before. Four panels were assigned different tasks: (1) evaluating the curricula of existing programs in light of graduates' experience; (2) exploring how genetic counselors' services could be reimbursed; (3) recommending ways of ensuring continuing education for genetic counselors; and (4) suggesting a means of evaluating the quality of programs and the competence of their graduates (Dumars et al., 1979). Of all the recommendations to come from the Williamsburg meeting, the guidelines that were established for the curricular content and structure of genetic counseling training had the most lasting impact. The Williamsburg curricular guidelines influenced planning for the many new training programs that started over the next decade. In 1989 yet another conference was held in Asilomar—this time under sponsorship of the NSGC as well as MCH. The purpose of this meeting was to reevaluate the Williamsburg recommendations for program curricula and clinical training and to explore innovative ways for addressing newer aspects of genetics practice, such as cross-cultural counseling and molecular genetics. Additional issues that were discussed included the pros and cons of instituting a doctoral degree in genetic counseling, and potential solutions for shortfalls in genetics "person-power"—including the possibility of more limited training for "genetics assistants" or "aides" who would assume routine tasks and perhaps bring more diverse cultural perspectives to counseling (Walker et al., 1990).

The National Society of Genetic Counselors

A milestone in the evolution of any profession is the formation of its own society. For genetic counselors, this came in 1979 when the NSGC was incorporated. The goals of the new society were "to further the professional interests of genetic counselors, to promote a network of communication within the genetic counseling profession and to deal with issues related to human genetics" (Heimler, 1979).[3] Over the years, the NSGC has, in fact, done this. In 1980, the newly formed NSGC—then numbering only about 200—lobbied successfully for genetic counselors to be included among subspecialties that would be certified by the ABMG. The NSGC has helped achieve representation by genetic counselors on the Boards of Directors of the American Society of Human Genetics (ASHG) and on numerous committees of the ASHG, the American College of Medical Genetics (ACMG), and various government advisory boards. The NSGC sponsors an annual meeting to provide continuing education for its members and a forum for discussing research and clinical issues of interest. Since 1992, it has published its own journal that is indexed in at least ten databases, including PubMed. By 1991, the NSGC had developed a code of ethics for the profession. Most importantly, the Society has become recognized as the voice of the profession and a resource for information about genetic counseling issues by the media, the public, and other health, public policy, and genetics professionals.

---

[3] Audrey Heimler provides a wonderful account of the early days of the NSGC and its contribution to the evolution of the genetic counseling profession in the *Journal of Genetic Counseling* (1997, 6:315–336).

Accreditation of Genetic Counseling Training Programs

In 1993, the ABGC was incorporated with the goal of certifying genetic counselors; this had been the province of the ABMG since 1980. This change was necessary so that the ABMG could be eligible for recognition by the American Board of Medical Specialties, which does not allow member boards to certify non-doctoral-level professionals, but it required a majority vote of all ABMG diplomates, including counselors. The vote passed in 1992, following a year of rancorous debate, and the ABGC was incorporated in 1993. However painful, forming the ABGC was an important landmark in the evolution of the genetic counseling profession because it not only allowed for more autonomous decision-making about certifying genetic counselors, but also provided an opportunity to accredit genetic counseling *programs*. The ABMG accredits fellowships (and now residencies) for Ph.D. and M.D. geneticists, but these are not degree-granting programs. In regard to *genetic counselors'* training, the ABMG had chosen to limit its oversight to approving sites in which genetic counseling students got clinical experience and to graduates' case logbooks that they submitted to establish board eligibility. It did not review or accredit genetic counseling training programs, which were proliferating rapidly in the early 1990s. Given that potential programs were seeking guidance about program design and that potential students wanted reassurance about newer programs they might be considering, the ABGC felt that it should undertake the task of program accreditation.

The ABGC's newly formed accreditation committee explored with other boards that accredited allied health programs and with outside consultants how the ABGC might approach accreditation. From these investigations it became clear that flexibility, variety, and innovation in training were more likely to occur if the accrediting body were to evaluate a program's ability to develop various *professional competencies* in its graduates rather than simply determining how well it adhered to prescribed guidelines for curriculum and clinical experiences. However, no expectations for "entry-level" competencies in genetic counseling had ever been clearly defined. To this end, the ABGC sponsored a 1994 meeting that included directors of all existing genetic counseling programs, the ABGC Board, and consultants from outside the genetic counseling field who had expertise in clinical supervision and accreditation. The goal was to develop consensus about what new graduates should be able to do. By analyzing the counselor's role in various clinical scenarios, participants identified areas of required knowledge and skills (Fiddler et al., 1996), and from these analyses 27 "competencies" were described. Competencies were further refined by the ABGC (Fine et al., 1996) to form the basis of a document that would be used to guide nascent programs and those seeking accreditation (American Board of Genetic Counseling, 1996). The ongoing validity of these was affirmed at another small retreat sponsored by the ABGC Board in July 2005, when the competencies were revisited and thought to need minimal, if any revision. Participants observed that while the *knowledge base* for trainees has changed, expectations for *basic skills* remain the same. Since helping to develop these competencies is what this book is all about, their description is appended to this chapter. They are also posted on the ABGC's website.

Worldwide Genetic Counseling Training

The need for and potential in having professionally trained genetic counselors as part of the workforce delivering genetics services is now recognized in many different nations. Since 1995 at least 26 new programs have been started in 17 countries outside of North America, with genetic counselors now being trained on five continents (Transnational Alliance for Genetic Counselling, 2009)! Directors of many of these programs met as a group for the first time in Manchester, England in May 2006 to learn about each other's curricula and experiential training, genetics service delivery models, and mechanisms for genetic counselor credentialing. A transnational alliance of genetic counseling (TAGC) was born at this meeting, and one outcome is that information about training programs around the world can now be found on the TAGC website.

Not all countries with training programs award a master's-level degree; in some cases genetic counseling education results in a diploma or certificate that documents appropriate knowledge, clinical experiences, and counseling skills. During the 1980s and 1990s, Regina Kenen studied the emergence and evolution of the genetic counseling profession, both in the United States and in Australia, finding that it involved three identifiable stages (Kenen, 1986, 1997). She described an initial "emergent" phase with professional issues and rivalries about who should provide genetic counseling—their relative status, power, and requisite skills. This was followed by a "consolidation" phase in which the service delivery model was refined and professional roles clarified. The final "institutionalized" stage was one in which the model and profession had become established so that goals and standards were understood by all and there was minimal conflict between the various constituencies.[4] Discussions in Manchester found several countries still in the emergent stage, but also emphasized that even in countries such as the U.S. where training programs have existed for nearly four decades, it was still necessary to adjust to changes in health care delivery, advances in genetics, and, increasingly, excursions of genetic counselors into "nontraditional" roles in research, public health, policy, and areas of medicine in which genetics historically has not been prominent.

By the time of the first meeting in 2006, seven countries had developed a mechanism to identify who was qualified to provide genetic counseling. While the specific names for these mechanisms vary, the purpose is the same: to ensure a minimum standard of safe practice so as to protect the public, and to elevate and promote awareness of the profession. Different countries have different pathways to establish eligibility for recognition of professional competence. In the U.S., Australasia, and South Africa, the only route is via a master's degree or graduate diploma in genetic counseling. Other countries (e.g., the U.K., Canada, the Netherlands, and Japan) have a second potential pathway allowing those with a bachelor's degree (in nursing or another relevant field) AND postqualification clinical experience, and in some cases counseling

---

[4] Margaret A. Sahhar provides an insightful overview of the development of genetic counseling training in Australia—comparing their education and training requirements to those in the U.K., Canada, and the U.S., in the *Journal of Genetic Counseling* (2005, 14:283–294).

training, a route to credentialing.[5] In general, these alternate pathways are eventually phased out, as they were in the U.S., as an increasing proportion of genetic counselors have had formal academic training and earned a post-bachelor's degree in the field.

Professional Recognition of Competence in Genetic Counseling

ABGC Certification   The ABGC has certified genetic counselors in the U.S. and Canada since 1993. Achieving certification requires that a candidate's application be approved by the ABGC Credentials Committee (credentialing) to establish "active candidate status". Once approved, the candidate must pass a written examination. Starting in 2009, this will be a single, comprehensive, four-hour examination, developed and administered by the ABGC (American Board of Genetic Counseling 2009). Prior to 2009, certification required the candidate to pass both a general genetics examination–developed and administered by the ABMG, and a genetic counseling examination, created by the ABGC.

When the ABMG first offered certification in 1981, people doing genetic counseling came from a variety of training backgrounds. Many had graduated from genetic counseling programs, but others were nurses, social workers, or simply had a post-baccalaureate degree in genetics. The ABMG established that eligibility for certification in genetic counseling required at least a master's degree in a relevant discipline, provision of genetic counseling in 50 diverse cases documented in a logbook submitted with the application, and letters of reference from three other geneticists.

Since then, requirements for certification have become more stringent, with the ABGC now requiring applicants to have graduated from a genetic counseling training program that was accredited when they entered training. Through the 2009 examination cycle, logbook cases must have been acquired in clinical sites approved by the ABGC, either via accreditation of the training program(s) with which the sites are affiliated, or by Board review of an application submitted for an "ad hoc" site utilized by one particular trainee over a specified period. The logbook has required the nature of the candidate's involvement in each case to be clearly described, with cases demonstrating a participation in a variety of counseling roles and clinical situations. Cases must be supervised by an ABGC or ABMG certified individual. Starting with the 2010 examination, the ABGC will no longer require candidates to submit their logbooks. It will be incumbent on training programs to ensure that their training sites are approved and that their trainees have appropriate clinical supervision and obtain the necessary breadth and depth of cases. The ABGC publishes a bulletin describing current requirements and providing application forms and instructions for the examination, which will be given annually starting in 2010. The ABGC website should be relied on for up-to-date information.

---

[5] This information comes from a Manchester meeting workshop organized by Lauren Kerzin-Storrar and Anna Middleton to explore credentialing models and consider the possibility of transnational reciprocity for counselors credentialed in one country who wish to practice in another. Ms. Kerzin-Storrar kindly provided her draft summary of the proceedings to the author, who also participated in the workshop.

With the advent of more international training programs, increasing numbers of counselors who had trained and practiced outside North America expressed a desire to be qualified to practice in the U.S. or Canada. After receiving many requests for access to ABGC certification, the Board developed a mechanism for appropriately trained individuals to apply for 'International Genetic Counselor Certification' (IGCC). This mechanism was also available to graduates of a few Canadian programs that were not ABGC-accredited at the time the trainee matriculated. Eligibility criteria were strict; the person needed to have received at least a master's degree from a formal genetic counseling program outside the U.S., and must also have acquired a 50 case logbook under appropriate clinical supervision in an ABGC-accredited genetic counseling program over no less than a six-month period. For a variety of reasons, the ABGC discontinued the IGCC program in September 2008. The Canadian Association of Genetic Counselors (CAGC) and the Genetic Counseling Registration Board in the U.K. have, or may soon have, mechanisms for credentialing counselors trained outside their respective countries.

Licensure and Registration   In the U.S., these two terms refer to establishment of an individual's credentials and formal recognition as a member of a profession by a state governmental body, such as a licensure board, Department of Consumer Affairs, etc. Such agencies are charged with protecting the public by ensuring that specified professionals provide a minimum standard of care within their scope of practice. Hospitals and other health care organizations generally expect that providers who seek to work in their institutions will be licensed or registered, as do many "third-party payers" such as insurance companies and publicly funded medical programs. Usually, it is the state's legislature that decides whether a group needs to be licensed to protect the interests of the citizens it represents. The legislature's motivation to pass a law mandating licensure is influenced by *public demand* (both on the part of the group seeking to be licensed and the public at large), by the *potential for harm* from unqualified practitioners, by the *number of practitioners* in the state, and also by having *a committed legislator* willing to carry the bill. Passage of a law is usually only the first step; regulations must then be written to define who will be licensed and how, and a board must be established to review credentials and investigate complaints. In 2000, California became the first state to pass legislation for licensure of genetic counselors. The first state to actually *issue* genetic counseling licenses was Utah, whose law provides 'title protection' that bars an unlicensed individual from calling him- or herself a "genetic counselor" and requires genetic counselors to be licensed in order to practice. As of March 2009, genetic counselors in five additional states have been able to obtain licenses (NSGC 2009). A few other states are still developing regulations to *implement* a licensure law that has been passed, and several more have licensure bills introduced or pending.

Other Forms of Credentialing   The United Kingdom and South Africa use the term "registration" in the same way as "certification" is used in the United States and Canada, although registration may be required in order to practice. Some countries (e.g., U.S., Canada, Japan) require examination by a certifying board, while others (e.g., Australia, U.K.) require postqualification work experience and portfolios detailing clinical training in approved clinical genetics centers (Sahhar et al., 2005). In the U.S. and South Africa, nurses working in genetics have their own separate process for credentialing, although some U.S. nurses with a master's degree were certified in genetic counseling by the ABMG in the 1980s.

PROFESSIONAL GROWTH AND SKILL ACQUISITION

The entry-level genetic counseling competencies that were defined at the 1996 ABGC consensus development conference are used not only to guide and evaluate training programs but also to monitor the progress of students as they acquire the knowledge and skills they will need to be effective genetic counselors. Training programs use the competencies in planning the timing and content of classes and clinical experiences so that students will have been exposed to relevant coursework by the time that they need to use this knowledge in interacting with patients. The competencies also frequently form the basis of evaluation forms used in clinical rotations. They are more than just a checklist of skills and reflect a need for the student to be able to call upon and integrate knowledge about genetic mechanisms, inheritance patterns, disease manifestations, family dynamics, and coping mechanisms with skills in obtaining and interpreting histories, pedigree construction, risk assessment, interviewing, psychosocial evaluation, explaining technical information, etc., in order to manage a counseling session. Other competencies address areas such as the ability to find and synthesize information, identify community resources and advocate for clients, function as part of a team, manage and document a case, provide public and professional education, evaluate and participate in research, show cultural awareness, and behave according to the philosophical, ethical, and legal tenets of the profession.

The last two competencies have to do with recognizing the limits of one's own expertise and taking responsibility for life-long learning. While genetic counselors enter the field with an impressive armamentarium of skills and knowledge, there is no way that two years of training can prepare them for all counseling situations or for future developments in genetics that cannot even be imagined today. Ongoing self-education is critical, and counselors must stay abreast of the literature, routinely attend professional meetings, and communicate with genetics colleagues in order to provide quality service. The NSGC has special interest groups (SIGs) for many subspecialty areas. Many of these SIGs have active e-mail list-serves that provide invaluable information and a forum to learn, ask questions, and discuss issues of common interest. A number of the SIGs sponsor workshops at the NSGC Annual Education Meeting to update their members and other counselors on recent advances and changes in counseling practice. There are also other avenues to explore and develop competence in a rapidly expanding variety of related areas. Some counselors elect to obtain additional formal training to enhance their ability to do psychotherapy, research, or administration, or perhaps to enable them to function in a new domain, such as behavioral or clinical research or commercial genetics. Maintaining membership in professional societies and being active on their committees afford opportunities to work with colleagues from around the country and to develop leadership skills. Involvement in education, advocacy, and political activism can also bring personal rewards and lead to recognition in the community and beyond.

As members of a relatively small profession that deals with issues at the cutting edge of science, medicine, and ethics we are all required to continue to grow and to take responsibility for helping other health professionals, policy makers, and clients understand genetics and its implications. The challenges are many, but the personal and professional rewards are enormous.

APPENDIX

Practice-Based Competencies (ABGC, 1996)

"An entry-level genetic counselor must demonstrate the practice-based competencies listed below to manage a genetic counseling case before, during, and after the clinic visit or session. Therefore, the didactic and clinical training components of a curriculum must support the development of competencies that are categorized into the following domains: Communication Skills; Critical-Thinking Skills; Interpersonal, Counseling, and Psychosocial Assessment Skills; and Professional Ethics and Values. Some competencies may pertain to more than one domain. These domains represent practice areas that define activities of a genetic counselor. The italicized facet below each competency elaborates on skills necessary for achievement of each competency. These elaborations should assist program faculty in curriculum planning, development, and program and student evaluation.

Domain I: Communication Skills

a. Can establish a mutually agreed upon genetic counseling agenda with the client.

The student is able to contract with a client or family throughout the relationship; explain the genetic counseling process; elicit expectations, perceptions and knowledge; and establish rapport through verbal and non-verbal interaction.

b. Can elicit an appropriate and inclusive family history.

The student is able to construct a complete pedigree; demonstrate proficiency in the use of pedigree symbols, standard notation, and nomenclature; structure questioning for the individual case and probable diagnosis; use interviewing skills; facilitate recall for symptoms and pertinent history by pursuing a relevant path of inquiry; and in the course of this interaction, identify family dynamics, emotional responses, and other relevant information.

c. Can elicit pertinent medical information including pregnancy, developmental, and medical histories.

The student is able to apply knowledge of the inheritance patterns, etiology, clinical features, and natural history of a variety of genetic disorders, birth defects, and other conditions; obtain appropriate medical histories; identify essential medical records and secure releases of medical information.

d. Can elicit a social and psychosocial history.

The student is able to conduct a client or family interview that demonstrates an appreciation of family systems theory and dynamics. The student is able to listen effectively, identify potential strengths and weaknesses, and assess individual and family support systems and coping mechanisms.

e. Can convey genetic, medical, and technical information including, but not limited to, diagnosis, etiology, natural history, prognosis, and treatment/management of genetic conditions and/or birth defects to clients with a variety of educational, socioeconomic, and ethnocultural backgrounds.

The student is able to demonstrate knowledge of clinical genetics and relevant medical topics by effectively communicating this information in a given session.

f. Can explain the technical and medical aspects of diagnostic and screening methods and reproductive options including associated risks, benefits, and limitations.

The student is able to demonstrate knowledge of diagnostic and screening procedures and clearly communicate relevant information to clients. The student is able to facilitate the informed-consent process. The student is able to determine client comprehension and adjust counseling accordingly.

g. Can understand, listen, communicate, and manage a genetic counseling case in a culturally responsive manner.

The student can care for clients using cultural self-awareness and familiarity with a variety of ethnocultural issues, traditions, health beliefs, attitudes, lifestyles, and values.

h. Can document and present case information clearly and concisely, both orally and in writing, as appropriate to the audience.

The student can present succinct and precise case-summary information to colleagues and other professionals. The student can write at an appropriate level for clients and professionals and produce written documentation within a reasonable time frame. The student can demonstrate respect for privacy and confidentiality of medical information.

i. Can plan, organize, and conduct public and professional education programs on human genetics, patient care, and genetic counseling issues.

The student is able to identify educational needs and design programs for specific audiences, demonstrate public speaking skills, use visual aids, and identify and access supplemental educational materials.

Domain II: Critical-Thinking Skills

a. Can assess and calculate genetic and teratogenic risks.

The student is able to calculate risks based on pedigree analysis and knowledge of inheritance patterns, genetic epidemiologic data, and quantitative genetics principles.

b. Can evaluate a social and psychosocial history.

The student demonstrates understanding of family and interpersonal dynamics and can recognize the impact of emotions on cognition and retention, as well as the need for intervention and referral.

c. Can identify, synthesize, organize and summarize pertinent medical and genetic information for use in genetic counseling.

The student is able to use a variety of sources of information including client/ family member(s), laboratory results, medical records, medical and genetic literature and computerized databases. The student is able to analyze and interpret information that provides the basis for differential diagnosis, risk assessment and genetic testing. The student is able to apply knowledge of the natural history and characteristics/symptoms of common genetic conditions.

d. Can demonstrate successful case management skills.

The student is able to analyze and interpret medical, genetic and family data; to design, conduct, and periodically assess the case management plan; arrange for testing; and follow up with the client, laboratory, and other professionals. The student should demonstrate understanding of legal and ethical issues related to privacy and confidentiality in communications about clients.

e. Can assess client understanding and response to information and its implications to modify a counseling session as needed.

The student is able to respond to verbal and nonverbal cues and to structure and modify information presented to maximize comprehension by clients.

f. Can identify and access local, regional, and national resources and services.

The student is familiar with local, regional, and national support groups and other resources, and can access and make referrals to other professionals and agencies.

g. Can identify and access information resources pertinent to clinical genetics and counseling.

The student is able to demonstrate familiarity with the genetic, medical and social-science literature, and on-line databases. The student is able to review the literature and synthesize the information for a case in a critical and meaningful way.

Domain III: Interpersonal, Counseling, and Psychosocial Assessment Skills

a. Can establish rapport, identify major concerns, and respond to emerging issues of a client or family.

The student is able to display empathic listening and interviewing skills, and address clients' concerns.

b. Can elicit and interpret individual and family experiences, behaviors, emotions, perceptions, and attitudes that clarify beliefs and values.

The student is able to assess and interpret verbal and non-verbal cues and use this information in the genetic counseling session. The student is able to engage clients in an exploration of their responses to risks and options.

c. Can use a range of interviewing techniques.

The student is able to identify and select from a variety of communication approaches throughout a counseling session.

d. Can provide short-term, client-centered counseling and psychological support.

The student is able to assess clients' psychosocial needs and recognize psychopathology. The student can demonstrate knowledge of psychological defenses, family dynamics, family theory, crisis-intervention techniques, coping models, the grief process, and reactions to illness. The student can use open-ended questions; listen empathically; employ crisis-intervention skills; and provide anticipatory guidance.

e. Can promote client decision-making in an unbiased, non-coercive manner.

The student understands the philosophy of non-directiveness and is able to recognize his or her values and biases as they relate to genetic counseling issues. The student is able to recognize and respond to dynamics, such as countertransference, that may affect the counseling interaction.

f. Can establish and maintain inter- and intradisciplinary professional relationships to function as part of a health-care delivery team.

The student behaves professionally and understands the roles of other professionals with whom he or she interacts.

Domain IV: Professional Ethics and Values

a. Can act in accordance with the ethical, legal, and philosophical principles and values of the profession.

The student is able to recognize and respond to ethical and moral dilemmas arising in practice and seek assistance from experts in these areas. The student is able to identify factors that promote or hinder client autonomy. The student demonstrates an appreciation of the issues surrounding privacy, informed consent, confidentiality, real or potential discrimination, and other ethical/ legal matters related to the exchange of genetic information.

b. Can serve as an advocate for clients.

The student can understand clients' needs and perceptions and represent their interests in accessing services and responses from the medical and social service systems.

c. Can introduce research options and issues to clients and families.

The student is able to critique and evaluate the risks, benefits, and limitations of client participation in research; access information on new research studies; present this information clearly and completely to clients; and promote an informed-consent process.

d. Can recognize his or her own limitations in knowledge and capabilities regarding medical, psychosocial, and ethnocultural issues and seek consultation or refer clients when needed.

The student demonstrates the ability to self-assess and to be self-critical. The student demonstrates the ability to respond to performance critique and integrates supervision feedback into his or her subsequent performance. The student is able to identify and obtain appropriate consultative assistance for self and clients.

e. Can demonstrate initiative for continued professional growth.

The student displays a knowledge of current standards of practice and shows independent knowledge-seeking behavior and lifelong learning."

Genetic Counselors' Scope of Practice (NSGC, 2007)

"This 'Genetic Counselors' Scope of Practice' statement outlines the responsibilities of individuals engaged in the practice of genetic counseling. Genetic counselors are health professionals with specialized education, training and experience in medical genetics and counseling who help people understand and adapt to the implications of genetic contributions to disease.[6] Genetic counselors interact with clients and other healthcare professionals in a variety of clinical and non-clinical settings, including, but not limited to, university-based medical centers, private hospitals, private practice, and industry settings. The instruction in clinical genetics, counseling, and communication skills required to carry out the professional responsibilities described in this statement is provided in graduate training programs accredited by the American Board of Genetic Counseling (ABGC)[7] or the equivalent, as well as through professional experience and continuing education courses.

The responsibilities of a genetic counselor are threefold: (i) to provide expertise in clinical genetics; (ii) to counsel and communicate with patients on matters of clinical genetics; and (iii) to provide genetic counseling services in accordance with professional ethics and values. Specifically:

Section I: Clinical Genetics

1. Explain the nature of genetics evaluation to clients. Obtain and review medical and family histories, based on the referral indication, and document the family history using standard pedigree nomenclature.

2. Identify additional client and family medical information relevant to risk assessment and consideration of differential diagnoses, and assist in obtaining such information.

3. Research and summarize pertinent data from the published literature, databases, and other professional resources, as necessary for each client.

4. Synthesize client and family medical information and data obtained from additional research as the basis for risk assessment, differential diagnosis, genetic testing options, reproductive options, follow-up recommendations, and case management.

---

[6] NSGC Definition of Genetic Counseling. *Journal of Genetic Counseling* April 2006; 77–82.
[7] American Board of Genetic Counseling website.

5. Assess the risk of occurrence or recurrence of a genetic condition or birth defect, using a variety of techniques, including knowledge of inheritance patterns, epidemiologic data, quantitative genetics principles, statistical models, and evaluation of clinical information, as applicable.

6. Explain to clients, verbally and/or in writing, medical information regarding the diagnosis or potential occurrence of a genetic condition or birth defect, including etiology, natural history, inheritance, disease management and potential treatment options.

7. Discuss available options and delineate the risks, benefits and limitations of appropriate tests and clinical assessments. Order tests and perform clinical assessments in accordance with local, state and federal regulations.

8. Document case information clearly and concisely in the medical record and in correspondence to referring physicians, and discuss case information with other members of the healthcare team, as necessary.

9. Assist clients in evaluating the risks, benefits and limitations of participation in research, and facilitate the informed consent process.

10. Identify and access local, regional, and national resources such as support groups and ancillary services; discuss the availability of such resources with clients; and provide referrals, as necessary.

11. Plan, organize and conduct public and professional education programs on medical genetics, patient care and genetic counseling issues.

Section II: Counseling and Communication

1. Develop a genetic counseling agenda with the client or clients that includes identification and negotiation of client/counselor priorities and expectations.

2. Identify individual client and family experiences, behaviors, emotions, perceptions, values, and cultural and religious beliefs in order to facilitate individualized decision making and coping.

3. Assess client understanding and response to medical information and its implications, and educate client appropriately.

4. Utilize appropriate interviewing techniques and empathic listening to establish rapport, identify major concerns and engage clients in an exploration of their responses to the implications of the findings, genetic risks, and available options/interventions.

5. Identify the client's psychological needs, stressors and sources of emotional and psychological support in order to determine appropriate interventions and/or referrals.

6. Promote client-specific decision making in an unbiased non-coercive manner that respects the client's culture, language, traditions, lifestyle, religious beliefs and values.

7. Use knowledge of psychological structure to apply client-centered techniques and family systems theory to facilitate adjustment to the occurrence or risk of occurrence of a congenital or genetic disorder.

Section III: Professional Ethics and Values

1. Recognize and respond to ethical and moral dilemmas arising in practice, identify factors that promote or hinder client autonomy, and understand issues surrounding privacy, informed consent, confidentiality, real or potential discrimination and potential conflicts of interest.
2. Advocate for clients, which includes understanding client needs and perceptions, representing their interests in accessing services, and eliciting responses from the medical and social service systems as well as the community at large.
3. Recognize personal limitations in knowledge and/or capabilities and seek consultation or appropriately refer clients to other providers.
4. Maintain professional growth, which includes acquiring relevant information required for a given situation, keeping abreast of current standards of practice as well as societal developments, and seeking out or establishing mechanisms for peer support.
5. Respect a client's right to confidentiality, being mindful of local, state and federal regulations governing release of personal health information.

This Scope of Practice statement was approved in June 2007 by the National Society of Genetic Counselors (NSGC)—the leading voice, advocate and authority for the genetic counseling profession. It is not intended to replace the judgment of an individual genetic counselor with respect to particular clients or special clinical situations and cannot be considered inclusive of all practices or exclusive of other practices reasonably directed at obtaining the same results. In addition, the practice of genetic counseling is subject to regulation by federal, state and local governments. In a subject jurisdiction, any such regulations will take precedence over this statement. NSGC expressly disclaims any warranties or guarantees, express or implied, and shall not be liable for damages of any kind, in connection with the information set forth in this Scope of Practice statement or for reliance on its contents.

Genetic counseling is a dynamic profession, which undergoes rapid change with the discovery of new genetic information and the development of new genetic tests and treatment options. Thus, NSGC will periodically review and, where appropriate, revise this statement as necessary for consistency with current practice information."

REFERENCES

American Board of Genetic Counseling (1996) "Requirements for Graduate Programs in Genetic Counseling Seeking Accreditation by the American Board of Genetic Counseling." Bethesda, MD: American Board of Genetic Counseling.

American Board of Genetic Counseling (2009) accessed 3/19/2009 at http://www.abgc.net/english/View.asp?x=1733.

American Society of Human Genetics Ad Hoc Committee on Genetic Counseling (1975) Genetic counseling. *Am J Hum Genet* 27:240–242.

Bennett RL, Steinhaus KL, Uhrich SB, O' Sullivan CK, Resta RG, Lochner-Doyle D, Markel DS, Vincent V, Hamanishi J (1995) Recommendations for standardized human pedigree nomenclature. *Am J Hum Genet* 56:745–752.

Breathnach FM, Malone FD, Lambert-Messerlian G, Cuckle HS, Porter TF, Nyberg DA, Comstock CH, Saade GR, Berkowitz RL, Klugman S, Dugoff L, Craigo SD, Timor-Tritsch IE, Carr SR, Wolfe HM, Tripp T, Bianchi DW, D'Alton ME (2007) First- and second-trimester screening: detection of aneuploidies other than Down syndrome. *Obstetr Gynecol* 110:651–657.

Broca PP (1866) *Traite des Tumeurs. Vol. 1.*, p. 80. Paris: P. Asselin.

Carr-Saunders AM (1929) Eugenics. p. 806. In: *The Encyclopedia Britannica* (14th ed.), Vol. 8. London: Encyclopedia Britannica Co.

Childs B, Zinkham W, Browne EA, Kimbro EL, Torbert JV (1958) A genetic study of a defect in glutathione metabolism of the erythrocyte. *Bull Johns Hopkins Hosp* 102:21–37.

Dumars KW, Burns J, Kessler S, Marks J, Walker AP (1979) *Genetics Associates: Their Training, Role and Function. A Conference Report.* Washington, DC: U.S. Department of Health, Education and Welfare.

Edwards JH, Harnden DF, Cameron AH, Crosse VM, Wolff OH (1960) A new trisomic syndrome. *Lancet* I:787–790.

Fiddler MB, Fine BA, Baker DL, and ABGC Consensus Development Consortium (1996) A case-based approach to the development of practice-based competencies for accreditation of and training in graduate programs in genetic counseling. *J Genet Couns* 5:105–112.

Fine BA, Baker DL, Fiddler MB and ABGC Consensus Development Consortium (1996) Practice-based competencies for accreditation of and training in graduate programs in genetic counseling. *J Genet Couns* 5:113–121.

Ford CE, Jones KW, Polani PE, de Almeida JC, Briggs JH (1959) A sex-chromosome anomaly in a case of gonadal dysgenesis (Turner's syndrome). *Lancet* I:711–713.

Garrod AE (1899) A contribution to the study of alcaptonuria. *Proc R Med Chir Soc*, n.s., 2:130.

Garrod AE (1902) The incidence of alkaptonuria: a study in chemical individuality. *Lancet* 2:1616.

Harper PS (2004) *Practical Genetic Counselling* (6th ed.). Oxford University Press, p 4.

Heimler A (1979) From whence we've come: a message from the president. *Perspect Genet Couns* 1:2.

Heimler A (1997) An oral history of the National Society of Genetic Counselors. *J Genet Couns* 6:315–336.

Hsia DY, Huang I, Driscoll SG (1958) The heterozygous carrier in galactosemia. *Nature* 182:1389–1390.

Jacobs PA, Strong JA (1959) A case of human intersexuality having a possible XXY sex-determining mechanism. *Nature* 183:302–303.

Jacobson CB, Barter RH (1967) Intrauterine diagnosis and management of genetic defects. *Am J Obstet Gynecol* 99:795–805.

Kenen RH (1986) Growing pains of a new health-care field: Genetic counselling in Australia and the United States. *Aust J Soc Issues*. 21:174–182.

Kenen, RH (1997) Opportunities and impediments for a consolidating and expanding profession: genetic counseling in the United States. *Soc Sci Med* 45:1377–1386.

Kunkel HG, Cappellini R, Müller- Eberhard U, Wolf J (1957) Observations on the minor basic hemoglobin component in the blood of normal individuals and patients with thalassemia. *J Clin Invest* 35:1615.

Lejeune J, Gautier M, Turpin R (1959) Etude des chromosomes somatiques de neuf enfants mongolien. *Compt Rend* 248:1721–1722.

Marks JH, Richter ML (1976) The genetic associate: a new health professional. *AJPH* 66:388–390.

Miller OJ and Therman E (2001). *Human chromosomes* (4th ed.). New York: Springer, p. 4.

National Society of Genetic Counselors' Definition Task Force: Resta R, Biesecker BB, Bennett RL, Blum S, Hahn SE, Strecker MN, Williams JL (2006) A new definition of genetic counseling: National Society of Genetic Counselors' Task Force Report. *J Genet Couns* 15:77–83.

National Society of Genetic Counselors, Inc. Professional Status Survey (2006) accessed August 10, 2007 at http://www.nsgc.org/client_files/career/2006_PSS_RESULTS.pdf.

National Society of Genetic Counselors, Inc. States currently licensing genetic counselors. Accessed March 19, 2009 at http://www.nsgc.org/members_only/licensure/licensure6.cfm.

National Society of Genetic Counselors, Inc. (2007) Genetic Counselors' Scope of Practice. Accessed October 21, 2007 at http://www.nsgc.org/client_files/SOP_final_0607.pdf.

Neel JV (1994) *Physician to the Gene Pool. Genetic Lessons and Other Stories.* New York. John Wiley & Sons.

Patau K, Smith DW, Therman E, Inhorn SL, Wagner HP (1960) Multiple congenital anomaly caused by an extra autosome. *Lancet* I:790–793.

Reed S (1955) *Counseling in Medical Genetics*. Philadelphia: W.B. Saunders.

Resta RG (1997) Eugenics and nondirectiveness in genetic counseling. *J Genet Couns* 6:255–258.

Resta R, Biesecker BB, Bennett RL, Blum S, et al. (2006) A New Definition of Genetic Counseling: National Society of Genetic Counselors' Task Force Report. *J Genet Couns* 15:77–83.

Sahhar MA, Young MA, Sheffield LJ, Aitken M (2005) Educating genetic counselors in Australia: developing an international perspective. *J Genet Couns* 14:283–294.

Serr DM, Sachs L, Danon M (1955) Diagnosis of sex before birth using cells from the amniotic fluid. *Bull Res Council Israel* 5B:137.

Sharma G, McCullough LB, Chervenak FA. 2007. Ethical considerations of early (first vs. second trimester) risk assessment disclosure for trisomy 21 and patient choice in screening versus diagnostic testing. *Am J Med Genet C Semin Med Genet* 145C:99–104.

Smith DW, Patau K, Therman E, Inhorn SL (1960) A new autosomal trisomy syndrome: multiple congenital anomalies caused by an extra chromosome. *J Pediatr* 57:338–345.

Steele MW, Breg WR Jr. (1966) Chromosome analysis of human amniotic fluid cells. *Lancet* I:383–385.

Therman E, Susman M (1993) *Human Chromosomes. Structure, Behavior, and Effects* (3rd ed.). New York: Springer, p. 1.

Transnational Alliance for Genetic Counselling, accessed March 19, 2009 at http://tagc.med.sc. edu/pg2.htm.

Tjio JH, Levan A (1956) The chromosome number in man. *Hereditas* 42:1–6.

Volk BW, Aronson SM, Saifer SM (1964) Fructose-1-phosphate aldolase deficiency in Tay-Sachs disease. *Am J Med* 36:481.

Walker AP, Scott JA, Biesecker BB, Conover B, Blake W, Djurdjinovic L (1990) Report of the 1989 Asilomar meeting on education in genetic counseling. *Am J Hum Genet* 46:1223–1230.

Weatherall DJ (1963) Abnormal haemoglobins in the neonatal period and their relationship to thalassemia. *Br J Haematol* 9:625–677.

Wooldridge A (1997) Eugenics: the secret lurking in many nations' past. *Los Angeles Times*, Sept 7, 1997.

2

The Ultimate Genetic Tool: The Family History

Jane L. Schuette, M.S., C.G.C. and Robin L. Bennett, M.S., C.G.C., D.Sc. Hon.

...as so often happens in medicine, new developments do not eclipse the tried-and-true method; instead, they give it new meaning and power.

—A. Guttmacher et al., 2007

Genetic counseling is dependent on the gathering of accurate, detailed, and relevant information. The family history, which is essentially a compilation of information about the physical and mental health of an individual's family, is a *fundamental component* of this process. Obtaining a family history provides a basis for making a diagnosis, determining risk, making recommendations for medical management, and assessing the needs for patient education and psychosocial support. The family history has long been regarded as essential to the care of patients at risk for relatively uncommon Mendelian disorders. However, the family history has been shown to help predict the risk of more common, multifactorial disorders as well. These include such varied health concerns as heart disease (Morales et al., 2008), colorectal cancer (Maradiegue et al., 2008), breast cancer (Nelson et al., 2005), ovarian cancer (Pharoah and Ponder, 2002), osteoporosis (Yoon et al., 2002), asthma (Cole Johnson et al., 2004), type 2 diabetes (Harrison et al., 2003; Valdez et al., 2007), glaucoma (Green et al., 2007), and clotting disorders (Dietrich et al., 2007), among many others.

A Guide to Genetic Counseling, Second Edition, Edited by Wendy Uhlmann, Jane Schuette, and Beverly Yashar
Copyright © 2009 by John Wiley & Sons, Inc.

It is therefore of utmost importance that genetic counselors possess the skills necessary to gather and record an accurate and relevant family history.

The pedigree is the diagram that records the family history information, the tool for converting information provided by the client and/or obtained from the medical record into a standardized format. It demonstrates the biological relationships of the client to his or her family members through the use of symbols and vertical and horizontal lines and the presence and/or absence of disorders through shading, hatching, and abbreviations. When complete, the pedigree stands as a quick and accurate visual record that assists in providing genetic counseling and disease risk assessment. An analysis of the pedigree reveals the number of family members affected and ages at diagnosis and at death, and may suggest the pattern of inheritance of a disorder within a family. It may provide information that aids in making a diagnosis, as well as information about the natural history of a disorder and its variable expression among family members. The pedigree offers a means of identifying family members at risk for being affected with a disorder as well as estimating risks for recurrence in future offspring. The pedigree may also indicate a history of other conditions for which an evaluation and/or genetic counseling are recommended.

The process of obtaining a family history and constructing a pedigree may reveal the social relationships of the client to his or her family members. Information about adoption, divorce, separation, and "blended families" may be obtained. Pregnancy loss, infertility, or death of family members is also recorded. The family history may provide information that suggests the extent of the medical, emotional, and social impact of a disorder for a family. Myths developed by family members, explaining who in the family is at risk and why, may be revealed. And finally, because the family history is often obtained at the beginning of the genetic counseling process, it is a critical mechanism for establishing a productive relationship with the patient and family.

This chapter reviews the components of gathering a family history and constructing a pedigree. In addition, we explore opportunities for psychosocial assessment and patient education that present themselves during the process of taking a history.

THE EVOLUTION OF THE PEDIGREE

> A complete pedigree is often a work of great labour, and in its finished form is frequently a work of art.
>
> —Pearson, 1912

Interest in family origins has existed for thousands of years as evidenced in many historical texts, the Bible being a prime example. The pedigree, as a diagram using lines to connect an individual to his or her offspring, was developed in the fifteenth century as one of several techniques for illustrating ancestry (Resta, 1993). However, the use of the pedigree to demonstrate inheritance of traits is a more recent convention, dating back to the mid-nineteenth century, when the inheritance of colorblindness was documented in a publication by Pliny Earle and the "inheritance" of genius and artistic ability was demonstrated by Francis Galton. Earle's pedigree utilized anonymous symbols (circles and squares) to represent the members of a family, while Galton's included the names of family members (Resta, 1993).

Throughout the history of the pedigree, a variety in styles and symbols has been commonplace, reflecting differences in individual preferences, professional training, and national styles. The use of squares and circles for males and females, respectively, by American geneticists and the astronomical symbols for Mars and Venus by English geneticists was one major difference in symbols evident in the early twentieth century (Resta, 1993). In the 1990s, surveys of pedigrees recorded in clinical practice and in professional publications demonstrated the persistence of extensive variation in the use of pedigree symbols and nomenclature. A survey of genetic counselors published in 1993 showed discrepancies even in common symbols such as those used to indicate pregnancy and miscarriage (Bennett et al., 1993). A review of medical genetics textbooks and human genetics journals also identified inconsistencies in the use of symbols (Steinhaus et al., 1995). Since the value of the family history in establishing an accurate diagnosis and risk assessment is diminished if symbols and abbreviations cannot be interpreted, a Pedigree Standardization Task Force (PSTF) was formed in 1991 through the National Society of Genetic Counselors in con-junction with the Pacific Northwest Regional Genetics Group (PacNoRGG) and the Washington State Department of Health. Recommendations for standardized human pedigree nomenclature were developed and subjected to peer review. These recom-mendations, which have helped to set a more universal standard, were published in the *American Journal of Human Genetics* (Bennett et al., 1995a) and the *Journal of Genetic Counseling* (Bennett et al., 1995b) and have been adopted internationally (Bennett et al., 2008). The NSGC adopted the following Standard Pedigree Symbol Position Statement in 2003.

> Standardized pedigree symbols offer a consistent method of recording and interpreting family history, increasing uniformity of medical information and enhancing quality control in clinical genetics, medicine, genetic education and research (NSGC, 2003).

In 2008 the task force (now called the Pedigree Standardization Work Group) proposed some minor changes to pedigree symbols, and importantly, determined that the nomenclature was the only consistently acknowledged standard for con-structing a family medical history (Bennett et al., 2008).

The pedigree has also been an invaluable research tool, historically providing evidence for the establishment of the inheritance pattern of particular disorders and then as an essential component of linkage analysis, assisting in the identification of disease loci. More recently, the family history has been touted as the penultimate public health tool for screening the population at large for many preventable, chronic conditions (Guttmacher et al., 2004; Bendure and Mulvihill, 2006). In a 2003 study comparing the documentation and quality of risk assessment between a questionnaire, a pedigree, and a chart review, it was found that approximately 20% of patients in an internal medicine practice were at an increased risk for disorders with known genetic components that were not documented in reviewed chart notes. A targeted family history analysis reveals patients who require increased medical surveillance, preventive measures, or genetic counseling and testing referral (Frezzo et al., 2003).

The recognition of the power of the family history and pedigree has occurred on the national level as exemplified by the U.S. Surgeon General's Family History Initiative, a collaborative effort involving multiple agencies, including the National Institutes of Health and the Centers for Disease Control and Prevention. The initiative plans to attain the goals of reminding health professionals and patients about the value of family history and making the process of collecting and analyzing data easier for health professionals and individuals through a web-based tool. The initial focus is on heart disease, diabetes, stroke, breast, and ovarian and colon cancers. The tool organizes family history information and prints out a pedigree and a report, and was made available in November 2005 (http://www.hhs/gov/familyhistory/2008). The goal is to encourage people to bring their family history to their health care provider for further discussion and action.

FAMILY HISTORY BASICS

A family history should be obtained from all clients seeking genetic evaluation and/or counseling. This includes the construction of at least a standard three-generation pedigree containing information on the client, the client's first-degree relatives (children, siblings, and parents), second-degree relatives (half-siblings, aunts, uncles, nieces, nephews, grandparents, and grandchildren), and, ideally, third-degree relatives (first cousins).

The first considerations when gathering family history information are Who, What, Where, When, and How.

Who?

In general the pedigree begins with the individual for whom an evaluation is being performed or for whom genetic counseling is being provided. The consultand (or client) is the individual(s) seeking genetic evaluation, counseling, or testing, who may or may not be affected. "Proband" is the term that designates the affected family member who brings the family to medical attention (Bennett et al., 1995a, 1995c; Marazita, 1995). Consultand and proband may be the same person, and there may be more than one consultand seeking genetic services.

What?

The nature of the referral or the reason for the visit should be clarified. Is this a referral for genetic counseling because of a family history of a particular disorder? Is this a diagnostic evaluation, and, if so, for what reason? Or is this a reproductive genetics consultation, and what is the indication?

The nature of the visit to the genetics clinic provides a focus for the process of obtaining a family history. During a consultation for advanced maternal age, for example, the counselor would obtain a standard three-generation pedigree and would use questioning directed at determining whether there are additional risks that need to be addressed or considered. Typical questions might include the following:

Are there any individuals in your family with cognitive impairment, birth defects, and/or inherited disorders?

Is there any history of stillbirth, multiple pregnancy losses, or infant death?

During a diagnostic evaluation triggered by findings suggesting the diagnosis of neurofibromatosis type I (NF 1), the counselor would obtain a standard three-generation pedigree that includes a series of focused questions about the presence of symptoms and signs of neurofibromatosis, especially in first-degree family members. This information is extremely important to the patient's evaluation because the presence of a first-degree family member is one of the criteria considered in establishing a diagnosis of NF 1 (Gutmann et al., 1997). This example of a targeted family history includes questions that focus on the gathering of information that weighs in favor of or against a particular diagnosis. It could be argued that all family histories are targeted, based on the indication for the genetics evaluation. The distinction probably relies more on the specificity of the indication for the evaluation and the degree of confidence that is given to the differential diagnosis provided. For example, a referral for a family history of cognitive impairment is fairly nonspecific, whereas a referral for a family history of tuberous sclerosis is very specific. Certain general questions should be asked during the course of obtaining any history, while more specific questions depend on the reason for genetic evaluation and counseling.

Inquiring about the presence of physical features *associated* with a particular diagnosis is also important when one is obtaining a family history; this may help to establish a diagnosis, and information about potentially affected family members may be revealed. In the case of NF 1, for example, asking about scoliosis and/or learning disabilities, problems *associated* with NF 1, may indicate a family member who may be affected. Or, if the indication for the visit is a history of fetal loss, the counselor would inquire specifically not only about fetal loss, but also about infant death, infertility, cognitive impairment, and birth defects in extended family members, seeking clues about the possibility of an inherited chromosome translocation, X-linked condition associated with male lethality, or other inherited conditions.

Where?

The family history should be obtained in an environment that is comfortable and free of distractions. It should also be obtained in a setting that preserves confidentiality.

When?

The pedigree is usually drawn in the presence of the client(s). Alternatives to the traditional face-to-face method include the family history questionnaire sent to patients in advance of their appointment and the telephone interview. Questionnaires and phone interviews offer the advantages of saving time and enabling advanced case preparation on the part of both the client and the counselor. For example, when there is a history of cancer in a close family member, it may be of particular importance to obtain medical records pertaining to the cancer diagnosis, in order to provide the client with an accurate risk assessment. If this is done in advance, the initial appointment is generally more productive. However, the face-to-face interview is an opportunity for the counselor to make important observations, obtain psychosocial information from the client, and set the stage for a relationship of trust. Complex relationships, such as marriages between biological relatives (consanguinity) or a history of multiple partners, may more likely be revealed in person. The family history and pedigree may be more accurate when the client is present during the recording; in fact, the details of a family history obtained through a questionnaire or phone interview should always be confirmed with the client in person.

In most instances, the family history is obtained during the information-gathering portion of the genetic counseling visit, before the examination, risk assessment, and/or counseling. In some instances, however, the family history may be deferred until the end of the visit, or even until the time of a follow-up appointment. This may be the case when there is a newly established diagnosis such as trisomy 21 in a newborn or in an ongoing pregnancy in which the counseling issues are given precedence.

A pedigree is part of a client's medical record. Pedigrees should be drawn on official paper or specific forms designated by the institution for inclusion in the medical record. Preprinted forms that serve as a template on which to construct the pedigree can be useful because they are efficient. Space constraints in the recording of a large family history can be a disadvantage, however.

All medical documentation including the pedigree, if recorded on paper, should be in black pen. This permits reproducibility and scanning into an electronic format. Taking a pedigree in pencil can sometimes be useful, since it is not unusual for the client to remember additional information after the form has been completed. The penciled pedigree can be redrawn in ink later. Although redrawing a pedigree originally done in pencil or one that is simply messy improves clarity, there is the potential for omitting important information in the transcription. The most efficient method is to master the skill of drawing an accurate and legible pedigree in ink the first time. A hint for fixing mistakes before the pedigree is placed or scanned into the medical record is to use a fine-point white correction fluid pen. Plastic drawing templates with varying sizes of squares, circles, triangles, and arrows are useful for keeping symbols neat and uniform, although some genetic counselors find the use of templates to be awkward, preferring instead to draw them freehand. Templates are available through many genetic testing companies and well as art supply stores. Pedigrees can also be generated via computer programs for publication, presentation, or the patient's medical record.

GATHERING THE INFORMATION AND CONSTRUCTING A PEDIGREE

The National Society of Genetic Counselors advocates the use of pedigree symbols as presented in "Recommendations for Standardized Human Pedigree Nomenclature," (Am J Hum Genet 56: 745-752, 1995), both in clinical practice and in medical/scientific publications.

Gathering the family history and constructing a pedigree is a process best conducted in step-by-step fashion. Standardized symbols and nomenclature should be used, as they offer a consistent method of recording and interpreting family history information.

Overview of Pedigree Construction and Standard Symbols

Some of the commonly used pedigree symbols, definitions, and abbreviations are summarized in Table 2-1. A male is designated by a square and, if possible, placed to the left of the female partner; a female is designated by a circle. A diamond can be used to represent an individual whose sex is not specified.

The proband or consultand is identified with an arrow (Table 2-1); the proband is distinguished from the consultand by the use of the letter P. It is extremely important to identify the consultand; otherwise, someone looking at a large pedigree may be unable to determine to whom the pedigree pertains.

There are four "line definitions" to orient generations within a pedigree (Table 2-2) (Bennett et al., 2008). A **relationship line** connects two partners (conventions for same-sex relationships are discussed shortly, in connection with assisted reproductive technology). A break in the relationship line (a double slash) indicates separation or divorce. The **line of descent** extends vertically (or sometimes diagonally if there are space constraints) from the relationship line and connects to the horizontal **sibship line**. Each sibling (including each pregnancy whether or not it is carried to term) is attached to the sibship line by an **individual line**. Twins share the same line of descent but have different individual lines. If twins are known to be monozygotic, a horizontal line is drawn above the symbols (not between the symbols, since it is a relationship line).

A number placed inside a symbol is an indication of how many males or females are in a sibship. For example, a square with a 5 inside means five males. If a person has had children with multiple partners, it is not always necessary to show each partner, especially if such information is not relevant to the family history. For example, a line of descent can extend directly from a parent without including the partner (Table 2-2).

A pregnancy is symbolized by a "P" inside a square or a circle if the fetal sex is known or inside a diamond if unknown. The "age" of the pregnancy is recorded by listing the first day of the last menstrual period (LMP), gestational age (e.g., 20 wk), or estimated date of confinement (EDC). Triangles represent pregnancies not carried

TABLE 2-1. Common Pedigree Symbols, Definitions, and Abbreviations

Instructions:
— Key should contain all information relevant to interpretation of pedigree (e.g., define fill/shading)
— For clinical (non-published) pedigrees include:
  a) name of proband/consultand
  b) family names/initials of relatives for identification, as appropriate
  c) name and title of person recording pedigree
  d) historian (person relaying family history information)
  e) date of intake/update
  f) reason for taking pedigree (e.g., abnormal ultrasound, familial cancer, developmental delay, etc.)
  g) ancestry of both sides of family
— Recommended order of information placed below symbol (or to lower right)
  a) age; can note year of birth (e.g., b.1978) and/or death (e.g., d. 2007)
  b) evaluation (see Figure 4)
  c) pedigree number (e.g., I-1, I-2, I-3)
  d) limit identifying information to maintain confidentiality and privacy

	Male	Female	Gender not specified	Comments
1. Individual	b. 1925	30y	4 mo	Assign gender by phenotype (see text for disorders of sex development, etc.). Do not write age in symbol.
2. Affected individual				Key/legend used to define shading or other fill (e.g., hatches, dots, etc.). Use only when individual is clinically affected.
			With ≥2 conditions, the individual's symbol can be partitioned accordingly, each segment shaded with a different fill and defined in legend.	
3. Multiple individuals, number known	5	5	5	Number of siblings written inside symbol. (Affected individuals should not be grouped).
4. Multiple individuals, number unknown or unstated	n	n	n	"n" used in place of "?".
5. Deceased individual	d. 35	d. 4 mo	d. 60's	Indicate cause of death if known. Do not use a cross (†) to indicate death to avoid confusion with evaluation positive (+).
6. Consultand				Individual(s) seeking genetic counseling/testing.
7. Proband	P	P		An affected family member coming to medical attention independent of other family members.
8. Stillbirth (SB)	SB 28 wk	SB 30 wk	SB 34 wk	Include gestational age and karyotype, if known.
9. Pregnancy (P)	LMP: 7/1/2007 47,XY,+21	P 20 wk 46,XX	P	Gestational age and karyotype below symbol. Light shading can be used for affected; define in key/legend.

Pregnancies not carried to term	Affected	Unaffected	
10. Spontaneous abortion (SAB)	17 wks female cystic hygroma	< 10 wks	If gestational age/gender known, write below symbol. Key/legend used to define shading.
11. Termination of pregnancy (TOP)	18 wks 47,XY,+18		Other abbreviations (e.g., TAB, VTOP) not used for sake of consistency.
12. Ectopic pregnancy (ECT)		ECT	Write ECT below symbol.

Source: Reprinted, with permission, from Springer Science & Business Media: Bennett et al., *J Genet Couns* 17:427. Copyright 2008 by the National Society of Genetic Counselors, Inc.

TABLE 2-2. Pedigree Line Definitions

1. Definitions	Comments
1. relationship line 2. line of descent 3. sibship line 4. individual's line	If possible, male partner should be to left of female partner on relationship line. Siblings should be listed from left to right in birth order (oldest to youngest).

2. Relationship line (horizontal)

a. Relationships		A break in a relationship line indicates the relationship no longer exists. Multiple previous partners do not need to be shown if they do not affect genetic assessment.
b. Consanguinity		If degree of relationship not obvious from pedigree, it should be stated (e.g., third cousins) above relationship line.

3. Line of descent (vertical or diagonal)

a. Genetic		Biologic parents shown.

- Multiple gestation	Monozygotic	Dizygotic	Unknown	Trizygotic	The horizontal line indicating monozygosity is placed between the individual's line and not between each symbol. An asterisk (*) can be used if zygosity proven.
- Family history not available/ known for individual	?	?			
- No children by choice or reason unknown		vasectomy or tubal			Indicate reason, if known.
- Infertility		azoospermia or endometriosis			Indicate reason, if known.

b. Adoption	in	out	by relative	Brackets used for all adoptions. Adoptive and biological parents denoted by dashed and solid lines of descent, respectively.

Source: Reprinted, with permission, from Springer Science & Business Media: Bennett et al., *J Genet Couns* 17:428. Copyright 2008 by the National Society of Genetic Counselors, Inc.

to term, for example, miscarriages or elective terminations (a diagonal line is drawn through the symbol to represent an elective termination). Rarely is the sex known in a miscarriage, but if it is, "male" or "female" should be written below the symbol (Table 2-1).

A diagonal line drawn through a symbol indicates that the person represented is deceased. This is a visual way of recording who is alive or deceased on a pedigree, although some clients may find it offensive to have a deceased relative "slashed out" when a genetic counselor is recording the pedigree in their presence. When obtaining a family history from a client who is adopted, it is essential to distinguish between the adoptive (nonbiological) family and the biological or birth family. In either situation, brackets are placed around the symbol for the adopted individual. If the nonbiological family is included, a dotted line of descent is used. Otherwise, a solid line of descent is used, just as for any other biological relationship (Table 2-2).

The need to represent pregnancies conceived through assisted reproductive technology (ART), such as artificial insemination by donor, has become more common. The conventions for symbolizing the biological and social relationships involved in ART within a pedigree are outlined in Table 2-3. Some general rules include placing a "D" inside the symbol for the egg or sperm donor. An "S" inside the female symbol denotes a surrogate. If this female is both the ovum donor and a surrogate, she is referred to only as a donor (in the interest of genetic assessment). The relationship line is between the couple (same-sex or heterosexual), and the line of descent extends from the woman who is actually carrying the pregnancy. By using these rules, any method of ART can be clearly illustrated (Bennett et al., 2008). Documenting elective sterilization (e.g., tubal ligation or vasectomy) is useful if reproductive counseling is considered and as a factor in assessing risks for recurrence.

A double horizontal relationship line is drawn to represent a consanguineous couple. If the degree of relationship is not obvious from the pedigree (e.g., third cousins), it should be indicated above the relationship line.

A shaded symbol indicates an individual affected with a condition that is known or suspected to be genetic. More than one genetic condition can be shown by partitioning the symbol into three or four sectors and filling in the sectors or using different patterns of fill. As long as the shading is defined in a key (see below), any pattern can be used.

Even when standardized pedigree symbols are used, it is essential to include a key (also called a legend). The key provides information that is vital to interpreting the pedigree. It is used to identify less commonly used symbols (e.g., adoption) or to identify shaded symbols, particularly when several disorders are represented by different symbols within a family.

The Standard Information Recorded on the Pedigree

The counselor should record ages and/or year of birth of the client and family members (especially first-degree relatives) on the pedigree, below the symbol or to the right if necessary, regardless of whether these individuals are reported to be affected or unaffected with a disorder. The age reached by an apparently unaffected family member may have important implications not only for that particular family member but for the client as well. For individuals reported to be affected with a particular disorder, the age of onset or age at diagnosis should be obtained. This is particularly important for many adult-onset conditions. For example, a client whose maternal

TABLE 2-3. Assisted Reproductive Technologies (ART) Symbols and Definitions

Instructions:
— D represents egg or sperm donor
— S represents surrogate (gestational carrier)
— If the woman is both the ovum donor and a surrogate, in the interest of genetic assessment, she will only be referred to as a donor (e.g., 4 and 5)); the pregnancy symbol and its line of descent are positioned below the woman who is carrying the pregnancy
— Available family history should be noted on the gamete donor and/or gestational carrier

Possible Reproductive Scenarios		Comments
1. Sperm donor		Couple in which woman is carrying pregnancy using donor sperm. No relationship line is shown between the woman carrying the pregnancy and the sperm donor.
2. Ovum donor		Couple in which woman is carrying pregnancy using a donor egg and partner's sperm. The line of descent from the birth mother is solid because there is a biologic relationship that may affect the fetus (e.g., teratogens).
3. Surrogate only		Couple whose gametes are used to impregnate a woman (surrogate) who carries the pregnancy. The line of descent from the surrogate is solid because there is a biological relationship that may affect the fetus (e.g., teratogens).
4. Surrogate ovum donor		Couple in which male partner's sperm is used to inseminate a) an unrelated woman or b) a sister who is carrying the pregnancy for the couple.
5. Planned adoption		Couple contracts with a woman to carry a pregnancy using ovum of the woman carrying the pregnancy and donor sperm.

grandmother and maternal aunt developed breast cancer before menopause may be at greater risk for breast cancer than the general population. A client whose mother was reported to be unaffected at age 65, however, may have a lifetime risk of breast cancer similar to that of the general population.

The units used to measure ages should be included after each number, using standard abbreviations [e.g., 35 y (years), 4 mo (months), 20 wk (weeks), 3 dy (days)]. It is important to note that the ability of clients to recall dates of birth or ages is variable, especially with respect to information on extended family members. Unless precise information is required, the counselor may wish to encourage the client to provide close estimates by asking, for instance, whether the family member is in her 50s, 60s, or 70s.

The health status of the client and each family member (or pregnancy) must be recorded succinctly. This includes information about the presence of birth defects, developmental delay and cognitive impairment, inherited disorders, mental health, and chronic illness. Specific and accurate information is best. For example, if a family member is reported to be affected with "muscular dystrophy," the type of muscular dystrophy should be specified. In most circumstances, if a family member at age 70 is reported to have had "heart problems requiring medication, multiple hospitalizations, and triple bypass surgery," it is adequate to record coronary artery disease or heart disease.

Although information recorded on a pedigree should not be too wordy, the use of multiple abbreviations can be confusing. For example "CP" may be an abbreviation for cleft palate or cerebral palsy, and "TS" is sometimes used for Tay–Sachs disease as well as tuberous sclerosis. If abbreviations are used, they should be defined in a key.

If a family member is deceased, cause and age at death are recorded on the pedigree. It is also important to inquire whether any family members, especially first-degree relatives, have had pregnancies that resulted in miscarriages, stillbirths, or infant deaths. Often clients will omit information about unsuccessful pregnancies, as well as data on siblings and other relatives who are not living or who died at or around the time of birth. It is also important to distinguish whether individuals who have no children have remained childless by choice or because of a known biological reason (infertility).

The Step-by-Step Process

The counselor should begin by providing a brief explanation to the client about the purpose and process of gathering the family history information. The counselor then asks sequential questions while, at the same time, drawing the pedigree. Usually the counselor begins with the client, drawing him or her on the pedigree, and obtaining the information described above (e.g., health status, age). If the client is an adult and has a partner, the partner may also be placed on the pedigree at this point, which helps with the positioning of the pedigree appropriately on the paper (usually in the center).

During questioning, use language and terms that are likely to be familiar to your patient or client. It is appropriate to use medical terminology if it is clearly understood by your patient. However, be prepared to use descriptive terms if your patient appears unlikely to comprehend. For example, ask about the presence of muscle weakness rather than a myopathy. Also consider the manner in which your questions are formulated. Rather than leading your client with a question like "Your brothers and sisters are in good health, right?", ask instead, "Do your brothers and sisters have any health problems?" It is also courteous and compassionate to acknowledge recent events such as miscarriage, the death of a close family member, or a recent serious diagnosis (Bennett, in press).

It is easiest to obtain family history information in chronological order. The counselor guides the client by proceeding through each first-degree relative, usually by first asking whether the client has had children and/or pregnancies. As a rule, it is easier to obtain information on the children before finding out about any siblings, simply because of the practical consideration that offspring are drawn on the pedigree on a line below the client. (If a child is the patient, it is usually easier to obtain information on his or her siblings before information on the parents is requested). Ages and information about the physical and mental health of each living child should be obtained. Cause of death, health problems, and age at death should be obtained for those who are deceased.

It should be ascertained consistently whether all pregnancies were conceived with the same partner and whether all brothers and sisters within a sibship have the same parents. Otherwise, such information may not be revealed until the pedigree is complete. The counselor needs to indicate on the pedigree any pregnancies conceived with different partner(s) or any siblings who have a different parent (Table 2-2).

The counselor then asks whether the client has brothers or sisters and whether such siblings have had any children or pregnancies; if so, information about their ages and health is elicited. The counselor should next inquire about the client's mother and father (whether living or deceased; their physical and mental health status), continuing through each family member until a three-generation pedigree has been constructed. When constructing a pedigree for adult-onset disorders, two generations of ascent (parents and grandparents) and two generations of descent (children and grandchildren) should be included.

It is important to obtain both the maternal and paternal sides of a family history, even if the visit is for risk assessment and counseling regarding a history of a particular disorder on one side of the family. A full family history allows the counselor to determine whether there are additional factors that may influence risk assessment, for psychosocial considerations (a focus on only one side of the family may unintentionally support the client's sense of responsibility or guilt for the disease in the family), and for completeness. Not uncommonly, additional risks are identified during the course of obtaining a family history, necessitating discussion and/or evaluation (Holsinger et al., 1992; Frezzo et al., 2003). A question mark is placed above the line of descent in instances in which little is known about the family history to indicate the appropriate inquiries were made.

A three-generation pedigree is usually adequate and is considered standard. Error rates in diagnosis, in age at diagnosis, and even in the existence of relatives increase as the degree of relationships increases (Ziogas and Anton-Culver, 2003). For many common diseases, having an affected close relative is the strongest predictor of an individual's lifetime risk for developing the disease (Walter and Emery, 2006). This is true for most single-gene disorders as well, although at times, especially for conditions with reduced penetrance and variable expressivity, information on extended family members may be useful. For example, a family history obtained for a patient in whom physical findings suggest the diagnosis of Marfan syndrome may include pertinent information beyond three generations. A positive history of sudden death in early adulthood in one or more distant family members may contribute toward the establishment of a diagnosis.

When the pedigree appears complete, many counselors ask a series of general questions about the presence of birth defects, cognitive impairment, and inherited disorders. More specific questions about the existence of associated anomalies or specific signs and symptoms may be asked when warranted, as in a targeted family history. This effort may seem redundant, but often clients recall additional important information after the pedigree has been completed, especially if the counselor makes a final extra attempt to elicit such recollections.

Additional Considerations

Several key points for gathering a family history and constructing an accurate pedigree bear highlighting. All have an impact on genetic risk assessment and counseling.

Ethnic Background   The counselor must inquire about the ethnic background of the client's paternal and maternal sides of the family, including the family's country of origin and religion. Responses to these inquiries may yield information that is useful for diagnostic purposes as well as for identifying couples at increased risk for being carriers of certain autosomal recessive disorders such as cystic fibrosis, Tay–Sachs disease, sickle cell anemia, and thalassemia that are more common in certain ethnic groups. In some disorders the sensitivity and specificity of genetic testing vary by ethnicity. This is true for cystic fibrosis, in which specific mutations occur with varying frequency among different populations (Grody et al., 2001; Richards et al., 2002; Watson et al., 2004), and for hereditary breast and ovarian cancer, in which three founder mutations are responsible for the majority of mutations among individuals of Ashkenazi Jewish ancestry (Nanda et al., 2005). The assessment of ethnicity is also important for identifying increased risk for chronic conditions due to multifactorial inheritance. For example, the prevalence of some disorders is higher in certain ethnic groups, such as glaucoma in African Americans and in Caribbeans of African descent (Fleming et al., 2005) and type 2 diabetes among Native Americans and Pacific Islanders (Eriksson et al., 2001).

The question about ethnic background should be posed in a manner that is clear to the client(s). The counselor may need to use alternative words or phrases such as "country of origin," "family's nationality," or "family's traditional religion," to ensure that clients thoroughly understand what information is sought. It may also be necessary to briefly explain the purpose of the inquiry as being related to accurate risk assessment, diagnostic, and/or screening considerations.

Consanguinity   The counselor should inquire whether key family members are related to one another. Determining whether consanguinity is present is important for the biological parents of the patient for whom an evaluation is being performed. Inquiring about consanguinity is also important for purposes of preconception counseling and when there are concerns about an ongoing pregnancy.

When asking about consanguinity the counselor may need to pose the question in a variety of ways:

Are you and your partner blood relatives?

Is there any chance that you and your partner are related to one another other than by marriage?

Were your parents or grandparents related to each other; for example, were they cousins?

In some instances (e.g., when a rare autosomal recessive disorder is a diagnostic consideration), it may be necessary to obtain additional information related to the possibility of consanguinity. The counselor may wish to obtain maiden names and surnames of the biological mother and father, and both sets of grandparents, as well as the city, town, or village (in addition to country) of origin to search for possible distant consanguinity or to document a lack of any evidence. It is also important to note that clients sometimes describe biological relationships inaccurately, and therefore the counselor must carefully establish the exact nature of every relationship that is a potential source of ambiguity. For example, a client may report that she and her partner are second cousins when, in fact, they are first cousins once removed (Fig. 2-1). Culture also plays a role in how clients describe their degree of relationship, and again care must be given to accurately determine individuals' common ancestry. (See Chapter 11 on Multicultural Counseling).

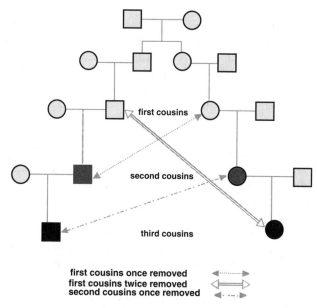

FIGURE 2-1. *Relationships*

Adoption Adopted persons are often frustrated when entering the genetics realm, which often begins with the collection of family history information; some have even sought genetic counseling and testing because of their anxiety surrounding their lack of knowledge about their biological family's medical background. However, the availability of DNA testing does not obviate the usefulness of a family history, because testing is often performed and interpreted in the context of established risk factors.

Recognition of the importance of family history, including known medical history of the adoptee and his or her biological parents, has resulted in legislation to require the collection and disclosure of nonidentifying social, medical, and psychological information in many states (Venne et al., 2003). The American Society of Human Genetics (ASHG) states that the genetic history should be included in an adoptee's record. The ASHG recommends that "when medically appropriate, genetic data may be shared among the adoptive parents, biological parents and adoptees" (ASHG, 1991). There is no uniformity in the extent and type of medical and family history information collected at the time of adoption, or mechanisms to confirm the validity of the information (Bennett, in press). There may be little information of value known by the birth parent(s) and/or collected by the adoption intermediaries. The ages of biological parents may be such that later-onset diseases in the birth parents and relatives may not be apparent, and there is often no mechanism for updating information on the health status of relatives. Genetic counselors should familiarize themselves with their state's laws regarding the collection and disclosure of information in order to assist their adopted clients and their families with obtaining family history information.

Identifying Information It is critical that the pedigree include the name and professional background (e.g., M.S., R.N., M.D.) of the person who recorded the pedigree. It is also important to identify the historian, the person providing the family history information. Information about the extended family provided by a foster parent may be more subject to questions of accuracy than information provided by a close biological relative. Recording the date the pedigree was obtained or updated is also important, particularly if the pedigree includes ages of family members instead of years of birth.

The Pedigree Standardization Work Group has recommended that the indication for obtaining the family history be recorded on the pedigree, for example, "cancer risk assessment," "abnormal ultrasound" (Bennett et al., 2008). This will serve to clarify the purpose, relation, and significance of the information reported.

Efficiency and Time Constraints Obtaining a family history can be a lengthy undertaking, especially in instances of large, extended families, multiple affected individuals, or numerous disorders or health problems. If the client is an overly enthusiastic participant with an affinity for details, the completion of this task could potentially occupy most of the time allotted for the clinic visit. Although no shortcut will be able to elicit equivalent information, there are several tips to consider for streamlining this process.

1. **Be prepared.** This refers to some of the first considerations of obtaining a family history: the who and what. The counselor needs to be prepared for each case.

2. **Prepare the client.** Explain the purpose of obtaining a family history to the client and indicate clearly the kind of information needed. This will assist the client in reporting relevant data.

3. **Control the process; keep the client focused.** The counselor needs to provide guidance to the client and refocus questioning as needed. The counselor should ask direct and specific questions.

4. **Be aware of time.** It can be helpful to communicate time constraints to a client at the start of the visit.

5. **Listen.** Listening is a complex skill, and it must be done efficiently in a multitasking environment: The counselor has to listen attentively while simultaneously drawing an accurate pedigree, framing directed questions, sorting though family history data, and interpreting information. Listening carefully is important for accuracy.

6. **Be aware of accuracy issues.** The counselor needs to develop the ability to quickly assess what information is relevant, what information is suspect, and what information is likely to be inaccurate. The more distant a family member, the more likely the medical information provided about him or her is unreliable. For example, a report of a second cousin who is mentally impaired as a result of birth trauma should not be taken as a definitive diagnosis. See further accuracy concerns below.

7. **For the novice: Practice!** Many genetic counseling students acquire facility in obtaining family histories and constructing pedigrees by practicing on friends and fellow students.

8. **Know when to use shortcuts.** For large families that include little relevant history, use abbreviation symbols for drawing sibships and extended family members (Table 2-1).

Verification of Pedigree Information and Documentation of Affected Status

Documenting which family members are known to be affected in a pedigree is essential. This may require verifying family history information for ensuring an accurate diagnosis and providing counseling. Verification can be accomplished by obtaining the medical records of the proband or other affected family member(s), genetic tests or other laboratory results, pathology reports, and autopsy results and, in some instances, by performing examinations of key individuals. For example, when a couple is counseled regarding a family history of cystic fibrosis (CF), it is important to obtain documentation of the diagnosis and DNA studies of the affected family member (if performed). The accuracy of risk assessment depends on confirmation of the diagnosis; the information regarding the sensitivity and specificity of CF mutation analysis depends on whether the affected family member's CF mutations are known. If the affected family member has had testing that revealed identifiable CF mutations, then negative carrier studies in the client would have greater predictive value. For a client who is concerned about a family history of cancer, pathology reports that document tumor types and medical records that confirm diagnoses are critical components of an accurate risk assessment. If the family member of interest is deceased and the medical records are not available, then sometimes a death certificate can provide useful information.

When the pedigree is being constructed, information about affected status that has not been documented (e.g., diagnoses reported by the client) should be distinguished from a diagnosis that was established by an examination, a laboratory study, and/or a review of medical records. A diagnosis documented by an evaluation is indicated by an E and an asterisk (*) (Table 2-4). If more than one evaluation has been done (e.g., MRI and DNA test) subscripts can be used (E_1, E_2) and defined in a key. If results of an evaluation are not known or unavailable, a "?" can be used.

As Table 2-4 shows, the situation of a client who has a high likelihood of developing a condition, because of a positive DNA test for example, but was asymptomatic at the time the family history was obtained, is represented by a vertical line down the center of the symbol. If the client develops symptoms, the symbol is shaded when the pedigree is updated. This designation is different from that of an individual who is known to carry a gene mutation by virtue of family history or through DNA testing but is not expected to develop symptoms.

Accuracy   An inaccurate family history is a reality of genetic counseling. Possible errors include incorrect diagnoses, wrong ages at diagnosis and/or symptom onset, errors in paternity, and lack of knowledge about the existence of certain relatives who do not have a disease (leading to overestimates of risk) and lack of knowledge about those who do have disease (leading to underestimates of risk) (Katki, 2006). There is also variability in accuracy depending on the disease being reported (Bennett, in press; Wolpert and Speer, 2005). For example, patient-reported positive family cancer histories for first-degree relatives are accurate and valuable for breast and colon cancer risk assessments (Murff et al., 2004), whereas underreporting has been noted to be a limitation for such histories of colon polyps or colorectal cancer in first-degree and second-degree relatives (Stark et al., 2006; Mitchell et al., 2004). Negative family history reports for ovarian and endometrial cancers are also less useful (Murff et al., 2004). Verification of information, particularly in more distant relatives, is often difficult or impossible. Cultural factors and patients' educational levels may also be barriers to obtaining complete/accurate health history (Carmona and Wattendorf, 2005). Clearly, family history information should be interpreted with caution.

Pedigree Updating   Updating the family history is an essential component of a follow-up evaluation for clients with or without an established diagnosis. Additional information may be obtained that provides further clues about a possible diagnosis;

TABLE 2-4. Pedigree Symbolization of Genetic Evaluation/Testing Information

Instructions:
— E is used for evaluation to represent clinical and/or test information on the pedigree
   a. E is to be defined in key/legend
   b. If more than one evaluation, use subscript (E_1, E_2, E_3) and define in key
   c. Test results should be put in parentheses or defined in key/legend
— A symbol is shaded only when an individual is clinically symptomatic
— For linkage studies, haplotype information is written below the individual. The haplotype of interest should be on left and appropriately highlighted
— Repetitive sequences, trinucleotides and expansion numbers are written with affected allele first and placed in parentheses
— If mutation known, identify in parentheses

Definition	Symbol	Scenario
1. Documented evaluation (*) Use only if examined/evaluated by you or your research/clinical team or if the outside evaluation has been reviewed and verified.		Woman with negative echocardiogram. E– (echo)
2. Carrier—not likely to manifest disease regardless of inheritance pattern		Male carrier of Tay-Sachs disease by patient report (* not used because results not verified).
3. Asymptomatic/presymptomatic carrier—clinically unaffected at this time but could later exhibit symptoms		Woman age 25 with negative mammogram and positive BRCA1 DNA test. 25 y E_1– (mammogram) E_2+(5385insC BRCA1)
4. Uninformative study (u)	Eu	Man age 25 with normal physical exam and uninformative DNA test for Huntington disease (E_2). 25 y E_1– (physical exam) E_2u (36n/18n)
5. Affected individual with positive evaluation (E+)	E+	Individual with cystic fibrosis and positive mutation study; only one mutation has currently been identified. E+(ΔF508) Eu E+(ΔF508/u)
		10 week male fetus with a trisomy 18 karyotype. 10wk E+(CVS) 47, XY,+18

or, in the instance of an established diagnosis, the births of additional family members may indicate other at-risk individuals for whom evaluations are indicated. Additionally, the health status of family members may have changed, affecting the risk assessment provided to the patient.

When the pedigree is updated, the date and recorder should be noted. When imaging updated pedigrees into the electronic medical record, the most current version should be identified.

Issues of Confidentiality The pedigree is a record of sensitive information, including family relationships, the health status of family members, dates of birth, marriages, and pregnancies. Notably, data are usually gathered from an individual patient and recorded without family members' consent or knowledge. Confidentiality is an issue because family members may not be aware that personal health information has been recorded, and privacy is an issue because individuals may learn unwanted information about themselves if this information is made available. For example, if the medical records, including the pedigree, of an individual are shared (with appropriate authorization), a relative could learn previously undisclosed information such as adoption, nonpaternity, or disease risk. It could be argued that an implicit consent exists because the information has been shared within the family, and therefore written consent for documentation and inclusion in an individual's medical record is not required (Lucassen, 2007).

It is generally not advisable to record family members' names on the pedigree, although if necessary first names or initials can be included to make it possible for the counselor to refer by name to a family member when asking questions. Use of birth year or age, year of death or age at death, rather than complete birth dates or dates of death of relatives, is compliant with Health Insurance Portability and Accountability Act (HIPAA) guidelines, in which exact dates are considered private and protected information (Bennett et al., 2008).

Additional confidentiality concerns arise when it is necessary to release information (with a signed medical record release) to a third party: an extended family member, insurer, or employer. Not all the information recorded in a pedigree may be necessary or appropriate for other individuals or parties to obtain. Full names of family members should not be imaged into the patient's electronic medical record without obtaining consent from these individuals, because of the possibility that the information will be released. A pedigree may also contain information about pregnancy termination, pregnancies conceived through assisted reproductive techniques, or presymptomatic carrier status that is not relevant to the purpose of the request for information. Genetic counselors need to carefully limit what information to include on a pedigree, or review the contents before sending it to a third party, since it may be appropriate to omit information deemed irrelevant or potentially stigmatizing. One alternative, especially if the pedigree was not specifically included in the request for information, is to provide the clinic chart note and genetic counseling letter without the pedigree, as these documents generally contain a summary of the pertinent family history information. This, however, may not be an option that can be exercised by the counselor. If pedigrees are routinely imaged into a patient's electronic record or included in the hospital chart, the decision to include the document will be made according to the institution's policies. The safest course is to discuss potential areas of concern with one's institution and one's clients before releasing pedigrees to third parties.

The American Health Information Community's Family Health History Multi-Stakeholder Workgroup is a component of the U.S. Department of Health and Human Services' Personalized Health Care Initiative charged with the creation of a core data set for family health history information and determination of the requirements for promoting incorporation of such information in electronic health records (Feero et al., 2008). This group is also considering a range of issues related to this information, including confidentiality, privacy, and security. The Workgroup has described how genetic/genomic data access should likely be treated as similar to other "sensitive" information in the electronic health record, with required disclosure considerations and controlled access (Glaser et al., 2008). Such sensitive information (psychiatric, drug and/or alcohol abuse, HIV/AIDS, reproductive information, and sexual abuse information) is accessed via *special* authorization, and such authorization must specifically refer to the information that is to be released.

Care should be taken if the names and contact details of family members are needed to facilitate verification of information. One method for tracking information is a number system: Each generation is recorded with a Roman numeral to the far left of the pedigree, and each individual within a particular generation is then assigned an Arabic numeral, from left to right, in ascending order (e.g., I-1, I-2). When this identification method is used, the names of family members for whom medical records have been requested can be recorded separately, allowing the pedigree number to serve as a means of identifying the family member on the pedigree. Spouses or partners may be given the same number with a different lowercase alphabetical letter (e.g., I-2a and I-2b). This method of identification is particularly useful for large research pedigrees and for pedigrees that will be published.

INTERPRETING THE FAMILY HISTORY AND PEDIGREE ANALYSIS

The pedigree should be an accurate and easily interpretable diagram from which risk information can be derived (see Table 2-5 for "red flags"). DNA analysis in many instances may define risks for patients and clients in absolute terms, but decisions to undertake testing in the first place may still be based partly on an assessment of the family history data. In other instances, where DNA analysis is not feasible, risk information is based solely on the analysis of the pedigree. It is therefore critical for the genetic counselor to carefully evaluate the data and to consider all possible modes of inheritance when providing risk information. Three important considerations in the interpretation of the family history data are the variable expressivity of inherited disorders, reduced penetrance, and the value of a negative family history.

Variable Expressivity

The concept of variable expression of inherited conditions, especially those that are dominantly inherited, should always play a role in determining what questions to ask the client when obtaining a family history. Already noted is the need to ask not only about the presence of a given disorder in relatives but also about the presence of associated physical features. For example, the proband in the pedigree in Figure 2-2 was referred for a diagnostic evaluation because of cleft palate and micrognathia. It was also reported that there was a family history of cleft palate in two first-degree relatives, the mother and a sibling. The differential diagnosis for these anomalies and

TABLE 2-5. Red Flags in a Family History Suggestive of a Genetic Condition

- Multiple closely related individuals affected with the same condition, particularly if the condition is rare
- Individual or couple with three or more pregnancy losses (e.g., miscarriages, stillbirths)
- Medical problems in the offspring of parents who are consanguineous (first cousins or more closely related)
- Sudden cardiac death in a person who seemed healthy
- Bilateral disease in paired organs (e.g., eyes, kidneys, lungs, breasts)
- Multiple common disorders in related individuals, especially if occurring at earlier age of onset than is typical
- An individual or individuals with:
  - Two or more medical conditions (e.g., hearing loss and renal disease, diabetes and muscle disease)
  - Two or more major birth anomalies
  - Three or more minor birth anomalies
  - One major birth defect with two minor anomalies
  - A cleft palate, or cleft lip with or without cleft palate
  - Congenital heart disease
  - A medical condition and dysmorphic features
  - Developmental delay with dysmorphic features and/or physical birth anomalies
  - Developmental delay associated with other medical conditions
  - Progressive cognitive impairment and/or loss of developmental milestones
  - Autism (particularly with dysmorphic features)
  - Progressive behavioral problems
  - Unexplained hypotonia
  - Unexplained ataxia
  - Unexplained seizures
  - Progressive neurological condition, movement disorder, and/or muscle weakness
  - Unexplained cardiomyopathy
  - Hematological condition associated with bleeding or clotting abnormalities
  - Unusual birthmarks (particularly if associated with seizures, learning disabilities, or dysmorphic features)
  - Hair anomalies (hirsutism, brittle, coarse, kinky, sparse, or absent)
  - Congenital or juvenile deafness
  - Congenital or juvenile blindness
  - Cataracts at a young age
  - Primary adrenocortical insufficiency (male)
  - Primary amenorrhea
  - Ambiguous genitalia
  - Proportionate short stature with dysmorphic features and/or delayed or arrested puberty
  - Disproportionate short stature with dysmorphic features and/or delayed or arrested puberty
  - Premature ovarian failure
  - Proportionate short stature and primary amenorrhea
  - Male with hypogonadism and/or significant gynecomastia
  - Congenital absence of the vas deferens
  - Oligozoospermia/azoospermia

- A fetus with:
  - A major structural anomaly
  - Significant growth retardation
  - Or multiple anomalies

Adapted from Bennett, *The Practical Guide to the Genetic Family History* (2nd edition). In press.

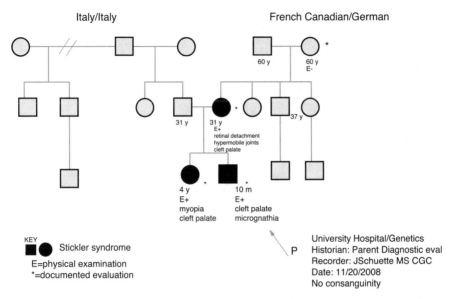

FIGURE 2-2. *Pedigree showing family history of physical features associated with stickler syndrome*

family history includes a condition known as Stickler syndrome, an autosomal dominant condition involving cleft palate, micrognathia, myopia, retinal detachment, hypermobile joints, and degenerative arthritis. When obtaining the family history, the genetic counselor inquired about the presence of physical features associated with this condition in other family members in an effort to compile data that would support or refute the diagnosis and provide evidence for other affected family members. As indicated in the pedigree, the patient's mother reported a history of bilateral retinal detachments and hypermobile joints in addition to the cleft palate. The patient's sister was reported to have early-onset myopia in addition to cleft palate. This information, along with the diagnostic evaluation, helped to confirm a clinical diagnosis of Stickler syndrome in the proband as well as in the mother and sibling.

It is important to remember that disorders may present diversely within a family, and in some instances the sum of varying manifestations among multiple family members will suggest the diagnosis of a particular disorder. Figure 2-3 is a pedigree illustrating such a family. The proband in this family was initially referred at age 1 year for an evaluation for U-shaped cleft palate, micrognathia, and multiple minor dysmorphic features. Multiple diagnostic studies including a karyotype, biochemical analyses, skeletal survey, renal ultrasound, and MRI were normal. The proband was seen again at age 2 and then at age 4, at which time global cognitive impairments were noted. In addition, when updating the family history, the proband's younger sister was reported to have recently been given the diagnosis of autistic spectrum disorder. The patient's mother reported premature ovarian failure, and the maternal grandfather was recently diagnosed with a Parkinsonian-type disorder with ataxia and tremor. This history strongly suggested the possibility of fragile X syndrome,

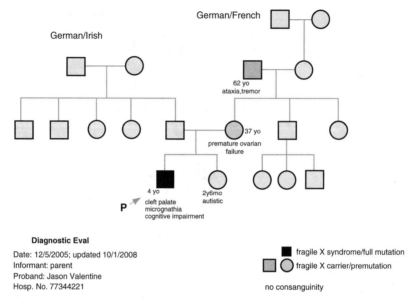

FIGURE 2-3. *Pedigree demonstrating features in multiple family members contributing to the diagnosis of fragile X syndrome*

which was later confirmed. Fragile X syndrome had not initially been a consideration in view of the patient's presenting features of multiple congenital anomalies, but became a likely consideration when the pedigree was updated during a follow-up visit.

Reduced Penetrance

A number of autosomal dominant disorders demonstrate reduced penetrance in which a family member known to carry a gene mutation (because the person has an affected parent and child) has no apparent symptoms. It is important to identify such relatives and recommend evaluation and genetic counseling since the potential implications for their health and medical care should be addressed. The pedigree in Figure 2-4 shows a patient referred for genetic counseling and risk assessment for a personal and family history of breast cancer. The penetrance of *BRCA1* or *BRCA2* cancer-predisposing mutations or the likelihood of cancer when a cancer-predisposing mutation is present is a significant clinical consideration. The penetrance is uncertain and probably variable (King et al., 2003; Antoniou et al., 2003). Clearly, several family members within the pedigree are mutation positive and would benefit from consultation to discuss recommendations for surveillance and health care management.

The penetrance of some disorders is age dependent, as in the case of breast and ovarian cancer as well as other conditions such as Huntington disease. Therefore, the ages of family members are an important consideration in an assessment of risks.

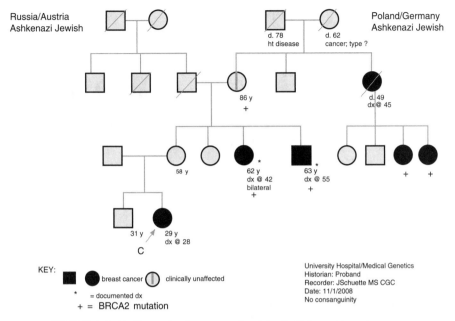

FIGURE 2-4. *Pedigree showing personal and family history of breast cancer*

Value of an Extended Negative History

An extended negative family history provides information that is often as important as a history of a genetic disorder in multiple relatives in several generations. For example, the pedigree in Figure 2-5 includes family history information for a client referred for genetic counseling because of a family history of Duchenne muscular dystrophy (DMD), an X-linked recessive disorder. Several of the client's distant relatives were reported to have died from complications of DMD. Of significant value is the presence of multiple unaffected males in the client's pedigree: She has two unaffected brothers and three unaffected maternal uncles. Such a history provides valuable information in arriving at an estimate of the patient's risk for being a carrier. In fact, a Bayesian analysis would significantly reduce the client's risk from her a priori risk of 1/8 to 1/138. This information may be a significant factor in her exploration of testing options.

Additional Points

Other important factors in pedigree analysis and risk assessment include ethnicity, presence of consanguinity, and a family history of a common chronic disorder. Ethnicity contributes to the consideration of disorders known to occur at a higher frequency within a particular ethnic group. Consanguinity contributes to the likelihood of an autosomal recessive condition, being biallelic for an autosomal dominant condition, or a multifactorial disorder. A positive family history of a common chronic

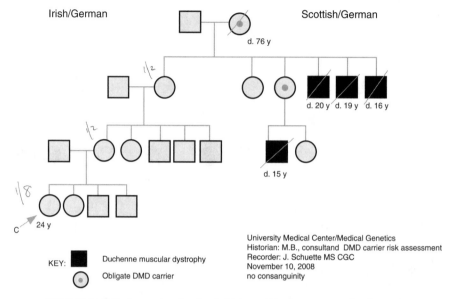

FIGURE 2-5. *Pedigree showing family history of Duchenne muscular dystrophy*

disease is generally associated with relative risks ranging from two to five times those of the general population; an even greater increase in relative risk is associated with an increasing number of affected relatives and earlier ages of disease onset (Bennett, in press; King et al., 1992). Examples of such common diseases include the following:

- Breast cancer occurring at less than age 45–50 years (premenopausal)
- Colon cancer occurring at less than age 45–50 years
- Prostate cancer occurring at less than age 45–60 years
- Vision loss occurring at less than age 55 years
- Hearing loss occurring at less than age 50–60 years
- Dementia at age 60 years or less
- Heart disease at age 40–60 years or less
- Stroke occurring at less than age 60 years (Bennett, in press; AMA, 2004).

Additionally, a strong family history of common chronic diseases may suggest a diagnosis of a Mendelian disorder. It is therefore critical to recognize different combinations of diseases within a pedigree, including the suggested pattern of inheritance, for facilitating a diagnosis in a potentially high risk family. There are over 150 Mendelian disorders that include such common conditions as coronary artery disease, myocardial infarction, stroke, thrombosis, sudden death, arrhythmia, aneurysm, arteriovenous malformations, cardiomyopathy, and diabetes in adulthood (Scheuner et al., 2004).

PSYCHOSOCIAL ASPECTS OF OBTAINING A FAMILY HISTORY

Gathering family history information provides the counselor with an excellent opportunity for engaging the client in a relationship that promotes mutual trust. It is an activity that requires participation of all parties—the client, the partner, the counselor, and perhaps extended family members. It can be an "ice breaker," an opportunity to establish an ongoing dialogue and interaction with the family. And, because many intimate family events and details are reported, such as death and loss, abortion, infertility, and consanguinity, the counselor can use these exchanges to set the tone for unqualified acceptance.

During the time spent obtaining family history data, there is an opportunity to make observations about the client and his or her family that may ultimately assist the counselor in coming to know the family. Interactions between couples and family members as information is gathered often provide clues about family dynamics. Does one member of the couple or family provide most or all of the information because he or she apparently has the most knowledge and is the family historian? Is he or she the dominant partner, or is there another reason? Does one family member consistently interrupt, correct, or contradict another? Is there tension or stress, or does the exchange between family members appear relaxed and mutually supportive?

Assessments about the level of family stress can sometimes be made during the gathering of family history information. The client and family may appear anxious when identifying members of the family as affected with disorders. A sense of guilt may also be apparent. For example, the counselor obtaining a family history from a patient who may be a carrier for an X-linked disorder has an opportunity to observe as the client provides information about potentially affected family members and carriers. When there is a positive history, the counselor should watch for clues that might provide an indication about the level of the family's sensitivity to this information. (See Chapter 18, for an illustration of a case that includes stress and anxiety related to the transmission of an X-linked condition).

A family's assumptions about the presence of a disorder in a family member often become apparent during the process of gathering the history. For example, the client may state that the cause of cognitive impairment in a sibling was "lack of oxygen" or "the cord was around the neck" during delivery. This may be an explanation that makes sense to the family and is "the story" that has been recounted over and over again. A sensitive counselor will understand that the suggestion of an alternative explanation for the cognitive impairment could be disruptive. Families may also have myths that have served to explain why certain members are affected with a disorder while others are not. For instance, some assume that sharing a family resemblance has predictive value in determining who will inherit a particular disorder. In other instances, a family may assume that only the females or only the males are at risk, even though the disorder in question is autosomal dominant. The genetic counselor needs to be cognizant of family assumptions and myths that may present themselves while the history is being recorded, as these may impact the client's understanding of genetic principles.

In addition to the subjective observations that can be made during the process of gathering the family history, the counselor can benefit from the objective information contained in the pedigree itself. Information about the nature of relationships (e.g., whether there has been a marriage, multiple marriages or partners, separation, or divorce) is valuable in assessing the client's experiences. The emotional and psychological impact of living with an illness in the family, particularly if sudden, premature, or fatal, and the nature of family relationships can contribute toward a sense of emotional closeness and personal likeness with an affected relative (Walter and Emery, 2005). Sex and/or age of disease onset or death of the affected family member may also contribute to a patient's perception of disease imminence.

Discussing a patient's understanding and beliefs about personal vulnerability due to their family history is important when communicating risk and facilitating decision making. Different beliefs about the roles of nature and nurture in contributing to disease can affect patients' sense of personal control and whether they feel empowered to exert such control over their risk (Walter and Emery, 2005). It is easy to anticipate how these family history factors might contribute to the complex nature of decision making for presymptomatic testing for such conditions as hereditary breast and ovarian cancer or Huntington disease. In the prenatal setting, when a family history of cognitive impairment in a sibling (regardless of whether there is a known diagnosis) is obtained from a client being counseled for advanced maternal age, this information is potentially useful. Despite the obvious potential impact on the patient's risks for having a similarly affected child, this personal experience is likely to have had an impact of some sort on the client's life, search for meaning and perspectives about disability, and hopes and dreams for the pregnancy. Exploration of this information is often useful for patients for whom the decision of whether to have prenatal testing is difficult.

SUMMARY

There are many methods of drawing pedigrees and describing kinship, but for my own purposes, I still prefer those that I designed myelf.

—Galton, 1889

The family history and pedigree are the basis for providing clients referred for genetic evaluation and counseling with a diagnosis, risk assessment, education, and psychosocial support. Accuracy, detail, and relevance are paramount. The genetic counseling student must develop a mastery of this fundamental task and employ standardized pedigree symbols and nomenclature that enhance the utility of the information obtained. The family history and pedigree have come a long way since the era of Francis Galton. An accurate and complete family history and pedigree lay the foundation for the highest standards of patient care and genetic counseling. They are tools now clearly viewed as having an essential role in all aspects of health care.

REFERENCES

American Medical Association (2004) Family medical history in disease prevention. http:// www.ama-asn.org/ama1/pub/upload/mm/464/family_history02.pdf. Accessed 12/2008.

American Society of Human Genetics Social Issues Committee report on genetics and adoption: points to consider (1991). *Am J Hum Genet* 48:1009–1010.

American Society of Human Genetics family history law: a guide for health care providers. http://www.ashg.org/press/healthprofessional.shtml#6. Accessed 12/2008.

Andrews LB, Elster N (1998) Adoption, reproductive technologies, and genetic information. *Health Matrix* 8:125–151.

Antoniou A, Pharoah PD, Narod S, Risch HA, Eyfjord JE, Hopper JL, Loman N, Olsson H, Johannsson O, Borg A, Pasini B, Radice P, Manoukian S, Eccles DM, Tang N, Olah E, Anton-Culver H, Warner E, Lubinski J, Gronwald J, Gorski B, Tulinius H, Thorlacius S, Eerola H, Nevanlinna H, Syrjäkoski K, Kallioniemi OP, Thompson D, Evans C, Peto J, Lalloo F, Evans DG, Easton DF (2003) Average risks of breast and ovarian cancer associated with BRCA1 or BRCA2 mutations detected in case series unselected for family history: a combined analysis of 22 studies. *Am J Hum Genet* 72:1117–1130.

Bendure WB, Mulvihill JJ (2006) Perform a gene test on every patient: the medical family history revisited. *J Okla State Med Assoc* 99:78–83.

Bennett RL, Steinhaus KA, Uhrich SB, O'Sullivan C (1993) The need for developing standardized family pedigree nomenclature. *J Genet Couns* 2:261–273.

Bennett RL, Steinhaus KA, Uhrich SB, O'Sullivan CK, Resta RG, Doyle DL, Markel DS, Vincent V, Hamanishi J (1995a) Recommendations for standardized human pedigree nomenclature. *Am J Hum Genet* 56:745–752.

Bennett RL, Steinhaus KA, Uhrich SB, O'Sullivan CK, Resta RB, Doyle DL, Markel DS, Vincent V, Hamanishi J (1995b) Recommendations for standardized human pedigree nomenclature. *J Genet Couns* 4:267–279.

Bennett RL, Steinhaus KA, Uhrich SB, O'Sullivan CK, Resta RG, Doyle DL, Markel DS, Vincent V, Hamanishi J (1995c) Reply to Marazita and Curtis (Letter to editor). *Am J Hum Genet* 57:983–984.

Bennett RL (1999) *The Practical Guide to the Genetic Family History*. New York: Wiley-Liss.

Bennett RL, Motulsky AG, Bittles AH, Uhrich SA, Doyle DL, Silvey KA, Cheng E, Steiner RA, McGillivray B (2002) Genetic counseling and screening of consanguineous couples and their offspring: recommendations of the National Society of Genetic Counselors. *J Genet Couns* 11:97–119.

Bennett RL (2004) The family medical history. *Prim Care* 31:479–495.

Bennett RL, Byers PH, Harrison T, Doyle DL (2007) Core elements of a genetic family history in the era of electronic medical records. Presented Paper, NSGC, AEC, Kansas City, MO, 10/07.

Bennett RL, French, KS, Resta RG, Doyle DL (2008) Standardized human pedigree nomenclature: update and assessment of the recommendations of the National Society of Genetic Counselors. *J Genet Couns* 17:424–433.

Bennett RL (in press) *The Practical Guide to the Genetic Family History* (2nd ed.). New York: Wiley-Blackwell.

Botkin JR, McMahon WM, Smith KR, Nash JE (2008) Privacy and confidentiality in the publication of pedigrees: a survey of investigators and biomedical journals. *JAMA* 279:1808–1812.

Burke W (2005) Taking family history seriously. *Ann Intern Med* 143:388–389.

Carmona RH, Wattendorf DJ (2005) Personalizing prevention: the U.S. Surgeon General's family history initiative. *Am Fam Physician* 71:36–39.

Chang ET, Smedby KE, Hjalgrim H, Glimelius B, Adami H (2006) Reliability of self-reported family history of cancer in a large case-control study of lymphoma. *J Natl Cancer Inst* 98:61–68.

Cole Johnson C, Ownby DR, Havstad SL, Peterson EL (2004) Family history, dust mite exposure in early childhood, and risk for pediatric atopy and asthma. *J Allergy Clin Immunol* 114:105–110.

Dietrich JE, Hertweck SP, Perlman SE (2007) Efficacy of family history in determining thrombophilia risk. *J Pediatr Adolesc Gynecol* 20:221–224.

Dudley-Brown S (2004) The genetic family history assessment in gastroenterology nursing practice. *Gastroenterol Nurs* 27:107–110.

Eriksson J, Lindström J, Tuomilehto J (2001) Potential for the prevention of type 2 diabetes. *Br Med Bull* 60:183–199.

Federal Register, 45 CFR, Aug 12, 2002. Standards for privacy of individually identifiable health information, Final Rule 160–164.

Feero WG, Bigley MB, Brinner KM (2008) New standards and enhanced utility for family health history information in the electronic health record: an update from the American Health Information Community's Family Health History Multi-Stakeholder Workgroup. *J Am Med Inform Assoc* 15:723–728.

Fleming C, Whitlock EP, Beil T, Smit B, Harris RP (2005) Screening for primary open-angle glaucoma in the primary care setting: an update for the US preventive services task force. *Ann Fam Med* 3:167–170.

Foster, RL (2005) Exploring web-based resources to support the family history public health initiative. *JSPN* 10:45–47.

Frezzo TM, Rubinstein WS, Dunham D, Ormond KE (2003) The genetic family history as a risk assessment tool in internal medicine. *Genet Med* 5:84–91.

Galton F (1889) *Natural Inheritance*. London: Macmillan, quoted by Resta (1993).

Glaser J, Henley DE, Downing G, Brinner KM (2008) Advancing personalized health care through health information technology: an update from the American Health Information Community's Personalized Health Care Workgroup. *J Am Med Inform Assoc* 15:391–396.

Green CM, Kearns LS, Wu J, Barbour JM, Wilkinson RM, Ring MA, Craig JE, Wong TL, Hewitt AW, Mackey DA (2007) How significant is a family history of glaucoma? experience from the Glaucoma Inheritance Study in Tasmania. *Clin Exp Ophthalmol* 35:793–799.

Grody WW, Cutting GR, Klinger KW, Richards CS, Watson MS, Desnick RJ (2001) Laboratory standards and guidelines for population-based cystic fibrosis carrier screening. *Genet Med* 3:149–154.

Gutmann DH, Aylsworth A, Carey JC, Korf B, Marks J, Pyeritz R, Rubenstein A, Viskochil D (1997) The diagnostic evaluation and multidisciplinary management of neurofibromatosis I and neurofibromatosis 2. *JAMA* 278:51–57.

Guttmacher AE, Collins FS, Carmona RH (2004) The family history-more important than ever. *N Engl J Med* 351:2333–2336.

Hall MJ, Dignam JJ, Olopade, OI (2008) Family history of pancreatic cancer in a high-risk cancer clinic: implications for risk assessment. *J Genet Couns* 17:365–372.

Harrison TA, Hindorff LA, Kim H, Wines RC, Bowen DJ, McGrath BB, Edwards KL (2003) Family history of diabetes as a potential public health tool. *Am J Prev Med* 24:152–159.

Holsinger D, Larabell S, Walker AP (1992) History and pedigree obtained during follow-up for abnormal maternal serum alpha-fetoprotein identified additional risk in 25% of patients. *Clin Res* 40:28A.

Katki HA (2006) Effect of misreported family history on mendelian mutation prediction models. *Biometrics* 62:478–487.

Kendler KS (2001) Family history information in biomedical research. *J Cont Educ Health Prof* 21:215–223.

King MC, Marks JH, Mandell JB (2003) Breast and ovarian cancer risks due to inherited mutations in BRCA1 and BRCA2. *Science* 302:643–646.

King RA, Rotter JI, Motulsky AG (eds) (1992) *The Genetic Basis of Common Diseases.* New York: Oxford University Press.

Lemonick MD (2004) The new family tree: the holidays are a perfect time to gather your family's medical history. *Time* 164:100.

Lucassen A, Parker M, Wheeler R (2007) Implications of data protection legislation for family history. *BMJ* 332:299–301.

Malin, B (2006) Re-identification of familial database records. *AMIA 2006 Symp Proc* 524–528.

Marazita M (1995) Standardized pedigree nomenclature (Letter to editor). *Am J Hum Genet* 57:982–983.

Maradiegue A, Edwards QT (2006) An overview of ethnicity and assessment of family history in primary care settings. *J Am Acad Nurse Pract* 18:447–456.

Maradiegue A, Jasperson K, Edwards QT, Lowstuter K, Weitzel J (2008) Scoping the family history: assessment of Lynch syndrome (hereditary nonpolyposis colorectal cancer) in primary care settings-a primer for nurse practitioners. *J Am Acad Nurse Pract* 20:76–84.

McGuinness TM, Noonan P, Dyer JG (2005) Family history as a tool for psychiatric nurses. *Arch Psychiatr Nurs* 19:116–124.

Mitchell RJ, Brewster D, Campbell H, Porteous ME, Wyllie AH, Bird CC, Dunlop MG (2004) Accuracy of reporting of family history of colorectal cancer. *Gut* 53:291–295.

Morales A, Cowan J, Dagua J, Hershberger RE (2008) Family history: an essential tool for cardiovascular genetic medicine. *Congest Heart Fail* 14:37–45.

Murff HJ, Spigel DR, Syngal S (2004) Does this patient have a family history of cancer? An evidence-based analysis of the accuracy of family cancer history. *JAMA* 292:1480–1489.

Nanda R, Schumm LP, Cummings S, Fackenthal JD, Sveen L, Ademuyiwa F, Cobleigh M, Esserman L, Lindor NM, Neuhausen SL, Olopade OI (2005) Genetic testing in an ethnically diverse cohort of high-risk women. *JAMA* 294:1925–1933.

Nelson HD, Huffman LH, Fu R, Harris EL; U.S. Preventive Services Task Force (2005) Genetic risk assessment and BRCA mutation testing for breast and ovarian cancer susceptibility: systematic evidence review for the U.S. Preventive Services Task Force. *Ann Intern Med* 143:362–379.

NSGC Standard Pedigree Symbol Position Statement (adopted 2003) http://www.nsgc.org/about/position. Accessed 12/2008.

O' Donnell CJ (2004) Family history, subclinical atherosclerosis, and coronary heart disease risk: barriers and opportunities for the use of family history information in risk prediction and prevention. *Circulation* 110:2074–2076.

Pearson K (ed) (1912) *The Treasury of Human Inheritance (Parts I and II)*. London: Dulau and Co. Quoted in Resta (1993).

Pharoah PD, Ponder BA (2002) The genetics of ovarian cancer. *Best Pract Res Clin Obstet Gynaecol* 16:449–468.

Quereshi N, Bethea J, Modell B, Brennan P, Papageorgiou A, Raeburn S, Hapgood R, Modell M (2005) Collecting genetic information in primary care: evaluating a new family history tool. *Family Pract* 22:663–669.

Reid G, Emery J (2006) Chronic disease prevention in general practice-applying the family history. *Aust Fam Physician* 35:879–885.

Resta RG (1993) The crane's foot: the rise of the pedigree in human genetics. *J Genet Couns* 2:235–260.

Rich EC, Burke W, Heaton CJ, Haga S, Pinsky L, Short P, Acheson L (2004) Reconsidering the family history in primary care. *J Gen Intern Med* 19:273–280.

Richards CS, Bradley LA, Amos J, Allitto B, Grody WW, Maddalena A, McGinnis MJ, Prior TW, Popovich BW, Watson MS (2002) Standards and Guidelines for CFTR Mutation Testing. *Genet Med* 4:379–391.

Scheuner MT, Wang SJ, Raffel LJ, Larabell SK, Rotter JI (1997) Family history: a comprehensive genetic risk assessment method for the chronic conditions of adulthood. *Am J Med Genet* 71:315–324.

Scheuner MT, Yoon PW, Khoury MJ (2004) Contribution of Mendelian disorders to common chronic disease: opportunities for recognition, intervention, and prevention. *Am J Med Genet* 125C:50–65.

Schwartz AG (2006) Lung cancer: family history matters. *Chest* 130:936–937.

Stark JR, Bertone- Johnson ER, Costanza ME, Stoddard AM (2006) Factors associated with colorectal cancer risk perception: the role of polyps and family history. *Health Educ Res* 21:740–749.

Steinhaus KA, Bennett RL, Uhrich SB, Resta RG, Doyle DL, Markel DS, Vincent V (1995) Inconsistencies in pedigree nomenclature in human genetics publications: a need for standardization. *Am J Med Genet* 56:291–295.

U.S. Department of Health & Human Services (2006) U.S. Surgeon General's Family History Initiative [Internet]. http://www.hhs.gov/familyhistory/. Accessed 12/2008.

Valdez R, Greenlund KJ, Khoury MJ, Yoon PW (2007) Is family history a useful tool for detecting children at risk for diabetes and cardiovascular diseases? A public health perspective. *Pediatrics* 120:S78–S86.

Venne VL, Botkin JR, Buys SS (2003) Professional opportunities and responsibilities in the provision of genetic information to children relinquished for adoption. *Am J Med Genet* 119A:41–46.

Walter FM, Emery J (2006) Perceptions of family history across common diseases: a qualitative study in primary care. *Fam Pract* 23:472–480.

Walter FM, Emery J (2005) "Coming down the line"—patients' understanding of their family history of common chronic disease. *Ann Fam Med* 3:405–414.

Watson MS, Cutting GR, Desnick RJ, Driscoll DA, Klinger K, Mennuti M, Palomaki GE, Popovich BW, Pratt VM, Rohlfs EM, Strom CM, Richards CS, Witt DR, Grody WW (2004) Cystic fibrosis population carrier screening: 2004 revision of American College of Medical Genetics mutation panel. *Genet Med* 6:387–391.

Wattendorf DJ, Hadley DW (2005) Family history: the three-generation pedigree. *Am Fam Physician* 72:441–448.

Wolpert CM, Speer MC (2005) Harnessing the power of the pedigree. *J Midwifery Womens Health* 50:189–196.

Yoon PW, Scheuner MT, Gwinn M, Khoury MJ, Jorgensen C, Hariri S (2004) Awareness of family health history as a risk factor for disease—United States 2004. *MMWR* 53:1044–1047.

Yoon PW, Scheuner MT, Peterson-Oehlke KL, Gwinn M, Faucett A, Khoury MJ (2002) Can family history be used as a tool for public health and preventive medicine? *Genet Med* 4:304–310.

Ziogas A, Anton- Culver H (2003) Validation of family history data in cancer family registries. *Am J Prev Med* 24:190–198.

3

Interviewing: Beginning to See Each Other

Kathryn Spitzer Kim, M.S., C.G.C.

The interview is a fundamental component in the genetic counseling process. When many of us think about an interview, we think about being asked questions as a means of screening for a job or acceptance into a school. Yet the derivation of the word interview is from the French, *entre voir*: to see each other (Encarta, 1999). In clinical work, we use an interview to begin to see our patients, to learn about them as individuals, and to let them see us, to learn about us as helping professionals.

GETTING STARTED

The process of genetic counseling starts long before you begin the actual interview. First there has to be recognition of the need for genetic counseling. Either a referring physician or the client must conclude that the problem facing the client is one that a genetic counselor might be able to address, for example, advanced maternal age, cleft lip and palate in a child, or history of cancer in the family. Then a request for an appointment is made (Kelly, 1977).

The initial contact sets the tone for what follows. It is important that everyone, including the first person to whom the client speaks, be professional, competent, and compassionate. If this is a member of the office staff, the genetic counselor will want to work with this individual to sensitize him or her to some of the issues in working

A Guide to Genetic Counseling, Second Edition, Edited by Wendy Uhlmann, Jane Schuette, and Beverly Yashar

with patients in a genetics clinic. Patients calling a genetic counseling office may be feeling anxious, they may feel urgency or a reluctance to schedule an appointment, or they may be vague or confused about what type of appointment they need. Sensitive handling and guidance may put patients at ease and help them enter into the genetic counseling process comfortably and cooperatively.

Because of this, in some practices genetic counselors schedule their own appointments or make follow-up phone calls to patients soon after an appointment is made by the office staff. During this phone call the genetic counselor might explain the genetic counseling process, take a pedigree, arrange to gather records, and take other steps needed to prepare for the patient's visit. Other preparations might include mailing educational information to the patient and arranging the meeting space and seating in a welcoming manner (Kessler, 1979; Weil, 2000).

While interviewing can refer to the entire counseling session with a client, in this chapter we consider the initial meeting between the genetic counselor and the client. We will use the model of face-to-face counseling with an individual, although the principles also apply to meeting with couples and families and to other types of counseling such as telephone or videoconferencing. Every meeting with a client will contain some of these elements even if the client has had a previous appointment. This chapter is not intended to give a script for a genetic counseling encounter, but only to outline some guiding principles. Every counselor will develop a personal style for working with clients, and every session will have its own flavor.

BREAKING THE ICE

When the genetic counselor first meets the client, they usually engage in some small talk or social banter. This allows the counselor and client to begin to formulate an image of one another, helping the client relax and laying the foundation for the counseling relationship. The counselor can use this conversation productively to start assessing the client's level of comfort, mood, language skills,* and a variety of other factors that can influence the subsequent interaction. Counselors often ask clients about the ease of finding the office, parking the car, or other matters related to their arrival at the appointment. While it is important not to stray into chitchat of a personal nature, there may be some value in using a more personal approach at times (Kessler, 1979; Weil, 2000; Baker et al., 1998).

One way of breaking the ice with a male client might be to ask about the sports jersey he is wearing and talk for a few minutes about that team or sport. This would present the counselor as a real person able to share in the client's life and interests.

A teenage girl is listening to an iPod while waiting for her genetic counseling appointment. The counselor might ask what she was listening to as a way to start the conversation about something the girl finds interesting and easy to discuss.

---

*The majority of genetic counselors in the United States conduct sessions in English only.

More often than not, genetic counseling clients come to the appointment with other people. Ideally, the client should have some control over who is present during the counseling. Children are usually seen with their parents, but they may need some private time depending on their age. Conversely, parents may need time to talk to the counselor without children listening. The people who accompany the client, or the absence of other people, is one additional piece of information that the counselor uses to assess the situation. A client who is accompanied to an appointment by a spouse, a sibling, or a parent may rely on that family member for support or help in decision-making. Conversely, a person who comes to clinic with a close friend rather than a family member may use different sources of support.

At the start of the session, the counselor will want to greet everyone present, establish how they are related to the patient, and determine what each person wants to be called. If a name is unfamiliar, asking how to pronounce it properly shows respect. This is a situation where cultural factors may play a significant role. The number of family members who attend clinic, the preference for use of first names vs. last names, who makes decisions in the family, and the expectations of the counselor will all vary from one family to another. Some clients will not be comfortable calling the counselor by a first name even when invited to do so. Counselors need to respect all these differences as much as possible without violating ethical behavior. Since cultural differences may play a significant role, this is addressed further in Chapter 11.

SETTING THE STAGE: CORE QUALITIES

Carl Rogers and colleagues are credited with describing some key attributes of the counselor that correlate with successful counseling sessions. (Weil, 2000) These attributes are respect, genuineness, and empathy. They create an atmosphere that allows for the subsequent counseling and sets a genetic counseling session apart from a medical examination or an information session. If education alone was the goal, then genetic counselors could be replaced by interactive CD-ROM or videotapes. Instead, it is the relationship between the counselor and client that allows the patients' needs to be met.

Respect

A couple brought their two children to clinic for assessment of their developmental and behavioral problems. The children became rowdy and disruptive. The father stated that he would "spank" the children so that they would behave. This is a difference in parenting styles that the clinic staff could not support. The staff decided it was important to address this behavior without disrupting the relationship with the family. The pediatrician involved in the exam intervened, politely assuring the father that the staff was capable of working with the children. The session continued, and the staff was able to provide the family with a diagnosis and follow-up plan for the children including early intervention and increased support from social services such as parenting classes.

Respect, sometimes described as unconditional positive regard, can be defined as acceptance of clients as they are. This does not mean accepting every action or behavior displayed by the client. It means finding a way to focus on the client and to work with the client even when you have differing views. It also means setting aside your personal feelings about a client. This may sound simple, but at times it is difficult to attain in the real world (Coulehan and Block, 2001).

In the book *The Spirit Catches You and You Fall Down*, the author, Anne Fadiman, tells the true story of a Hmong girl named Lia. Lia's parents believe a spirit is responsible for her epilepsy, and it is extremely frustrating to Lia's doctors that the parents do not always give Lia her prescribed medicines. One of the biggest challenges these care providers face is trying to see the parents as loving, caring, good parents despite the enormous cultural differences and approaches to health and illness (Fadiman, 1997).

Genuineness

> Be careful what you pretend to be because you are what you pretend to be.
> —Vonnegut

The second key attribute of good counselors is genuineness. As it sounds, this means being yourself even within your professional role. A genetic counselor needs to be honest about his or her role, the limits of his or her knowledge, and personal feelings. For example, a student genetic counselor would introduce herself as a student and enlist the help of her supervisor as needed during a session.

One aspect of genuineness is the counselor's awareness and appreciation of his/her own inner feelings and attitudes during the counseling session. These feelings are usually not conveyed verbally to the client, but are used by the counselor to increase understanding of the situation and increase empathy toward the client. Allowing yourself to feel the emotions associated with the client's story enables you to listen with a sense of appreciation for his/her experience. Thus some counseling theorists think of genuineness and empathy as forming a feedback loop. Genuineness can be viewed as a way of being that underlines providing true empathy (Cochran and Cochran, 2006; Donoghue and Siegel, 2005).

The match between the counselor's inner process and the response to it is called congruence. For example, if there is a difference between what is said and what is expressed nonverbally there is a lack of congruence. It may not be possible to understand the feelings of a client if you cannot tap into some inner response of your own. Therefore, counselors need to be humble in order to be genuine. It might be more effective to tell a client that you do not understand but that you would like to do so than to mutter, "I understand" when they tell you about a difficult experience or something outside of your experience (Donoghue and Siegel, 2005).

> Eyes shining with unshed tears as a father relates the story of his child's death and the subsequent grief he has endured would alert the father to the counselor's genuine response to his tragedy.

> Telling a patient that testing is a personal choice and that you will support any decision that she makes in a tone of voice that implies criticism and disapproval would not be a genuine response irrespective of the selection of words.

Most counselors refrain from sharing personal experiences with clients since the focus of the session needs to stay on the client. However, counselors draw on personal experience to attempt to understand the situations of their clients. There are even times when personal experience can get in the way of being genuine or empathic. It is highly valuable to self-reflect on how your client's experiences are the same as and different from your own. This personal reflection is one of the ongoing tasks of a counselor (Matloff, 2006).

Genuineness, as the name implies, cannot be imitated. Students will find that their genuine voice increases as they gain experience. It is easier to sound confident or reassuring when you have been down a similar path many times before. Students must learn to find their own voices through observation of various styles and self-reflection. Merely copying the words or behaviors of a supervisor will not be sufficient. This is an area in which mentoring from a supervisor can be of enormous help to a student. Supervisors need to give students opportunities to explore different modes of working with patients. Effective supervisors model counseling and provide suggestions, but do not require students to mimic their sessions (Swietzer and King, 2004).

Empathy

This leads to the final component of a successful counseling atmosphere: empathy. Nearly every model of counseling starts with empathy as a necessary condition for beginning to work with clients. Empathy can be described as the ability to accurately understand the client's experience as if it were your own and to communicate this understanding to the client. "Empathy requires a constant shifting between my experiencing 'as you' what you feel and my being able to think 'as me' about your experience." (Murphy and Dillon, 2003, p. 88).

Empathy can be viewed as a feedback loop. The counselor's attempts to demonstrate understanding will increase or decrease the empathic connection with the client. The client's response to the counselor will indicate whether the counselor is on-target and should do more of the same or is off-target and should change direction.

One of the simplest demonstrations of understanding is reflection. Using reflection, the counselor restates what the client has said. The trick of doing this well is to express the client's sentiments without sounding like a parrot. As a student gains counseling skills the reflections often go to a deeper level, expressing unstated sentiments that the counselor has "heard."

If you appropriately and accurately capture the client's view, the client will feel understood. This has the dual effect of increasing the client's self-esteem and encouraging the client to say more about the topic. It also makes the client more receptive to further interaction with the counselor. If you only approximate the client's thoughts and feelings but do so in a genuine and respectful way, the client will probably correct you and continue. Missing the mark altogether or failing to respond suggests to the client that his or her comment was not relevant to genetic counseling. Because it is so central to the ethos of genetic counseling, the topic of empathy is explored in much greater detail in Chapter 5 (Coulehan and Block, 2001; McCarthy Veach et al., 2003).

Consider the situation of taking a pedigree. Your client reveals that her grandfather died last week. The genetic counselor has several choices about how to respond. The counselor may reflect what has been said responding with, "Oh, he died very recently."

On a somewhat deeper level, the counselor who hears sadness in the client's voice responds by expressing sympathy and concern for the family.

A counselor who doesn't reflect anything before asking the age and cause of death would seem cold and uncaring. This would decrease any empathic connection between the client and the counselor. It would also send a signal that the counselor is only interested in facts and not feelings.

The follow-up to these reflections will depend on the circumstances. If this grandfather's death is most likely unrelated to the current visit and the client does not seem to be in distress at this time, a simple reflection and expression of sympathy may be all that is needed.

If the grandfather's death is related to the reason for the genetic counseling appointment or if the client is overcome with grief, it may be important to explore the meaning of this death for the family and how his passing will affect the counseling session.

CREATING A WORKING AGREEMENT

To proceed with the genetic counseling session, the counselor must develop a working agreement with the client. A working agreement is a shared vision of what is to come. Since many clients come to genetic counseling with only a vague understanding of the service, it behooves the counselor to start by eliciting the goals of the client and attending to the psychological needs expressed by the client surrounding these issues. This often takes the form of asking the client why s/he has come or what s/he was told about the appointment with the genetic counselor. Typically, the counselor tries to assess what the client hopes to achieve by attending the appointment. (See discussion of contracting and open and close ended questions below.) If the client seems unsure, the counselor may state his/her understanding of the appointment, for example, "I believe you were referred by your doctor to discuss your history of . . . ." Once this basic reason for meeting has been established, the counselor will want to show confidence that there is a plan for the session and that the counselor will work to meet the client's goals. While showing this leadership, it is still important to emphasize that the client will have input on the process and direction and that together they will shape the session.

Genetic counselor: What are you hoping to gain from genetic counseling?

Client: I need to know I won't get cancer.

Genetic counselor: As important as that is, no test can determine that. We could talk about the tests there are, what you could learn from them, and strategies you could use to lower your risk of developing cancer. How does that sound to you?

Many beginning counselors worry about the time needed to address the client's psychological needs. Often, acknowledging an issue and tailoring comments in this direction is sufficient. If the genetic counselor feels there are large unmet needs, an additional session with the genetic counselor or a referral for more counseling with another provider may be warranted.

From this assessment, the counselor can help the client formulate realistic goals for the session. For example, a prenatal client might say that her goal is to learn that her unborn baby is healthy. The counselor might help her to understand that a more realistic goal is that she will learn about tests available to determine whether certain conditions are present in her pregnancy. During this process, it is of paramount importance that the starting point is the needs of the client. Models of counseling that value the client as a partner or expert in care are favored.

A woman who has undergone BRCA testing and has been found to carry a mutation that confers high risk for cancer has come to the genetic counselor to discuss her options. When the word mastectomy is first uttered, a look of panic crosses the woman's face. The counselor needs to explore why this is. It could be that the patient has some misinformation about mastectomy that she got from reading outdated articles. However, it could also be that the last memory the patient has of her mother is that her mother went to the hospital for a mastectomy and was never well again. The patient's needs in these two different scenarios will probably be very different.

Goal setting can be complicated when there are multiple people involved in a session. If your "client" is actually a couple or a family, then the goals should be mutually constructed. If an individual client has brought others to the appointment, then the influence of these others may need to be considered; for example, a woman considering presymptomatic testing for a familial BRCA1 mutation might be strongly influenced by an at-risk sister or an affected family member in the room.

Balancing the needs of family members can be challenging. In most medical systems following a western perspective, the patient's individual autonomy is the primary consideration. However, in genetics, the family is sometimes the "client." By involving other family members, we may get a broader perspective of the problem, identify resources or barriers, and develop a more realistic set of goals. The counselor may have to consider individual needs and balance them against the needs of other individuals or the family as a group. This may mean arranging time to speak to individuals apart from their family as well as in a group (Barnett, 2007; Murphy and Dillon, 2003). This is another area where the counselor needs to be especially sensitive to family and cultural norms.

Consider the case of a client who does not seem to know why she has been sent to genetic counseling. Asking, "Can you tell me what you hope to gain from our meeting today?" will not be a productive line of questioning. It may be necessary to take a more structured approach: "My understanding is that your doctor wanted us to discuss the genetic testing that is available to you. Would it be OK with you if we start with that?"

Once the client and counselor have formulated goals for the session, they can create a contract for achieving these goals, a process sometimes referred to as "contracting." A contract is usually a verbal statement about how the goals will be met. Using the same prenatal example, the counselor might explain that a family history will be taken to assess risks, that prenatal testing options and limitations will be explained, and that the counselor will enable the client to choose the course of action that seems most in line with the client's beliefs and desires. Both parties have responsibilities in this model. Each agrees to contribute to the session, and they share responsibility for the session being successful.

It is key to remember that this contract is a plan to be negotiated between the counselor and the individual client and not a preformed plan that the counselor imposes on all clients. The plan should take the individual client's preferences into consideration. This will require flexibility on the part of the counselor: The counselor must be willing and able to deviate from his/her plan for the session. For example, in a pediatric setting the contract would include a description of the physical and laboratory examinations that are planned and the personnel this will involve. Consideration for the individual might dictate that the fewest number of people possible will be in the room when a teenage girl needs to disrobe and that, within reason, the girl might have a choice about who is there.

One exception to this ideal of flexibility would be if the case is substantially different from what the counselor had expected or prepared for. If, for example, the client reveals a history that had previously been unknown to the counselor, the counselor might not be prepared to counsel about that issue on the spot. It might be necessary to initiate a break in the session to look up information or to reschedule the appointment in order to give the counselor adequate time to prepare and gather records. An example of this would be a prenatal patient scheduled as an advance maternal age case who additionally has family members with birth defects and mental impairments that were not communicated to the genetic counselor in advance.

The flexibility of the session refers not only to the topics to be covered but also to the order in which they will be discussed. Counselors usually have an outline in mind for a session; beginning counselors are often wed to completing the outline in order. This helps them feel more in control. It often throws them off course if the client asks a question or makes a statement that takes the session in an unplanned direction. However, continuing with the session without addressing the question will be unsatisfying to the client: The client will not feel understood and cared for. Sometimes it is OK to tell a client that the question will be answered a bit later, but in doing so, there is a risk that the client will not be able to focus again until the question is answered.

When possible, adjust the order of the session to accommodate the client's inquiries. If it seems more appropriate, the counselor can give a brief answer at the time the question is asked, promise to say more later, and then resume with the session. Ideally, the counselor will remember to ask if the client is satisfied with the answer after coming back to this topic later in the session.

At the start of a pre-amniocentesis session, the patient asks how big the needle is. If the genetic counselor does not address the issue now, it is quite possible that the patient's fear will prevent her from participating in the session in any meaningful way.

Finally, it is the responsibility of the counselor to periodically stop and check whether the goals are being met; for example, the counselor might say, "I know you wanted to learn about your testing options today. Do you feel like your questions have been answered?"(Murphy and Dillon, 2003; McCarthy Veach et al., 2003).

Contracts may need to be revised as new information comes to light in a session. For example, if a family history reveals substantial new information that needs to be discussed, it may be necessary to suggest a second appointment or referral to another genetics clinic to cover all the important topics. This could come up when a pediatric or prenatal patient has a family history of cancer. Another problem that can arise is the realization that you will not be able to meet the goals as expected. For example, if it becomes apparent that the counselor and client do not speak a mutual language sufficiently well for the client to give informed consent for a procedure, it may be necessary to delay the appointment until an interpreter can be located or to reschedule.

Typically, contracts include a time component. The client will want to know approximately how much time will be needed for the appointment and whether follow-up appointments may be needed. Ideally, some of this will be done at the time of scheduling so that the client can make appropriate arrangements for child care, transportation, parking, time off from work, and other logistical issues. It is the counselor's responsibility to stay on time. This may mean redirecting or focusing the client's comments to more effectively meet goals. All counselors have had the experience of a client raising an important issue as time is running out—the so-called hand on the doorknob comment. One way to attempt to avoid these moments is to tell the client explicitly when you have about 5 minutes left in the session and to invite questions or comments at this time. This may give the client the encouragement s/he needs to raise an issue.

Contracts also need to spell out potential costs of visits and testing. Although this is never a popular subject for genetic counselors, it does not serve the client well if a test is explained in detail and the client decides to undertake the testing only to find out that a payment that the client cannot afford is expected at the time of service. Counselors need to be informed about the fees and insurance coverage associated with genetic counseling and testing.

> While this may seem like a very detailed approach to initiating a visit, many clients are unfamiliar with genetic counseling services and will be grateful for this information. It may allow them to relax and more fully participate in the important work that is to follow.

VERBAL AND NONVERBAL COMMUNICATION

> There are no facts, only interpretations.
> —Friedrich Nietzsche

A genetic counselor and client use both verbal and nonverbal clues to gain knowledge about the other and to demonstrate that understanding. Counselors use attending behaviors and active listening as tools for this communication. Attending behaviors include head nodding, smiling, and facing the client. Attending behavior is increased by eliminating distracting movements such as fiddling or wiggling.

Active listening can be as simple as indicating that you are paying attention. Sometimes all a client needs is some encouragement to continue speaking ("I see," "Uh huh"). At other times, the client will need more prompting. ("Tell me more about. . . ," "Can you give me an example of what you mean by. . .") A counselor can also redirect a client to talk about something the counselor sees as important ("You were talking about your uncle who has learning issues.") Active listening can also involve the use of reflection, that is, paraphrasing, repeating, or summarizing the client's words (McCarthy Veach et al., 2003).

> **Client:** There is no good answer. I can't believe I am faced with these decisions. This is difficult.
> **Genetic counselor:** Yes, this really is truly difficult. (Repeating)

> **Client:** I feel like I gave this disease to my son.
> **Genetic counselor:** It seems like you feel responsible for your son's condition. (Paraphrasing)

> **Client:** I can't begin to tell you how upsetting this is. I never expected to be in this position. I keep thinking I'll wake up and find out it was all a dream.
>
> **Genetic counselor:** Clearly this is very upsetting and it can be hard to accept this type of information. (Summarizing)

The genetic counselor will want to be careful to use language and word choices that convey acceptance and respect and do not communicate judgments or bias. One important way to do this is to use people-first language, for example, to say "a child with cystic fibrosis" or "a man using a wheelchair" rather than "a cystic fibrosis child" or "a wheelchair-bound man." This conveys a respect for the person and views the person as more important than a diagnosis or condition. (Hodgson et al., 2005).

Medical personnel, including genetic counselors, often get caught up in the use of jargon. For genetic counselors, the word "mutation" may simply mean an alternative gene form, but to a client that word may conjure up images of science-fiction "mutants." Words such as "risk" connote more danger than more neutral words such as "chance." Beginning genetic counselors may sometimes feel tongue tied by trying to avoid potentially problematic words; however, with practice counselors will find that the words will flow more naturally. If a good working rapport has been established, most clients will overlook an occasional faux pas.

A counselor can often get cues about language choices from the client. If a mother refers to her child as having "special needs," the counselor may choose that language rather than referring to the child's "development delays." The counselor can also model language for the family; a counselor would speak about a child with Down syndrome even though a family might report that they have a relative with mongolism.

The counselor will also want to be sensitive to factors such as acceptability of eye contact or the expectations about handshakes that can vary from one culture to another. The counselor should actively examine his or her own culture and cultural expectations since these will be the starting point for assessing others. Please refer to Chapter 11 for more discussion of this important topic.

When the counselor observes a behavior in the client, the counselor should not make a speedy judgment about the meaning of that behavior. Instead, the counselor needs to adopt a questioning attitude that allows for several alternative interpretations. Drawing a conclusion prematurely could lead the counselor to a false understanding of the situation. Acting on this false assumption could break down the support and empathy that the counselor is trying to convey. For example, a patient who is quiet might be shy, tired, bored, or upset. The counselor would want to use several strategies to differentiate these. Has the patient demonstrated any body language such as a yawn that would provide a clue? Is the patient's posture tense or distraught, such as closed fists or wringing hands? Sometimes reflection on a hunch may help, such as, "It is hard to talk about such personal matters." The more tools a counselor has to unravel the situation, the more likely that the counselor will be able to make a more genuine connection with the patient. These tools are acquired from experience and practice.

Consider a situation in which a prenatal counselor observes that a patient being seen before ultrasound and amniocentesis has her legs crossed and is jiggling one foot. It could be that the patient is bored. It could be that the patient is impatient or nervous about the upcoming procedures. It could be chilly in the room, and the client might be cold. Or it could be that the patient had been instructed to consume a large quantity of water and not to use the restroom before the ultrasound!

When the client's verbal and nonverbal behaviors do not match, the counselor will want to take particular note. Research has shown that nonverbal behaviors are often more telling than verbal ones. An example would be a client who says she has no concerns but is on the verge of tears or a teenager who is laughing at odd times. The counselor may choose to respond to this as it is observed or may file the discrepancy away for a time in the session when it may become relevant or when a deeper counseling relationship has been established (Okun and Kantrowitz, 2008).

The counselor also needs to be aware of the impact of his or her own body language. A large portion of what we communicate to others is done through our posture and facial expressions. This is a constant, largely unconscious, process. The goal for the counselor is to use nonverbal behavior more deliberately to communicate focus on the client, a process referred to as physical attending. This is usually achieved by midlevel eye contact (looking at the patient without staring), an attentive, open seated stance (leaning somewhat toward the patient with arms and legs uncrossed), and the attitude that almost nothing can distract you from paying attention to the patient (ignoring noises from the hallway, not looking at the clock as if you are out of time). Since gestures can have specific meaning to clients, they should be kept to a minimum or at least monitored for impact (McCarthy Veach et al., 2003; Coulehan and Block, 2001).

It is also important to think about what is NOT being said. Clients may avoid certain topics that are painful, embarrassing, or otherwise uncomfortable. A counselor should listen for clues that there may be unexpressed questions. For example, if the answer to "Are there any more questions?" is "I guess not," you might suspect that the client is reluctant to broach a subject. Also, if experience tells you that certain questions are common, but your client has not asked, you may want to raise the subject first. For instance, families faced with a diagnosis of a sex chromosomal difference such as Klinefelter syndrome (47, XXY) often worry about homosexuality, but may be afraid to ask about this sensitive subject.

Adjustments will be needed when more than one person attends clinic. It is important to look at each individual as he or she speaks and to position yourself so you can be attentive to everyone. When using an interpreter, the counselor should look at the client rather than the interpreter. It is the client's body language and expressions that are significant, and it is the client who needs to feel the counselor's empathy.

It is also important to monitor the pace and volume with which you speak. Because many counselors feel a need to cover large amounts of information with clients, there is a tendency especially among novice counselors to speak too rapidly or to introduce new topics too frequently. This heightens the tension in the session and decreases comprehension and comfort for the client. A puzzled expression on the client's face would be an immediate clue that the pace is too fast. It is the counselor's responsibility to make sure the client can follow the conversation: The counselor pauses and asks the client what she makes of the information presented thus far. This allows the counselor to see whether the client has understood and whether the information has been relevant to the client. Since it can be difficult for counselors to self-evaluate, the use of a tape recorder or having an experienced counselor observe may be useful additional tools to get feedback on these behaviors.

The counselor should speak in a comfortable, conversational speed and tone that can be easily heard and followed by the client. While it is natural and appropriate to speak more quietly when a sad subject is under discussion or a patient is grieving, the counselor should be careful not to adopt a tone that might convey shame or embarrassment when discussing sensitive information such as elective pregnancy termination, domestic violence, or disease symptoms such as incontinence (McCarthy Veach et al., 2003).

A genetic counselor stumbles over her words while explaining a pattern of inheritance to a client. She says, "Oops! I guess I should have had that second cup of coffee this morning. Let me try that again." The hope is that the client will see the counselor as a real person with strengths and weaknesses just like everyone else.

Humor plays an interesting role in the genetic counseling process. As has been mentioned before, inappropriate displays of humor should be noted, but clients sometimes use humor as a defense mechanism, perhaps as a way of lowering tension or as a coping strategy. Generally, counselors will want to respect this, but not allow the session to get off track by following the clients' lead away from important feelings. (Weil, 2001) However, there may be a role for the judicious use of humor as a rapport-building technique and a way of appearing more human and less intimidating.

Humor is very dependent on nonverbal cues such as facial expression and tone of voice. It is much harder to use over the telephone or online than in person. Humor is also very culturally dependent and often does not translate well. An example like the one described in the text box relies on the listener's ability to relate to drinking coffee as a way of becoming more alert in the morning, a habit common in the United States but not everywhere.

SPECIFIC INTERVIEWING TECHNIQUES

Questioning

Genetic counselors need to have several strategies for gathering information and generating discussion. The method selected should match the type of information that is needed (Table 3-1). Asking questions is one of the primary tools. Students will

TABLE 3-1. Interviewing Techniques

Questioning
Open-ended: Invites broad responses
Focused: Guides response toward specific circumstances
Closed-ended: Asks for yes/no answers or for specific details; does not encourage elaboration
Rephrasing: Restate your understanding of what the client has said
Reflecting: Repeat the last phrase of a client's statement as a question

From Baker et al. (1998) p. 59, Table 3.1

sometimes tell supervisors that certain questions are difficult to ask because the student perceives the question as personal. Students need to develop the ability to ask personal questions in calm, nonjudgmental ways. It will help to remember that as long as the answer to the question will be useful in helping the client, then it is a valid question. Counselors should have specific reasons for asking the questions they do and should ask questions in systematic and purposeful ways.

Closed-ended questions are questions that typically can be answered with one or two words (often yes or no). These questions are useful for obtaining specific information. They tend to keep discussion to a minimum and do not encourage expression of emotion. Open-ended questions invite a client to say more about a subject and give a more nuanced response. These questions can be the starting point for discussion.

It might seem that open-ended questions are preferable. This is not always true. Sometimes a brief specific answer is desired ("How old are you?"). At other times, clients may be confused, wary, or reluctant to participate, and closed-ended questions can be used as a starting point. The most important guidepost when questioning a client is this: Don't make assumptions. If you're unclear about an aspect of a client's experience or perception, or if you perceive that a particular issue is significant to a client, ask about it.

Closed-ended question: Do you have children?
Closed, but somewhat more inviting: How many children do you have?
Open-ended question: Please tell me about your children. (Although this is worded as a command, it serves the function of a question.)

Closed-ended question: Do you understand the information I have just provided?
Open-ended question: What questions do you have about the information provided?
More inviting of discussion: What are you thinking about the information we just went over?
Most inviting: How are you feeling about the information that we just went over?

The intent of focused questioning is to create opportunities for the client to identify specific experiences or insights that may be related to the current circumstances or decision-making process. Focused questions can also be used as a prompt to continue a discussion the client many have truncated because s/he had said enough or was unsure whether the counselor wanted to hear more. The simple question "Can you tell me more about that day/conversation/experience?" allows the client to share more about his or her experiences and for you as the counselor understand what is important to the client.

As the counselor, it is important for you to evaluate the client's responses. For many, it will be the first time that they have been invited to tell a story by a professional. Are they intrigued by your question but unsure if they believe that the counselor really wants to hear the response, or are they hesitant because they don't yet feel ready to discuss the topic at this time? If the latter is your assessment you may want to provide a summary of your thoughts as a counselor ("I asked about this because it may be relevant to your current situation and I want to understand more about what you think").

Generally when a mutually respectful relationship has been established with the counselor, a client not only will respond to questions but will welcome them as an opportunity to explore relevant experiences and consider how they have shaped their views. However, if a client provides a general unfocused reply to your query, assess the reasons for this reaction. Might you have been unclear? Is the client trying to avoid the interaction, or did you as the counselor make a wrong turn—for example, by unwittingly acting on an incorrect assumption about the client or misinterpreting certain cures or responses. If the counselor's line of questioning is unfounded, it is necessary to stop and correct the direction of the conversation.

It is not always necessary to ask a question to get more information. Sometimes counselors use reflections, follow-up, or silence to encourage elaboration on a topic (McCarthy Veach et al., 2003). It is also important to remember that some clients, most notably men and teenagers, will not be comfortable with a question about their feelings. A question about what they are "thinking" is a good way to open discussion with people who are reluctant to discuss emotions.

Rephrasing

Rephrasing involves stating in your own words what the client has just told you. It is a valuable tool for demonstrating to the client that s/he is being listened to and ensuring that you have understood what s/he intended to convey. It reinforces for the client that you have understood a part of his or her experience. It is especially valuable when you and your client have different language skills or when a client uses a great deal of slang or colloquial speech that is unfamiliar to you.

Suppose your client, the mother of two children who is now pregnant by a new partner, states: "So I just don't know if he [i.e., the new partner] is gonna disappear or what." What she has just said seems to be a clear and fairly frank assessment of the strength of her current relationship. The counselor may feel that this statement can be taken at face value, or she may choose to rephrase it to ensure that she fully understands the woman's meaning. The counselor may reply with something like, "So, you don't think that he's very committed to the relationship?" and pause (i.e., is she nodding in agreement?) and then proceed to inquire about the basis for her statement ("Why do you think that is?"). The counselor will have ensured that she indeed understood what the client was saying and will have laid the groundwork for ongoing clarification of her understanding as they cover topics such as risk assessment, prenatal testing, pregnancy termination, and other areas in which an understanding of the client's personal relationships and beliefs is essential to providing quality care.

Reflecting

Reflecting involves repeating the last phrase of a client's statement in the form of a question to encourage further exploration of the topic. It is also used to maintain the direction of a conversation. Its uses are demonstrated in the following exchanges:

> **Client:** Well, since my nephew was diagnosed with muscular dystrophy, my husband just seems scared about another pregnancy
>
> **Counselor:** He seems scared?
>
> **Client:** Well, I guess we're both a little scared, you know, that it might happen to us?

> **Client:** So that's my decision—a mastectomy is better than cancer
>
> **Counselor:** Better than cancer?
>
> **Client:** Well sure, that way I don't have to worry any more.

Reflecting encourages the client to amplify his or her thoughts and ideas in a way that more clearly identifies the significance of his or her feelings or observations. This also gives the counselor more information regarding the basis for the client's thoughts and beliefs, so that s/he can respond without making assumptions. In the second example, the client's comments about a mastectomy may indicate that she believe surgery will permanently protect her from cancer.

Redirecting

Redirecting is used by the counselor to manage the rate of information exchange—to direct the introduction and flow of topics, or to refocus the discussion when the client has gone off on a tangent. The following are examples of statements that can be employed to redirect the counseling interaction:

> That's an important issue, but first I'd like to go back to. . . .
>
> We will get to that, but first I think it would be helpful to hear. . . .
>
> Before moving on, let me ask you a little more about. . . .
>
> How about that other matter you mentioned regarding. . . .
>
> I'd like to slow down here a bit. Do you think what you just said about . . . is relevant to the decision you're facing today?

That's an important question, which is best answered by your cardiologist. So, could we come back to. . . .

Promoting Shared Language

One technique that can enhance client comfort and understanding is an effort by the counselor to mirror the client's language or communication style (to an appropriate degree). The counselor should not abandon his or her own style, but convey to the client that s/he is being heard and understood as an individual. The counselor might say, "Well, what I call the 'nonworking' gene and you call the 'bad' gene are really the same thing," and from this point on you would use the client's term. Additionally, the counselor might model or invite the client to use alternative terms that could be helpful in the future. For example, "Neurofibromatosis is a mouthful, isn't it? It is also called 'NF,' which is what you'll hear me use today." However, if a client refers to herself as handicapped, then the counselor would use this term instead of the word disabled. Finally, using shared language, similar terminology and phrasing as the client can also increase the empathetic connection with your client.

Communication style is a broad area and includes word usage, speaking tempo, and the use of colloquial terms. The counselor's ability to echo the client's communication style, if appropriate and comfortable, can facilitate communication. For instance, if your client has a deliberate manner of speaking, while you are naturally a rapid talker, you might choose to slow down your tempo to be more in step with your client. Likewise, if certain colloquial terms the client uses are comfortable for you, you might want to include them in your conversation throughout the session.

> A client reports that she has come for genetic counseling because she had a cousin who had Mongolism. After asking a few questions about this cousin, the counselor might say, "It does sound as if this cousin had what some people call Mongolism. Most people now call this Down syndrome or trisomy 21." During the rest of the counseling session, the counselor would use the term "Down syndrome" as an example for the client.

Silence

Silence is a particularly effective technique that is often difficult for beginning counselors. Most Americans are conditioned to fill silence. However, many clients use silence as a time to reflect on what has been said, to formulate what to say next, or to gain composure. A counselor who fills the silence too quickly does not allow for these processes and may communicate the message that the counselor will determine the direction of the session without input from the client. Clinicians may offer their own thoughts too quickly rather than waiting for the client; this is especially true of beginners who are trying to be helpful by appearing smart and having answers. We show respect for a client's story by pausing to take it in rather than rushing to comment on it. Some studies indicate that clients often will NOT mention their most important concern first. A longer pause may allow them to get to their deeper concerns. A good rule of thumb for someone who is working on this skill is to count to ten before speaking. (Murphy and Dillon, 2003; McCarthy Veach et al., 2003; Sharf, 1990).

OBTAINING PEDIGREES

Most genetic counseling sessions will involve constructing a pedigree. The pedigree not only provides a succinct pictorial representation of the family, it can also be a tool for learning more about the client. Some counselors systematically gather information about health and illness beliefs, family patterns of relating, or experiences with loss in the form of genograms (Eunpu, 1997). Even without such a system, all genetic counselors can use the pedigree as a counseling tool. By listening to the way a client describes family members, you can begin to formulate a mental awareness of how close-knit a family is, how medically sophisticated they are, whether the client approaches problems with optimism or skepticism, and what impact the disease in question has had on the family. Clients will often make seemingly off-hand remarks about speaking to a family member recently ("When I spoke to my sister yesterday, she said"), where family members live ("I don't see them as often. They live in California."), and other bits of personal data that the genetic counselor can use to form an image of the family even if specific questions about these matters are not asked.

The other interesting aspect of taking a pedigree is that the client is the expert and the counselor is the one who is learning—a reverse of the way things often are in a medical setting. This can be empowering to the client, especially if the genetic counselor conveys respect for the partnership that is forming and the client's contribution to the success of the session. (Baker et al., 1998) For more on pedigrees, see Chapter 2 by Schuette and Bennett in this text.

Although a pedigree can reveal some aspects of a family's experience with a disease, the genetic counselor will want to ask more about this. This is often done through narrative, or getting the client to tell the story.

A man with Tourette syndrome came for genetic counseling. He expressed his goal as learning the odds that his children would be affected with the syndrome. As the pedigree was taken the following story emerged: It seemed that the symptoms were more of a problem for family members such as his mother than they were for him. As he talked about his marriage and the possibility of children, he seemed happy, not reluctant or anxious. The counselor expressed to him that he seemed eager to be a parent and that he did not seem very worried about having a child with the syndrome no matter what the odds were. He agreed with this assessment, and the counselor and he were able to have a very productive discussion. The man left feeling very satisfied with the information that was presented and validated for his feelings.

ASSESSMENT

Assessment is an ongoing process throughout the session. Genetic counselors are looking for a client's assets, that is, strengths and resources. Questions might be asked about how past problems were solved, about support systems, about religious practices, and about a host of other factors that will shape how a client learns about or copes with a genetic issue.

Support systems are critical for most families facing genetic diseases or birth defects. As mentioned above, the pedigree may be one of the first assessment tools that is used to look at family structure and potential support. The counselor may also ask about school or early intervention, friends, insurance coverage and financial resources, work constraints or supports, and spiritual or pastoral supports. Looking at the client in his/her environment, a systems approach, may be useful for organizing your thinking about the case. (Spitzer Kim, 1999; Miller et al., 2006)

The genetic counselor needs to continually monitor the affect or emotional state of the client. Information imparted during sessions can be highly charged. A client who is experiencing a great deal of emotion may no longer be able to listen or engage during the session until these emotions have been vented. A child who is becoming less cooperative and more agitated during a session may be reacting to news that he will need to have his blood drawn at the end of the session. The parents supervising this child may also have stopped listening because they are wrapped up in memories of the last time a blood draw was attempted.

One area of genetic counseling that can become rote or cookie-cutter is the delivery of information. This is because the information has become very familiar to the counselor—almost like turning on a tape recorder. However, the counseling experience will be richer and more rewarding if this is not the case. The counselor needs to remember that this may be the first time that the client has heard this information or considered the personal consequences. Rather than launching into a preplanned discussion of information, the counselor should inquire about the client's knowledge on the subject. It is more comfortable for clients if the counselor approaches this obliquely and not as if it is a quiz. For example, framing the question as "What have you been told about. . ." rather than "What do you know about. . ." can give the patient the permission they need to reveal what they do and, more importantly, what they do not know.

It is particularly important that the counselor adjust the discussion based on this inquiry. Many beginning counselors will ask whether clients know anything about genetics and then will proceed to explain genes and chromosomes even if the client says she has a Ph.D. in molecular biology. However, even if the client does have a Ph.D. or M.D., the genetic counselor will still want to assess the client's comprehension of the information as it relates to his or her own circumstances. If there are multiple people attending the session, each of them may have different experience and different levels of knowledge, so the counselor will want to include each of them in the discussion. This may be of particular importance when one member of a couple has personal (family) experience of a condition and the other partner does not.

It is also important to assess attitudes and beliefs and not to make assumptions. A person's profession, level of education, religion, ethnic background and other demographic data do not correlate one to one with particular decisions or beliefs. It would be presumptuous to assume that only certain options are open to someone based on the religious or ethnic background recorded in the history.

In her memoir, *Expecting Adam*, Martha Beck vividly describes how people had expectations about her behavior and attitude toward Down syndrome based on the fact that she was a graduate student at Harvard. Nearly everyone expected that she would terminate her affected pregnancy, and she felt enormously isolated from her community for making a different decision. (Beck, 1999)

SUMMARY

The process of interviewing is complex. However, successful navigation of this phase of the genetic counseling session sets the stage for the family and the counselor to enter into the medical, diagnostic, informational, psychosocial counseling, and follow-up phases of the genetic counseling appointment with the information, trust, and rapport that will be needed for a satisfactory visit.

This chapter provides a very brief introduction to interviewing. Creating an appropriate atmosphere through the use of respect, genuineness, and empathy underlies the process of genetic counseling. Genetic counselors use verbal tools like open- and closed-ended questions, reflections, and silence; effective counselors also are aware of nonverbal cues. Developing these skills and applying them in the clinical setting is an ongoing learning experience. More resources for continuing to explore this topic can be found in the bibliography.

ACKNOWLEDGMENTS

I would like to thank the faculty, staff, and students of the Arcadia, Berkeley, and Brandeis Genetic Counseling Programs for all they have taught me and all the support they have shown me over the past 25 years. A number of them generously gave their time and expertise to the editing of this chapter. And a special thanks to Seymour Kessler and the thousands of patients who have shaped my thinking and experience as a genetic counselor.

REFERENCES

Baker DL, Schuette JL, Uhlmann WR (eds) (1998) *A Guide to Genetic Counseling*. New York: Wiley-Liss.

Barnett RM (2007) Prenatal diagnosis for Huntington disease. *Perspect Genet Couns* 29(2). www.nsgc.org.

Beck M (1999) *Expecting Adam*. Crown.

Cochran JL, Cochran NH (2006) *The Heart of Counseling*. Belmont, CA: Thompson Brooks/Cole.

Coulehan JL, Block MR (2001) *The Medical Interview* (4th ed.). Philadelphia: FA Davis.

Donoghue DJ, Siegel ME (2005) *Are You Really Listening?* Notre Dame, IL: Sorin Books.

Encarta Dictionary (1999) New York: St. Martin's Press.

Eunpu D (1997) Systemically-based psychotherapeutic techniques in genetic counseling. *J Genet Couns* 6(1):1–20.

Fadiman A (1997) *The Spirit Catches You and You Fall Down*. New York: Farrar, Strauss and Giroux.

Hodgson J, Hughes E, Lambert C (2005) "SLANG" —Sensitive Language and the New Genetics—an Exploratory Study. *J Genet Couns* online 29 Dec.

Kelly PT (1977) *Dealing with Dilemma: A Manual for Genetic Counselors*. New York: Springer.

Kessler S (ed) (1979) *Genetic Counseling Psychological Dimensions*. New York: Academic Press.

Matloff E (2006) Becoming a daughter. *J Genet Couns* 15(3):139–143.

McCarthy Veach P, LeRoy BS, Bartels DM (2003) *Facilitating the Genetic Counseling Process*. New York: Springer.

Miller S, McDaniel S, Rolland J. Feetham SL (2006) *Individuals, Families, and the New Era of Genetics*. New York: Norton.

Murphy BC, Dillon C (2003) *Interviewing in Action. Relationship, Process, and Change* (2nd ed). Brooks/Cole.

Nietzsche F. Available at http://www.quoteland.com/author.asp?AUTHOR_ID=73. Accessed on 2007 May 20.

Okun B, Kantrowitz R (2008) *Effective Helping*. Belmont, CA: Thomson Brooks/Cole.

Sharf B (1990) *A Shared Understanding* (Videorecording). Chicago: Univ. of Illinois.

Spitzer Kim K (1999) Case Report: A Systems Approach to Genetic Counseling for Albinism. *J Genet Couns* 8(1):47–54.

Swietzer HF, King MA (2004) *The Successful Internship* (2nd ed). Belmont, CA: Thompson Brooks/Cole.

Vonnegut K (1966) *Mother Night*. New York: Harper and Row.

Weil J (2000) *Psychosocial Genetic Counseling*. New York: Oxford University Press.

4

Thinking It All Through: Case Preparation and Management

Wendy R. Uhlmann, M.S., C.G.C.

INTRODUCTION

The phone rings. The person calling is:

- *a 42-year old woman with breast cancer and a family history of early-onset cancer*
- *a 30-year old man whose father and several relatives have Huntington disease*
- *a pediatrician who has a 6-month-old patient with developmental delay*
- *a 26-year-old woman who has had three first-trimester spontaneous miscarriages*

Mastering the art of case preparation enables you to confidently provide genetic counseling to a patient for a condition that you cannot spell or pronounce and have never seen before. Mastering the art of case management enables you to provide genetic counseling and competently manage the different components of a case within the allotted time-frame and to effectively complete the necessary follow-up. The goal of this chapter is to provide an overview of case preparation and management that will

A Guide to Genetic Counseling, Second Edition, Edited by Wendy Uhlmann, Jane Schuette, and Beverly Yashar

be applicable regardless of clinical setting. It should be emphasized that clinics and genetic counselors will have varied ways of conducting case preparation and management and not all presented elements will be done for each case.

Case management begins when the appointment is scheduled and continues long after the patient has left your clinic. As the above phone calls illustrate, genetics clinics see patients for a wide variety of indications, requiring that the genetic counselor be able to modify case preparation and management accordingly. Even within a clinical genetics specialty, patients are referred for different indications and have diverse backgrounds. The abilities to think critically, research, assess, anticipate, and communicate are required for successful case preparation and management. While a genetic counselor can do his or her best to prep a case, one must be ready to handle the "surprises" that are learned when obtaining a family history or performing a physical examination. Fortunately, with online access to the medical and scientific literature and genetic databases and resources, information needed for a case is often just a few keystrokes away.

The extent of case preparation (Fig. 4-1) is somewhat unique to genetics and is critical for providing genetic counseling and ensuring that the information is accurate and current. It is because of the vast number of genetic conditions, combined with the rapid advances being made in molecular genetics and testing, that case preparation is an important and necessary component of a genetics clinic visit. Key Internet genetic resources are presented in this chapter and are highlighted in an article by Uhlmann and Guttmacher (2008). As with any medical specialty, effective case management, including follow-up, is also important for genetics patients. The different aspects of case management (Fig. 4-2) are presented in this and other chapters.

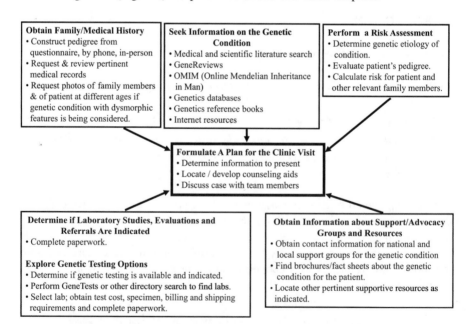

FIGURE 4-1. *Overview of case preparation. The extent of case preparation will depend on the indication for the clinic visit and not all of these components will be part of each case*

Manage the Clinic Visit

• Ascertain patient's questions and concerns
• Describe to patient what visit will entail and who will be involved
• Obtain family and medical history information
  - Share information with team members
• Assist with recording findings on physical exam (if done)
• Provide genetic counseling
  - Be aware of how patient is processing information and adapt
    genetic counseling as indicated.
• Be mindful of time constraints
  - For patients needing more time, determine if session can be
    extended or whether return visit is needed
• Facilitate decision-making
• Close session by summarizing key points and recommended follow-up

Coordinate Follow-up

• Communicate clearly with patient about recommended follow-up
• Establish with patient how results will be communicated (return visit, phone, letter)
• Provide consulting specialists with pertinent information about the patient's medical and family history and indicate the specific features associated with the genetic condition to assess
• Obtain and report results of tests and evaluations
• Send summary letters to referring physician and patient as indicated

---

FIGURE 4-2. *Components of case management*

Many details are included because successful case preparation and management depends on keeping track of details and balancing several tasks simultaneously. Given the amount of content and details in this chapter, it is recommended that you first skim the chapter to obtain an overview of case preparation and management. Then as you prepare for cases, you can go back and read sections and use the relevant tables to create "to do" lists.

THE INITIAL INTAKE

The most important information to ascertain during the initial intake is the indication for the clinic visit, which will be used to determine who sees the patient and will guide your case preparation. It is often a secretary or clinic scheduler who will have the first contact with a patient who calls to set up an appointment. Some patients may not understand why they need to be seen or may think just having a genetic test is all that is needed. The genetic counselor can help clinic schedulers understand what typically happens during a clinic visit so that they can effectively address patients' initial inquiries. Since genetics clinic visits are often an hour or more, it is helpful to inform patients of this in advance.

Even though just standard contact information needed to schedule the appointment is being obtained, important insights can be gained about the patient's state of mind (e.g., anxious, confused, angry, concerned, upset), whether there is cognitive impairment, whether there is a need for an interpreter, and whether the diagnosis is known or unknown, new or established. It is important for genetic counselors to encourage whoever is scheduling appointments to write brief notes and communicate their impressions if the patient intake was not routine. This "heads-up" can be beneficial when first meeting with patients.

If your clinic routinely sends patients forms to complete, it is helpful to include space for patients to share their concerns and questions and indicate who will be coming to the appointment. It is not unusual for other family members to come to the appointment, because the genetic information is also relevant for them and/or to be there to support the patient. If other family members are coming because the information has personal implications, they may require separate registration, particularly if a physical examination is involved. More time may also be needed for the appointment, along with larger or additional rooms. However, depending on the issues to be discussed and the time limitations of a visit, it is not always appropriate for other family members to be present, particularly young children if only their parent is being evaluated. Therefore, depending on the clinical indication, it may be preferable to see family members at a follow-up visit, and this is best determined and communicated before the initial appointment.

BILLING ISSUES FOR GENETICS CLINIC VISITS

"Will my genetics clinic visit be covered by my insurance?" is a question frequently asked by patients when scheduling their appointment. For insurance coverage of the clinic visit, generally a referral is needed from the patient's primary care physician. Even if a specialist has made the consult request, the visit will still likely need the primary care physician's approval. Depending on the patient's type of insurance and plan, there may be deductibles and copayments, and the genetics clinic visit may be fully, partially, or not at all covered. An additional referral may be needed for genetic testing or other evaluations and testing. You should take the time to learn how patients are billed in your clinic and who is responsible for handling billing questions and problems. Ascertain whether there are options for patients with limited funds and if payment plans can be arranged. If you work in a hospital, social workers may be able to help low-income patients and patients without health insurance identify where they can apply for state-funded insurance and obtain healthcare services. Keep a file with the names and contact information of individuals who have been helpful in addressing billing issues to use with future patients.

The National Society of Genetic Counselors has billing and reimbursement resources available at their website. The American College of Medical Genetics has published a manual on billing and reimbursement, and the Secretary's Advisory Committee on Genetics, Health and Society published a report on this topic in 2006, which also gives an overview of how health insurance works in the United States and the different types of insurance plans (SACGHS, 2006). Billing and reimbursement is addressed further in Chapter 10.

PREPARING A CASE

The extent to which you need to prep a case (Fig. 4-1) will depend on the clinical indication, your knowledge base, and what your clinic generally prefers to ascertain before seeing a patient. If you have previously seen a patient with the same genetic condition, you may be able to reach into your files or memory and be ready to counsel. However, given the rapid advances being made in genetics, it is important to make sure your information is current and not assume that case prep done for a previous patient with the same condition will suffice. In preparing a case, it is also important to balance what is needed to be sufficiently prepared with the possibility that the patient may not keep the appointment.

As you prepare a case, think about it from the patient's perspective. What questions would you have? What would you want to learn? Basic information to ascertain for cases is provided in Table 4-1. Some general questions to guide your case preparation are listed in Table 4-2. The specific information that is ascertained for cases will depend on

TABLE 4-1. Basic Information to Ascertain for Genetics Cases

- Incidence of genetic condition and carrier frequency
  - Ethnicity-dependent variation in incidence and carrier frequency
- Genetic etiology of condition
  - Mode(s) of inheritance
    - Percent of cases inherited versus *de novo* (due to new mutation)
    - Percent of cases due to germline (gonadal) mosaicism
  - Gene(s) and Chromosome location(s)
    - Genetic heterogeneity
    - Allelic heterogeneity
    - Function of gene(s)
    - Penetrance
- Clinical features
  - Types of symptoms and medical problems
  - Genotype-phenotype correlations
  - Variable expressivity?
  - Anticipation?
- Age of onset, natural history, prognosis, and lifespan
- Testing options
  - Diagnostic
  - Carrier
  - Presymptomatic/Predictive
  - Prenatal
  - Preimplantation genetic diagnosis
- Management and treatment options
- Prevention and surveillance options
- Support / Advocacy groups and other resources
- Research studies (if pertinent or requested)

TABLE 4-2. General Questions to Guide Your Case Preparation

- Why do you think the patient is seeking genetic counseling/evaluation at this time?
- What are some questions you think the patient likely will have?
- Given the clinical indication, what information needs to be obtained to provide genetic counseling?
- Can you back up the information you will present with reliable studies/references?
- What family and medical history information would be important to obtain? Are there specific medical records that should be requested from the patient? From relatives?
- Given the patient's family history and the inheritance of the genetic condition (if known), what risk figures would you provide the patient? His/her relatives?
- Are risk figures consistent across studies/references? If inconsistent, why is there variability and what are the limitations of the studies?
- Is genetic testing available? Is it clinically indicated? How good is the testing?
- Are there other tests that should be performed? Should the patient be referred to other specialists for evaluation?
- Are there support groups for the genetic condition and patient publications?
- In what order would you envision presenting information to the patient? What are the specific points that need to be emphasized?
- What visual aids do you plan to utilize? Are there visual aids that you need to develop?

the genetic condition, the clinical indication, and what is known/unknown. Obtaining this information can take time, as multiple articles and resources may be needed.

For patients with an unknown genetic diagnosis, you may be able to generate differential diagnoses to consider based on your review of family and medical history information and by entering clinical features into the search function in OMIM (Online Mendelian Inheritance in Man). Having some idea about different potential diagnoses in advance can help your team determine the patient information to ascertain, what to look for on physical examination, and whether there are genetic testing options to consider.

You also need to think globally and recognize other conditions in the family history, independent of the indication for the clinic visit, that pose a genetic risk. For example, a patient being seen for neurofibromatosis may have a family history of early-onset cancer, which will need to be addressed, deferred to another clinic visit, or referred to a cancer genetics clinic. If a patient being seen for Marfan syndrome is of reproductive age and taking medications, you may look up the medications to see whether they pose a teratogenic risk and/or note that this should be discussed with her gynecologist/obstetrician.

Prenatal questions come up, not just in prenatal genetics clinics but also with patients seen in pediatric, adult and specialty genetics clinics. Parents may inquire about recurrence risks and reproductive options. Adults with a personal and/or a family history of a genetic condition may be contemplating a pregnancy and likewise want similar information. For patients with a genetic condition who are of or are approaching reproductive age, you should be prepared to address whether the genetic condition would pose any health issues during pregnancy.

While you can anticipate certain questions patients likely will have during their genetics clinic visit, you should also think about questions patients may not even know to ask and be prepared to provide this information. Some patients come with lists of questions, while other patients feel inhibited asking questions. Anticipating patients' questions, asked and unasked, and preparing accordingly is key to successful case management.

Formulating a Plan for the Clinic Visit

As you prepare for a case, it is important to determine what information to present, the main points to emphasize, how information can be presented to facilitate the patient's understanding, and what counseling aids can assist in this process. Care should be taken not to overwhelm the patient with information, but sufficient information must be presented to allow a clear understanding of the genetic condition and risks and enable informed decisions to be made. In short, a key part of case preparation is envisioning the session and planning accordingly. The use of counseling aids (see section on "Locating and Developing Counseling Aids") can help you organize a session. Initially, it also may be helpful to prepare a brief outline for the session and key points. Such an outline will help you to formulate a "game plan," but is not to be seen as a rigid framework for the genetic counseling session. You have to be flexible enough to "go with the flow" of a session and modify as needed, while at the same time being sure to cover the necessary information. In addition, you need to be able to respond to both verbal and nonverbal cues as to how the patient is assimilating the information and adapt the counseling as indicated.

Obtaining Family History Information

The patient's family history is essential to providing genetic counseling. Family histories are obtained through questionnaires provided to the patient before or at the appointment, by phone or in person during the clinic visit. The benefit of sending family history forms in advance is that it allows patients the opportunity to talk with other family members, if needed, to obtain accurate information about ages, causes of death, and medical conditions. It is not unusual for information to be learned that was not known before. If constructing the pedigree from a questionnaire, it is helpful to use Post-it notes on the pedigree to identify family history information that still needs to be ascertained or clarified during the visit. Post-it notes on the pedigree can help prompt you to ask specific medical questions as well.

Telephoning a patient in advance for family history information does take time and can involve phone charges. Before you call a patient, you should first determine whether the call is needed and the minimum information that is required for your case prep. Asking a few targeted questions to identify the specific genetic condition(s), which family members are affected, and how these individuals are related to the patient can provide important information for your case preparation, risk assessment, and determination of medical records that would be helpful to review.

Even if you have seen other family members in your clinic, HIPAA (Health Insurance Portability and Accountability Act) privacy regulations prohibit you from acknowledging that you have information about the family. You will still need to obtain the family history from your patient. You cannot access or refer to these previous histories, even if they are more accurate, without authorization from these family members. Histories change with time, so even if the patient has been seen previously in your clinic, it is important to update family and medical history information. Obtaining a complete family history and constructing a pedigree are discussed in detail in Chapter 2.

Requesting Photographs

Sometimes it can be helpful to look at actual photographs of other family members (e.g., parents, siblings) to assist in establishing a diagnosis, particularly when evaluating patients who have dysmorphic features and an unknown diagnosis. Photographs of the patient at different ages are useful, as the features of a genetic condition can change over time and the diagnosis may be more evident at an earlier or later age. Viewing photographs of other family members can help to establish whether a feature that is consistent with a genetic condition (e.g., hypertelorism) is actually a familial trait. Letting patients know that they can just bring in photo albums may make it easier to fulfill your request for photographs. Photographs may also be taken of the patient during the genetics clinic visit, with a signed release, to aid in diagnostic discussions with other geneticists and for use in teaching conferences and publications. The American College of Medical Genetics has a practice guideline for medical photographs with a model informed consent form available at their website and you should also check your institution's policy on taking patient photographs.

Review of Medical Records

Reviewing medical records is a key component of case preparation and can provide information that is critical for genetic counseling. Table 4-3 has information on obtaining and reviewing medical records. Medical record review is important for learning about the patient's medical history, documenting clinical symptoms, confirming a diagnosis, establishing differential diagnoses, and providing an accurate risk assessment. Finding out what tests and evaluations have already been done can reduce the likelihood of unnecessary duplicate studies. This record review can also help determine whether additional tests or evaluations are needed. Given the pace of advances in testing, if a karyotype, chromosome microarray analysis, or genetic testing was done previously, reports will be useful in determining whether the test should be repeated or additional studies ordered and will be helpful to the laboratory, if more testing is done.

Depending on the genetic condition, medical records may also be needed from other family members. It may only be necessary to obtain medical record documentation of a diagnosis in a single affected individual, such as is the case for Huntington disease. However, in evaluating a patient to establish a diagnosis for a hereditary cancer syndrome, medical records may be needed from several affected relatives to confirm their types of cancer and ages of onset. A patient may have only vague information about a relative (e.g., "My grandmother had a female cancer") that can be clarified with medical records. In addition, when medical records are reviewed, it may become evident that inaccurate medical information about relatives has been passed down through the family. Confirmation of or ruling out a diagnosis in relatives can have significant implications in establishing a patient's diagnosis and performing a risk assessment.

Records may be difficult to obtain from family members, either because the patient is reluctant to make the request or because relatives may not wish to share them. For

TABLE 4-3. Obtaining and Reviewing Medical Records

- Patient or referring physician should be informed of need for medical records when appointment is scheduled
- Allow sufficient time to obtain medical records for a clinic visit
  - Records may be readily available or may take days to weeks to obtain
  - Some clinics and small hospitals may charge patient a fee, especially if beyond a certain page limit
  - Patients can sometimes expedite obtaining records by picking them up
- Authorization for release of medical records
  - Provide patient with medical records release form which can also be duplicated if records are needed from several doctors/hospitals and from other family members
  - Authorization needed from patient, parent (if patient is a minor) or legal guardian (will need documentation of guardianship); next of kin (if deceased)
- Specific medical records to request
  - Summary letters documenting the diagnosis/suspected diagnosis, symptoms, reason for referral
  - Relevant evaluations by other specialists, lab (especially genetic test results if available), radiology and pathology reports
  - General records related to routine medical care usually are not necessary
- Review of medical records
  - Highlight text or mark records with post-it notes to alert team members to relevant content
  - May be helpful to write brief timeline that summarizes patient's medical history. This can be useful for seeing the patient and dictating clinic letters.

deceased individuals with unavailable records, sometimes a death certificate can provide useful diagnostic information. If medical records cannot be obtained, it may limit the information that can be provided. In the absence of medical records, it should be noted in clinic visit documentation that family medical history information is "reported by the patient." In addition, if medical records are required for an accurate risk assessment, it should be noted that medical records would need to be reviewed to comment more specifically on recurrence risks.

Psychosocial Information Can Be Extracted from Medical Record Review

Medical records can also provide information about how the genetic condition has impacted the patient or family member. Looking at the number of hospitalizations, procedures, and tests and reading through the notes and summaries can provide a sense of what the course of the genetic condition has been, how long the patient has experienced symptoms, and whether the patient has been compliant with past medical recommendations. This information may form the basis for beginning an exploration of psychosocial issues (e.g., "I had a chance to review your medical records and can see that you have really been through a lot"). A notation in the medical records that a patient has not been compliant in the past may influence how you present medical recommendations. Sometimes medical records will allude to the patient's disposition (e.g., pleasant, angry, upset). It is important not to attempt to predict from these subjective comments how a patient might respond to a genetics clinic visit. Remember that a patient's disposition is largely influenced by what is occurring in his or her life and depends on the focus of an appointment (e.g., a patient may be angry because he/ she was just informed about a diagnosis).

FINDING INFORMATION ON GENETIC CONDITIONS

You have just been scheduled to see a patient for a genetic condition that you know absolutely nothing about. Genetic counselors frequently find themselves in this situation, given that there are several thousand genetic conditions. The unknown can easily become known if you know where to seek information. There are genetics reference books that provide overviews of genetic conditions, useful for background information; however, it is critical that you access the primary literature. The following online computer resources have been in existence for years and are considered the "bibles" in the field of clinical genetics and a starting point for case preparation. You can save time by bookmarking websites you frequently use for case preparation. With any resource, including the "bibles," it is important to check the publication date and to conduct a literature search, discussed below, to obtain the most up-to-date information.

GeneTests

The online computer resource GeneTests, funded by the National Institutes of Health and developed at the University of Washington, is considered to be a key resource for clinical genetics professionals and has the following resources:

- *GeneReviews* has expert-authored, peer-reviewed summaries of genetic conditions including clinical features, diagnostic criteria, differential diagnoses, management, prevalence, inheritance, molecular genetics, genetic testing, genetic counseling considerations, patient resources, and links to pertinent articles, policy statements/guidelines, and genomic databases.
- *GeneTests* is an international directory of laboratories offering clinical and research genetic testing, searchable by genetic condition, gene, protein, and clinical feature. It includes information on test methodology, whether prenatal diagnosis is offered, and laboratory certification.
- *GeneClinics* is a directory of national and international genetics clinics, searchable by state, zip code, country, and services (e.g., pediatric genetics).

In addition, GeneTests has educational resources about clinical genetics and genetic testing, including an illustrated glossary and case examples.

Online Mendelian Inheritance in Man (OMIM)

Online Mendelian Inheritance in Man (OMIM) is a comprehensive online database of genetic conditions, their patterns of inheritance, and a compendium of human genes. It originally appeared in book form as a single volume in 1966 as Victor A. McKusick's *Mendelian Inheritance in Man: Catalogs of Human Genes and Genetic*

Disorders. OMIM cites the seminal papers on a genetic condition, including clinical features, biochemical features, inheritance, mapping, molecular genetics, population genetics, pathogenesis, diagnosis, clinical management, animal models, and history. OMIM can be used to generate differential diagnoses by conducting a search with the clinical features; for example, "hearing loss, short stature, mental retardation" will yield a list of genetic conditions with these clinical features. You need to try your search with different terms—for example, for a condition with deafness, also search for "hearing loss," for epilepsy, also try "seizures," and for "developmental delay," additionally search for "mental retardation." OMIM also includes a clinical synopsis of the genetic condition, which lists the clinical features from head to toe, internal and external. The clinical synopsis is useful for physical examinations and for determining what features to inquire about when obtaining family and medical histories. It can also be used as a quick handout about the genetic condition for case conferences. OMIM has links to cytogenetic map locations, gene maps, sequences, and gene databases. The OMIM Help and FAQ sections provide useful information about searching and using OMIM effectively.

Conducting Literature Searches

Conducting literature searches is important for making sure that you have pertinent, accurate, and up-to-date information about a genetic condition. Literature searches are conducted with Medline (the online index to the medical literature, which can be accessed through PubMed), Google Scholar, and other medical literature review programs. You will need to conduct literature searches to obtain articles from both the medical and scientific literature to address the topics in Table 4-1. Try searching for the name of the genetic condition independently and then combined separately with such words as "genetic testing," "molecular genetics" and "genetic counseling." Word choices in a search can make a significant difference in yielding relevant articles, even using "genetic" versus "genetics." Critical thinking and evaluation skills and knowledge of reputable journals, resources, and authors are needed as you sift through the information you obtain and decide what information to present. There are tips and shortcuts to conducting searches, which you can learn by reading program instructions, asking a reference librarian, or talking with colleagues.

A search of the medical literature is an important part of case preparation, and it is helpful to share pertinent articles you find with team members. You may also consider informing patients about your literature search. Sometimes, patients are reassured when you let them know that you have searched the medical literature to obtain the most up-to-date information about their genetic condition, especially in cases of less common genetic conditions.

PRACTICE GUIDELINES

As part of case preparation, it is important to ascertain whether there are relevant practice guidelines for providing genetic services and genetic testing for the patient you are seeing. It is critical for genetic counselors to be knowledgeable and up-to-date on the standards of practice in genetic counseling. The National Society of Genetic Counselors has developed recommendations for practice guidelines and describes their intended clinical use (Bennett et al., 2003). In addition to knowing about practice guidelines for genetic counselors and geneticists, you should also be familiar with the practice guidelines pertaining to genetics in your medical specialty. For example, if you work in prenatal genetics, you should be familiar with the genetics practice guidelines developed for obstetricians-gynecologists and in cancer genetics, those developed for oncologists. Sometimes, a patient organization will put together guidelines for healthcare professionals caring for patients with the specific genetic condition. There are also practice guidelines and position statements that discuss general precepts in our work, including genetic testing of minors, prenatal and childhood testing for adult-onset conditions, testing of children being placed for adoption, professional disclosure of familial genetic information, and duty to recontact, among others.

You can find relevant practice guidelines from the websites of professional genetics and medical organizations, the National Guideline Clearinghouse, and the HumGen International database and by a search of the medical literature. In addition to helping guide case management, practice guidelines can be useful when a course of action is questioned to show the patient that you are following standards of care. Keep in mind that depending on the year the guideline was written, it may not be current, and for newer tests and aspects of care, a practice guideline may not yet exist.

FINDING SUPPORT/ADVOCACY GROUPS AND PATIENT RESOURCES

An important part of genetic counseling is helping patients to realize that they are not alone by providing contact information for support/advocacy groups and other helpful resources. Traditionally, patient organizations were referred to as "support groups," but generally the preferred term now is "advocacy groups," which reflect the increasing role of these patient organizations, particularly in policy issues and research (Terry et al., 2007). These groups provide patients with resources about the genetic condition and the opportunity to connect with other individuals who are dealing with similar issues and challenges. Often these groups have information about living with the genetic condition that may not otherwise be readily available. Support/ advocacy groups are not geared solely toward the individual with the genetic condition but often have informative resources for family members, caregivers, and healthcare professionals.

You can locate support/advocacy groups through online directories (Table 4-4) and by doing an Internet search for the genetic condition. Chapters in your state can usually be identified by accessing the organization's website, and your state genetics program may also have group listings. Many United States-based patient organizations have international members and chapters. Websites such as

TABLE 4-4. Some Resources for Locating Support/Advocacy Groups and Information about Genetic Conditions for Patients

Support group listings

- Genetic Alliance
- GeneTests—Search genetic condition and select "Resources"
- National Organization for Rare Disorders (NORD)

Patient information about genetic conditions and support group information

- Genetics Home Reference
- Genetic and Rare Diseases Information Center (GARD)
- March of Dimes (search Fact Sheets; also available in Spanish)
- Medline Plus
- National Human Genome Research Institute
- NIH-Health Information (National Institutes of Health)
- National Organization for Rare Disorders (NORD)
- Office of Rare Diseases, National Institutes of Health
- Orphanet

Information on inheritance and basic genetics concepts

- Genetics Home Reference
- Centre for Genetics Education
- GeneTests
- Genetic Alliance (e.g., "Understanding Genetics: A Guide for Patients and Professionals")
- National Human Genome Research Institute
- EuroGentest (has fact sheets translated into different languages)
- Genetic Information Group (has fact sheets translated into different languages)

International resources

- Orphanet
- EuroGentest
- Genetic Information Group
- International Genetic Alliance
- Australasian Genetic Alliance

Orphanet, International Genetic Alliance, Genetic Interest Group, Australasian Genetic Alliance, and Information for Genetic Professionals also have links to patient organizations in different countries, and some genetics professionals organizations' websites in other countries include support group links. In addition to providing patients with contact information for support/advocacy groups, it is also helpful to include this information in the clinic letter that is sent to the referring physician and/or patient.

While locating groups and organizations is relatively straightforward, determining whether the focus matches the patient's needs can take some thought. For example, a patient who electively terminates an affected pregnancy may not feel comfortable attending a group for patients with the specific genetic condition or a group for women

---

⸱ to Consider in Evaluating Support Group Literature

⸱ by a reputable group?

⸱ued audience for the publication (e.g., patients, family members, healthcare ⸱)?

⸱ublication appropriate for your patient? (You particularly need to think about this question ⸱oviding the publication to patients with a tentative diagnosis or a new diagnosis, a patient with an abnormal pregnancy, or a teen).

- Is the information accurate?
- Is the information up-to-date?
- Is the information clearly presented? Are there helpful visual aids?
- Is the content balanced? Too optimistic? Too discouraging?
- What is the readability of the publication? Is the writing technical? Are definitions of medical terms provided? Is the readability appropriate for a patient with limited education or cognitive impairment?
- Are there key topics that are not covered in this publication?
- How is the patient likely to feel after reading this publication?

---

who have experienced spontaneous pregnancy loss. An asymptomatic patient with a Huntington disease gene mutation may feel uncomfortable attending a group with symptomatic individuals. Through a group, patients may meet individuals who are more severely affected than themselves. It is helpful to give patients "a heads-up" about such considerations when providing support group information.

Patients generally welcome receiving information about their genetic condition that is written in understandable terms. Patients may in fact bring information from an Internet search to the appointment, which is helpful to discuss. You can locate patient information about a genetic condition using the resources in Table 4-4 and by Internet search. Fact sheets about patterns of inheritance, genetic testing, prenatal testing, and other basic genetic concepts, translated in different languages, can be obtained from websites such as EuroGentest and Genetic Interest Group. Questions to consider before providing patients with literature are listed in Table 4-5. Resources for developing and evaluating patient-focused information and materials are available at the Genetic Alliance website "Access to Credible Genetics Resources" section and by Internet search.

PERFORMING A RISK ASSESSMENT

Patients often seek information about the risk of a genetic condition for themselves, their children/future children, and other relatives. The steps and variables to consider in conducting a risk assessment are presented in Figure 4-3, and risk figures to provide are in Table 4-6.

A key step is to determine the pattern(s) of inheritance for the genetic condition. Make sure you know the hallmark features and risk figures for each pattern of inheritance so that you can readily assess pedigrees. Keep in mind that there can be factors such as variable expressivity, reduced penetrance, heterogeneity, and

Determine Genetic Etiology of Condition
• Mendelian or non-Mendelian inheritance?
• Consider possibility of: heterogeneity, gonadal
  mosaicism, new mutation

Evaluate Patient's Pedigree
Take into account:
• Penetrance
• Variable expressivity
• Anticipation
• Possibility of non-paternity

Perform Risk Assessment
• Derive risks based on established
  pattern(s) of inheritance
• Obtain empiric risk figures if
  non-Mendelian genetic condition

Perform Bayesian analysis (if indicated)
May be possible to modify patient's risk based on:
• Family history
• Age
• Absence of symptoms
• Gender (for X-linked recessive conditions)
• Test results

Determine Risk Figures to Provide
• Risk to patient
• Risk to children/future children
• Risk to relatives

FIGURE 4-3. *Risk assessment*

mosaicism with genetic conditions that can affect interpretation of the pedigree. In the back of your mind, think about whether non-paternity needs to be considered.

If the pattern of inheritance for a genetic condition is known, calculating the risks is usually straightforward. However, if the genetic condition can be inherited in different ways, it is important to take this into account when evaluating the pedigree and to recognize that a range of figures may need to be provided. While it is important to be global in considering different patterns of inheritance, you also need to be practical and think about the most likely pattern(s) of inheritance and the fact that certain patterns of inheritance are less common (e.g., X-linked dominant, mitochondrial, Y-linked). If the

TABLE 4-6. Risk Figures to Provide to Patients˙

Depending on pattern(s) of inheritance and health status of patient (affected/unaffected) provide:

■ Incidence of genetic condition and carrier frequency in the general population and patient's ethnic group (if indicated)
■ Percent of cases inherited versus *de novo* (due to new mutation)
  ■ Percent of cases due to germline (gonadal) mosaicism
■ Patient's risks to be: affected, carrier, unaffected
  ■ Penetrance of condition (risk to have symptoms) if inherit gene change(s)
■ Risk to children/future children to be: affected, carrier, unaffected
■ Risk to other relatives (particularly 1st-degree relatives)
■ Potential modification of risk figures based on test results (prior risk; risks if results are positive or negative)

˙Note: Not all of these risk figures will be provided to the patient, but you need to think about which risk figures are relevant and should be communicated.

TABLE 4-7. Tips for Evaluating Pedigrees

- *First step in evaluation of a pedigree:* Assess whether condition appears to be dominant or recessive; autosomal or X-linked. If individuals are affected in more than one generation, likely dominant inheritance; if both males and females are affected, likely autosomal.
- Consider most likely pattern of inheritance and remember that X-linked dominant, mitochondrial, and Y-linked conditions are rare.
- If only males are affected, think about X-linked inheritance.
- If there is male-to-male transmission, this rules out X-linked recessive, X-linked dominant, and mitochondrial inheritance.
- If transmission to affected males is only through females, think X-linked or mitochondrial inheritance.
- Remember that females can be affected with X-linked recessive conditions (manifesting females) if there is skewed X-inactivation or the female is the daughter of an affected father and a carrier mother. Generally, affected females will have milder symptoms if affected.
- Autosomal recessive conditions can appear to follow an autosomal dominant pattern of inheritance if there is consanguinity in more than one generation or if carrier frequency is high.
- If there are multiple pregnancy losses, consider a chromosome rearrangement (e.g., translocation, inversion).
- Be mindful of reduced (or incomplete) penetrance and also consider whether family members could have been affected but died before the onset of symptoms.
- Keep in mind whether there is variable expressivity, anticipation, heterogeneity, and mosaicism with the genetic condition and whether non-paternity would affect pedigree interpretation.
- Be cautious in interpreting the pedigree when the family size is small.

mode of inheritance is not known for the genetic condition, you will likely need to seek data from empiric studies. Some tips for evaluating pedigrees are in Table 4-7.

Make sure you ascertain general population risks and carrier frequencies for the genetic condition(s) so that you can present risk figures in a global context. It is helpful for patients to know whether their risk is the same, lower, or higher than the general population risk. If a carrier frequency is not specified, this generally can be derived using your knowledge of Hardy–Weinberg equilibrium [$p^2 + 2pq + q^2 = 1$; p and q are allele frequencies ($p + q = 1$), and for rare conditions p, the most common allele, will be approximately equal to 1 and the carrier frequency ($2pq$) will be equal to $2q$]. For example, for the autosomal recessive genetic condition, cystic fibrosis (CF), which has an incidence (q^2) of 1/2500, $q = 1/50$, p approximates 1, and $2pq$, the carrier frequency would be calculated as $(2)(1)(1/50) = 1/25$. Depending on the genetic condition, there may be specific risk models available to calculate carrier risk, likelihood of having a gene mutation, and other risk figures. When genetic testing is a consideration, it can be helpful to show calculations of risk before testing and how risk figures would be modified depending on test results.

Bayesian Analysis

Bayesian analysis, a calculation that takes into account the patient's baseline (a priori or prior) risk and modifies it based on his or her age, clinical status, family history, or test results (conditional probability), can be an important part of risk assessment. Performing a Bayesian analysis can significantly impact the risk figures you provide and potentially result in a risk reduction that negates the need for further testing. The case below illustrates how Bayesian analysis can be used to modify carrier risk based on family history (in this case, the number of unaffected male children for an X-linked recessive condition). Bayesian analysis is often used to derive the risk modification figures seen in genetic test reports.

Ann, age 35, comes to see you for preconception genetic counseling. She is concerned about her risk for having a son with hemophilia, given her family history of this condition (two maternal uncles, maternal aunt's son, maternal grandmother's brother, all deceased). Hemophilia is an X-linked recessive condition. Given this family history, Ann's maternal grandmother and maternal aunt would be obligate carriers. Ann's mother would have a 50% risk of being a hemophilia carrier, and therefore Ann would have a 25% carrier risk [50% chance mother is a carrier multiplied by 50% chance that Ann would inherit the X chromosome with the hemophilia gene mutation if her mother was a carrier = 25%]. However, Ann's mother's carrier risk for hemophilia is actually less than 50% because she has three unaffected sons. By performing a Bayesian analysis (Table 4-8), her carrier risk can be reduced from 50% to 11%. Ann's carrier risk would be half this risk, which is 5.5%. Ann's risk for having a child with hemophilia would be 1.4% (5.5% chance Ann is a carrier multiplied by $^1/_2$, the chance of having a son, multiplied by $^1/_2$, the chance a son would receive the X chromosome with the hemophilia gene mutation = 1.4%). The above example shows that by simply using pen and paper to perform a Bayesian analysis, Ann's risk for having a son with hemophilia was significantly reduced, without doing any genetic or other testing.

TABLE 4-8. Modification of Carrier Risk for Hemophilia by Performing a Bayesian Analysis Using Family History Information

Probability	Ann's Mother Carrier	Ann's Mother Non-carrier
Prior probability	$1/2^a$	$1/2^a$
Conditional probability (3 unaffected sons)	$1/8^b$	1^b
Joint probability[c]	1/16	1/2 (= 8/16)
Posterior probability[d]	(1/16)/(1/16 + 8/16) = 1/9 = 11%	(8/16)/(8/16 + 1/16) = 8/9 = 89%

[a] Ann's mother's prior probability of being a carrier of hemophilia is $^1/_2$ [the chance that she inherited the X chromosome with the hemophilia gene mutation from her mother, who is an obligate carrier]. Probability that Ann's mother is not a hemophilia carrier is also $^1/_2$ [the chance that she inherited the X chromosome without the hemophilia gene mutation from her mother].

[b] If Ann's mother is a carrier of hemophilia, each son would have a $^1/_2$ chance of receiving the X chromosome with the hemophilia gene mutation and a $^1/_2$ chance of being unaffected. The probability that all three sons would be unaffected if Ann's mother is a carrier is 1/8 [$^1/_2 \times {}^1/_2 \times {}^1/_2 = 1/8$]. If Ann's mother is not a carrier of hemophilia, she would have a 100% (=1) chance for having unaffected sons.

[c] Joint probability = prior probability multiplied by conditional probability.

[d] Posterior probabilities always add up to 1 (or 100%).

Performing a Bayesian analysis requires careful thought in terms of the numbers utilized in the calculations, and the reader is referred to medical genetics texts, books on risk calculation (e.g., Ian Young's book, *Introduction to Risk Calculation in Genetic Counseling*, Oxford University Press), and articles (e.g., Hodge, 1998; Ogino and Wilson, 2004; Ogino et al., 2007) to learn about this statistical tool.

Chromosome Rearrangements

Providing genetic counseling and risk assessment for patients referred because of a structural chromosome abnormality or rearrangement can be challenging. Any chromosome and any part of a chromosome can be involved. There may be a limited to non-existent number of patients with the identical chromosome abnormality or rearrangement reported in the medical literature. This can make it challenging to predict phenotype and determine recurrence risks. While you may be able to locate reports on patients who have similar chromosome abnormalities through database or medical literature searches, it is important to emphasize the limitations of drawing conclusions from a small patient sample and to consider bias of ascertainment issues.

Determining risks will depend on whether the chromosome rearrangement is *de novo* or inherited, balanced or unbalanced. For inherited balanced chromosome rearrangements, generally you can be reassuring. However, even if a chromosome rearrangement appears balanced, there remains the small possibility of gene disruption, which could result in abnormalities. OMIM cytogenetic and gene maps can be used to find genes that are in the region of the chromosome abnormality or rearrangement, but this does not predict whether gene function will be disrupted or what the outcome will be. Even if the chromosome rearrangement appears balanced, especially if there are phenotypic abnormalities, chromosome microarray analysis or other studies may need to be considered.

Risk assessment for chromosome rearrangements is complex and involves taking into account the chromosome breakpoints, reasoning through meiotic outcomes, and determining which possibilities might be viable. Often you will only be able to provide patients with a range of recurrence risk figures that will partially depend on whether the chromosome rearrangement was ascertained because of a history of pregnancy loss, after a child was born with birth defects, after a stillbirth, or during a workup for infertility. The recurrence risk is highest when the chromosome rearrangement is ascertained after the birth of a child with birth defects. *Chromosome Abnormalities and Genetic Counseling* (R.J. McKinlay Gardner and Grant R. Sutherland, Oxford University Press) provides an overview of chromosome rearrangements and recurrence risks. The information in Table 4-9 is typically provided to patients with a chromosome rearrangement. Table 4-10 has key cytogenetics databases and patient resources.

It is important to take the time to go through the report on the chromosome rearrangement and explain the terminology. A copy of the karyotype can help the patient understand terminology in the report and see the chromosome rearrangement, if it is visible. Exchanging pen caps to demonstrate translocations or rearranging letters (e.g., "ACBD" instead of "ABCD") for a chromosome inversion can simply be done to actively show a chromosome rearrangement. Developing counseling aids using

TABLE 4-9. General Information Provided to Patients with a Chromosome Rearrangement

- Incidence of chromosome rearrangement (e.g., 1 in 500 for balanced chromosome translocations)
  - Percent that arise *de novo* versus inherited (if known)
  - Etiology/how the chromosome rearrangement occurs
- Specific information about the patient's chromosome rearrangement
  - What is known in the literature about clinical features and prognosis from reported cases
- Implications
  - Risk for infertility (compared to baseline risks)
  - Risk for pregnancy loss (compared to baseline risks)
  - Risk to have child who is: unbalanced, carrier of chromosome rearrangement, non-carrier
  - Risk for relatives to have chromosome rearrangement
  - Gender differences (if any) for the above risks
- Reproductive and testing options
  - Prenatal testing
  - Preimplantation genetic diagnosis
  - Donor sperm or donor egg (depending on patient's gender)
  - Adoption

TABLE 4-10. Cytogenetics Databases and Patient Resources

Cytogenetic Databases

- Information for Genetics Professionals—Cytogenetics Resources
  Links to chromosome ideograms, karyotypes, FISH information, nomenclature, cytogenetic databases, resources, references, lectures
- Association for Clinical Cytogenetics
  Follow link to Cytogenetics Databases
- Chromosomal Variation in Man—Online Database
  Developed by Digamber S. Borgaonkar, Ph.D. Database of chromosome variations and anomalies, numerical anomalies, and chromosomal breakage syndromes
- European Cytogeneticists Association Register of Unbalanced Chromosome Aberrations
  Database of cytogenetic and clinical information on rare chromosomal disorders, including microdeletions and microduplications
- Chromosome Abnormality Database (CAD)
  Database of constitutional and acquired chromosome abnormalities
- Developmental Genome Anatomy Project (DGAP)
  Database searchable by chromosome breakpoint

Patient Resources

- Chromosome Deletion Outreach (CDO) [includes registry]
- Unique: Rare Chromosome Disorder Support Group [includes registry]
- Chromosome Help-Station
- Centre for Genetics Education—Fact Sheets
- Genetics Home Reference

TABLE 4-11. Communication of Risk Figures—Quick Tips

- Put risk figures in a global context
  - All of us are carriers of several non-working genes
  - Baseline 3% risk for birth defects/mental retardation
  - General population incidence and carrier frequency of the genetic condition
- Give risk figures in different ways (e.g., percentages; fractions; if there were 100 people, "x" would have the condition)
- Give both sides of risk figure (e.g., 20% risk to be affected; 80% chance not affected)
- Use pictures and diagrams

colored chromosome ideograms can be helpful to show both the normal chromosomes and the rearranged chromosomes. Such diagrams can also be helpful for the patient to use when explaining the chromosome rearrangement to other family members.

Risk Presentation

Equally important to performing an accurate risk assessment is effective risk presentation and communication; this topic is discussed in Chapters 6 and 7, and some tips are included in Table 4-11. You should be able to clearly explain to patients how a risk figure was derived. If you are using empiric studies and find that risk figures differ from study to study, try to determine the reasons for the differences and consider whether the studies have limitations. If more than one risk figure or a range is applicable, this information should be provided to the patient. The necessity for taking the time to perform an accurate risk assessment cannot be overemphasized. The risk figures you provide could significantly impact the decisions of patients and their family members. In summary, make sure that the risk figures you provide are accurate, clearly presented, and documented.

LOCATING AND DEVELOPING COUNSELING AIDS

An important part of case preparation is thinking about how you can make it easier for the patient to comprehend and retain information. In genetics clinics, you will generally find counseling aids such as *Counseling Aids for Geneticists* (Greenwood Genetic Center) and *Genetics Visual Aids for Educators and Health Care Professionals* (CCL Books). These counseling aids have karyotypes, diagrams of different patterns of inheritance, segregation of translocations and inversions, molecular testing methodologies, prenatal diagnostic procedures, cancer genetics, and helpful aids on other genetic concepts; currently, these aids are available in English, Spanish, and French.

Rather than relying only on available counseling aids, you also should think about creating your own aids to present the information in Table 4-1. To make counseling aids:

- Use Powerpoint or other computer program
- Search for images of clinical features at patient organization websites, Atlas of Developmental and Genetic Diseases and by Google image search. It can also be

TABLE 4-12. Benefits of Genetic Counseling Aids

- Facilitate provision of genetic counseling
  - Organize content
  - Clearly present complex information
  - Emphasize and summarize key points
- Facilitate patient understanding and reinforce information
  - Hearing and seeing information
  - Can review counseling aids after clinic visit
- Facilitate communication of information in a family
  - Can share counseling aids with other family members
- Facilitate letter-writing
  - Can efficiently dictate letter content directly from counseling aids
- Facilitate case presentations

helpful to find diagrams of human anatomy to show parts of the body affected by the genetic condition.

- List clinical features and place checkmarks next to features the patient has to show if diagnostic criteria are met.
- Show patient a diagram of the pattern of inheritance and review with patient's own pedigree to explain inheritance and risk figures.

Developing counseling aids for a case helps organize the session and takes the pressure off you to remember information about a condition that you have only just learned. The benefits of creating and using counseling aids for your cases and providing copies to patients are presented in Table 4-12.

GENETIC TESTING

Ordering a Genetic Test Requires:

- Pre-test counseling and informed consent
- Accurate pedigree analysis and risk assessment
  - Determination of who will be most informative for testing (particularly if patient is unaffected and an affected family member needs to be tested first)
- Knowledge of different genetic testing methodologies and their limitations
- Search of genetic testing databases for laboratories offering specific genetic test
- Assessment of the genetic testing offered by different laboratories
- Selection of laboratory
- Handling of logistics: complete requisition and billing forms, obtain and ship specimen
- Accurate interpretation of test results
- Post-test counseling

An important part of case management is exploring genetic testing options, determining applicability to your case, presenting test information in a manner that facilitates patients' understanding and decision-making, and coordinating testing logistics. This section on genetic testing focuses on the coordination of cases requiring DNA or biochemical analysis. Coordination of cytogenetic studies is not included since most genetics clinics either have a cytogenetics laboratory at their institution or an established contract with an outside laboratory. Your institution may do genetic testing in-house and/or have preferred laboratories to which specimens are sent for more commonly ordered genetic tests. Even if an institution/clinic has a contract with a laboratory, you may be able to make the case to send a patient's sample to another laboratory depending on testing methodology and sensitivity.

It is important to keep in mind that the availability of genetic testing does not obligate its use. Genetic testing is a "moving target" with evolving changes in methodology, detection rate, result time, and cost. Even if it is a laboratory that you have sent samples to previously, make sure there have not been any interim changes with the test. Genetic tests can be costly when introduced and become more affordable as testing advances are made. Likewise, detection rates can be lower at first and increase over time with improvements in testing methodology. It is for these reasons that consideration should be given as to whether it is best to order or defer testing, especially since insurance may not cover the same genetic test twice. If it has been a few years since the patient had genetic testing and testing has improved, it may be possible to convince the insurer to cover the genetic test a second time.

Critical to genetic testing is pre-test counseling, the informed consent process, and post-test counseling. Genetic test results often have implications for healthcare and life decisions of other family members, not just the patient. The limitations and implications of genetic testing need to be thoroughly discussed. It is not unusual for patients to assume that because a blood sample is provided, a result will be obtained. If genetic testing does not yield a result or is unavailable, the importance of keeping in touch with a genetics clinic to learn about advances in testing should be emphasized.

Pre-test Counseling and Informed Consent

Take time to **DISCUSS** the following:

Decisions (Will healthcare and life decisions change?)
Insurance implications
Sensitivity and other test parameters
Costs
Uses & limitations of test results
Siblings & other relatives at risk
Supportive resources

Finding and Selecting a Laboratory

Anna, age 18, was seen for genetic evaluation because of a suspected diagnosis of Friedreich ataxia. Friedreich ataxia, the most common inherited ataxia, follows an autosomal recessive pattern of inheritance and has a typical age of onset in the teens. Anna had balance problems, falling, and difficulty in walking starting at age 12. She did not have any dysarthria (thick or slurred speech), which is typically seen with this condition. A blood sample was initially tested for the common GAA repeat expansion in the FRDA1 gene. Results: 952 GAA repeats/18 GAA repeats (>67 GAA repeats—expanded range). According to the report, Anna was at least a carrier but unlikely to be affected with Friedreich ataxia. Given our concern about her neurological symptoms, we sent a second sample to a laboratory that did sequencing of the FRDA1 gene. Anna was found to have a point mutation in the FRDA1 gene, a "G" (guanine) to a "T" (thymine), which changed the coded amino acid from glycine to valine, G130V. This gene mutation had been previously reported in the literature and was associated with a milder course of Friedreich ataxia, with absence of dysarthria and cardiac involvement.

Laboratory selection is critical and can make a difference in making a diagnosis. Some laboratories have established reputations for testing for specific genetic conditions that you can learn about through your colleagues and by reading the genetics literature. There are online comprehensive databases of genetic testing laboratories including GeneTests, UCSD Biochemical Genetics, European Directory of DNA Diagnostic Laboratories, Orphanet, and directories in other countries. GeneTests and Orphanet also include international laboratories.

These directories of laboratories are listings only and do not provide information on test sensitivity and other variables for assessing a test and a laboratory as described in Chapter 9. You will need to review specific test information provided by the laboratory at their website or contact the laboratory directly. "Tiered testing," starting with the most common gene mutations or methodologies likely to identify mutations, may be offered. Additional genetic tests may need to be considered, particularly if the first methodology utilized does not identify a gene mutation.

You should evaluate what each laboratory offers in terms of test methodology, sensitivity, result time, and cost, in order to finalize laboratory selection. If the patient is of reproductive age, a laboratory that also offers the test prenatally is preferable, since the patient may later want this option. Result time can be a determining factor when results have implications for treatment or for a pregnancy. Cost and billing options can be key factors in final laboratory selection when there are no differences in test methodology and detection rate.

If you are seeing a patient who has a family history of a genetic condition but is unaffected, you may first need to coordinate genetic testing for an affected family member, and if unavailable, an obligate carrier may suffice. If an affected family member is known to have had genetic testing, you should ask the patient to request a report. Laboratories generally like to have documentation of a mutation before testing at-risk family members, and when possible, it is helpful to send a patient's sample to the same laboratory where a family member has been previously tested. If no affected family member is living, inquire whether genetic testing on tissue block samples, if available from a deceased affected relative, is an option.

Information to Obtain from the Laboratory About the Genetic Test

Table 4-13 lists the general information you will need to obtain before sending a sample. Through genetic testing databases (see "Finding and Selecting a Laboratory"), it is generally possible to directly link to laboratories' websites, which will usually have information about the test. If you need to call a laboratory and specifically have questions about the actual test rather than logistics, inquire if there is a genetic counselor or laboratory supervisor with whom you can speak.

TABLE 4-13. Information to Ascertain When Arranging Genetic Testing

Genetic Test	Considerations
Specific gene(s)	All known gene(s) for a genetic condition or most common gene(s) for genetic condition
Methodologies	Targeted mutation analysis [specific mutation(s), mutation panels]; mutation scanning (entire coding region or select exons); DNA sequencing (targeted exons or full sequencing); functional assays; other methodologies.
	Is stepwise/tiered testing available?
Accuracy and limitation of test results	Test sensitivity and specificity; ethnicity differences?

Specimens	Considerations
Type of specimens accepted	- Blood, cheek swab, mouthwash
	- Prenatal samples (chorionic villus sample—villi and/or cultured cells; amniocentesis sample—fluid and/or cultured cells)
	- Biochemical testing (blood, urine, cultured cells)
	- Skin biopsy/tissue, cultured cells
	- Tissue block
Type of tube, flask for specimen	Heparin (green top) for chromosome analysis, FISH; EDTA (lavender top) or ACD (yellow top) for DNA analysis; heparin and EDTA for chromosome microarray analysis
Amount of specimen needed	Minimum for child, adult, prenatal sample
Prenatal samples	Maternal or parental blood samples needed? Control sample(s) needed?
Affected family member	Need to be tested first? Consider sending sample to same laboratory where affected family member has been tested.
Retention of specimens after testing completed	Length of time samples retained? Future testing if no mutation identified with current methodologies?

Shipping Specimens	Considerations
Lab provision of test kits	Lab may provide test kits and pre-printed shipping labels. Lab may be able to send a test kit to the patient or physician if sample needs to be obtained locally.
Lab address and phone number	May use different address for weekend deliveries.

TABLE 4-13. (*Continued*)

Shipping Specimens	Considerations
Preferred courier service	Some labs may have preferred courier service (check lab's shipping instructions)
Temperature for shipping	Room temperature (usually); some tests may require that sample be sent on cold packs or dry ice.
Shipping	Standard overnight (delivery next business afternoon); priority overnight (delivery next business morning—extra charge). Priority overnight may be preferred by lab depending on when samples are set up or if sample is to be delivered on a Friday.
Days specimens accepted	Many labs do not accept weekend or holiday deliveries, especially academic labs.

Billing Options	Considerations
Institution/clinic/physician	May lower the cost of the genetic test, particularly if there is an established laboratory contract/volume discount.
Patient's insurance	Lab may require pre-authorization for testing from insurer in order to bill insurance directly; partial payment by patient with sample may also be required. Lab may offer service of checking patient's insurance for coverage of testing.
Patient	Lab may bill patient directly. Partial or full payment may be required with sample. Ascertain whether lab will accept credit card payment (and which ones are accepted), check from patient, or need cashier's check/money order.

Paperwork to Accompany Sample	Considerations
Requisition form	Can save time by making pre-printed labels with your clinic address and billing information (if done by institution) to use with requisition forms. Can make xeroxed copies of requisition forms with this information typed in for frequently ordered tests.
Consent form	If lab does not provide a consent form, consider adapting one of the template consent forms available at the NSGC website, "Tools for Your Practice" section.
Pedigree	Can save time by attaching copy of pedigree instead of drawing one on the form.

Results	Considerations
Time-frame for results	Ascertain expected time-frame for results. May inquire whether there is notification about result delays, particularly for prenatal testing.
Communication of results	Ascertain how results are communicated: FAX, mail, phone, secure website. Some labs will call when results are abnormal.

Genetic Testing for Prenatal Samples: Special Considerations

Making arrangements for genetic testing on prenatal samples requires special attention because of timing issues and the fact that the results could have significant implications for the pregnancy. When genetic or biochemical testing is requested for a prenatal sample, usually cytogenetic studies to rule out a chromosome abnormality will also be done. Even if your institution has a cytogenetics laboratory, the genetic testing laboratory may prefer to receive the entire sample to ensure that the sample size is adequate to complete both analyses. Depending on the genetic condition and type of testing, laboratories may also request a control sample, a maternal blood sample (to rule out the possibility of maternal cell contamination of a prenatal specimen), or samples from both parents (to confirm carrier status, determine inheritance of alleles).

Obtaining and Shipping Samples

Most samples for genetic testing will need to be sent by overnight courier at room temperature; usually, dry ice will be required with samples sent for biochemical testing. The airbill number should be noted so that the sample can be tracked if not received. Generally, labs are closed on holidays and many labs do not accept weekend deliveries. Some labs accept samples on Saturday but may use a different delivery address. It may be possible to send the sample on Friday and specify Monday delivery or keep the sample at room temperature or in a refrigerator and ship on Monday; check with the laboratory about these options.

Sending Samples Internationally

If genetic testing for a condition is not available in your country, you may consider sending a sample to a laboratory in a different country. In the United States, patient specific results may only be shared with clinicians or patients if they were performed in a CLIA (Clinical Laboratory Improvement Amendments)-certified laboratory, and few international laboratories have this certification. For US institutions that have a CLIA license, sending samples to a non-CLIA approved laboratory would be considered out of compliance with their certification. Payment for genetic testing is almost always required with the sample and generally is not reimbursable by insurance in the United States. Samples shipped outside and into the United States and from one country to another will need to go through customs. Therefore, declaration forms, usually two copies, one affixed to the outside of the package and one internal, specifying the contents (e.g., human blood sample, diagnostic testing) and value of the package (e.g., no value) will need to accompany the sample. For DNA testing, find out if just extracted DNA can be sent, which also makes it easier to maintain a backup sample. Coordinating arrangements to send a sample internationally takes time, and therefore before seeing a patient, you should make sure that you have worked out the logistics, including selection of a courier service that accepts international samples and making sure forms do not need to be translated into another language.

Required Paperwork for Genetic Testing

Ordering genetic testing is usually more involved than just checking off a box on a form. Paperwork sent with a sample typically includes a requisition form (including provision of pertinent family history and clinical information), a billing form, and a consent form. There are model consent forms at the members' section of the NSGC website, "Tools for Your Practice," if one is not provided. Be sure to note if a family member has an identifiable gene mutation(s) and provide the report if available. Given the time needed, it is helpful to complete the paperwork in advance if you think the patient will likely have genetic testing. Copies of all paperwork should be kept in case it becomes separated from the sample or the laboratory has questions.

Genetic Testing Fees and Insurance Coverage

"How much is the genetic test, and will it be covered by my insurance?" are questions frequently asked by patients. The content and the resources in the section on "Billing Issues for Genetic Clinic Visits" also apply to coverage of genetic testing. Often, genetic counselors are at the "front lines" dealing with patients' testing questions and providing information for insurance pre-authorization. Genetic counselors may also be at the "back end" of handling insurance problems, so it is best to address insurance issues up front to minimize complications. Knowledge of insurance issues will come from experience, learning how billing issues are handled for your clinic, reading available resources, and asking questions of your colleagues (medical and administrative).

Covered benefits for genetic counseling and testing depend on the insurer and the specific plan/policy that the patient has. Coverage is more likely when the genetic test is standard of care or when the results will directly influence a patient's treatment and management. Patients should be informed in advance if insurance authorization is needed or if partial/full payment must be sent with the sample. Even laboratories willing to bill the patient's insurance may require partial payment up front and if insurance does not fully cover the test, the patient would be held financially responsible. Genetic tests can range from a couple hundred dollars or less (low-complexity tests, e.g., single gene mutation) to several thousand dollars (high-complexity tests, e.g., DNA sequencing), and the following points should be kept in mind:

- Test cost and billing codes (CPT codes) may be posted at the lab website, or contact the lab.
- Confirm whether the provided price is for institution/clinic billing, insurance billing, or patient billing, as the cost for each may be different.
- Some institutions have lab contracts and receive volume discounts.
- Test cost may be lower if the institution/clinic/physician is billed or when full payment is sent with the sample.
  - Some institutions do not allow institution billing.
- Test fees can be modified at any time, generally at the beginning of the fiscal year (January or July).

Dealing with insurance issues can be time-consuming. Some laboratories offer the service of checking whether the patient's insurance will cover the genetic testing. The genetic counselor may be involved in providing patients with genetic testing costs and billing codes and helping patients with insurance issues. Given the time involved, generally it is helpful to have the patient take the first step to find out about their insurance coverage for the genetic testing and provide you with insurer contact information if follow-up is needed. When contacting the patient's insurer, you will need the patient's policy information, the test codes and cost.

- If genetic testing is approved, request the insurance authorization number or written confirmation of approval.
- If testing is denied and clearly clinically indicated, find out about the appeals process. Sometimes, it is helpful if the genetic counselor or staffing physician speaks directly with the insurance case manager or medical director.
- When an affected family member needs to be tested before testing at-risk family members and this testing is denied, you can raise the option of having family members cover the test costs.

Insurance coverage of genetic testing is particularly an issue for patients with Medicaid (state-funded) insurance because generally laboratories will only accept this insurance from patients who reside in their state.

Insurers may require a letter of medical necessity before providing authorization for genetic testing. Some laboratories provide insurance template letters at their website. The letter should focus on the benefit to the patient and generally should only include healthcare implications for other family members if covered by the same insurer. Keep the letters clear and short, generally less than one page. Keep copies of letters that were successful in obtaining coverage for genetic testing to use as a template for future letters. Sample letters and helpful recommendations can be found in an article by Shappell and Matloff (2001); tips are also included in Bombard (2002) and Table 4-14.

Implications of Genetic Test Results for Insurance Coverage

The possible impact that genetic test results could have on insurance coverage is an important issue to address before testing. For individuals considering presymptomatic or predictive genetic testing for hereditary conditions, particularly neurological conditions like Huntington disease, this is particularly a concern. It is generally recommended that patients make sure that they have the desired insurance coverage (health, life, long-term disability, long-term care) before testing. The Genetic Information Nondiscrimination Act (GINA), passed in 2008 after a 13-year effort, provides individuals with federal protections against genetic discrimination in health insurance and employment, but does not include protections for life, long-term disability, and long-term care insurance. The National Society of Genetic Counselors has downloadable resources on genetic discrimination, including a brochure for patients, and resources are also available at the Genetic Alliance, Coalition for

TABLE 4-14. Letter Content to Insurance Companies Requesting Coverage of Genetic Testing

- Patient information
  - Name, date of birth, insurance policy number
- First sentence of letter: State specific genetic test requested and why.
  - If primary care physician is also requesting this test, this should be noted.
- Genetic condition information
  - 1- to 2- Sentence summary of key clinical features and medical issues.
  - For genetic conditions with morbidity and mortality issues, this should be emphasized.
  - For asymptomatic patients, note inheritance of genetic condition and patient's risk.
- Genetic test information
  - Stress how genetic test results will impact patient's care (e.g., needed to make diagnosis; necessary for management, treatment, surveillance)
    - Particularly note if management will change based on test results.
    - If appropriate, emphasize needed surveillance and cost savings if patient is negative for gene mutation.
  - If test is standard of care, cite guidelines, professional societies' position/policy/consensus statements
    - Consider providing copies of key citations.
  - Note test sensitivity (likelihood of identifying gene mutation) if it is reasonable.
- Laboratory and billing information
  - Cost, billing codes (CPT codes)
  - Name of laboratory, phone number, website
- Close letter with thanking them in advance for considering the request and provide your phone number in case additional information is needed.

Genetic Fairness, and National Human Genome Research Institute websites. Patient organizations for specific genetic conditions may also have information on genetic discrimination issues. Searchable databases of state and federal laws on genetic information and insurance discrimination are available at the National Human Genome Research Institute and National Conference of State Legislatures websites; international laws, policies, and guidelines can be accessed through HumGen.

DNA Banking

DNA banking is the long-term storage of an individual's DNA. Genetic testing often relies on identifying a mutation in an affected individual before at-risk family members can be tested. Banking DNA on key affected family members who may not be alive when testing becomes available ensures that at-risk family members will have the option of testing in the future. DNA banking should be raised if the patient (or family member) with a genetic condition has a limited lifespan and (1) genetic testing is unavailable, (2) testing is available but has a low detection rate or is unaffordable, or (3) testing was done and no mutation was identified. It is particularly important to raise the option of DNA banking if a patient is participating in a research study since provided samples will likely be inaccessible. Some laboratories offer the option of sending DNA

TABLE 4-15. Information to Ascertain When Arranging DNA Banking

- Length of time samples are stored
  - Fixed time period or indefinitely
- Cost
  - One-time payment?
  - Annual or periodic storage fee?
  - Additional fees charged with each release of the sample?
  - Insurance coverage; method(s) of payment

    DNA banking is generally inexpensive and usually not covered by insurance.
- Type(s) of samples accepted and amount required
- Paperwork
  - Forms required for DNA banking
  - Forms required for future release of DNA sample
- Shipping requirements
  - Provision of test kits

banking test kits directly to patients (cheek swab or mouthwash kits). In selecting a laboratory for DNA banking, it is important to find out the information in Table 4-15.

Patients need to think globally about relatives who may benefit from having future access to their DNA sample and carefully document the names of these family members. The National Society of Genetic Counselors has produced downloadable resources for patients and healthcare professionals about DNA banking. Laboratories that do DNA banking can be located through GeneTests and other genetic testing databases and by doing an Internet search for "DNA Banking."

Genetic Test Results

Take time before clinic to review your patient's report and check the content for accuracy:

- Do you have the report for the right patient?
- Was the specific requested genetic test done?
- Are there any errors in the report? Is the patient's identifying information (e.g., name, birthdate) correct with no misspellings?
- Is the interpretation consistent with the patient's test result? Labs often use template text, and inadvertently, the text may not match the test results.

If there is incorrect information, request that the report be reissued. Make sure you fully understand the content of the report and, if needed, contact the laboratory for clarification.

The report should clearly specify the genetic test that was done and provide the results. It is important to establish whether a change in the DNA sequence is a disease-causing mutation, a common polymorphism, a rare sequence variant, or a variant of unknown significance (VUS). Generally, laboratories will include in their reports literature citations, if they exist, and it is helpful to read cited articles. While the laboratory will report a result and its significance, it is up to the clinician to determine clinical implications for the patient and whether additional studies, if available, are indicated. The interpretation is based on considerations such as the type of gene change, where the gene change occurs, how much of the gene is disrupted, whether the gene change occurs at an evolutionarily conserved site, and other factors.

Generally, a search of the literature and mutation databases is done. Gene structure (e.g., number of exons) and sequence can be ascertained at ENSEMBL and other database links in OMIM. Locus-specific mutation databases and gateways can be accessed through OMIM and identified through an Internet search. Copy number variants can be searched in the Database of Genomic Variants and other databases. Some laboratories maintain their own mutation databases and can inform you whether a sequence variation has been seen in other samples sent to their laboratory. For novel gene changes, samples may be requested from the parents to determine whether it is inherited and/or from other affected family members to help establish the significance. Another sample from the patient may be needed for additional studies. The American College of Medical Genetics has developed recommendations for interpreting and working up sequence variations (Richards et al., 2008) and interpreting copy number variants (Manning and Hudgins, 2007; Shaffer et al., 2007).

When no gene mutation is identified in a patient with a genetic condition and other testing methodologies exist, consideration should be given to additional genetic testing. Often, additional genetic testing can be done on the original submitted sample, but sometimes another sample from the patient will be required, especially if additional testing is done by a different laboratory.

Given the genetic test results, you should consider how the patient's risk is modified and determine whether Bayesian analysis is indicated. It is important to keep in mind that the genetic test result may not be the whole story and that genetics does not necessarily equal destiny. Genetic heterogeneity, variable penetrance, genotype–phenotype correlations, modifying genes, gene–environment interactions, and epigenetic and other factors may be considerations and may impact on result interpretation.

Communication of Genetic Test Results

It is Friday afternoon, and the laboratory has just called you with an abnormal test result. Should you call the patient or wait till Monday? Should you call the patient at work or wait till evening and call her at home? When you do call, what should you say?

There should always be a plan for communicating test results. At the clinic visit, you should discuss how results will be communicated—in person, by phone or by mail. Prenatal genetic test results are almost always phoned to patients because of timing issues and potential implications for the pregnancy. Other clinics may phone out results, particularly for a routine test or a known diagnosis. Presymptomatic testing protocols, such as the one established for Huntington disease, require that patients return to clinic to receive their test results (International Huntington Association and World Federation of Neurology Research Group on Huntington's Chorea, 1994). Scheduling a return clinic visit means that the patient will be prepared to receive results, "good" or "bad," on a specific day. The results of genetic testing can be complex, confusing to patients, and subject to misinterpretation, which is why it is often optimal to meet in person.

Patients should be informed about the normal time-frame for receiving results. You should make sure you have a copy of the report a few days before the appointment and, if it is not received, contact the laboratory. It is best to notify the patient in a timely manner if results will not be available. Since patients may assume that a delay means that the result is abnormal, it is important to explain the reason for the delay. One can also anticipate delays around the holidays, when laboratories may be closed or have fewer workers, and so inform patients in advance.

Results should only be disclosed to the patient (or their guardian), parents (if patient is a minor), and the referring physician, unless permission is specifically obtained to share the results with others. Permission should be obtained if the patient's results are to be released to physicians other than the referring physician and to family members.

If results are communicated by phone:

- Ascertain preferable times to call.
- Establish whether a work number goes directly to the patient or is a general line and how the call should be identified.
- Listen to voice cues since the patient cannot predict work circumstances in advance. If there is hesitancy, ask if you can call back at a better time or see if the patient wishes to relocate to a more private location.
- Keep the call brief and supportive when results are abnormal and arrange for in-person follow-up or another time to talk, if indicated.

It is helpful to provide the patient with a copy of the results for his or her records and potentially to share with family members. Try to anticipate ways of facilitating the patient's understanding of the results, such as using a highlighter on important parts of the report, using counseling aids, and creating diagrams/pictures to illustrate the result (Figure 4-4). Generally, the test report and/or a letter summarizing the results and their significance is provided to the patient and/or referring physician.

Test results can alter risk assessment and may have significant implications for the patient and family members. For patients who have undergone extensive workups and lived for years with speculation about an unknown diagnosis, genetic test results may result in a diagnosis to which the patient now needs time to adjust. For some patients, genetic testing just further confirms a known diagnosis and importantly enables other at-risk family members to now have the option of testing to determine their status.

MYH7(Myosin, Heavy Chain 7)

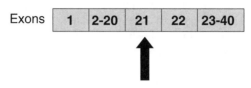

2389G>A
DNA Sequence Change:**G**CC to **A**CC
DNA Base Change:**G**uanine to **A**denine
Amino Acid Change:Alanine to Threonine

FIGURE 4-4. ***Diagram for patient illustrating gene mutation***. *Patient with hypertrophic cardiomyopathy has mutation in the MYH7 gene (myosin, heavy chain 7). Diagram shows where in the gene the change occurred (exon 21) and how a letter change in the DNA sequence, a "G" to an "A," changes the coded amino acid*

Depending on the genetic condition and indication for testing, if a mutation is not identified [unless true negative result for familial or known mutation(s)], it should be emphasized that testing did not identify a gene change with today's technology and the patient should be encouraged to remain in contact with a genetics clinic and consider retesting in the future.

MANAGING THE CLINIC VISIT

Genetic counselors often see patients as part of a team. Before you see a patient, it is important to determine your role and establish who will be responsible for specific parts of a case. This is particularly important for genetic counselors working in teaching hospitals, where there may also be other rotators assigned to see a patient in addition to the genetic counselor and/or physician. Such preparation makes for smoother transitions in a session and less duplication of information. If a physical examination is to be performed, it is important to establish what will be addressed before the exam (usually the family and medical history) and what counseling will be deferred until afterward. Risk figures and other pertinent information should be reviewed in advance with team members so that the genetic counseling provided will be consistent. It is already challenging for patients to understand information without having to deal with any discrepancies.

At the start of the clinic visit, let patients know:

- Who they will be seeing (names and roles)
- What will happen during the clinic visit, including whether a physical examination, tests/evaluations will be performed
- Who will receive documentation of the clinic visit (referring physician, patient, both)
- Time limitations for the visit

The flow of a session will depend on whether it is a counseling appointment only, counseling with a physical exam, or counseling with a prenatal diagnostic test or other procedure. Successful case management depends on being able to integrate the issues the patient wants addressed with the established components of a genetics clinic visit in the allotted time. When diagnosis is the focus, let the patient know at the outset that additional evaluations and follow-up visits may be needed and it is possible that a diagnosis will not be made. If the patient expresses that he wants genetic testing and you know it is unavailable or will not be done that day, it is helpful to acknowledge this at the start of the appointment so that the patient knows why his initial request will not be met, which will lessen his frustration. If you sense that the patient is very anxious about his risk for a genetic condition and you know the risk is low or lower than what the patient stated, you may consider sharing this information at the start of the session to ease his anxiety.

Key to managing a session is obtaining family and medical history information efficiently:

- Give a "heads-up" of information that is needed and why
- Ask clear, focused questions
- Put on a "detective hat" and think of questions you can ask quickly to obtain needed information (e.g., For a patient with a cardiovascular genetic condition, ask whether anyone else has the same condition or a heart condition)

The pace of asking questions can influence the pace at which patients respond. Probably one of the more challenging things to learn is how to politely cut off talkative patients and to bring them back to the question at hand. It can also be challenging to determine when a response to a question is not going to yield the desired information and needs to be redirected. Generally, the most pertinent information will be given within the first few minutes after a question is asked; however, it is not unusual for patients to remember important information and provide it later in the session.

If you are independently seeing a patient before being joined by other team members and have obtained information the others should know, you can sometimes convey this information while the patient is present (e.g., "Ms. Clayton was telling me about her son Jason's recent surgeries"). If issues have come up that you feel are best communicated without the patient present, you will need to initiate a break in the counseling session. This can be accomplished by telling the patient that you would like to go over all the information he/she has provided with your team. This effectively communicates to the other team members that you have important information to share and lets the patient know what you will be doing when you leave the room.

During the genetic counseling session, it is important to periodically "check in" with the patient about his/her understanding of presented information and to give bottom-line, summary statements to emphasize the "take-home messages." Managing a case also entails bringing a session to a close, reiterating key points, and making sure that the recommendations and plans for follow-up are clearly communicated. Overseeing case management is like being a guide in a museum. There will be a lot to see in a single room; you need to take in the highlights and then guide your patient to the next room.

Handling Time Constraints

- *The patient scheduled to see you at 10:00 A.M. has arrived at 11:00 A.M.*
- *Your patient keeps bringing up new issues, and you have yet to complete the family history information.*
- *Your patient is confused and having a difficult time understanding the information.*
- *Your patient is crying.*

What do you do when you have no time left but clearly there are issues that need to be addressed? As these examples illustrate, there are many patient circumstances that can impact the timing of the visit and affect the overall clinic schedule. When it becomes evident that more time is needed, you will need to do some triaging. Is it possible, given your clinic schedule, to extend the counseling session? Can another team member meet with your next patient? Can you meet with your patient later that same day, or is another clinic appointment needed? For example, if a patient is having prenatal testing and the information remaining to be discussed has no bearing on this decision, you can ask the patient to return to your office after the procedure.

It is important to recognize that you need to have sufficient time available to effectively provide genetic counseling. In addition, patients can take in only so much information at one time. When a follow-up appointment needs to be scheduled because the available time is insufficient to address issues, communicate this clearly to the patient. Disappointment over not having everything addressed in a single visit can be lessened by informing patients about this possibility when the appointment is scheduled and giving a reminder about time limitations at the start of the session. As genetic testing becomes available for more conditions, the issues of what can be accomplished in a single visit and the potential for "information overload" will need to be taken into consideration.

Working with Interpreters

Working with interpreters adds another layer of complexity to managing a clinic visit, and more time should be allotted for the clinic visit. It is helpful to brief the interpreter before the start of the session about the clinic visit. It is preferable to have an interpreter with a medical background, and hospitals often have listings of employees who can serve as interpreters; it will take some advance planning to make sure the interpreter is available. In addition, it is helpful to have an interpreter of the same gender as the patient, to lessen the chance of the patient feeling inhibited in discussing sensitive and intimate medical issues. Ideally, it is best to have an interpreter who is not a family member, to avoid possible censoring of communicated information and feeling pressured.

Even if you are using an interpreter, it is appreciated if you greet the patient in his/her native language; you can ascertain how to say "hello" and "welcome" either by an Internet search or by asking the interpreter. When working with an interpreter, it is important to maintain eye contact with the patient and assess his/her body language and response to presented information. Given the time needed to state information and have it translated and the comprehension issues, you should focus on presenting information that will impact patient care and decision-making. You should present information succinctly and clearly, minimize use of technical terms and abstract concepts, use pictures/diagrams, and make bottom-line summary statements; this should generally be the approach with any patient, but this is especially important with language and comprehension issues). There are many important considerations and issues in working with interpreters that are beyond the scope of this chapter, and you should refer to other resources.

REFERRALS TO OTHER SPECIALISTS

Patients who are diagnosed or are being seen to rule out a genetic condition will often need referrals to other specialists (e.g., cardiologists, neurologists, ophthalmologists, etc.). The genetic counselor is frequently an important link between the patient, the genetics clinic, and other specialists, making sure that pertinent information is communicated and follow-up initiated. It is helpful to be specific about the confirmed or suspected diagnosis and clearly communicate what needs to be evaluated. For example, "*Patient with suspected Marfan syndrome, rule out ectopia lentis*" would alert the ophthalmologist to look for this feature. If you suspect a genetic condition in a pregnancy for which there are associated ultrasound abnormalities, sharing this information with the ultrasound staff can help them do a more focused assessment. Providing specialists with pertinent medical records, test results, and relevant information about the genetic condition enhances patient care. Keep in mind that genetics clinics are specialty clinics and that often referrals to other specialists need to first be approved by the primary care physician for insurance coverage. Patients may also benefit from seeing a licensed therapist for short-term or long-term therapy. There may be therapists at your institution to refer patients. The patient can also find a local therapist by talking with his physician, clergy, and friends.

REFERRALS OF FAMILY MEMBERS TO GENETICS CLINICS

"Who is the patient?" is a question that frequently arises in genetics clinics. Genetic information has implications for other family members, and it is not unusual for other family members to accompany the patient to a clinic visit. It may be another family member, instead of the patient you are actually seeing, who in fact needs to be evaluated or tested first. Through the use of online clinic directories, genetics clinics can be identified for family members. Every state has one or more genetics clinics and/or provides periodic access to outreach clinics. Depending on location, a genetics clinic in a neighboring state may be closer for a patient. You can locate genetics clinics through GeneTests, Organization for Rare Diseases/GARD (Genetic and Rare Diseases Information Center), and Orphanet and through directories available at genetics professional organizations websites. A specific directory for Cancer Genetics Services is available through the National Cancer Institute.

CASE DOCUMENTATION

Documentation is important for both patient care and communication with team members about the status of a case. Genetic counselors working at hospitals and clinics with online medical records can readily document relevant phone calls and paste in patient e-mails. Sending letters to the referring physician and/or the patient that summarize the genetics clinic visit is a key component of case management. Medical documentation is discussed in Chapter 10.

Considering all there is to do for a single case, you will need to develop a system to keep track of your "active" cases. A tracking system is important because genetic studies often take a month or longer to complete, by which time you will already be involved in counseling other patients. Consult with your colleagues about computer database programs they have utilized to track test results and pending evaluations. The use of a computer database is also helpful for generating patient lists for case conferences, completing clinic surveys and reports, and thinking about potential research studies.

IS A GENETICS CASE EVER COMPLETE?

It is not unusual for several years to pass between an initial clinic visit and a return visit. A case that you may have considered complete may later reopen as a result of advances in knowledge about the genetic condition and genetic testing. Given how rapidly genetics is evolving, it is important to emphasize to patients the need to keep in touch with a genetics clinic. This is particularly important for cases where no diagnosis was made, no genetic testing is available, or testing was done and no mutation was identified with current technology. While ideally one would like to be able to inform patients when advances pertinent to their genetic condition are made, logistically this is not feasible. Encouraging patients to join support/advocacy groups and/or periodically check their websites is helpful since these groups often have publications through which they disseminate information about advances. Recommending that patients be seen for follow-up in a genetics clinic will ensure that there is genetics input in their medical care and make it possible to inform patients about advances that may impact their care and potentially other family members.

CONCLUSIONS

Mastering case preparation and management is key to providing effective genetic counseling. The ability to successfully prepare for and manage a case will directly impact the quality of care, education, and counseling provided. As this chapter illustrates, genetic counselors have a pivotal role in case preparation and management, tasks that have many important components and details to oversee. From just knowing the bare basics of a patient's indication for a clinic visit, the genetic counselor can seek out pertinent information and resources and successfully prepare to see a patient. Critical-thinking skills and the abilities to anticipate, research, evaluate, prioritize, present, coordinate, and triage are needed for successful case preparation and management. You will become more efficient and learn "shortcuts" as you prep more cases and develop the ability to do abbreviated case prep when genetic conditions are first ascertained during the clinic visit. Your case preparation and management skills will continue to evolve throughout your clinical experiences, and each case will provide a new opportunity to implement, refine, and master these skills.

REFERENCES

Bennett RL, Pettersen BJ, Niendorf KB, Anderson RR (2003) Developing standard recommendations (guidelines) for genetic counseling practice: A process of the National Society of Genetic Counselors. *J Genet Couns* 12:287–295.

Bombard AT (2002) Letter to the editor: Insurance justification letters. *J Genet Couns* 11:75.

Gardner RJM, Sutherland GR (2004) *Chromosome Abnormalities and Genetic Counseling* (3rd ed.). Oxford: Oxford University Press.

Hodge SE (1998) A simple, unified approach to Bayesian risk calculations. *J Genet Couns* 7:235–261.

International Huntington Association and World Federation of Neurology Research Group on Huntington's Chorea (1994) Guidelines for the molecular genetics predictive test in Huntington's disease. *Neurology* 44:1533–1536.

Manning M, Hudgins L (2007) Use of array-based technology in the practice of medical genetics. *Genet Med* 9:650–653.

Ogino S, Wilson RB (2004) Review: Bayesian analysis and risk assessment in genetic counseling and testing. *J Mol Diagnostics* 6:1–9.

Ogino S, Wilson RB Gold B, Flodman P (2007) Bayesian risk assessment in genetic testing for autosomal dominant disorders with age-dependent penetrance. *J Genet Couns* 16:29–39.

Online Mendelian Inheritance in Man, OMIM (TM). McKusick-Nathans Institute of Genetic Medicine, Johns Hopkins University (Baltimore, MD) and National Center for Biotechnology Information, National Library of Medicine (Bethesda, MD), URL: http://www.ncbi.nlm.nih.gov/omim/ Accessed 2008 Dec 11.

Richards CS, Bale S, Bellissimo DB, Das S, Grody WW, Hegde MR, Lyon E, Ward BE; Molecular Subcommittee of the ACMG Laboratory Quality Assurance Committee (2008) ACMG recommendations for standards for interpretation and reporting of sequence variations: Revisions 2007. *Genet Med* 10:294–300.

Secretary's Advisory Committee on Genetics, Health and Society (2006) Coverage and reimbursement of genetic tests and services: Report of the Secretary's Advisory Committee on Genetics, Health and Society. Available at http://oba.od.nih.gov/SACGHS/sacghs_documents.html. Accessed December 3, 2008.

Shaffer LG, Beaudet AL, Brothman AR, Hirsch B, Levy B, Martin CL, Mascarello JT Rao, KW; a Working Group of the Laboratory Quality Assurance Committee of the ACMG. (2007) Microarray analysis for constitutional cytogenetic abnormalities. *Genet Med* 9:654–662.

Shappell HL, Matloff ET (2001) Writing effective insurance justification letters for cancer genetic testing: a streamlined approach. *J Genet Couns* 10:331–341.

Terry SF, Terry PF, Rauen KA, Uitto J, Bercovitch LG (2007) Advocacy groups as research organizations: the PXE International example. *Nat Rev Genet* 8:157–163.

Uhlmann WR, Guttmacher AE (2008) Key internet genetics resources for the clinician. *JAMA* 299:1356–1358.

Young I (2006) *Introduction to Risk Calculation in Genetic Counseling* (3rd ed.). New York: Oxford University Press.

5

Psychosocial Counseling

Luba Djurdjinovic, M.S.

INTRODUCTION

This chapter offers you an opportunity to understand the importance of psychosocial assessment and counseling skills in genetic counseling. Psychological perspectives and theories offer models by which a genetic counseling session can be framed and understood. There is no single practice theory that defines genetic counseling, yet psychological and family systems dynamics are evident in our practice and assist us every day. Central to our practice are skills of listening and empathy, which are part of all major counseling approaches. Your evolution as a genetic counselor will ask you to develop these essential skills and simultaneously will bring into focus personal values and views that will inform as you are invited to understand the counselee. Case examples, theories, and practical approaches are offered to assist you in your ongoing refinement of creating psychologically meaningful connections that enrich the genetic counseling experience.

In my earliest days as a genetic counselor I struggled to understand what genetic counseling was all about. What did I have to offer that other professionals could not? The cognitive challenge of appreciating the medical and genetic variables in a case was very exciting, but these technical elements took a different shape when I sat with a patient. It was when I recognized that my empathic attunement with patients and families brought the science to life that I really understood the genetic counseling experience. My wish to "know" more fully the meaning of a genetic concern for

A Guide to Genetic Counseling, Second Edition, Edited by Wendy Uhlmann, Jane Schuette, and Beverly Yashar
Copyright © 2009 by John Wiley & Sons, Inc.

individual counselees has led me to provide a genetic counseling experience that is both a scientific and a psychological practice.

The earliest definers of genetic counseling understood the need for psychologically based discussions of genetic concerns (Reed, 1955; Kessler, 1979). The counseling aspect of genetic counseling has evolved in the last several decades to a more recognizable structure through which it embraces a number of psychological perspectives. In the last decade in particular there has been increased focus on the psychological needs of counselees, including a new definition of genetic counseling and numerous calls to ensure that the genetic counseling experience is psychologically rich (Lerman, 1997; Matloff, 1997; Eunpu, 1997a; Weil, 2000; Resta et al., 2006). Yet emerging evidence about the practice styles and content of genetic counseling sessions raises professional questions (Roter et al., 2006). What are the components of the counseling in our routine session? Do we understand what is effective? How do we develop and refine our counseling skills?

Almost all genetic counseling sessions contain competing priorities between the medical and psychological considerations of genetic conditions. How these priorities are set, and to what extent they are addressed, are matters that vary with clinical setting and clinical experience. The increasing emphasis in genetics on one-time visits has a limiting effect on what can realistically be addressed, but regardless the experience will be psychologically significant to the counselee. We have a responsibility to be sure that we understand what that psychological response may be and facilitate the use of genetic information. Our understanding of the psychological dimension ensures an optimal genetic counseling experience and will guide the genetic counselor in framing the session.

Genetic counseling sessions involve a context that is complex in verbal and nonverbal communication between counselee and genetic counselor. The psychological content of this communication forms a stratum at which perspectives, experiences, beliefs, emotions, and expectations of counselor and patient overlap. A family therapist once described the dynamics in such an encounter as being like a dance (Gratz, 1997). The dance is initiated through an articulated, or sometimes assumed, understanding of the individuals in the session and what each wishes to gain. The dance is set against a backdrop of the community of each participant. The counselee brings into the room, actually or more often figuratively, her family and their socio-ethnic communities. The genetic counselor also brings a socio-ethnic perspective and also represents an institutional medical structure. The willingness of all parties to join in the dance will have its moments of unfamiliarity, awkwardness, and adjustment, as each person communicates information and gradually comes to a mutual acceptance of style.

The interweaving of sociocultural strata with the psychological allows the genetic counselor to consider the counselee in his or her fullest complexity. Understanding this complexity is as cognitively challenging and rewarding as our discussions about the genetic issues. The counselor's challenge is to provide an experience that offers opportunities to consider the client's concerns and questions in the fullest manner. It thus requires us to be cognizant of, and facile with, psychological dynamics.

The counselor is engaged in a complex psychodynamic process that involves the lessening of denial, the relief of guilt, lifting of depression, the articulation of anger, and gradual, rational planning for the future. Everyone who has provided genetic counseling has witnessed these processes.

—Hecht and Holmes, 1972

Recent literature provides support for a psychologically oriented genetic counseling experience (Michie et al., 1996; Pieterse et al., 2005; Aalfs et al., 2006). Many genetic counselors will agree that a classic question raised by the counselee is "Why did this happen?" This question frequently directs conversation to a didactic explanation, yet it may represent a more existential concern ("Why did this happen to me?") (Levine, 1979). So, how should we consider the wishes and needs of the counselee? Or, as the family therapy theorist Virginia Satir asks, "What is the message about the message?" (quoted in Kessler, 1979). The answer is in part a willingness to attend to the psychological dimension of the discussion and the development of a personal evaluation process that supports the development of skills over time and monitors patterns of use.

PSYCHOSOCIAL ASSESSMENT AND THE STRUCTURE OF A SESSION

There is no prescribed process nor identifiable tools common to all counselors. However, the tool most central to all genetic counseling sessions is the family history. It is through the construction of this familial diagram that medical and social information is revealed. This provides "an important opportunity to assess and address psychological issues" (Weil, 2000). The pedigree in its simplest form offers us critical clues to understanding our patient's existing relationships as well as absent relationships due to divorce, death, or adoption. The counselee's ability to provide information can suggest the level of connectedness in a family (Eunpu, 1997b). More recently, it has been suggested that the traditional pedigree can be expanded to consider extrafamilial relationships that influence individual and family dynamics to enhance the conversation about the meaning of the genetic counseling information (Peters et al., 2004).

Counselees provide information about themselves in a number of ways. A counselee's available social support, and ability to avail him/herself of it, is sometimes revealed by whether a given patient attends a session alone or with a partner or other family member. Counselees also can provide hints at the burden they may be carrying by statements such as "It's really up to me," "I need to know," "It's my fault." Counselees give direct information about themselves that a genetic counselor can utilize to form a psychosocial answer to the question "Who is this person?" It also helps to address the counselor's question, "Can I understand this patient, and what can I offer beyond the didactic information?" Further, can I "create a process, regardless of time, that facilitates the client's ability to use genetic information in a personally meaningful way that minimizes psychological distress and increases personal control" (Biesecker and Peters, 2001)?

By eliciting information to the following questions, we come to understand the counselee and begin to elucidate the meaning of their concern. This evolves through a directed process of learning who the counselee is.

1. How do you "know" the client?
   a. Review of chart or intake sheet
   b. Demographic information
   c. Pedigree construction process
   d. Presenting concern
   e. Ethnocultural community
2. What does the patient disclose about him/herself and how?
   a. Social support
   b. Narrative surrounding this issue
   c. Attitudes and beliefs
3. What variables may influence the genetic counseling session?
   a. Level of anxiety or distress
   b. Depression
   c. Issues of education
   d. Language
   e. Evidence of a working relationship between counselor and counselee
4. How do you as the genetic counselor feel about this client and their situation?

THE PATIENT'S STORY

A powerful tool in assessment is asking the counselee to tell us what brings them to genetic counseling. Our wish to know the patient's circumstances and experience begins to form a relational context for the genetic counseling session. It is the patient telling a personal story and our attuned listening that allows for assessment of concerns and emotional issues. The counselee's narrative is increasingly valued in the psychological community as practitioners seek to have the patient's voice be as central as the theoretical construction (Belenky et al., 1986; Miller, 1976; Gilligan, 1982; Kleinman, 1988; Rosenwald and Ochberg, 1992). The story tells us which ethnocultural perspective is identified and how religious affiliation and beliefs are described by the counselee (Kenen and Smith, 1995). Through the narrative we can begin to appreciate the meaning of the issue that has led to the appointment. Paying close attention to the narrative keeps us from making assumptions about what personal concerns a genetic risk presents and what brings people to see us. Further, the narrative "knits together...recollected past with a wished-for future" (Brock, 1995, p. 152). The meaning of an event can be intergenerationally constructed ("it skips generations"), and it is often attached to perceptions of risk ("I know I'm a carrier"; "I think I inherited that gene"). This meaning from the counselee's perspective provides an invitation to the emotional content of the session. It is common for there to be a tension between the counselor's need to present the medical genetic information and the patient's need to explore existential questions of "why." The tension is a reminder that we need to facilitate a session to ensure that needs are met.

ACHIEVING DYNAMIC PSYCHOLOGICAL ENGAGEMENT: THE WORKING ALLIANCE

Most genetic counselors will agree that we share a genuine wish to be of assistance. This alone will not ensure that the concerns and needs of the counselee will be attended to. It is the emergence of a working alliance that provides a dynamic process for information exchange and exploration of meaning. The process of initiating rapport usually begins with delineation of mutual expectations and goals. The transformation of rapport into a psychologically based experience requires attending and ensuring that a "working alliance," "working relationship," or "therapeutic alliance" will evolve. The concept of a working alliance has its origin in early psychodynamic theory, which has been generalized into other counseling perspectives. Bordin (1979) deconstructed the analytic definitions and offered a definition in which the alliance grows out of a mutual agreement on goals and tasks. Further, these expectations are set within a relational milieu of client and counselor that includes understanding and empathy. It is this relational context *that ensures the counselee is "heard" and the "hopes" of the session are most likely to be achieved.*

A number of psychological scales have been used to evaluate working alliances in various counseling settings. Some of the measures include the patient's perception of the counselor's willingness to help, the level of agreement between counselor and patient clinical goals, and the level of mutual respect (Tichenor and Hill, 1989). These measures nicely define the minimal parameters required to initiate and maintain psychologically driven engagement in the genetic counseling session.

The working alliance is central to the genetic counseling process. It begins to emerge through the knowledge that we acquire in our initial assessment and the first statements between the counselor and patient: "What brings you to our office today?... What do you hope we will discuss today?... We would like to use some of our time today to review your family medical history." The genetic counselor's ability to facilitate a balanced discussion of everyone's agenda further shapes this working relationship. Forming this alliance is only one part of the process; maintaining its integrity can be a more challenging aspect. It is important to recognize that the alliance develops through an iterative process that draws from listening to direct words and indirect clues throughout the session. This will build trust and confidence that the counselor understands (Donahue and Siegel, 2005). Facilitating this alliance encourages mutual understanding and offers the potential for the best outcome.

The emerging alliance is maintained and enhanced through an active commitment to ensuring that the following elements are practiced throughout the genetic counseling session.

Self-Awareness and Self-Attunement

Practicing genetic counselors recognize that personal actions, feelings, behaviors, experience, and language play a role in the trust building phase of the session. We cannot assume that we are always the "same" with each counselee. Genetic counselors are witnesses to complex difficult decisions and a wide range of emotions, all of which can trigger personal reminders, anxiety, disappointment, or strong feelings. As the working relationship emerges it is important that the genetic counselor have a self-attunement process to respond to inner dialogue and adjust so as to remain fully present and attend to the conversation with the counselee. This ability to become momentarily aware and to refocus is a learned and practiced skill.

Our roles require us to be able to be self-aware of our vulnerabilities, counter-transference triggers, and abilities to take in the experience of others (Weil, 2000). It is essential that each counselor commits to self-reflection, discussion with colleagues, and/or personal counseling to fully experience and understand all that is presented in a genetic counseling session.

Confidentiality and Boundaries

The working relationship is strongly influenced by issues of confidentiality and respect for physical and emotional boundaries. The ability to fully share personal and family information requires an understood agreement that the information will not be disclosed beyond the clinical genetics experience without permission from the counselee. This includes a clinical setting that limits what can be overheard. It is only when this parameter is in place that we can expect and invite patients to disclose difficult issues and emotions. Similarly, note-taking during the session can be alarming if the content and purpose are not disclosed in advance. Sometimes the issue of confidentiality is not related to persons in the room but involves family members seen earlier or scheduled for future visits. It can also involve issues of paternity and previous pregnancy terminations, matters commonly kept secret within families. Therefore, anxiety about disclosure of these events may result in less than satisfying discussions.

Emotional and physical boundaries make patient and counselor alike feel "safe" in an intimate discussion. The need for boundaries is central to all forms of connection. Boundaries can be defined as those safeguards that do not impinge on patient autonomy, self-expression, confidentiality, and physical safety. The degree of physical and emotional boundary enforcement is influenced by the nature of the experience, previous experience (e.g., sexual abuse) in which boundaries have not been respected, and cultural perspectives. The emergence of a working relationship requires that boundaries are respected. In forming connections, for example, it is sometimes necessary to be able to shift a boundary. A familiar example is when a counselee needs a more rigid boundary and appears to resist efforts on the part of the genetic counselor to engage in the clinical genetics process. This can be due to generalized anxiety about possible outcomes of the session or it may be in response to the genetic counselor's eagerness and enthusiasm in forming a working alliance.

Sometimes it is "too much, too fast." Raising or maintaining boundaries does not necessarily dampen the emotional content, it ensures that there is "safety" in its expression.

As a general rule, physical contact with the counselee, other than a hand shake, must be limited. Only when permission is given should there be limited physical contact with a patient. We may choose to comfort a patient during a moment of intense grief or despair if a supportive gesture is invited, but appropriate occasions for such contacts are not common. Physical comforting of the patient such as hugging and touching is well understood in psychological circles as disruptive, as well as disrespectful to the patient. Physical contact between counselor and patient can be counter to the cultural practices of the patient. For instance, what might seem like an innocent touch of a child's head can be experienced as threatening by parents of Asian background.

On a final note, it is also important to remember that the issues of boundaries are central to the counselor as well. Unless the counselor can feel safe, the process she directs will be fragmented and may not serve the needs of the patient. It is appropriate for the counselor to create and, at times, define the boundaries that will allow for her full participation.

Patient Autonomy

Patient autonomy is a central tenet in genetic counseling, ensuring that the counselee acts in a personally congruent manner. Historical pressures shaped early genetic counseling discussion and definitions with assurances that autonomy was preserved through a practice of "nondirectiveness" (Resta, 2006).

In the 1970s Seymour Kessler defined nondirectiveness in the practice of genetic counseling as "procedures aimed at promoting the autonomy and self-directedness of the client" (Whipperman-Bendor, 1997). The common usage of this term in our professional discourse often blurs our understanding and stirs conflict in some genetic counselors in providing information or recommendations related to health protective behaviors (Rees et al., 2006). At times, challenging questions from our counselees, "What should I do?" or "What would you do in my situation?", can lead the counselor to retreat into the arms of nondirectiveness with statements about his/her value-neutral position. There appears to be some confusion about the role of nondirectiveness in our professional practice.

It is important to consider the origins of the nondirective concept and the influence of Carl Rogers', client-centered theory on promoting patient autonomy and appreciate the influences of both on our definitions and practice. As the genetic counseling profession has expanded and addressed many new clinical areas, professional confusion about the term appears to impact "critical discussion of both the psychological and the societal implications of genetic knowledge" (Wolff and Jung, 1995). There have been numerous efforts to disentangle the issues of non-directiveness and autonomy (Kessler, 1979, 1992, 1997; Weil, 2003; Resta, 2006, Weil, 2006).

If we understand that "nondirectiveness" is not a theory but an essential ethical principle of our practice, then we should value and embrace the opportunity that emerges in genetic counseling discussions to affirm our patients as their own moral agents. So, when questions arise. "What should I do?", this is simply an invitation for the counselor to fully appreciate the counselee's dilemma and to seek exploration of issues involved. A simple and genuine inquiry on the part of the counselor, "I would like to understand your question better," sets aside the question and returns the focus on to the counselee. Request for direction for a decision from a genetic counselor is primarily an effort on the part of the counselee to weigh options, to seek validation about a choice or decision, and seek some information of how others made a decision. As a general rule, a direct request for direction (other than review of clinical care guidelines) is an invitation to the counselor to empathically understand and guide a discussion where the best decision emerges; it is not a request for your decision. It is always important to recognize that in some cultures there may be an invitation for the counselor's input in decision-making, challenging the tenet of patient autonomy in genetic counseling (Rolland, 2006; Weil and Mittman, 1993).

Patient autonomy is the outcome of a counseling experience where an enhanced decision-making climate is promoted through information, empathic attunement, and professional guidance. The genetic counselor embraces nondirectiveness as an ethical principle, not a psychological theory.

Listening

The working alliance evolves as the counselor actively listens to the need and concern of the counselee. Listening is the "mortar" of the evolving alliance (Graybar and Leonard, 2005). The first step is a willingness by the counselor to understand through careful listening to what brings the counselee to the appointment (Donahue and Siegel, 2005). There is much to learn and understand from our counselees' experience. Much has been written to inform the genetic counselor of the complexity and challenges that individuals and families with genetic risk face (Smith et al., 2006, Etchegary, 2006, Kay and Kingston, 2002, Tercyak et al., 2001, Barbain and Christian, 1992). So, it is important that the counselor "brackets" his or her beliefs and biases and avoids presumptions to ensure that attunement with the lived experience of the counselee can be achieved (Spinelli, 2001).

The nature of the genetic counseling process requires the counselor to provide information that can be lengthy, and often time constraints risk limiting or prematurely terminating an invitation to understand the counselee's narrative. A discourse that does not have pauses for input from the counselee will limit psychosocial participation and encourage assumptions on the part of the counselor, which can result in a less than satisfactory experience for all involved. It is a common struggle for genetic counselors to create a balance in each session between the didactic and supporting a discourse about the meaning of the information provided. The first step to ensuring an interpersonal milieu is to invite and listen carefully to the counselee's narrative.

Empathy

The working relationship emerges from careful listening and the presence of empathy. The presence of empathy in the genetic counseling session will ensure that the needs of the counselee will be central to the process and that an interpersonal psychological infrastructure will grow to assist in discussion of the meaning of genetic risk. Empathy can be difficult to define. Many authors have attempted to capture the complex nature of this specific form of connection.

> "The capacity to understand what another person is experiencing from within the other person's frame of reference," "it is the accepting, confirming and understanding human echo," and "comprehending the momentary psychological state of another person"
> —Bellet and Maloney, 1991; Jordan, 1991

Empathy is thought of as having both affective and cognitive functions that provide the ability to deeply appreciate the counselee's experience and simultaneously consider how this must be understood. The counselor's emotional attunement is simultaneously understood through a cognitive process and results in the "fullest appreciation" of the counselee "at that moment" in the session (Surrey, 1991). This empathic attunement can be achieved through spoken and unspoken content (Kohut, 1984; Wolf, 1988; Basch, 1980; Jordan et al., 1991).

The practice of empathy in the genetic counseling session requires that the genetic counselor is willing to attend to the counselee by providing required information and the psychological opportunities for empathic attunement. The role of empathy in the genetic counseling encounter has been strongly supported as a central element in a client centered approach to genetic counseling (McCarthy Veach et al., 2003; Weil, 2000; Evans, 2006). Empathy and empathic attunement in a genetic counseling session evolve through three phases of information analysis. The first phase attempts to integrate the content of the patient's story, identifying the patient's affective state and appreciating our own response to the story. The second phase requires a careful consideration of the significance of the patient's story and the messages within. The final phase involves a decision as to how to effectively acknowledge what has been discerned (Basch, 1980). It is the genetic counselor's goal to foster a continuum of empathic connection to allow the emergence of a working alliance, so as to invite personal reflection and a fostering of trust in genetic counseling (Bovee, 2007).

It is through the counselor's empathic stance that a counselee begins to feel understood. Being understood provides a platform for the formation of self-empathy and, in so doing, enhances the patient's ability to personally appreciate the complexity of presented information, choices, and the clinical course of a condition. This is believed to be central to one's ability to make decisions or take actions (Jordan, 1991b; Jordan et al., 1991; Miller, 1991a; Surrey, 1991).

Empathy is an ability that comes to some more easily, yet maintaining the empathic connection or attunement is an evolved skill. The learning begins within our own life experiences and relationships. For counseling professionals empathic attunement is explored and developed in case supervision. Essential to this skill is

[handwritten notes:]
I. Integrate content of story
II. Consider significance of story
III. Decide how to acknowledge what you've learned from pt's story

"a well-differentiated sense and an appreciation of, and sensitivity to, the differences as well as the sameness of another person" (Jordan, 1991a). It is essential that a counselor develop the skill to stay aware of dynamics within the session as well as her own feelings, intuition, and personal experiences.

A common challenge in maintaining empathic attunement is to not "take on" the counselee's feelings. This can be very difficult at times. In cases where empathic attunement converts to a moment of sympathy, the counselor must have the personal psychological agility to return to an empathic position with awareness that one's personal experience may influence the genetic counseling discourse. It is crucial that a counselor be able to differentiate feeling sympathy from feeling empathy. The counselor's sympathetic experience of a patient involves an emotional response based in the counselor's personal life. When we feel moved to tears by despair in our counselee, for example, it is important to differentiate between a personal identification with the counselee (remembering a similar experience) as opposed to having, in that moment, deeply appreciated their pain. The sympathetic response on the part of the genetic counselor is real. Yet, it needs to be put aside and attention refocused on the responses of the counselee.

An essential extension of this skill is to regain an empathic connection or attunement after one is disrupted. (I discuss common disruptions later in this chapter.) It is essential to recognize a disruption or anticipate the impact of a counselor's inattention, or such action in the session may shift the focus and an empathic attunement may be dropped. The shift could be brought to the attention of the counselor by a change in topic, body language, and/or the counselor feeling that something is different. This then requires a quick assessment by the counselor and an effort to move back into empathic attunement. Sometimes, the counselor may have experienced a concern that creates a barrier that is limiting the attunement. It often requires a conscious effort on the genetic counselor's part to reach out to the counselee and reestablish the empathic attunement. This act of refocusing on the counselee and achieving an empathic connection is termed "raising one's empathy" (Wolf, 1988). Maintaining empathic attunement ensures that the needs and experiences of the counselee are central throughout the session and not limited to the initial rapport-building phase.

The following case illustration describes how a working relationship forms through empathic connections in a genetic counseling session. I have selected a case that involves a one-hour session and demonstrates the unfolding of a session with an uncertain agenda.

A family was referred for genetic counseling after the birth of a son with bilateral coronal craniosynostosis. At the time the appointment was scheduled, the mother of the child explained that the child's surgeon had recommended genetic counseling. The parents arrived for the appointment with their infant son and their 6-year-old son. After I settled the parents and the children into the consultation room and made appropriate introductions, I opened the session, "I understand your son was born with a form of craniosynostosis and you were referred by Dr. W. How can we help you?" The father responded, "We don't know, the doctor thought we should come here." This response was somewhat unexpected. It was an awkward beginning since nothing was identified as a common goal. I proceeded to briefly describe what kinds of issues we might discuss in relation to their son's diagnosis. The mother interrupted, "They gave us a booklet about craniosynostosis.... The doctors told us that we have a 4% chance that this will happen again." (The mother reached into her purse and handed me the booklet). I experienced the mother's response as having a tone of anger and defensiveness. I will admit that I was a bit put off by the mother's response. I almost instantaneously reminded myself that the mother was telling me something important here and it did not necessarily mean that they had the facts and the appointment was scheduled in error. I asked the parents to tell me how they felt about this risk. This was the question that truly opened the session.

The session progressed with my inviting the couple to tell me "their story." The parents did not hesitate to share their experience. As the parents told the story they looked at each other frequently. At one point I observed that the mother looked very teary. In that moment I began to more fully appreciate the experience for the mother. I said to her, "The feelings are still with you after all these months." She nodded and went on. I believe this early empathic connection formed the path to what unfolded later in the session. As an aside, the telling of "the story" was frequently interrupted by the older son. There were many requests for items in the mother's purse and requests to me for drawing paper. Interruptions were also initiated by the mother, who frequently turned to her sons and spoke to them. I understood these interruptions as a tool to diffuse parental anxieties about the content of the session and what still might be said. I made every effort to respect the defense that I understood to be stimulated by anxiety. I also experienced my own anxiety when I considered the remaining time in the session, the still unformed goal for the session, and my clinical appreciation of the heterogeneous etiology and resulting risk. I was committed to introducing my concerns about the risk figure but, at that point in the session, I had no idea how I would do that.

I asked the parents to tell me how they had explained their son's condition to family and friends. The mother quickly responded with a clear description and added, "It's no one's fault." I asked the couple if they had looked for possible causes. The mother quickly responded, "I thought I was responsible, but the doctor helped me understand I was not. The baby and I have a flatness here (pointing to the midface). I was stuck to my mother's spine in the uterus, the doctor had to turn me and pull, then I was born. I am worried because we are planning to start trying again." I became aware that this statement made me feel better since I had a direction and potentially something to offer. I guessed that a possible unspoken agenda for this couple could be prenatal testing options. I asked the couple if they were interested in discussing their future pregnancy and what options may be available to them. The mother forcefully stated, "We are Christians and accept what is given." I nodded in acknowledgment. This was followed by the mother turning to her husband and telling him what she had thought of ultrasound studies for reassurance. She turned to me and said, "We have not discussed it, but is it possible?" I understood this to be the concerns that led to the appointment. After my discussion about ultrasound, she shared that she very much wanted another child but was afraid. This was followed by, "My older son is not from this marriage, and the baby was conceived before we got married. I would love to tell people I am pregnant without a reaction of shock." The mother had told me something she felt burdened by, and I accepted her need to share this.

As I was approaching the final ten minutes of the session, I realized that I needed to make a transition to a closure of the session and find a way to encourage the couple to initiate an evaluation process that would offer diagnosis and risk assessment specific to their circumstances. It was my sense that the mother carried guilt from more than one source, one of which may be her own belief that the craniosynostosis is familial.

I offered the following statement to bring the session to a close: "I can see that your plan to have another child carries a lot of meaning for you. What you have told me today allows me to understand what has made this decision important and difficult. As I think about our conversation today, I have the sense that you are still trying to understand why this happened and how this may affect your future children." The father said, "It was just a fluky thing," but the mother said, "Yes (pause) I'm not sure." The session concluded with my offering a formal genetic evaluation process as a way to assist in answering some of their questions. The couple and the children left, with the mother thanking me "for listening." This was for her the unstated but, perhaps, primary goal of this session.

It is not unusual that counselees cannot articulate their questions or agenda. This is in part because they may not understand the reason for the referral by their medical provider or, as in this case, because of guilt and a possible understanding by the mother that her shared appearance with her son had recurrence implications. This case had a number of instances in which I questioned where I was going and why I did not even construct a pedigree. The counselees never gave me permission to engage in a more formal genetic evaluation process. But, without the conversation that did unfold, the possibility of risk assessment might never have been identified by the couple.

DISRUPTIONS IN THE WORKING ALLIANCE

The working relationship, as illustrated in the above case report, emerges relatively quickly by attending to emotions, beliefs, and memories that form associations for the patient. These associations occur in varying degrees and can be positive or negative. The ability to observe, hear, and understand them can be critical to maintaining the integrity of the working relationship. The most common disruptions to the working relationship can be categorized into three areas: transference, countertransference, and empathic breaks.

Transference and Countertransference

The concepts and experience of transference and countertransference are about imposing an invalid understanding and a response to someone through an unconscious template. This template is superimposed on a person. Sometimes it can be correct, but most of the time it is simply a projection of a belief or a wish on the part of the person who creates this understanding for another. For example, consider the basis of our first impressions about others, "I like her" or "There is something odd about her." Usually, this can be attributed to a historical imprint. It is often difficult to sort out what has stimulated our assumptions or beliefs. This imprint can happen on the part of the counselee or the genetic counselor. What genetic counselors can take from this psychological dynamic is that we all can have an unconscious response to another.

The counselor's responsibility in the genetic counseling session is to make oneself aware of such dynamics. The value of this knowledge is not to provide a therapeutic intervention to eliminate the response but to be aware that a response may emerge to defend against the imprint. It is the response that can have disruptive effect on the session. Depending on the time frame of a genetic counseling session, it may be possible in some cases to invite a discussion that may allow for the unconscious to become conscious.

The term transference has its roots in psychoanalytic theory, and it describes patterns of expectations that interfere with relationship building. These expectations are unconscious and are not easily observable to the patient or counselor. Transference is a ubiquitous phenomenon in which one brings old patterns of expectation to new situations in attempts to create familiar structure for the event (Basch, 1980). This psychoanalytic concept can be generalized to all counseling experiences. It is further argued that "Transference phenomena emerge in all relationships.... We bring experience with important relationships in the past into current interaction with people—particularly through the relational images we carry with us" (Miller and Stiver, 1997).

Most genetic counseling sessions do not evidence unconscious psychodynamically driven transference responses as seen in psychoanalysis. Yet it does occur, in a more conscious way, where the counselor or counselee becomes aware of a belief and experiences discomfort. When the genetic counselor has this experience, it often informs the dynamics in the session. When the counselee superimposes a belief, expectation, or feeling and it is recognized by the counselor as possibly transferential, one should not be quick to correct the imprint. A hasty decision to correct can be disruptive to the working relationship, and if the counselee is unaware of the distortion, the resulting confusion may elicit a more intense response from the counselee. The challenge for the genetic counselor is not to unconsciously respond to the counselee's transference.

Countertransference is commonly defined as the reaction or response to transference. It is generally the counselor's reaction to the counselee's story, her defenses and emotions or transference (Weil, 2000). The countertransference reactions in genetic counseling practice are most often of two types, associative and projective (Kessler, 1992a). Associative countertransference arises in that empathically attuned moment in a session when a patient shares an experience, a loss, a wish, or a story that carries the counselor (usually for a short time) into his inner self. This introspection is often accompanied by a review of mental images and a recall of conversations. These remembered emotions may rise to the surface. "Such associations may lead to others, and before the counselor knows it, she may no longer be attending to what the counselee is saying and feeling but to her own internal voice and possibly a personal suffering. In such an event, the distraction may impede or interfere with a full understanding of the counselee" (Kessler, 1992a). It is important to distinguish between an association that allows us to more deeply appreciate a patient's experience and one that takes up time and emotional space within the session. The patient may detect the counselor's distractedness or recognize that the counselor's comments are about herself and not the patient. It is here that the empathic connection fails and often fractures a discussion, often shifting the focus back to the didactic content of the session.

Projection and Projective Identification

Projection is a type of countertransference in which a counselor has made assumptions about the experience of the patient. These assumptions are based on a parallel past experience for the counselor such as loss, suffering, fear, or panic. Usually, the counselor does not recognize these as one's own and instead assumes the feelings are originating from the counselee (Peters, 1997). This type of countertransference carries the potential risk that the counselor will make assumptions about a patient's experience and truncate the empathic attunement, thus disrupting the working relationship.

We attempt to understand the counselee and his or her story with a genuineness that requires us to have our affective states accessible to us. On occasion, a counselor may be "hooked" by a perception or transference of the patient because of his/her own unresolved issues. This is less common. However, this type of disruptive dynamic is one of the major reasons why it is important that counselors identify transferential beliefs and behaviors through a personal counselor or supervision.

On occasion, we meet a counselee who directs a projection onto the counselor. This is an unconscious defense mechanism to block or disavow a feeling or a meaning onto the counselor. A familiar example is when a counselee will repeatedly inquire whether their decision has angered the genetic counselor. In such cases of projection, the counselee is angry with his/her decision or with the necessity of having to make a decision.

Another more subtle form of projection, not always simple to recognize, is projective identification. This complex psychodynamic experience can occur when a situation is extremely challenging to the counselee and he/she is not able to bring forward adequate psychological defenses to respond. What is confounding about this defense mechanism is that the counselor, who is the "object" of the projected feeling, finds some congruence in the feeling. Unexpectedly, the counselor has a feeling experience that she attributes to herself and not the counselee. Therefore the counselor becomes a temporary repository of the feeling that is unacceptable to the counselee.

In summary, unconscious and conscious processes occur in the counselor as well as the counselee. The challenge is to appreciate psychodynamic clues to reduce the risk of disrupting the working relationship. The following case offers a glimpse into a possible transference reaction, one that could easily evoke a countertransference.

The genetic counselor is meeting with a couple who has just learned through the use of ultrasound that their 23-week fetus has a cystic hygroma. The genetic counselor attempts to provide information about cystic hygromas and the areas of uncertainty that surround this finding. The father insists, "You are not telling us everything you know." The counselor is taken aback by this comment and attempts to frame the areas of uncertainty again. The father presses the counselor for detailed information about all possible scenarios, and whenever the counselor attempts to remind the couple that these are the only possible scenarios, the father becomes more suspicious that the counselor is withholding information. He continues to repeat, "You know more than you're telling!"

The father appears to be bringing a historical experience or expectation that is interfering with his ability to participate in the counseling session. The experience could have had its origins in a previously frustrating medical visit. It is possible that the father had early life experiences that resulted in poor information disclosure to him with resulting trauma around unexpected news. We can imagine that the counselor could feel an increasing level of anger at the father's response. As a committed genetic counselor there would be a natural vulnerability to a suggestion that her counseling agenda was to withhold information. The tensions that are created limit the ability to maintain a relationship with the father and continue the session.

A possible intervention could be to consider transference as playing a part in the father's reaction and to ask the father to explain what he believes has not been disclosed. The instinctual response is to attempt to reassure the father of her commitment to full disclosure. This may be a useful statement to make, but it does not remove the barrier of distrust that is being enforced by the father. Attempts to appreciate and acknowledge the father's reactions are more likely to be helpful in changing the dynamics and shifting the transference.

An Empathic Break

An empathic break is a common dynamic in most psychologically driven discussions. This terms describes a shift or a change in the interpersonal dynamics or what feels like a loss of focus that usually signals a disruption or loss of an empathic connection. This may have a potentially serious impact on the process and goals set at the beginning of the session. It is, in my opinion, critical to rapidly recognize and address an empathic break in a session. Breaks can result from many factors: conscious and unconscious perceptions that are not addressed including issues of boundaries, autonomy, confidentiality, lack of cross-cultural sensitivity, or simple interruptions in the counseling session (phone calls, a knock on the door, hallway noises, etc.). The recognition of an empathic break can sometimes be difficult, as it is often a momentary experience. It can result from the actions of the counselor as well as the counselee. The counselor may suddenly remember an issue that has not been explored and conversationally thrust it into the session. The counselee may feel that the counselor has minimized the counselee's concern or that an emphasis has been placed on some information, giving it greater significance than intended by the counselor. This may result in feeling confused and stimulate the need to create distance. At this point, the counselee may not be psychologically available to continue with the session.

Sometimes the counselee will, in the telling of his/her story, share some information that may be challenging to the values or perspective of the counselor. The counselor's need to reassess her perspective (even if it takes only a few moments) could signal disapproval or confusion to the counselee. This perception could lead to an empathic break, precluding a psychologically driven discussion. It is not uncommon for counselees to make attempts to shift from a point of discussion. It sometimes is a test of what is possible or not possible to share.

The counselor's ability to return to the empathically attuned position after an empathic break may assist in the reconnection. Sometimes the counselor finds it difficult to reconnect at the point at which the disconnection occurred. It is here that the counselor should attempt to "raise her empathy," that is, quickly make a genuine effort to understand and return to the patient and the story. This skill of "raising one's empathy" comes with practice. It is my opinion critical to recognize and address an empathic break in a session. Sometimes acknowledging that a shift has occurred can assure the counselee that his vulnerabilities are being attended to and that a sincere effort to understand is offered. In a final note, we should not minimize the importance of disruptions of the session (noise, children in the room needing attention from the counselee) and how such events trigger an empathic break. There is also evidence that these same disruptions that shift the counselee or the genetic counselors from "the moment" appear to impact information recall (Dillard et al., 2007).

DISCUSSING DIFFICULT ISSUES AND GIVING BAD NEWS

One of our most important roles as genetic counselors is to sit with a person or family and announce that a genetic evaluation has identified a risk, and that this risk carries implications that can change their understanding of themselves or a loved one, as well as their future. These conversations are frequently experienced as bad news. The psychological response to difficult news varies from person to person. It is, in part, influenced by the gap between what the counselee believes and what is now being presented (Buckman, 1992). The following brief case illustrates such a gap.

> The genetic counselor met with a 38-years-old woman of Ashkenazi descent who was referred by her physician after a discussion of a paternal family history of breast cancer. She is the mother of two boys, 8 and 10. After a review of medical records and risk assessment counseling, the woman elected to undertake testing for the Ashkenazi mutations in BRCA 1 and BRCA 2. Testing revealed that she had one of the common mutations identified in persons of Ashkenazi descent. Upon receiving the information, the woman expressed disbelief and sadness. When this reaction was explored, she explained that she assumed that since she resembled her mother's side of the family, the chances for her being mutation positive were less. Confrontation with the gap between what she believed and what was subsequently identified had left her unprepared and very shaken.

One of the most critical steps for genetic counselors to manage is the assessment of what counselees believe and understand about the risks they face. This insight allows for structuring a discussion that honors the "gap" and provides adequate time to assist each counselee in her recognition of the issues surrounding the assumed and the real risks.

At the moment of our announcement to the patient or family that we intend to disclose the clinical findings or test results, two reactions are set in motion: The patient awaits the news, and the counselor anticipates a response. The counselor needs to appreciate the ways that someone may need to defend against overwhelming feelings and to recognize that whatever styles of coping are selected, it is an effort by the counselee to emerge intact from the discussion and experience. In this moment, the genetic counselor must strive to achieve empathic attunement. This is not always easy since we may experience sympathy and feel our own emotions. A quick recovery and return to attending to the feelings and comments of our counselee is critical. There are always situations in which the news we are presenting will bring forth emotion, alarm, and disbelief. We need to practice caution in these moments and not prematurely disrupt the emotional tension to relieve our own discomfort. Most often, the counselee will seek to regain emotional equilibrium and signal to you to continue in your explanation. Proceed cautiously with the explanation and stop periodically to seek what is needed from the counselee: "Tell me, what are you feeling?" "Should we take a short break?" "What is most important for you to know now?" The goal is to find a balance between information and witnessing the impact of the news. Achieving this balance is part intuition, part experience, and mostly driven by taking direction from the counselee. Giving "bad news" is not easy, but genetic counselors have a unique opportunity to introduce troubling information in a manner that will be viewed over time as caring and supportive.

The approach we use in presenting difficult information must be sensitive to the patient as well as to our own experience of the case. Central to giving bad news is providing information directly and empathically. It is difficult to achieve a balance here: "It is an art to do both at the same time. It is common for medical providers to choose one over the other, the idea is to be straightforward without sacrificing empathic attunement" (Peters, 1997). The context in which we give this information is equally critical. The material that follows, which attempts to guide the counselor in this challenging task, draws from the work of several authors (Ives et al., 1979; Goodman and Abrams, 1988; Buckman, 1992; Guest, 1997).

1. Prior to meeting with the counselee and/or family, delineate the goals and information that needs to be provided. Consider what may assist the counselee in understanding and formulate a plan of action.
2. Familiarize yourself with the patient's available support structure if possible.
3. Determine who should be present at the time of disclosure.
4. Identify the room or setting where the meeting will occur. It is essential that the setting provides privacy. There should be adequate seating for all present.
5. In giving the difficult information it is important to introduce the subject quickly: "I have news about ——." Attempt to give the most critical information

in two to three sentences, using limited genetic/medical terms, Then STOP and allow quiet time for the patient to absorb what you have just said.

6. Ask if the counselee would like you to provide more detail. Be aware of word choices, so that a balance between honesty and compassion is achieved. It is very important not to respond to the anxieties or sadness in the counseling room by giving facts. Information does not comfort everyone.

7. Look to the counselee to determine the pace of the discussion. Avoid excessive reassuring statements. The counselee must be able to cognitively and emotionally integrate the experience before reassuring statements (which are more often an attempt to reassure the counselor than the counselee) can be accepted.

8. Ask, "Do you have questions?" Listen for "buried" questions.

9. Ask, "How can I be helpful?... Do you want some one here with you?"

10. Ask who will be available to offer support after the counselee leaves the session.

11. In bringing the session to a close, ask the counselee to tell you what she understood about the information received. Ask what she will do after leaving the session. Make a plan to follow up on this conversation. Agree on a next step.

12. Finally, consider who is available to you to review the experience of giving difficult news (Mast et al., 2005).

Giving difficult information can be particularly challenging when the patient is cognitively delayed. The challenges most often lie in our own concern that the information we see as important may not be understood or appreciated for its significance. It is important for all who work with patients with cognitive limitations to remember that the counselees' ability to discuss feelings and their experience of a situation is not impacted by their particular difficulty in understanding medical or genetic information. This lack of convergence can sometimes make the counselor feel less confident in the session, since what aids our feelings of mastery is often our role of information giver. Here our role may be limited to supporting the counselees in their feelings. Further, it may be helpful to remind ourselves that such counselees, being categorized into a stigmatized group, may be "highly motivated to dissociate themselves from outward signs of incompetence" (Finucane, 1997). In other words, they may not acknowledge their lack of understanding. Some of the suggestions provided below for giving difficult news to children may be applied when informing counselees with cognitive delays.

1. Consider the child's age and developmental ability to appreciate the information. Structure the information content appropriate to the level. This may require follow-up appointments.

2. Discuss with guardians privately the objectives of the meeting with the young counselee. Also identify who will be included in the session.

3. Information must be presented in clear, simple statements. Repeat information more than once in the session. Be prepared to have the same questions raised by the counselee throughout the session.

4. Listen for "magical thinking" on the part of the counselee.

5. Appreciate the psychological challenges the information may have on self and/ or sexual identity. Be available to discuss issues of sexuality (Money, 1994).

6. Make plans to have the conversation continue with you or an appropriately trained professional.

Another area entailing special considerations is work with counselees for whom English is a second language. This is challenging especially when interpreters are inadequate or when there are family members who are also affected by the information (Ho, 2008; Preloran et al., 2005). Additionally, some patients with a psychiatric diagnosis can pose difficulty in forming a working relationship, or it may be difficult to assess their ability to integrate the information provided in the session (Peters, 2007; Pealy et al., 2009).

REACTIONS AND PSYCHOLOGICALLY CHALLENGING EXPERIENCES

The information that patients learn in the genetic counseling process has the potential to be psychologically overwhelming and to result in an emotional response. Among the many responses to unexpected news, the most common are denial, anger, fear, despair, guilt, shame, sadness, and grief. These responses elicit in the patient an emotional rather than a cognitive understanding of the implications of the information. The role of the genetic counselor is to provide what can be called "a holding environment," where there is appropriate support, empathy, and time for a response to be expressed and understood.

Denial, the inability to acknowledge to oneself certain information or news, is a common response when the information elicits shock and fear. This defensive psychological position emerges when other defenses no longer work. The reaction of denial is usually short term and is part of a coping strategy applied to impending or actual loss (Kubler-Ross, 1969). The patient's failure to acknowledge some aspect of external reality that is apparent to others has been further delineated into the constellation of disbelief, deferral, and dismissal (Lubinsky, 1994). The careful delineation of these denial experiences can assist the counselor in choosing more appropriate interventions. To allow for a process that is respectful of any such defense, interventions should be considered only after the counselee has had adequate time to assimilate the news.

Anger is a complex and universal emotion that seeks to blame; in its most extreme form, there can be a wish to achieve revenge. Anger can be directed at others or at oneself (Lazarus, 1991). It can be subtle or overt. It may be that there are gender differences in the construction of anger (Miller, 1991b). The patient with an angry response to information is probably experiencing fear, powerlessness, guilt, shame, or extreme anxiety. Anger is also a critical step in the resolution of loss, as the counselee seeks meaning in the need to abandon the hope of a wanted or expected outcome (Kubler-Ross, 1969; Bowlby, 1980).

Counselees need the opportunity to express and understand their anger. Assisting the counselee to explore the underpinning of his or her anger will invariably reveal other feelings, usually sadness. For some, anger is a "safer" emotional expression than sadness or grief. Providing the counselee with an opportunity to share their anger is the first step in transforming a feeling into deeper understanding.

A useful intervention is to invite the patient to discuss the anger. "You sound angry." "Can you tell me more?" It is very important that the counselor remain nondefensive, and especially crucial, not trivialize the anger (Peters, 1997). Anger can appear in the form of blame and may be focused on objects (e.g., a lab test), on persons in the past or future, or on the counselor, who represents the medical community. Anger can sometimes take other forms; one form is crying. I have found tears to be more common in women, probably reflecting the social unacceptability of anger for women. The inability to shift anger in the genetic counseling session can impede counseling goals or decisions that are being made (Smith and Antley, 1979). Interventions should include witnessing the feeling, honoring its role, and providing a working relationship that through empathic attunement lifts anger (usually for a short time), making it possible to address immediate issues.

Working with angry patients frequently evokes our own reactions that need to be temporarily quelled. If the counselor's feelings continue to be present after the session, it is important to speak with a colleague to understand the meaning of the interaction for the counselor.

Parents of children with genetic conditions frequently report feelings of **guilt and shame** (Antley et al., 1984; Weil, 1991; Chapple et al., 1995). The emotions of guilt and shame have different origins and can provide the counselor with information about the patient and possible approaches for discussing the issue. In some families the recognition of the mode of inheritance can trigger feelings of guilt and blame (James et al., 2006). Patients who hold themselves responsible for what they perceive as a negative outcome will frequently attempt to correct their guilt through self-blame, rationalizations, or other intellectualizations. Patients who express shame are offering you an opportunity to appreciate that events have placed "a burden of the self" (Kessler et al., 1984). Patients experiencing shame will often attempt to reduce the psychological challenges to the self by means of denial and withdrawal. The counselor's ability to witness the guilt and shame response of the patient provides the first step in offering an intervention that shifts the patient from a position of guilt and shame to one of more self-empathic understanding (Kessler et al., 1984). Genetic counselors should be cautious to not rapidly offer reassurances and instead should consider offering an opportunity for exploration (Weil, 2000). It is the process of exploration that can offer some relief.

Grief and despair are common responses to loss or anticipated loss. Families who learn that their child has a genetic disorder or that a pregnancy has elicited abnormal prenatal test findings will experience a grief process like that of families in which a neonatal death has occurred (Antley et al., 1984). The unexpected loss often results in feelings of shock, anger, yearning, and sadness that may be experienced in phases or concurrently (Kubler-Ross, 1969). Over time, several weeks and sometimes several months, resolution takes the form of gradual acceptance and a personal meaning is created. It is useful to appreciate that sadness or sorrow may be revisited at critical life cycle junctures. This does not necessarily suggest that the grief is unresolved (Hobdell and Deatrick, 1996). Yet, if the process is interrupted or blocked by disenfranchising the emotion, individuals and families retreat and lose resiliency, and this can lead to depression, anxiety, fear, and anger resulting in protracted grief.

Psychological interventions can be beneficial for some (Leon, 1990). For the majority, resolution of grief takes the form of being "able to make the loss seem meaningful and to gain a renewed sense of purpose and personal identity" (Shapiro, 1993). Our role as genetic counselors is to be open to listening to the pain. This act of witnessing and telling of their personal loss, even for a short time, offers a psychic comfort to the counselee (Greenspan, 2003). Grief resolution is a process, and the genetic counselor's invitation to understand the loss is a step (in some cases the only steps available to the counselee) to move through the phases of grief and loss.

The genetic counseling experience brings into focus many personal perspectives on loss, a range of responses and needs of our counselees. It is helpful to consider the unique aspects of loss that may emerge after susceptibility testing. It has been proposed that some families benefit from hope as a strategy for living with risk and through testing of at-risk family members there can be a "loss of uncertainty" (the challenge of now knowing who is at risk) and grief and sadness because of missed opportunities (Quaid et al., 2008; Sobel and Cowan, 2003). On a self-care note, witnessing your counselee's sadness may trigger your own recall of a loss experience. It is important to take a few minutes and have some self-empathy for your own personal experience.

Questions in the genetic counseling session may be vehicles for expression of feelings. By asking "Why me?" or just "Why?", the counselee is attempting to share an emotional reaction and discover the meaning of the event. If emotion is what drives the question, the counselor's efforts to provide information rather than addressing the emotion behind the question will disrupt the "holding environment," and a facilitative moment for appreciating the patient's experience will be lost.

On occasion, this questioning is an attempt to temporally distance oneself from the psychologically painful moment. A psychologically painful moment is not always visible to the counselor. This may occur when the "self" feels challenged and experiences feelings of shame, guilt, and, not too infrequently, anger.. The question may be a request to repeat some information ("Tell me again what will happen"), or it may be directed at the counselor ("Do you have time to explain this to me?"). Multiple questions may be asked, one immediately after another, without allowing time for a complete answer. Questionning can also seem confrontational, challenging the expertise of the counselor by inquiring about the certainty of the diagnosis and/or accuracy of testing. It is necessary to respect such expressions of the counselee's need to reduce the psychological tension and/or the release of intense feelings of anger and frustration.

In rare cases, questions may become barriers between the counselor and counselee. It is useful to attempt to understand what stimulated the barrier: Was it an empathic break, or is the counselee simply letting you know that she is tired and needs to stop? It is natural for the counselor, recognizing the emerging barrier and resulting disruption in the working relationship, to try to limit a flow of disruptive questions. The counselor needs to rely on her evolving understanding of the counselee and the emotional content of the session to determine what to do next. There must be a balance: Open acknowledgement of the barrier needs to be accompanied by an offer of assistance to explore the emotional tensions that led to the questions. Ability to achieve this balance comes primarily from experience. One frequently employed intervention is to directly ask the counselee to elaborate on the present experience. One can generally assume that an attempt to describe the emotion is permission for the counselor's assistance. When a patient appears to be inarticulate, or says, "I can't put it into words," the counselor should refrain from information giving and start looking at support options. For example, the counselor may perceive a need to allow adequate time for the patient to choose the next step. If this turns out to mean taking a break or scheduling a return visit, it is important to assess the patient for risk factors (level of support, suicide) and to contract for continuation of the discussion.

COUNSELEES' COPING STYLES

Psychologists have studied coping patterns and styles from different perspectives: psychodynamic, cognitive-behavioral, and neurophysiological. They have observed that most people have one or two primary coping styles, which they employ throughout their lives. Coping strategies are employed for problem solving or to change the meaning of what has been experienced (Pargament, 1997). A set of coping styles identified by Lazarus 1991 is summarized as follows:

Confronting: Trying to change the opinion of the person in charge
Distancing: Going on as if nothing happened
Self-controlling: Keeping feelings to oneself
Seeking social support: Engaging in conversation in the hope of learning more
Accepting responsibility: Criticizing oneself
Escape-avoidance: Hoping for a miracle
Plan: Identifying and following as action plan
Positive reappraisal: Identifying existing or potential positive outcomes

---

Coping strategies are not defined by a specific emotion, but are adaptive responses to psychologically challenging situations. Recognizing a coping reaction is helpful in guiding the genetics counseling session and identifying how best to assist the counselee in seeking support regarding a decision or adjusting to information provided in the genetic counseling session. Psychologically based intervention may be required when a counselee's coping strategy does not work and is disruptive to the counselee and his/her family. A simple and often effective intervention is asking the patient to describe how he or she has managed other difficult situations. This may bring awareness and may allow you to validate the personal experience and challenge that is now eliciting this coping strategy. This type of approach will not eliminate the strategy, but by possibly establishing empathic understanding the counselee may recognize the initial feeling that is triggering the response. The objective in this process is to bring some awareness, but not to eliminate the coping strategy, since the coping strategy may be required for assisting the counselee in adjustment to or resolution of the experience that triggered the response.

THEORIES THAT SURROUND OUR WORK

The psychological dynamics within a genetic counseling session can be considered from many theoretical perspectives. Some basic principles of psychological theory have been placed at the foundation of genetic counseling practice to guide the genetic counselor in appreciating the psychological concerns that emerge within a counseling session. In recent years a number of efforts to appreciate the dynamics within the genetic counseling session have led to a call to define and describe the genetic counseling process. Recently, a consensus conference met to consider the elements of the genetic counseling process (McCarthy Veatch et al., 2007). They affirmed the following tenets of genetic counseling that ensure that a psychological milieu is achieved:

1. The relationship is integral to genetic counseling.
2. Patient autonomy must be supported.
3. Patients are resilient.
4. Patient emotions make a difference.

I will describe a set of theories and some clinical material from my and others' practice to share my appreciation of the psychological dynamics in a genetic counseling session. The theories I have selected have been helpful to me. It is important that each counselor identify and develop his or her own set of clinical perspectives through experience and continuing education. I offer these only to demonstrate the rich psychological dynamics that exist in a session. Each genetic counselor must decide the degree to which she chooses to employ a theoretical framework or engage the genetic counselee in discussions that may shift a psychological barrier or tension. An important consideration is that most formal theories of psychology were constructed from a western cultural perspective. Furthermore, the common paradigm is white, middle-class, heterosexual, and patriarchal in experience. It is for these reasons that the psychological constructions we use will be limited. Not every template will fit every situation or work for the duration of the counseling relationship. Our choice of theory will be influenced by the case, our own skill level, and the constraint of time available.

I have found that looking through a psychological "lens" has enhanced my appreciation of the complexity of issues that a genetic concern raises for the counselee. This deeper understanding of the counselee only strengthens the essential working relationship.

The metaphor of taking a photograph offers a way to consider how to choose and work with a theoretical perspective. For photographers, the process is dynamic, as is the meeting with our counselee. The case that is presented to us is like the composition that draws our attention and engages us to take the photo. The combination of lens and aperture that we choose determines what will be in focus at that moment and what will remain in the background. This parallels what we choose to facilitate as discussion points in a session, and when we change the focus throughout the session. The lens we choose can also be fitted with filters that provide the cultural tones to the composition. The click of the shutter captures the image, just as in a counseling session we attempt to fully and empathically understand the counselee on different levels.

Central to all genetic counseling encounters are the principles defined by Carl Rogers, which provide the framework of practice for the genetic counselor. Rogers pioneered a form of psychotherapy that is described as "nondirective," "client-centered," or "person-centered approach." The central hypothesis is that "a climate of facilitative psychological attitudes" promotes self-understanding and changes in attitude and behavior (Kirschenbaum and Henderson, 1989). Carl Rogers argued that for change to occur three attitudes need to exist in the therapeutic relationship: genuineness, empathic understanding, and unconditional regard of the counselee.

Carl Rogers published his description of this counseling approach. In addition to stressing the critical role of facilitative experience, he also argued for the centrality of a "nondirective" approach: "The non-directive viewpoint places a high value on the right of every individual to be psychologically independent and to maintain his psychological integrity." He went on to add, " In the field of applied science, value judgments have a part, and often an important part, in determining the choice of technique"(Rogers, 1942).

The historical influences of the eugenics movement and other sociopolitical events led to a quick acceptance of this theoretical framework. The willingness of the genetic counseling community to embrace this approach assisted in the greater public acceptance of genetic testing and counseling. There have been many numbers of papers attempting to remind us of the origin and true meaning of nondirectiveness within the genetic counseling context (Kessler, 1992; Fine, 1993; Wertz, 1994; Wolff and Jung, 1995; Michie et al., 1997; Bernhardt, 1997; Whipperman-Bendor, 1997; Weil, 2003; Resta, 2006; Weil, 2006).

It is important to restate again that the client-centered model seeks to assist a counselee through a therapeutic relationship that is formed by genuineness, empathic understanding, and unconditional regard of the counselee. It is these three elements that must be developed and maintained in the genetic counseling practice model. "When any of these three is missing, a message is given that emotional issues are not relevant to the counseling process" (Weil, 2003).

Other theoretical perspectives (the various "settings" on the psychological lens) offer the counselor a way to appreciate who this counselee is, as an individual, within his or her family, and as a member of the larger community. I prefer to develop my understanding of the counselee from the smallest "aperture" to the panoramic perspective. The smallest aperture is the psychological makeup of the counselee. In the process of the counseling session, a broader view is required that includes relational issues, family dynamics, and sociocultural context. In using this approach with many families over the years, I have experienced an understanding that might not have emerged without a theory-based perspective. Looking through these lenses does not imply that we are initiating a psychotherapeutic relationship with a counselee. A decision to engage in a psychotherapeutic dialogue requires mutual consent and process.

I have selected the three most useful clinical perspectives that I employ in my daily practice. The self-psychological perspective provides a way to consider someone's psychological integrity. The relational model offers an understanding of how connections foster coping and relational skills. The family systems approach describes families in action. Each theory offers a way to "see" the genetic counseling patient.

Self-Psychology

This psychoanalytic approach (derived from Freud's theory and methods) was formulated by Heinz Kohut in the 1960s. His writings, and the contributions of many others, have offered a clinical perspective on the emergence of a "self" and what is required for the "self" to thrive. Kohut departed from classic analytic theories that identified the origin of behaviors in biological drives. He was convinced that the early childhood relational context with the parent or caregiver (object) forms the structure of the self. He referred to these experiences as "self objects." Unlike other analytic theories of the time, he argued that the lifelong vigor of the self is dependent on maintaining a relational context and having experiences that fortify the self. He believed that the psychological challenges that face us can be traced back to self object experiences.

Kohut's self-psychology theory has provided a way to appreciate the psychological cohesion of the counselee. This can be useful in anticipating responses to difficult news and evaluation of suicide ideation. This is well demonstrated in the following 1994 case report by June Peters:

> The patient (V.B.) was a 36 year old married Caucasian woman who had extreme distress about her abnormal maternal serum-alpha fetoprotein. V.B. expressed ambivalence about the pregnancy, identified marital conflicts, and was preoccupied with bodily sensation. She reported difficulty concentrating at work and lack of sleep. In an attempt to appreciate the psychological tensions of V.B., the counselor's exploration of past and present relationships was troubling. V.B. identified herself as a child as withdrawn, isolated, unattractive, and a failure. Her social support was minimal. On direct inquiry about suicide ideation, V.B. revealed that she had considered killing herself and the fetus if amniocentesis detected anything seriously wrong
>
> —Green-Simonsen and Peters, 1992; Peters, 1994

In the aforementioned case depression and extreme anxiety is not solely attributable to a genetic diagnosis. Rather, it is more descriptive of the counselee and her psychological makeup. V.B.'s feelings of unattractiveness, sense of failure, and focus on bodily sensation could suggest to us a "self" that may have had limited self-object experiences. The genetic counselor appropriately appreciated that the "self" cohesion may not be strong. News of a fetal aneuploidy could shatter a fragile cohesion. The "self" attempts to regain cohesion through stages of rage. It is difficult to know how the rage will be expressed (verbally or through an act that places the person at risk). Direct questioning of this distressed counselee revealed a fantasy of suicide.

To promote shifts in self understanding and enhancing psychological cohesion the self-psychologist uses the classic psychoanalytic tool of interpretation. What distinguishes Kohut's work is that the interpretations are, in part, derived from empathic attunement with the counselee. The treatment process employs the psychoanalytic concepts of "working through the transference." This step in the analytic process requires long-term counseling during which the counselee begins to see the therapist through transference, a series of interpretations, some of which are empathically derived bring the therapist back into focus. This process aims to bring psychological relief and to increase cohesion of the self (Kohut, 1971, 1977, 1984).

The classic psychoanalytic process does not fit a genetic counseling session, since the sessions are limited. However, Kohut's contributions offer evidence that the counselor's commitment to empathic listening and understanding can lead to a more effective experience. The theory also can assist the counselor in gaining deeper appreciation for the psychological construction of personalities.

Self in Relation Theory

The theoretical work that has emerged since the 1970s from Jean Baker Miller and her colleagues at the Stone Center (Wellesley College, Massachusetts) has had a strong influence on my ability to appreciate what psychological events can promote change within the counselee. The theory presented is derived from the experiences of women. The 1970s and 1980s saw a criticism of psychological theories that attempted to generalize across gender lines and cultural perspectives. The writings of Miller, Gilligan, Belenky, Clinchy, Goldberger, and Tarule set the stage for collaborative discussions on learning from women about their psychological development and dilemmas. What emerged was an evolving theory of "self in relation" that allows for greater appreciation of relational context for women and, not surprisingly, for men as well (Bergman, 1991).

The Stone Center writers argue that the development of "self" emerges from relational interactions with early caregivers and later with others in adult life. Central to their thinking is a de-emphasis of individuation and separation as psychological requirements for ego formation. Further, the ability to respond to critical life events can be influenced by the level of connectedness with self and others. The genetic counselor's ability to "connect" and understand the counselee's connections and disconnections enhances the counseling session. It is through the counselor's empathic understanding of events that led to the disconnections that the counselee begins to experience self-empathy. Self-empathy is a requirement for change or action. In other words, psychological vulnerabilities can be reduced through a process that explores connectedness. This exploration is done from a position of empathic attunement and mutuality. The shifts in psychological tensions are often evidenced in what Jean Baker Miller has termed "zest"; the actions and attitudes that once could not be considered or accomplished become more possible.

In the genetic counseling setting, relational theory assists in appreciating the psychological barriers of men and women who seem to have difficulty determining a course of action. I have also found this work to be very useful in assisting counselees with protracted grief reactions or feeling that they could not participate in a decision process.

The following case is an illustration.

A 33-year-old woman with Treacher Collins syndrome had been followed by the local craniofacial evaluation team since she was 18 years old. At that time she requested surgery to make her feel better. She quickly convinced the medical group with her numerous stories of stares and comments from the public as she rode the bus to work. Susan and her sister made an appointment to see me. The appointment began with Susan reminding me of my role on the craniofacial team and she recalled my discussions with her about Treacher Collins. I asked Susan and her sister what their expectations were from this appointment. I was a bit surprised to learn that they wanted me to provide psychological support to Susan. Susan has been given a diagnosis of mild mental retardation. They were approaching me after not being able to identify a therapist or counseling program in the community that worked with persons with a diagnosis of mental retardation.

After describing our program limitations (during which Susan cried and asked repeatedly why it was so), I made an attempt to understand the basis of Susan's distress. Susan was able to tell me that she had been experiencing what I understood as anxiety and obsessive compulsive behaviors. She also added that she had been having difficulty swallowing so she had been limiting her diet to pudding and mashed potatoes.

I then asked the obvious question, "Have you discussed this with your doctor?" Susan's sister quickly volunteered that Susan would not go to the doctor. I asked Susan to tell me why she did not want to go to the doctor. "She refuses!" added the sister. Her explanations merged her experiences during her complicated cranio-facial surgery, a hysterectomy for dysmenorrhea, and increasing frustrations that her concerns were not being addressed. As she said, "He won't listen!" Susan's sister interrupted with a description of family frustrations with Susan's behavior. It was evident that they were angry. The sister, who is closest in age to Susan, felt that "maybe if she talked to someone it might help."

I concluded the session with an attempt to bridge Susan's medical distrust and the need to offer her some relief from her complaints. I agreed to see Susan again.

The second session did not include the sister. The session was primarily devoted to hearing and appreciating Susan's experience. This was not always simple, as she would find herself in the middle of a story and not be able to complete it. I repeatedly acknowledged how helpful her stories and memories were in understanding why it is so hard to get medical guidance now. Whenever possible, I would introduce the need to make a referral for medical evaluation and the possible role of a medication that might assist in alleviating the symptoms, Susan would cry. She would ask me to promise that I would not make her go. I continued to remind her that she was the person that would make the appointment. The session led to two more. The third session focused on her feeling of "being different" and her sense that "no one listens." I explored with her what would be required for her to make an appointment with her doctor, specifically, social support. The session ended with her saying "Maybe I will go."

The fourth session involved Susan calling the doctor's office and asking that the doctor call her at home first. She thought that she could explain it better if she spoke to him ahead of time. Susan attended that appointment and was given some relief for her symptoms.

This case demonstrates that in the face of family disconnection around her increasing anxiety about medical appointments, Susan's sense of difference and abandonment were heightened. I accepted the challenge of "no one listens" and within several sessions was able to provide empathic attunement that decreased, to some degree, her sense of stigma. This allowed her to appreciate that it was hard to go to her medical appointments and ask for help. This could only be achieved once her self-empathy was encouraged. Susan's request to call for an appointment came out of a sense of connection in the relational context. Finally, this case only hints at the complexity involved in working with counselees with an intellectual impairment. Persons with mild mental retardation "are highly motivated to dissociate themselves from outward signs of incompetence." Until recently, little has been published about the developmental, cognitive, and cultural aspects of persons with mental retardation (Finucane, 1997)

Family System Theories

> Families comprise persons who have a shared history and a shared future
> —McGoldrick and Carter, 2003

The counselee and his/her family are central to all genetic counseling sessions. Our efforts to appreciate the counselee's family bring an important dimension to the genetic counseling process. Families are often complicated in structure, affiliations, boundaries, and relational cohesion. Additionally, the variables in a family change and reconstitute into equally complicated forms. Families also are part of other systems, ethnic, racial, religious, that directly influence construction of meaning of genetic risk and disease (Rolland, 2006). The "family of origin" of our counselee offers lessons of adaption to personal and family challenges. The genetic counseling experience can at times bring into focus family interpersonal dynamics, family systems, and family belief systems that will guide the counselee in decision-making and/or creating meaning for information provided through the genetic counseling experience.

Family systems theories help us "keep in focus" the adaptations of families to critical life events (Feetham and Thomson, 2006). A number of family theorists have offered tools to understand how families respond to normal and critical life events. Having an appreciation of family systems theory offers the counselor a lens to understand communication patterns, responses, and adaptations to events in a family. On occasion, the genetic counseling process and expected decisions may initialize shifts in family patterns and disruptions in communication. Most families are able to restore their functional state; generally, families are resilient.

Family is conceptualized "as an open system that functions in relation to its broader sociocultural context and that evolves over the life cycle" (Walsh, 1982, p. 9). The diversity of family structures and norms requires the counselor to learn about each particular family. It is when hearing their story that an assessment can be made if a family is experiencing a loss of function. This assessment must include an appreciation of family norms that are influenced by society or an ethnic subculture (Walsh, 1982).

Our consideration of the family begins with those present in the room and expands with the pedigree. Families freely share developmental challenges of a child with a recognized genetic condition as families with adult-onset genetic condition share personal meaning about the implications of genetic risk. Our pedigree process illuminates relationships, community, disconnections, and intergenerational interactions. Bringing forth family context into the genetic counseling session informs empathic connections and guides discussion.

In recent years a new way of thinking about families has emerged that assumes that families have the ability to find equilibrium after a disruption. Family resilience theory is based on "a deep conviction in the potential for family recovery and growth out of adversity" (Walsh, 2003). This perspective invites practitioners and families to appreciate that families have inherent strengths in their belief systems, communication and problem solving approaches, patterns of connection and access to community support that foster adaptive responses to challenging events.

Families facing genetic risk and disease share challenges and often demonstrate resilience through adaption, information and family cohesion (Vermaes et al., 2007; Packman et al., 2007; McCubbin et al., 1998; McCubbin et al., 1998; Fanos, 1999; Parker, 1996; Hilbert et al., 2000; Forrest et al., 2007) For most families, resilience is an emergent process, and it is important that genetic counselors appreciate that they may be meeting a family in this process (Patterson, 2002).

Some families require therapeutic interventions when there is a loss of function in the family system. Family therapy theorists such as Murray Bowen, Gregory Bateson, Carl Whitaker, Nathan Ackerman, Virginia Satir, Jay Haley, and Salvador Minuchin emerged in the late 1940s and over the next 50 years described numerous approaches to treating families. More recently, models have merged to assist families with chronic illness, genetic illness, and disease (Mikesell et al., 1995; Rolland and Williams, 2005). All major theories and models of family therapy are based on a central belief that individuals are best understood through family dynamics. In addition, families are viewed as "rule-governed, homeostatic systems". Family rules essentially organize family interactions and maintain stability by prescribing members' behaviors (McGolderick et al., 1989). The family is also considered from a life cycle and hierarchical perspective.

Family systems models have been applied to families seen in genetic counseling practice (Heimler, 1990; Thayer et al., 1990; Eunpu, 1997a; Eunpub; Rolland and Williams, 2005). As the practice of genetic counseling evolves, so do our efforts to apply a broad range of family systems models to understanding our counselee and their families. Additionally, models of family therapy have been adapted for families facing genetic concerns.

Most family therapy models fall into one of three approaches, although some combine approaches.

1. **Strategic Approach**. This approach finds its roots in the work of Milton H. Erickson and Jay Haley, who describe the use of directive therapeutic interventions with families to address current concerns. The therapist determines corrective actions with the goal of changing behavior in the family system (Nichols and Schwartz, 2004).

2. **Structural Approach**. This approach focuses on family structure as the key organizing tenet of functionality and essential to the well-being of family members. Families in crisis can lose their structure and break into subsets. The subsets need to be restructured to return to original family function. Salvador Minuchin argued that families respond to stressors through the support of interfamilial boundaries and the arrangement of power (Nichols and Schwartz, 2004).

3. **Multigenerational Approach**. Family system theorist Murray Bowen described interlocking concepts that include differentiation of the self, family dynamics, and emotions. Relationships to others and to the family are disrupted through unresolved issues within the family of origin and the experience of loss, often intergenerational (Freeman, 1992). The tenets of Bowen's theory are frequently incorporated in new emerging models of family systems.

In the mid-1980s the writings of John Rolland began to describe the family as it addressed the issue of illness over time. Today, this work is known as the **Family Systems-Illness Model.** The model provides a perspective on the interactive processes of psychosocial demand of the illness, family beliefs, and family functioning. The inclusion of belief systems in a family response is essential to facilitate effective coping and adaptation to illness (Kleinman, 1988; Rolland, 1994). This model also considers anticipation of future loss, an experience common to families faced with genetic disease. More recently, this model has been expanded to consider the unique challenges presented by genetic and genomic conditions and the issues that families face with "at-risk" and pre-symptomatic phases of genetic illness. This approach is called the **Family Systems Genetic Illness Model** (Rolland and Williams, 2005). The following case presentation attempts to highlight this.

Lori and Richard were referred to the genetics clinic by her obstetrician after her fourth first-trimester miscarriage. This young couple worked together in her family-owned business. The genetic counseling session identified that Lori's mother had seven successive miscarriages, gave birth to Lori, and then went on to adopt a son. Lori's mother was an only child. Her mother had several miscarriages.

Information was provided about miscarriages and the possible role of a chromosome translocation for the family history. The couple refused chromosome testing since it was evident to them that a pattern existed. As Lori confidently stated, "My mother had seven and then I was born."

Several months passed, and the clinic was contacted to arrange chromosome testing on products of conception for Lori. The analysis revealed an unbalanced translocation. At this point, the couple agreed to testing for themselves. Tests identified Lori as carrying a balanced translocation. The couple continued their optimism since they felt the family pattern had been demonstrated.

Several more miscarriages occurred (with normal karyotypes). The total number of pregnancy losses came to seven. Lori entered her eighth pregnancy with optimism. She would attempt to reassure her less confident husband with statements like "It makes sense that all 'unbalanced' would end in a miscarriage, it already happened to us" and "That's what miscarriages are for." As the pregnancy approached the 16th week of gestation, Lori and Richard requested prenatal testing. The test result identified the fetus as carring an unbalanced translocation. "It wasn't supposed to happen like this: the eighth was going to be okay" (Shapiro and Djurdjinovic, 1990).

"In the face of possible loss, creating meaning for an illness that preserves sense of competency is a primary task for families. In this regard, a family belief about what and who can influence the course of events is fundamental" (Rolland, 1990). Lori's family normalized the multiple, successive pregnancy losses as the pattern that occurs before the birth of a child. There is also a suggestion that after the birth of this child, no other pregnancies are sought. Families are expanded through adoption. As Lori experienced each of her seven losses she could turn to the family belief to find some meaning for her sadness. After the prenatal determination that the eighth pregnancy included an unbalanced translocation, Lori's disbelief went beyond grief into feelings of failure.

Deborah Eunpu presented a model of case formulation, **Systemically Based Psychotherapeutic Technique**, that linked individual, interactional, and intergenerational issues as they may apply to a family with a genetic concern. She advocates that the combined use of the genogram with an intersystem case formulation provides "a thorough psychosocial assessment of the individual and family" (Eunpu, 1997a; p. 10). In utilizing this approach the counselor is able to identify intergenerationally based beliefs and attitudes about a genetic condition. The counselor's knowledge about patterns of communication and relational dynamics offers a genetic counseling experience that is relevant to that family structure and honors their belief system.

Amy is 24 years old and has been followed by the local breast disease center because of fibrocystic breast disease and a family history of early breast cancer. At her last visit with her physician she requested prophylactic mastectomies. A genetics consult was arranged.

Amy attended the first session with an unaffected maternal aunt. The genetic counseling session explored the reason that promoted her request for surgery and her family history. In brief, Amy had three of five maternal aunts who were reported to have breast cancer in their mid 30s. One of the maternal cousins also had been diagnosed in her 30s. The maternal grandmother was initially reported to have had "stomach cancer." Review of medical records confirmed ovarian cancer. Amy's mother was in her 50s and had no history of cancer diagnosis.

In applying the intersystem genogram guidelines to assess health and illness beliefs and attitudes, consider the following:

THE HEALTH/ILLNESS BELIEFS AND ATTITUDES GENOGRAM: APPROPRIATE WHEN THERE IS AN AFFECTED FAMILY MEMBER

1. Who was reported as affected (sick/ill) in your family?
2. Who believed him/herself to be affected?
3. What messages did you receive from family members about the diagnosis?
4. What were the attitudes of family members to those who were/are affected?
5. What obligations or loyalties were created by the presence of an affected family member?
6. What is the meaning of doing something different regarding the genetic risk in your family? (Eunpu, 1997a; p.15)

Pedigree discussions revealed that Amy and her aunt believed that the only way to escape "cancer" was to have the breast removed. Amy went on to report that her mother had prophylactic mastectomies at 34 years of age (this was not disclosed when I asked "has your mother had any history of cancer?") and that the aunt attending the session had prophylactic mastectomies last year when she turned 30 years of age. The aunt told numerous stories of caring for her dying sisters who were 12 to 16 years older than she. She said that "it was stupid not to do this." Amy's mother was the first to take a prophylactic step and they believed that's why she is "cancer free" at 50 years of age. This led the remaining aunts to seek surgery, and now Amy was being encouraged to take this step.

This partial glimpse into this family tells us about an emerging belief about protecting against cancer. The decision to have surgery also protects family ties of survivors. The influences on Amy's decision in part will be based in the unfolding sessions that will explore genetic etiology and testing. The trauma of the surviving sisters (Amy's mother and aunts) has influenced her. This case argues for the value of bringing the "family" together in family cancer discussions. The genetic counselor's ability to engage the survivors in the discussions that are yet to unfold may offer options not yet considered in this family. This case supports the effectiveness of blending the pedigree with principles of the genogram through an intersystem case formulation. Most recently, the pedigree as tool to appreciate a counselee's relational affiliations within family and outside has been offered through the work of Peters et al. (Peters et al., 2004). They demonstrate that the pedigree offers many opportunities to learn about the counselee and family. The roles of genetic counselors and the nature of familial risk invites all genetic counselors to develop an approach to understand "the family" in genetic counseling. To understand your counselee is to "recognize the interdependence among the roles and functions of all family members" (Parke, 2004, p. 366).

MEN IN OUR PRACTICE

Until recently, women and/or children were the primary consultants in our genetic counseling practice. Fathers and husbands have always been valued attendees in a genetic counseling session, but not the primary consultand. Until recently, little has been written to assist genetic counselors in appreciating the "man" in the room. As a result of susceptibility risk assessment and testing and emergence of cardiovascular genetics, men are likely to more often be the primary counselee. In a profession in which the great majority of practitioners are women, it may serve us well to consider what we can learn from our male counselees and what is understood about men seeking help, men in families, men and psychological disposition.

Men's psychological development has been described as development of "self" with goals of autonomy, separation, and individuation. Men in western cultures must also assimilate conflicting social messages about men (Faludi, 1999). The dominant social culture has historically asked men to maintain emotional stoicism and demonstrate autonomy, yet men are raised and function within relational contexts, families, and communities. Some argue that men in western culture, in particular, are asked to take on traditional roles of masculinity and simultaneously challenged to participate more fully in emotional and relational experiences (Englar-Carlson and Shepard, 2005, 2006). As genetic counselors, we need to consider our beliefs about men, men and health, and men in relation to others. A common belief is that men do not ask for help. There is evidence that help seeking has been intertwined with concepts of masculinity. Value is placed on enduring symptoms and not readily seeking medical assistance. Additionally, it appears that the influence of others (partners and spouses) often provides a needed drive to seek help (O'Brien et al., 2005). Little is understood about men in health care settings and their responses to genetic risk and genetic conditions. Men are sometimes experienced by the genetic counselors as "bystanders" or appear to be distant or ambivalent about attending the genetic counseling session. Are they? And if so, what is the reason for this? (Locock and Alexander, 2006; Robson, 2002; Hovey, 2005).

Men of nonwestern dominant cultures can take on roles in the genetic counseling session that can be confusing or unfamiliar as decision makers for their wives, whom we see as our primary counselee (Awwad et al., 2004) We have much to learn about our male counselees. As more men seek genetic counseling for cancer or cardiovascular assessment we need to be skilled in attending to men's risk conceptualization, help seeking skills, ambivalences, adaptions to information, and changes in intrafamilial communication and understanding why (d'Agincourt-Canning, 2006; Metcalfe et al., 2002; Wylie et al., 2003; Liede et al., 2000; Feldman and Broussard, 2006; King et al., 2006). In addition, genetic counselors need to consider personal beliefs about men, masculinity, gender roles, and the counselor's personal ability to find empathic attunement with male counselees.

SUPERVISION: REFINING THE PSYCHOLOGICAL LENS

> Supervision is an essential component of genetic counseling student's professional preparation, providing a vehicle for their clinical skill development and for insuring a standard of patient care. The role of supervision for post graduate counselors is less apparent.
>
> —Zahm et al., 2008

The ability of counselors to master the lens, aperture, and filters of the psychological issues within each session requires an organized analysis of content and experience. All professionals experience an evolution in their skill base and set standards that sometimes cannot be immediately achieved. We all want to feel competent and comfortable. To achieve this goal there needs to be a process by which we confront our awkwardness and our anxiety; "I want to say just the right thing—what is the right thing?" Genetic counselors who are drawn to the psychological aspects of our practice are invited to seek additional reading and training. One learning method that is underutilized in our profession is case supervision. The supervision process ensures a continuing education experience as well as an ongoing dialogue of self awareness about vulnerabilities, tensions, and frustrations that may impact the counselee (Kennedy, 2000; Middleton et al., 2007). These discussions can occur on an individual basis with a clinician recognized to have more experience than the counselor, a colleague, or group supervision (leader or peer). The aim of such a discussion is to guide the counselor to a deeper and more complex understanding of the issues that are presented by the counselee and the personal meaning of the issues to the counselor. It will enhance appreciation of questions raised and responses to them and the conscious or unconscious interpersonal or family dynamics and finally allow counselors to acknowledge themselves as part of the psychological milieu that stimulates a response from the counselee.

Ideally, participation in case discussions should involve many sessions. This allows for extended analysis of a case as well as an opportunity for the counselor to fully appreciate how one's own psychological needs and tensions impact on the cognitive tasks of the genetic counseling session.

In recent years, postgraduate "peer supervision" has emerged with an overall positive response by participating genetic counselors. Genetic counselors seek supervision for a range of reasons that include need for support and need to share a counseling experience with a counselor with more experience, " to dig further"

(Zahm et al., 2008). As our profession matures and as we seek to offer exemplary psychologically attuned genetic counseling, we will need to learn from other psychologically trained professionals. Seeking a supervision group outside of our community of genetic counselors is another way to broaden our perspectives and skill. We could look at other professions that utilize postgraduate supervision and promote use of supervision with an experienced leader and adherence to common group dynamic rules of confidentiality and commitment to explore issues over a period of time. This ensures growth professionally and personally through guidance from group members and an experienced leader in a climate of trust.

Recently, we have been introduced to a concern of "compassion fatigue" among genetic counselors. It has been proposed that this personal struggle can be a by-product of empathic connection in our daily work. Supervision can be a very important tool in fine-tuning our skills in finding "the delicate balance between empathic connection and detachment" (Benoit et al., 2007).

CONCLUSION

A common criticism of psychologically directed genetic counseling is that the growing reality of the "one-time session" prohibits this type of practice. I am troubled by this perspective. Regardless of how often we are able to engage with a counselee, each connection forms the foundation for a psychological dynamic. The degree to which a counselor and patient choose to explore the psychological content within the session will depend on the goals that were mutually set and the skills of the counselor. It is a disservice to the patient to not be fully cognizant of the psychological framework that surrounds the genetic counseling discussions. In a medical climate in which other professionals are seeking roles with families facing genetic testing and diagnosis, it becomes more imperative that genetic counselors demonstrate and remain committed to the full scope of genetic counseling. Time constraints and the role expectations set in the definition of genetic counseling force some counselors to attend to the psychological aspects last, if time is remaining. To see genetic counseling as linear steps in a process inaccurately deconstructs an interactive dynamic where the psychological is parallel to the genetic and medical discussions. In settings in which counselors have the opportunity to meet families with social workers and psychologists, for example, multidisciplinary clinics, genetic counselors must still continue attending to the psychological dynamic. Our mental health colleagues can bring a special richness to the genetic counseling session. But it is only the genetic counselor who provides the unique knowledge base that allows for the unfolding of genetic and medical information in a psychologically attentive way. To distance ourselves from the psychological skills we bring is to lose the core of our professional role.

I am committed to the belief that the vitality and longevity of the genetic counseling profession is very much tied to psychological practice. I am not proposing that we should see ourselves as therapists, only that we remain committed to the earliest visions of our profession, which supports a relationally based process and honors psychological attunement as a tenet of the genetic counseling experience.

REFERENCES

Aalfs CM, Oort FJ, de Haes JCJM, Leshot NJ, Smets EMA (2007) A comparison of counselee and counselor satisfaction in reproductive genetic counseling. *Clin Genet* 72:74–78.

Antley RM (1979) The genetic counselor as facilitator of the counselee's decision process. *Birth Defects Orig Artic Ser* 15(2).

Antley RM, Bringle RG, Kinney KL (1984) Downs syndrome. In: Emery AH, Pullen IM (eds), *Psychological Aspects of Genetic Counseling*. London: Academic Press, pp. 75–94.

Awwad R, McCarthy Veatch P, Bartels DM and LeRoy BS (2008) Culture and acculturation on Palestinian perception of prenatal genetic counseling. *J Genet Couns* 17(1):101–116.

Barbain O A, Christian M (1999) The social and cultural context of coping with Sickle Cell Disease: I. A review of biomedical and psychosocial issues. *J Black Psychol* 25(3)277–293.

Basch MF (1980) *Doing Psychotherapy*. New York: Basic Books.

Basch MF (1988) *Understanding Psychotherapy*. New York: Basic Books.

Bellet PS, Maloney MJ (1991) The importance of empathy as an interviewing skill in medicine. *JAMA* 266(13):1831–1832.

Belenky MF, Clincy BM, Goldberger NR, Tarule JM (1986) *Women's Ways of Knowing: The Development of Self, Voice, and Mind*. New York: Basic Books.

Benoit LG, Veach McCarthy P, LeRoy BS (2007) When you care enough to do your very best: Genetic counselor experiences of compassion fatigue. *J Genet Couns* 16(3)299–312.

Bergman SJ (1991) Men's psychological development: A relational perspective. *Work in Progress, Stone Center Working Paper Series*, Wellesley, MA.

Bernhardt BA (1997) Empirical evidence that genetic counseling is directive: Where do we go from here? *AM J Hum Genet* 60:17–20.

Biesecker BB, Peters KF (2001) Process studies in genetic counseling: Peering into the black box. *Am J Med Genet* 106:191–198.

Blumenthal D (1990/91) When reality differs from expectations. *Perspect Genet Couns* 12(4):3.

Bordin ES (1979) The generalizability of the psychoanalytic concept of the working alliance. *Psychother Theory Res Prac* 16(3):252–260.

Bordin ES (1982) A working alliance based model of supervision. *Couns Psychologist* 11:35–42.

Bovee A (2007) *Personal Communication*. Binghamton, NY: Ferre Institute.

Bowlby J (1980) *Loss, Sadness and Depression*. New York: Basic Books.

Brock SC (1995) Narrative and medical genetics: On ethics and therapeutics. *Qual Health Res* 5(2):150–168.

Buckman R (1992) *How to Break Bad News*. Baltimore: Johns Hopkins University Press.

Chapple A, May C, Campion P (1995) Parental guilt: The part played by the clinical geneticist. *J Genet Couns* 4(3):179–192.

Charles S, Kessler L, Stopher JE, Domcheck S Hughes Halbert C (2006) Satisfaction with genetic counseling for BRCA1 and BRCA2 mutations among African American women. *Patient Educ Couns* 63:196–204.

Corgan RL (1979) Genetic Counseling and parental self-concept change. *Birth Defects Orig Artic Ser* 15(5C):281–285.

d'Agincourt-Canning L (2006) A gift or a yoke? Women's and men's responses to genetic information from BRCA1 and BRCA 2 testing. *Clin Genet* 70:462–472.

Dillard JP, Shen L, Tluczek A, Modaff P, Farrell P (2007) The effect of disruptions during counseling on recall of genetic information: The case of cystic fibrosis. *J Genet Couns* 16(2):179–190.

Djurdjinovic, L (1997) Generations lost: A psychological discussion of a cancer genetics case report. *J Genet Couns* 6(2):177–180.

Donahue PJ, Siegel ME (2005). *Are You Listening? Keys to Successful Communication.* Norte Dame, IN: Sorin Book, p. 196.

DudokdeWit AC, Tibben A, Frets PG, Meijers-Heijboer EJ, Devilee P, Kiljn JG et al. (1997). BRCA 1 in the family: A case description of psychological implications. *Am J Med Genet* 71:63–71.

Englar-Carlson, M., & Shepard, D.S. (2005) Engaging men in couples counseling: Strategies for overcoming ambivalence and inexpressiveness. *The Family Journal,* 13, 383–391.

Englar-Carlson, M., & Stevens, M. (Eds.). (2006) *In the room with men: A casebook of therapeutic change.* Washington, DC: American Psychological Association.

Etchegary H (2006) Discovering the family history of Huntington's Disease. *J Genet Couns* 15(2):105–117.

Eunpu DL (1997a) Generations lost: A cancer genetics report commentary. *J Genet Couns* 6(2):176.

Eunpu DL (1997b) Systemically-based psychotherapeutic technique in genetic counseling. *J Genet Couns* 6(1):1–20.

Faludi S (ed) (1999) *Stiffed: The Betrayal of the American Man.* Harper Collins.

Fanos JH (1999) "My crooked vision": The well sib views ataxia-telangectasia. *Am J Med Genet* 87(5):420–425.

Feetham SL, Thomson EJ (2006) Keeping the Individual and family in focus. In: Miller SM, McDaniel SH, Rolland JS, Feetham SL (eds), *Individuals, Families, and the New Era of Genetics: Biosychosocial Perspectives.* New York: WW Norton and Co.

Feldman BN, Broussard CA (2006) Men's adjustment to their partners' breast cancer: A didactic coping perspective. *Health Soc Work* 31(2):117–127.

Fine B (1993) The evolution of nondirectiveness in genetic counseling and implications of the Human Genome Project. In: Bartels DM, LeRoy BS, Caplan AL (eds), *Prescribing Our Future. Ethical Challenges in Genetic Counseling.* Chicago: Aldine De Gruyer, pp. 101–117.

Fine BA, Baker DL, Fiddler MB,ABGC Consensus Development Consortium (1996) Practice-based competencies for accreditation of and training in graduate programs in genetic counseling. *J Genet Couns* 5(3):113–121.

Finucane B (1997) Acculturation in women with mental retardation and its impact on genetic counseling. *J Genet Couns* 7(1):31–47.

Forrest Keenan K, Miedzybrodzka Z, van Teijlingen E, Mckee L, Simpson SA (2007) Young people's experience of growing up in a family affected by Huntington's disease. *Clin Genet* 71:120–129.

Fox M, Weil J, Resta R (2007) Why we do what we do: Commentary on a reciprocal-engagement model of genetic counseling practice. *J Genet Couns* 16:729–730.

Frans J. M. Grosfeld, Cees J. M. Lips, Frits A. Beemer and Herman F. J. ten Kroode (2000) Who Is at Risk for Psychological Distress in Genetic Testing Programs for Hereditary Cancer Disorders? *Journal of Genetic Counseling* 9(3):253–266.

Frazer FC (1976) Current concepts in genetics: Genetics as a health care service. *N Engl J Med* 295:486–488.

Freeman D.S (1992) *Multigenerational Family Therapy*. Haworth Press, New York.

Gilligan C (1982) *In a Different Voice: Psychological Theory and Women's Development*. Cambridge, MA: Harvard University Press.

Goffman E (1963) *Stigma*. Englewood Cliffs, NJ: Prentice-Hall.

Goldstein WN (2000) The transference in psychotherapy: The old vs. the new vs. dynamic. *Am J Psychotherapy* 54(2):167–171.

Goodman JF, Abrams EZ (1988) Giving bad news to parents. In: Ball S (ed), *Strategies in Genetic Counseling*, Vol 1.New York: Human Sciences Press, pp. 137–154.

Gratz H (1997) Personal communication.

Graybar SR, Leonard LM (2005) In defense of listening. *Am J Psychotherapy* 59(1):1–18.

Greene-Simonsen DM, Peters J (1992) A successful blending of genetic counseling and psychotherapy. *Perspect Genet Couns* 14(2):5.

Greenspan M (2003) *Healing Through the Dark Emotions: The Wisdom of Grief, Fear and Despair*. Boston: Shabhala Publications.

Guest F (1997) Giving bad news. Presented at Trends I Health Care, Scottsdale, AZ.

Hand-Mauser ME (1989) Techniques in systemic family therapy: Application for genetic counseling. In: Ball S (ed), *Strategies in Genetic Counseling*, Vol 2.New York: Human Sciences Press, pp. 93–120.

Hecht I, Holmes LB (1972) What we don't know about genetic counseling. *N Engl J Med* 287:464.

Heimler A (1990) Group counseling for couples who have terminated a pregnancy following prenatal diagnosis. *Birth Defects Orig Artic Ser* 26(3):161–167.

Hilbert G, Walker M., Rinehardt J (2000). " In it for the long haul": Responses of a parents caring for children with Sturge-Weber syndrome. *J Fam Nurs* 6:157–179.

Ho A (2008) Using family members as interpreters in the clinical setting. *J Clin Ethics* 19(3):223–233.

Hobdell E, Deatrick JA (1996) Chronic sorrow: A content analysis of parental differences. *J Genet Couns* 5(2):57–68.

Hovey J (2005) Fathers parenting chronically ill children: Concerns and coping strategies. *Issues Comprehensive Pediatric Nurs* 28:83–95.

Hughes C, Lerman C, Schwartz M, Peshkin B, Wenzel L, Narod S, Corio C, Tercyak K, Hanna D, Issac C, Main D (2002) All in the family: Evaluation process and content of sister's communication about BRCA 1 and BRCA 2 genetic test results. *Am J Med Genet* 107:143–150.

Ives EJ, Henick P, Levers MI (1979) The malformed newborn: Telling the parents. *Birth Defects Orig Artic Ser* 15(5C):223–231.

James CA, Hadley DW, Holtzman NA, Winklestein JA (2006) How does the mode of inheritance of a genetic condition influence families? A study of guilt, blame, stigma, and understanding of inheritance and reproductive risks in families with X-linked and autosomal recessive diseases. *Genet Med* 8(4):234–42.

Jordan JV (1991a) *Empathy and self boundaries*. In: Jordan JV, Kaplan AG, Miller JB, Stiver IP, Surrey JL (eds), *Women's Growth in Connection*. New York: Guilford Press, pp. 67–80.

Jordan JV (1991b) Empathy, mutuality, and therapeutic change: Clinical implications of a relational model. In: Jordan JV, Kaplan AG, Miller JB, Stiver IP, Surrey JL (eds), *Women's Growth in Connection*. New York: Guilford Press, pp. 283–289.

Jordan JV, Surrey JL, Kaplan AG (1991) Women and empathy: Implications for psychological development and psychotherapy. In: Jordan JV, Kaplan AG, Miller JB, Stiver IP, Surrey JL (eds), *Women's Growth in Connection*. New York: Guilford Press, pp. 27–28.

Kay E, Kinsgton H (2002) Feelings associated with being a carrier and characteristics of reproductive decision making in women known to carriers of X linked conditions. *J Health Psychol* 7(2)169–181.

Kenen RH, Smith ACM (1995) Genetic Counseling for the next 25 years: Models for the future. *J Genet Couns* 4(2):115–124.

Kennedy A (1997) Personal communication.

Kennedy AL 2000 Supervision for practicing genetic counselors: An overview of models. *J Genet Couns* 9:379–397.

Kessler S (1979) *Genetic Counseling*. New York: Academic Press.

Kessler S (1992a) Psychological aspects of genetic counseling. VII. Thoughts of directiveness. *J Genet Couns* 1:9–17.

Kessler S (1992b) Psychological aspects of genetic counseling. VIII. Suffering and countertransference. *J Genet Couns* 1(4):303–308.

Kessler S (1992c) Process issues in genetic counseling. *Birth Defects Orig Artic Ser* 28(1):1–10.

Kessler S, Kessler H, Ward P (1984) Psychological aspects of genetic counseling. III. Management of guilt and shame. *Am J Med Gent* 17:673–697.

Kessler S (1996) Presentation to the annual education meeting of the National Society of Genetic Counselors, San Francisco, CA.

Kim KS (1999) A systems approach to genetic counseling for albinism. *J Genet Couns* 8(1):47–56.

King KM, Thomlinson E, Sanguins J, LeBlanc P (2006) Men and women managing coronary artery disease risk: Urban-rural contrasts. *Soc Sci Med* 62(5):1091–102.

Kirschenbaum H, Henderson VL (eds) (1989) *The Carl Rogers Reader*. Boston: Houghton Mifflin.

Kleinman A (1988) *The Illness Narratives*. New York: Basic Books.

Knafi KA, Knafi GJ, Gallo AM, Angst D (2007) Parents perception of functioning in families having a child with a genetic condition. *J Genet Couns* 16(4):481–492.

Kohut H (1971) *The Analysis of the Self*. New York: International Universities Press.

Kohut H (1977) *The Restoration of the Self*. New York: International Universities Press.

Kohut H (1984) *How Does Psychoanalysis Cure?* Chicago: University of Chicago Press.

Kubler-Ross E (1969) *On Death and Dying*. New York: Macmillan.

Lazarus RS (1991) *Emotion and Adaptation*. New York: Oxford University Press.

Leon IG (1990) *When a Baby Dies*. New Haven, CT: Yale University Press.

Lerman C (1997) Psychological aspects of genetic testing: Introduction to the special issue. *Health Psychol* 16(1):3–7.

Levine C (1979) Genetic Counseling: The client's viewpoint. *Birth Defects Orig Artic Ser* 15(2):123–135.

Liede A, Metcafe K, Hanna D, Hoodfar E, Snyder C, Durham C, Lynch HT, Narod SA (2000) Evalauation of the needs of male carriers of mutations in BRCA 1 or BRCA 2 who have undergone genetic counseling. *Am J Hum Genet* 67:1494–1504.

Locock L, Alexander J (2006) "Just a Bystander"? Men's place in the process of fetal screening and diagnosis. *Soc Sci Med* 62(6):1349–1359.

Lubinsky MS (1994) Bearing bad news: Dealing with mimics of denial. *J Genet Couns* 3(1):5–12.

Marteau T, Richards M (eds) (1996) *The Troubled Helix: Social and Psychological Implications of the New Human Genetics.* Cambridge: Cambridge University Press.

Marteau, TM., Croyle, RT (1998). The new genetics psychological responses to genetic testing. *BMJ* 316(7132):693–696.

Mast MS, Kindlimann A, Langewitz W (2005) Recipents' perspective on breaking bad news: How you put it really makes a difference. *Patient Education and Counseling* 58:244–251.

Matloff ET (1997) Generations lost: A cancer genetics case report. *J Genet Couns* 6(2):169–180.

McCarthy Veatch P, Bartels DM and LeRoy BS (2007). Coming full circle: a reciprocal-engagement model of genetic counseling practice. *J Genet Couns* 16:713–728.

McCubbin H, Thompson E, Thomson A, Futrell J (eds) (1998) *Resiliency in Ethnic minority Families: African American Families.* Thousand Oaks, CA: Sage.

McCubbin H, Thompson E, Thomson A, Fromer J (eds) (1998) *Resiliency in Ethnic Minority Families: Native and Immigrant American Families.* Thousand Oaks, CA: Sage.

McDaniel SH, Campbell TL (1999) Genetic testing and families (editorial). *Fam Syst Health* 17(1)1–3.

McDaniel SH (2005) The psychotherapy of genetics. *Fam Process* 44(1):25–44.

McGoldrick M, Gerson R (1985) *Genograms in Family Assessments.* New York: Norton.

McGoldrick M, Anderson CM, Walsh F (eds) (1989) *Women in Families.* New York: Norton.

McGoldrick M, Carter B (2003) The family life cycle. In: Walsh F (ed)., *Normal Family Process* (3rd ed). New York: Guildford Press.

Meiser B (2005) Psychological impact of genetic testing for cancer susceptibility: An update of the literature. *Psychooncology* 14:1060–1074.

Metcalfe KA, Liede A, Trinkaus M, Hanna D, Narod SA (2002) Evaluation of the needs of spouses of female carriers of mutations in BRCA 1 and BRCA2. *Clin Genet* 62:464–469.

Michie S, Mareau TM, Bobrow M (1996) Genetic Counseling: The psychological impact of meeting patients' expectations. *J Med Genet* 34(3):237–241.

Michie S, Bron F, Bobrow M, Marteau TM (1997) Nondirectiveness in genetic counseling: An empirical study. *Am J Hum Genet* 60:40–47.

Middleton A, Crowley L, Clarke A (2007) Reflections on the experience of counseling supervision by a team of genetic counselors from the UK. *J Genet Couns* 16:143–155.

Mikesell R.H, Lusterman D.D, McDaniels S.H. (eds) (1995). *Integrating family therapy: Handbook of family psychology and systems theory* Washington DC, American Psychological Association.

Miller JB (1976) *Towards a New Psychology of Women.* Boston: Beacon Press.

Miller JB (1991a) The development of women's sense of self. In: Jordan JV, Kaplan AG, Miller JB, Stiver IP, Surrey JL (eds), *Women's Growth in Connection*. New York: Guilford Press, pp. 11–26.

Miller JB (1991b) The construction of anger in women and men. In: Jordan JV, Kaplan AG, Miller JB, Stiver IP, Surrey JL (eds), *Women's Growth in Connection*. New York: Guilford Press, pp. 181–196.

Miller JB, Stiver IP (1997) *The Healing Connection: How Women Form Relationships in Therapy and in Life*. Boston: Beacon Press.

Miller SM, McDaniel, SH, Rolland JS and Feetham SL (2006) Individuals, Families and the New Era of Genetics New York W. W. Norton and Co.

Money J (1994) *Sex Errors of the Body and Related Syndromes: A Guide to Counseling Children, Adolescents and Their Families* (2nd ed). Baltimore: Paul H. Brookes.

Nichols, M., & Schwartz, R. (2004) *Family therapy: Concepts and methods*, (7th edition). Allyn and Bacon, Boston.

O'Brien RO, Hunt K, Hart G 2005 "Its caveman stuff, but that is to a certain extent how guys still operate": men's accounts of masculinity and help seeking. *Soc Sci Med* 61:503–516.

Packman W, Henderson SL, Mehta I, Ronen R, Danner D, Chesterman B, Packman S (2007) Psychological issues in families affected by maple syrup urine disease. *J Genet Couns* 16:799–809.

Pargament KI (1997) *The Psychology of Religion and Coping: Theory, Research, Practice*. New York: Guilford Press.

Parker M (1996) Families caring of chronically ill children with tuberous sclerosis complex. *Fam Commun Health* 19:73–84.

Parke Ross D (2004) Development of the family. *Annu Rev Psychol* 55:365–399.

Parkes CM, Laungani P, Young B (1997) *Death and Bereavement Across Cultures*. London: Routledge.

Pealy HL, Hooker GW, Kassem L, Biesecker BB (2009) Family risk and related education and counseling needs: perceptions of adults with bipolar disorder and siblings of adults with bipolar disorder. *Am J Med Genet A*. 149(3):364–71.

Peters J (1993) Interface of genetic counseling and psychotherapy: Take back the hour! Unpublished.

Peters J (1994) Suicide prevention in the genetic counseling context. *J Genet Couns* 3 (3):199–213.

Peters J (1997) Personal communication.

Peters JA, Kenen R, Guisti R, Loud J, Weismman N, Greene MH (2004) Exploratory study for the feasibility and utility of colored eco-genetic relationship map (CEGRM) in women at high genetic risk for developing breast cancer. *Am J Med Genet* 130A(3):258.

Petterson JM (2002) Understanding family resilence. *J Clin Psychol* 58(3):233–248.

Pieterse AH, Ausems MG, Van Dulmen AM, Beemer FA, Bensing JM (2005) *Am J Med Genet A* 137(1):27–35.

Preloran HM, Browner CH, Lieber E (2005) Impact of interpreter's approach on Latina's use of amniocentesis. *Health Education Behavior* 32(5):599–612.

Quaid KA, Sims S I, Swensom MM, Harrison JM, Moskowitz C, Stepanov N, Suter GW, Westphal BJ (2008) Living at risk: Concealing risk and preserving hope in Huntington disease. *J Genet Couns* 17(1):117–128.

Reed SC (1955) *Counseling in Medical Genetics.* Philadephia PA: WB Saunders.

Rees G. et al. (2006) A Qualitative Study of Health Professionals' Views Regarding Provision of Information About Health-Protective Behaviors During Genetic Consultation for Breast Cancer. *Journal of Genetic Counseling,* Vol.15, No. 2, pp. 95–104.

Resta RG (ed) (2000) Psyche and helix: psychological aspects of genetic counseling. In: *Essays by Seymour Kessler.* New York: Wiley-Liss.

Resta RG (2006) Defining and redefining the scope and goals of genetic counseling. *Am J Med Genet C Semin Med Genet* 142C:269–275.

Resta RG, Biesecker BB, Bennett RL, Blum S, Hahn SE, Strecker MNet al. (2006). A new definition of genetic counseling: National society of genetic counselors' task force report. *J Genetic Couns* 15(2):77–83.

Robson F (2002) "Yes! A chance to tell my side of the story": A case study of a male partner of a woman undergoing termination of pregnancy for foetal abnormality. *J Health Psychol* 7:183–193.

Rogers CR (1942) *Counseling and Psychotherapy: New Concepts in Practice.* Boston: Houghton Mifflin.

Rolland JS (1990) Anticipatory loss: A family systems developmental framework. *Fam Process* 29(3):229–244.

Rolland JS (1994) *Families, Illness, and Disability.* New York: Basic Books.

Rolland JS, Williams JK (2005) Toward a biopsychosocial model for the21st century genetics. *Fam Process* 44(1):3–24.

Rolland JS (2006) Genetics, family system and multicultural influences. *Fam Syst Health* 24(4):425–442.

Rosenwald GC, Ochberg RL (eds) (1992) *Storied Lives.* New Haven, CT: Yale University Press.

Roter D, Ellington L, Hambey Erby L, Larson S, Dudley W (2006). The genetic counseling video project: Models of practice. *Am J Med Genet C Semin Med Genet* 142C:209–220.

Shapiro HC (1993) *When Part of the Self Is Lost: Helping Clients Heal After Sexual and Reproductive Losses.* San Francisco: Jossey-Bass.

Shapiro HC, Djurdjinovic L (1990) Understanding our infertile genetic counseling patient. *Birth Defects Orig Artic Ser* 26(3):127–132.

Smith JA, Brewer Hm, Eatough V, Stanley CA, Glendinning NW, Quarrell OWJ (2006) The personal experience of juvenile Huntington's disease:an interpretative phenomenological analysis of parents' accounts of the primary features of a rare genetic condition. *Clin Genet* 69:486–496.

Smith RW, Antley RM (1979) Anger: A significant obstacle to informed decision making in genetic counseling. *Birth Defects Orig Artic Ser* 15(5C):257–260.

Sobel S, and Cowan CB (2003) Ambiguous loss and disenfranchised grief: the impact of DNA predictive testing n a family as a system. *Fam Process* 42(1)47–57.

Sorenson JR, Swazey JP, Scotch NA (1981) Effective genetic counseling: Discussing client questions and concerns. *Birth Defects Orig Artic Ser* 17(4):51–77.

Spinelli E (2001) Listening to our clients: A dangerous proposal. *Am J Psychotherapy* 55(3):357–363.

Surrey JL (1991) The self-in-relation: A theory of women's development. In: Jordan JV, Kaplan AG, Miller JB, Stiver IP, Surrey JL (eds), *Women's Growth in Connection.* New York: Guilford Press, pp. 51–66.

Swinford A, Phelps L, Mather J (1988) Countertransference in the counseling setting. *Perspect Genet Couns* 10(3):1–4.

Targum SD (1981) Psychotherapeutic considerations in genetic counseling. *Am J Med Genet* 8:281–289.

Tercyak KP, Johnson SB, Roberts SF, Cruz AC (2001) Psychological response to prenatal genetic counseling and amniocentesis. *Patient Educ Couns* 43:73–84.

Thayer B, Braddock B, Spitzer K, Irons M, Miller W, Bailey I, Rosenbaum B, Blatt RJR (1990) Development of a peer support system for those who have chosen pregnancy termination after prenatal diagnosis of a fetal abnormality. *Birth Defects Orig Artic Ser* 26(3):149–156.

Tichenor V, Hill CE (1989) A comparison of six measures of working alliance. *Psychotherapy* 26(2):195–199.

Vermaes Ignace P.R., Gerris JRM, Janssens JMAM (2007) Parent's social adjustment in families of children with spina bifida: A theory driven review. *J Pediatric Psychol* 32(10):1214–1226.

Wachbroit R, Wasserman D (1995) Clarifying the goals of nondirective genetic counseling. *Rep Inst Philos Public Policy* 15(2,3):1–6.

Walsh F (1982) *Normal Family Processes*. New York: Guilford Press.

Walsh F (2003) Family resilience: strengths forged through adversity. In: Walsh F (ed), *Normal Family Process* (3rd ed) New York: Guildford Press, p. 401.

Walsh F (2003) Family resilience: A framework for clinical practice. *Fam Process* 42(1):1–18.

Weil J (1991) Mother's postcounseling belief about causes of their children's genetic disorders. *Am J Hum Genet* 48:145–153.

Weil J, Mittman I (1993) A teaching framework for cross cultural genetic counseling. *J Genet Couns* 2(3):159–169.

Weil J (2000) *Psychosocial Genetic Counseling*. New York: Oxford University Press.

Weil J (2003) Psychosocial genetic counseling in the post-non directive era: A Point of view. *J Genet Couns* 12:199–211.

Weil J, Ormond K, Peters J, Peters K, Biesecker BB, Leroy B (2006) The relationship of nondirectiveness to genetic counseling: Report of a workshop at the 2003 NSGC Annual Education Conference. *J Genetic Couns* 15(2):85–93.

Whipperman-Bendor L (1996/1997) Nondirectiveness: Redefining our goals and methods. *Perspect Genet Couns* 9(4):1, 9.

Wolf ES (1979) Transferences and countertransferences in the analysis of disorders of the self. *Contemp Psychoanal* 15(3):577–594.

Wolf ES (1988) *Treating the Self*. New York: Guilford Press.

Wolff G, Jung C (1995) Genetic counseling in practice: Nondirectiveness and genetic counseling. *J Genet Couns* 4(1):3–26.

Wylie JE, Smith KR, Botkin JR (2003) Effect of spouces on distress experienced by BRCA I mutation carriers over time. *Am J Med Genet* 119 C(1)35–44.

Zahm KW, Veatch McCarthy P and LeRoy BS (2008) An investigation of genetic counselors experiences in peer group supervision. *J Genetic Couns* 17(3):220–233.

6

Patient Education

Ann C.M. Smith, M.A., D.Sc.(Hon), C.G.C. and Toni I. Pollin, M.S., Ph.D., C.G.C.

Ours is an era in which patients seek greater engagement in health care choices, increasing the demand for high-quality information about clinical options.
—Woolf, 2005

It is often said that knowledge is power. For individuals affected by or at risk for a genetic condition, having adequate knowledge or access to knowledge about a specific diagnosis, including its etiology and management implications, gives one the power to respond to one's own life situation. Patients who are struggling with basic questions, uncertainties, and/or confusing information may have difficulty understanding their situation and seeking help.

Genetic counselors are often the health care professionals who first begin the discussions of the underlying genetic basis for a condition and provide insight about implications for the individual and other family members regarding current health concerns and future reproductive planning. *What* is said and *how* information is presented during the early genetic counseling sessions can have a significant impact on a person's or a family's ability to process, understand, and assimilate information into their own personal life circumstances. However, the very nature of genetic counseling often places the counselor in the role of delivering "bad news" or information that families want but are also apprehensive of hearing. The challenge is to communicate such genetic information in a climate that is supportive and culturally sensitive and encourages individual autonomy in decision-making.

A Guide to Genetic Counseling, Second Edition, Edited by Wendy Uhlmann, Jane Schuette, and Beverly Yashar
Copyright © 2009 by John Wiley & Sons, Inc.

Communication is the cornerstone of genetic counseling, as outlined in its early definition in 1975: "Genetic counseling is a *communication* process which deals with the human problems associated with the occurrence or risk of occurrence of a genetic disorder in a family" (ASHG Adhoc Committee, 1975). A variety of media are used to communicate—the spoken word, writing, graphics, pictures, video, and the Internet.

Inherent to communicating about genetics is overcoming a number of barriers that can interfere with a client's understanding of the genetic information. By its very nature, genetic information is often complex and highly technical, with a lexicon or vocabulary of its own. Individuals and families dealing with genetic disease must assimilate large amounts of new information that is often complicated and abstract. Many late-onset genetic conditions, such as cancer and Huntington disease, evoke a variety of feelings of fear, anxiety, or depression that may hinder the genetic counseling process itself. Similarly, the unexpected birth of a child with birth defects often precipitates a cascade of psychosocial reactions (e.g., denial, anger, grief) that affect not only the parents' readiness to hear but also how much they can hear. Culture, beliefs, and traditions also impact a person's perception and understanding of biology and genetics and may conflict with long-held personal beliefs.

In 2003, the National Society of Genetic Counselors adopted a new definition of genetic counseling, "Genetic counseling is the process of *helping* people understand and adapt to the medical, psychological, and familial implications of genetic contributions to the disease" (NSGC Definition Task Force, 2006). This chapter focuses on how the genetic counselor serves as an instructor during the genetic counseling process, highlighting the essential tools used to communicate technical information in a way that ultimately fosters informed decision-making. An understanding of the ways in which adults learn and the use of effective tools for communication can enhance the education process. When coupled with compassion, empathy, and sensitivity to ethnocultural values, the genetics encounter moves from a simple educational contact to the multifaceted practice of genetic counseling.

SHARING EXPERTISE

The practical definition of *expertise* according to Wlodkowski (1993) involves three essential elements: We know something beneficial; we know it well; and we are prepared to convey it through an instructional process. As instructors, genetic counselors are uniquely trained to integrate knowledge from the fields of medicine, human genetics, and psychology. This skill permits them to communicate their knowledge about genetic conditions in terms that can be more clearly understood and are likely to have practical applications for the family.

There is no substitute for knowing a topic inside and out. However, experts in many fields often make the classic mistake of believing that knowing a lot about a subject means they can automatically teach it effectively. Before sharing your expertise with your patients, consider the following:

- We should ask ourselves if we understand WHAT we are going to educate families about.

- Can we explain it in our own words?
- Is there more than one example—a story, fact, research finding, or analogy—that would be useful in explaining a particular genetic concept?
- Are there any visual aids (pictures, diagrams, etc.) that are effective in demonstrating the concept?
- Do we know what we don't know and feel comfortable admitting it?

Counselees don't expect us to know everything—but they desire an honest explanation of what is known. Human genetics is rapidly changing, requiring counselors to continually keep abreast of new information of relevance to their patients. Given the rarity of many genetic conditions, maintaining up-to-date knowledge of every possible condition is virtually impossible; however, having the skills and ability to access the most current information is critical and essential!

Four characteristics of a skilled and motivating instructor that help to enhance adult learning are defined by Wlodkowski (1993): expertise, empathy, enthusiasm, and clarity. These have particular relevance to genetic counselors and can be learned and improved upon through continued practice and effort. Just as musicians perfect their singing repertoire or orchestral talents through dedicated training and practice, genetic counselors can also perfect these four skill areas.

Wlodkowski (1993) views *empathy* as the most important psychological process inherent in communication. In the context of genetic counseling the counselor must not only have a realistic understanding of the counselee's needs and expectations, but also be able to provide information in a context that is appropriate to the counselee's level of experience and skill development and respects the learner's perspective. Building on a foundation of *expertise* and empathy, the *enthusiastic* instructor values the subject matter and demonstrates her commitment to the topic with appropriate degrees of emotion, animation and energy, which in turn serve to motivate the learner. *Clarity* reflects the language used and how it is organized to ensure that the counselee can comprehend the information being presented.

Information should be conveyed through an instructional process preceded by intensive preparation and organization of materials. A well-prepared counselor can display a relaxed familiarity with a specific genetic condition or area of information. Preparation permits us to spend most of our time looking at the learner/couple and talking with them—not to them! Rather than lecturing to the client, the counselor seeks to facilitate a two-way give-and-take communication flow. For novice genetic counselors this may feel awkward, given the amount of information that needs to be gathered and shared. Yet the ability to do several things at once (think, observe, ask questions, construct a pedigree, give feedback, etc.) must be mastered. Student genetic counselors may tend to keep their eyes glued to intake sheets, notes, and/or templates for pedigree construction, rather than on the patient.

ADULT LEARNERS

In communicating about genetics, genetic counselors take on the role of instructors, sharing their expertise with patients, parents, and other family members. The methods of educating adults differ from those of teaching children. In contrast to younger students, who are motivated by external pressures from parents and teachers, adult learners are motivated by internal factors such as self-esteem, recognition, and better quality of life (Knowles, 1973; 1980). Adults are generally motivated to learn and seek out information for specific reasons; they are often goal-oriented and pragmatic, seeking information to solve problems, build new skill sets, pursue job advancement, or make decisions (Cross, 1981). Recognition and understanding of different learning styles is critical for counselors to be successful instructors. Learning styles, which are typical ways of feeling, behaving, and processing information in a learning situation, change over a person's life span (Hyman and Rosoff, 1984; Kuznar et al. 1991).

Individual learning styles differ from person to person and are influenced by education level, intelligence, personality, personal experiences, culture, and sensory and cognitive preferences (Collins, 2004). These styles can be conceived of as different "learning intelligences," which include: linguistic, logical and mathematical, spatial (perception of objects via senses), kinesthetic, intrapersonal, interpersonal, musical, and naturalistic (Collins, 2004). Another conception considers the experience of learning as analogous to the six strings of a guitar, representing six learning capabilities: (1) rational; (2) emotional; (3) relational; (4) physical; (5) metaphoric; and (6) spiritual."Activation" or playing more than one string (a chord) is likely to have a more significant impact on the learning experience than a single string (Boud and Griffin, 1987).

Instructors working with adults should consider what the learner's motivation is for seeking information and what the learner already knows. Failure to connect the knowledge or information to the daily needs and life of the learner does not permit a bridge for common understanding.

MODELS OF ADULT LEARNING

We are all guilty of trying to teach as we have been taught—and in the historical pedagogical model, it is the teacher who decides what will be taught and delivers the lecture; the student is expected to be ready to listen, absorb, and learn what the instructor lectures about. A parallel can be drawn between this model of learning and the biomedical model of physician-patient interaction. For both, the relationship is asymmetrical, with the teacher/physician taking a dominant role, controlling the interaction by asking questions and initiating topics for discussion. In the context of the biomedical model, emphasis is placed on communicating technical information rather than on how it is understood or acted upon.

Educators have suggested at least three better ways to instruct adults: (1) treating the adult student as a partner in the learning process; (2) building and placing value on previous learning and life experiences; and (3) promoting personal direction and control of learning. Malcolm Knowles, considered by many to be the grandfather of adult education, has written extensively about the adult as a self-directed learner and offers the androgogical or adult model of learning (Knowles, 1973, 1980). Contrary to the traditional or pedagogical model in which the learner is dependent, with little experience of value, Knowles' model is characterized by a learner who is self-directed and whose experience becomes a resource to be used, valued, and accepted. The "readiness" to learn stems from a need to know or do something rather than a requirement for advancement. Genetic counseling practice adheres to the principles of Knowles' model of adult learning, viewing the counselee's life experience, attitudes, and needs as important to the genetic counseling process.

Kenen and Smith (1995) suggest two models stemming from the sociological literature with major relevance to this discussion: the life history or narrative model and the mutual participation model. Under the **life history/narrative model** described by Mishler (1986), counselor and counselee possess dual roles: The counselor is both interviewer and listener, and the counselee is both respondent and narrator. The main focus for the counselor is to listen actively to the stories that the counselee narrator is telling. The interaction recognizes and values the client's beliefs and cognitive perceptions and fosters client power. Under this model, the counselor is interested in *themal* coherence, that is, how utterances express a client's recurrent assumptions, beliefs, and goals or cognitive world (Mishler, 1986). The counselor—as interviewer and listener—actively enters the counselee's storytelling by the form and intent of questions asked, assessments made, acknowledgments, and silences.

The **mutual participation model** (Szasz and Hollender, 1956) is premised on the idea that the counselor and counselee have approximately equal power as adults; are mutually interdependent; and engage in activity that will be satisfying to both. Under this model, the counselor assists the patient/counselee to help him/herself, thereby enhancing rather than narrowing autonomy. Counselor and counselee work as equal partners in seeking solutions, with free give and take, permitting clarification of information about genetic facts as well as the psychological, social, and cultural determinants. The interaction is of one adult with another. These two models complement each other during the natural flow of the counseling session. As the genetic counselor seeks to develop rapport with the counselee during the information-gathering phase, the life history/narrative model may have primacy in the counselor's approach, yielding later to a mutual participation model as the counselor seeks to promote the counselee's autonomy.

GENETIC COUNSELING IN THE INFORMATION AGE

The role of genetic counselors in the provision of information has shifted in the past decade. Whereas previously patients lacking a medical background were likely to receive information in the clinical setting, the availability of the Internet has made it possible for patients to have unprecedented access to an overwhelming abundance of information from a variety of sources from lay-authored publications to peer-reviewed.

This information availability is an opportunity in that it has the potential to create informed consumers, but also a challenge in that it has the potential to spread misinformation that could be useless or even harmful. Importantly, patients have access to original research, with many journals providing free access to some material and authors encouraged to make final manuscripts of all NIH-funded projects available online in accordance with the NIH Public Access Policy (http://publicaccess. nih.gov/).

To embrace the growing challenges and opportunities provided by increasingly universal access to the Internet, counselors need to expand their role from empowerment via the *provision* of information to empowerment via the *navigation* of information. By encouraging patients to bring their findings from the Internet, counselors can model the gathering of information and the discriminating of sources and information. This is essential in a field in which the information is ever-changing. Thus an emerging educational role of a genetic counselor might be to review the information brought by the patient with him/her, critically evaluating its content and concluding whether the information is accurate/useful. Thus the patient learns how, whether, and why the specific information is or is not useful and is also introduced to methods for evaluating future information.

THE GENETIC COUNSELING SESSION—A VEHICLE FOR PATIENT EDUCATION

By its relatively structured organization and logical progression, the typical genetic counseling visit serves as a vehicle for patient education and is divided into seven major components or phases: (1) information gathering, (2) diagnosis, (3) risk assessment, (4) information giving, (5) psychological assessment and counseling, (6) help with decision-making, and (7) ongoing client support (Walker, 1996). During each of these phases, educational opportunities exist to present new information, correct misconceptions, reinforce information, or lay the foundation for future patient education and counseling. The genetic counselor must be alert to these opportunities and take advantage of teachable moments as they present themselves.

A **teachable moment** is defined as "the point(s) at which an individual, couple or family is most able to comprehend and absorb the information being given" (Andrews et al., 1994). Ideally, genetic counseling is most effective when provided after the initial shock and denial of learning a genetic diagnosis has diminished, and the client is able to listen and fully comprehend the information presented. However, this ideal is often not achievable because of scheduling, insurance, or managed care requirements. Follow-up counseling over a series of appointments to reinforce previous discussions has tremendous merit but has become less feasible in today's era of cost containment.

The subsections that follow present several of the major components of genetic counseling, with examples of teachable moments that might typically occur.

Information Gathering

During the information gathering phase, it is important to establish and understand what the patient's perception of the problem or reason for coming is before moving on to setting the agenda for the remainder of the visit (Riccardi and Kurtz, 1983;

Walker, 1996). Patient perception may be enhanced or complicated by information gathered before the session. This may include a combination of medically correct and incorrect information.

In a large consumer survey of 5915 individuals/families affected by genetic conditions about providers' knowledge of genetics, 64% reported receiving no genetics education materials from their primary care providers. Instead, they sought genetics-related information from other sources, including websites (89%), literature (61%), advocacy support groups (59%), one-on-one discussion (41%), and classes (14%) (Harvey et al., 2007).

Thus part of the initial assessment is to find out what information the patient has gathered, what his/her perception of the information is, and how this perception impacts on the presenting situation. It is important not to give into the possible temptation to dismiss all previously gathered information but instead to use it as part of the foundation of the information giving phase.

In the context of patient education, learning is tied to clearly understood expectations. Hence, clarification of counselor and counselee expectations, problem identification, and contracting with the patient about the organizational plan and content of the visit provide the foundation for a logically sequenced and well-organized session. Similar to the teacher who follows a logical course outline or instructional plan, the counselor has the responsibility for providing overall structure and ensuring smooth transitions, thereby setting the stage for the educational aspects of the genetic counseling session. Jumping from topic to topic can be extremely confusing and disorienting for the counselee. A logical sequence with smooth transitions is beneficial; however, the counselor must maintain flexibility and be ready to diverge from the established action plan when it is prudent to do so. The dynamic is what makes genetic counseling a process tailored to the counselee's needs rather than a standard, rote instruction. For example, a parent who becomes emotionally over-whelmed upon learning the nature of the inheritance pattern of her child's condition and the role of her own genes likely requires as the next step not risk figures for having future affected children but instead attendance to possible feelings of guilt and shame for having passed on a genetic mutation.

Obtaining the family pedigree can also provide an instructional opportunity. The pedigree, which serves as a visual generation-to-generation "tool" with which to build later discussions of inheritance mechanisms, also provides an opportunity to correct prior misconceptions related to proneness in the family (Kenen and Smith, 1995). The concept of **proneness** refers to lay beliefs about inheritance, and the nature and extent to which people feel prone to a genetic disease or feel that other family members are subject to have or acquire the condition (Richards, 1993). Each counselee's concept of proneness merits further exploration, since it may interfere with the counselee's understanding of general genetic principles. Green et al. (1993) found that many individual's views of proneness differ substantially from that of Mendelian inheritance, especially among families with a history of a genetic condition. Often the phrases "in the family," "inherited," and "genetic" are used idiosyncratically (e.g., "Well, of course, I know that hereditary things can't run in the family.") The recognition of such teachable moments permits the counselor not only to identify potential misconceptions or family "myths," but also to lay the foundation for future discussions. Just introducing certain genetic concepts (e.g., dominant inheritance and variable expressivity), albeit briefly and simply, serves as a prelude to the more detailed discussion of inheritance during the information giving phase.

Diagnosis

During the physical examination, opportunities exist to educate the patient about the diagnostic process. It is often helpful to explain that a genetics exam includes the usual general review of systems, height, weight, and head circumference measurements, as well as a more detailed assessment and series of measurements for normative comparison checking for minor findings of the head, face, neck, trunk, skin, and extremities. Care should be taken to ensure that patients understand that generally no one finding is diagnostic, but that geneticists look for patterns of findings that suggest a specific diagnosis or syndrome. Technical descriptors or terms (e.g., hemihypertrophy, hypertelorism, brachycephaly; microcephaly, etc.) can sound frightening, and the counselor can assist the patient and family by providing explanations. Pointing out pertinent findings as well as normal variations to patients can also make the physical examination more understandable and hence less threatening. Furthermore, such introductory remarks open the door for future discussions of physical features relevant to a specific diagnosis.

In cases of presymptomatic or carrier testing, adequate pretest information must be provided that addresses the risks, benefits, efficacy, potential test results, and alternatives to testing; it is also essential to furnish information about variability in symptoms and age of onset and about decisions that will likely become necessary if the test is positive (Andrews et al., 1994).

Information Giving

During the *information giving* phase, the focus is on providing factual data and information in a culturally sensitive and individualized fashion tailored to the client/ counselee. Often this centers on helping families to comprehend the medical facts related to diagnosis, natural history, and management and/or treatment options; causation and recurrence risks; available reproductive options; and available support resources.

The counselor must now bring together all the information elicited and observations made during each of the phases of the genetics visit, capitalizing on any groundwork laid during previous teachable moments. The counselor weaves the information together with counseling and support in a fashion that is easily understandable and relevant to the needs and concerns of the counselee. It is important for the counselor to:

- Distill complex information down into clear, understandable concepts.
- Restrict the use of complex terminology and medical jargon.

- Refrain from equating the patient/client to the diagnosis; use of words such as diabetic, hemophiliac, etc., can demean the patient and detract from his/her own individuality.
- Provide information, beginning with the general then moving on to more specific information. For example, it is fairly common when reviewing basic genetic concepts to begin with a brief explanation of chromosomes (in all cells of our body) and then move from a normal karyotype to a pair of chromosomes (usually the pair in question if the gene has been linked) to a specific band area to genes to DNA.
- Promote a two-way mutual exchange of information, especially with respect to the patient's understanding of the problem and diagnosis, expectations and requests for the session, and participation in the choice and discussion of treatment and/or action plans.
- Encourage counselees to restate the information in their own words.
- Correct and clarify potential misunderstandings or incorrect information.
- Offer ample opportunities for questions and answers.
- Provide summary statement(s) and restate risk figures.
- Be attentive to both verbal and nonverbal cues, providing adequate reassurance and messages of support.

In this way, the counselor goes beyond simply educating about the genetic and medical facts, using a decision-support model, and recognizes that before making decisions, the counselee must "process and personalize facts effectively and cognitively" (Walker, 1996).

Communication of Risk

One of the major focuses of genetic counseling is risk assessment and the provision of recurrence risk information to the client in an understandable fashion. The term **risk** refers to the probability that an event will happen. For the public, this term has an inherent negative connotation, imparting a sense of danger (e.g., risk of being struck by lightning, hit by a car, or dying of cancer). Everyday words like "chance" and "likelihood" are more neutral. Families may also have preconceived beliefs about their risk status (proneness).

Several factors should be considered when providing risk information to clients/ counselees. While there is no one correct way to present risk information, the presentation must be balanced, accurate, and tailored to the client. Individuals vary in how they understand risks numerically (i.e., **objective risk estimate**) and in their interpretations (i.e., **subjective risk estimate**). While studies have found no numerator bias in the manner in which a risk is *framed* (e.g., 4/100 or 40/1000), almost a third of women with less than a college education failed to recognize that 1/1000 is equivalent to <1% (Chase et al., 1986). For many, the fraction 1/800 *sounds* higher than 1/400 because of the larger denominator. The numeric equivalent that individuals attach to non-numeric phrases of probability (e.g., *often, rarely, never*) is also highly subjective, and the use of such nonnumeric phrases by the counselor introduces a potential for bias. Many people have difficulties interpreting abstract probabilities and evaluating what they mean; they frequently perceive chance in a binary fashion—all or nothing.

An individual's estimate of the likelihood that a given outcome will occur is affected by the ease with which he or she can think of actual or "concrete" examples of the instance, a concept referred to as the availability heuristic (Tversky and Kahneman, 1973). In the availability heuristic, actual or dramatic instances of certain outcomes will increase the perceived likelihood that the outcome will occur. How many times have the parents asked, "If it was one in a million before—how could the risk be only 1%?" Families who have experienced a rare event may perceive their future risk as 100% (since it has happened already). Similarly, a woman undergoing prenatal diagnosis who knows someone who has also undergone the procedure is likely to be influenced by that personal encounter—or concrete instance—in her perception of the procedure, its risks, and the likelihood of the test leading to a "good" outcome (birth of a normal baby). If the friend's experience involved complications (e.g., multiple taps; miscarriage), this concrete instance may affect the counselee's own perception of the risks of the procedure for herself. Women undergoing amniocentesis for advanced maternal age tend to overestimate failure, both in terms of perceived probabilities of procedural complications and with respect to the chances that the test will reveal a problem with the fetus (Adler et al., 1990).

Another heuristic often used is the representativeness heuristic, in which a judgment of probability is made based on how well the items being judged match a prototype or idealized example, such as assuming that the probability of the birth of three girls in a row is lower than that of an assortment of boys and girls. The use and misuse of heuristics, including the availability heuristic, was recently explored among undergraduate students, genetic counseling students, and genetic counselors (Dewhurst et al., 2007). Genetic counselors outperformed genetic counseling trainees, who in turn outperformed undergraduate students, in correct application of probability rules rather than incorrect use of heuristics. Nevertheless, some genetic counselors did use heuristics to arrive at incorrect answers, highlighting the importance of appropriate awareness by genetic counselors of probability rules (Dewhurst et al., 2007).

Ultimately, it is the counselee's perception of risk rather than the actual risk that is meaningful. It is important, therefore, to explore the counselee's own impression or perception of risk figures compared to the actual or objective risk given. Families view risks differently, depending on their own experience with the condition in question and their view of any attendant problems. For example, the perceived burden of the outcome associated with 1% risk to have a child with Down syndrome may be higher for the couple who already has a child with Down syndrome than for the couple at risk because of advanced maternal age alone. In a family counseled by one of the authors in which one parent had neurofibromatosis and the other had a dominant connective tissue disorder, the couple viewed the 25% risk for having a child with both conditions as "lower" compared to the 100% they originally anticipated.

Explaining Mendelian inheritance can, at first glance, appear relatively straight-forward, but issues such as genetic heterogeneity, variable expressivity, anticipation, nonpenetrance, gonadal mosaicism, new mutations, sex-limitation, imprinting, phenocopies, and genocopies can introduce great confusion. Add to this the nontraditional forms of inheritance, for example, uniparental disomy, mitochondrial inheritance, and trinucleotide repeats, and the counselor is truly challenged to make these concepts understandable.

Ideally, counselors should provide risk information in several different ways. Rather than refining the risk to the fraction of a percent, it is more important to consider *how* to present recurrence risks in a manner that will have meaning for the family. Thus it is important to frame risks by providing the likelihood of an unfavorable outcome balanced by the likelihood of a favorable outcome. A 1% risk for complications may be perceived as much higher if its corollary—the 99% chance of no complications—is not also presented. The manner in which risks are presented or framed also impacts the client's subjective perception. In prenatal counseling, major information to be provided pertains to risk: procedure-related risks, the likelihood of detecting a fetal abnormality with available techniques, the patient's individual risks based on age or other factors, and background population risks. Walker (1997) suggests that it is more helpful to present prenatal risks to the counselee in terms of *how* the specific risk factor (e.g., age, maternal serum screen result, or exposure) *changes* his/her chances from what it would have been without that factor. Stating number data both as fractional risks (1 in 4 chance) and percentages (25%) can also improve client understanding.

The use of metaphors, such as tossing a coin, can provide concrete examples of probability. However, it should also be remembered that in some cultures this activity is seen as a form of gambling and hence may have negative connotations. In the case of Mendelian inheritance, tactile or visual examples illustrating patterns of inheritance can prove extremely beneficial. Standard diagrams illustrating dominant, recessive, and X-linked inheritance not only help the counselor explain the different possible genotypes, but can also be given to the parent or counselee to take home as added reinforcement of these concepts. Encouraging the counselee to restate what has been said in his/her own words is also effective in ascertaining his/her level of understanding of the concepts and information discussed. Often, asking counselees how they might explain the inheritance to a relative or friend encourages them to restate what they have learned and offers the counselor an opportunity for clarification. Additional discussion of the application and use of instructional aids is found later in this chapter.

Facilitating Ongoing Client Support

In supportive counseling, the counselor tries to facilitate the counselee's ability to cope and deal with presented information. By encouraging the counselee to discuss what the information means for him or her (e.g., exploring feelings about raising a child with a disability, reactions to learning a diagnosis, personal values or previous experiences with handicapping conditions, etc.), the counselor seeks to foster counselee adaptation and self-efficacy.

Information and resources constitute one of the most critical needs of individuals, parents, and/or families of a child or family member newly diagnosed prenatally or postnatally with a birth defect or a chronic medical or genetic condition. For some individuals and families, the need to seek as much information as possible and network with other families can be intense and immediate; others may feel somewhat threatened by these activities. A patient or family with a newly diagnosed birth defect or genetic condition may have no idea how to identify resources. Ideally, the counselor knows what an agency or group can offer families and should be able to provide primary contact information. While families vary in how much additional information they want and when they want to seek peer support, they generally gladly accept the ready accessibility of such information. Some parents express a strong desire for parent-to-parent referrals.

During the 1980s, in the midst of the self-help era, many voluntary genetic support groups were established to provide information, peer support, and advocacy for their respective populations, both locally and nationally. Given the rarity of many genetic conditions, not every condition will have an established support group, thereby challenging the counselor to identify other resources in the community or nationally that may have relevance to the family. Families and patients affected by the specific disorder themselves are an extremely practical and rich source of information. Ideally, an organized parent support group is best. Some genetic conditions are so rare, however, that families may have to fall back on informal networking with other parents who have had the same experience. This option, nevertheless, can be extremely beneficial. Counselors can play a role in ensuring access to quality information by directing counselees to trusted sources, particularly the Genetic Alliance, the National Organization for Rare Disorders, and Genetics Home Reference, portals to information sources and accessible to consumers at various levels of health and scientific literacy.

ADDITIONAL ASPECTS OF PATIENT LEARNING

Barriers to Client Learning

There are both internal and external barriers to client understanding of genetic information. Internal barriers include a client's personal and cultural beliefs and education level. External barriers prevent access to services for largely economic reasons in today's health care marketplace.

Bad News

In a study that examined parental experiences and preferences related to communicating medical bad news (e.g., communicating a diagnosis of Down syndrome), a difference was found between what parents *desired* and what they actually *experienced* from physicians. Parents preferred significantly more communication of information and feelings by their physician. They expressed strong preferences for the physician to show caring (97%), to allow parents to talk (95%), and to allow parents to show their own feelings (93%)(Sharp et al., 1992). Families often feel lost, inadequate, fearful, and/or even angry at learning "bad news." Genetic counselors seek to develop a climate of support that encourages patients to express their feelings and emotions, simultaneously promoting a mutual exchange of information between counselee and counselor.

Patient/Client Expectations

It is useful to consider outcome-based research about genetic service delivery and expectations about services from the client's perspective. One study (Middelton et al, 1996) examined consumer expectations about and satisfaction with the genetics services among individuals receiving pediatric or prenatal genetic coun-seling services in the Mid-Atlantic region. Clients were asked to prospectively rank the "importance" of discussing a series of issues before their initial genetics visit. After the visit they ranked the "level" to which these same issues were discussed during the counseling session. Table 6-1 summarizes pediatric and prenatal clients' expectations based on a ranking of the five most and least important issues to be discussed. In general, pediatric clients desire information that assists them in learning about the impact of the genetic condition on themselves and/or their child, specifically as it relates to medical treatment, management, and diagnosis. Prenatal clients, on the other hand, appear to place primacy on the administrative details about prenatal testing (e.g., how they will learn about results; test accuracy; and procedural risks). Relationship issues were among the least important issues for both groups. While limited, these results are worthy of further study because they offer a consumer-based perspective about expectations for the content of genetic

TABLE 6-1. Consumer Perspectives on the Most and Least Important Issues for Discussion Before to Pediatric or Prenatal Genetics Visit

Pediatric Genetics Patients	Prenatal Genetics Patients
MOST Important Issues to Discuss or Learn About	*MOST Important Issues to Discuss or Learn About*
Available medical treatment/management	How I will learn test results
What is wrong with me/my child	Accuracy of prenatal testing
Learning coping skills	Risks of prenatal testing
If the condition can be cured	Find out chance of genetic condition occurring in me, my child, or other family members.
Chance of the condition occurring in me or my child	What to expect when having prenatal testing
LEAST Important Issues	*LEAST Important Issues*
My relationship with my partner or spouse	Talk about my/my partner's pregnancies
Plans for future pregnancies	Pregnancy termination options
Availability of prenatal testing	Discuss my feelings about pregnancy
My or my partner's/spouse's pregnancies	Decide if I should have another child
Alternative reproductive options	Discuss reproductive options

Source: Middelton et al., 1996.

information to be discussed. At the very least, such findings stress the importance of understanding what the client's expectations are and how they relate to patient satisfaction and improved genetic service delivery.

In a study by Roter et al., important differences in genetic counselors' ability to engage clients through the use of active facilitation skills and lowered verbal dominance were linked with more positive "simulated client" ratings. These results were interpreted to suggest that counseling behaviors are valued by clients (Roter et al., 2006). An exploratory study conducted by Bernhardt et al. found that while most counselors and clients agreed that the provision of information was a goal and increased knowledge an outcome of genetic counseling, provision of support and assistance with decision making were highly valued. Other benefits reported by clients included more interpersonal factors such as having their concerns listened to and being understood (Bernhardt et al., 2000).

Recall

Experience has shown that patients, like students, forget almost half of what they are told. In genetic counseling, when the information being communicated is technical and new, comprehending and remembering a series of new terms, genetic concepts, and risk information can present a formidable task. Recall can be significantly improved, however, when information is organized and categorized verbally (Riccardi and Kurtz, 1983). Studies of physician-patient communication have shown that patients recall best what they are told first and what they consider important (Ley, 1972). The most effective means of increasing long-term patient recall is to couple patient restatement with ample opportunities for feedback from the physician or professional (Kupst et al., 1975).

Riccardi and Kurtz list several factors that influence patient recall, compliance, and satisfaction. Important information should be "categorized" or highlighted verbally (e.g., "I am going to tell you what we think your son has and what tests we want to perform to confirm this diagnosis."). Then the counselor might continue, "First, we feel that both his delay in development and the birth defects may be caused by an abnormality of his chromosomes. To determine this, we need to study his chromosomes by getting a blood sample." Important information should be given first: "It's important for you to remember that". Encouraging patients to restate the "message" in their own terms is extremely beneficial. Potential misunderstandings or incorrect information should be immediately clarified. Providing the patient with ample opportunities to ask questions is critical and has been shown to improve understanding and recall. Try to restrict the use of technical and medical jargon, using everyday language to permit increased comprehensibility. Provide an appropriate level of reassurance and messages of support, and be attentive to both verbal and nonverbal cues.

Ethnocultural Barriers to Health and Genetic Services

The US population is becoming increasingly multicultural, with an ever increasing influx of new immigrants, many of whom do not speak English as their first language.

Since the early 1990s, 600,000 legal immigrants have been added to the US population each year, the majority arriving from Latin American and Pacific Asian countries (see Chapter 11, Multicultural Counseling). Ethnocultural differences in the perception of health and disease, disability, and disease burden, as well as interpretation of risk factors, pose formidable barriers to those attempting to deliver adequate and quality health and genetic services to this diverse population.

Finding genetics instructional materials for the non-English-speaking patient is becoming easier. Simple translation of English text into another language (Spanish, French, etc.) is generally not satisfactory. The Genetic Alliance has many available materials in European and non-European languages. Numerous websites offer health information in various languages. Of course, as with any other resource, it is up to the counselor to vet the English language version of the materials for accuracy and sensitivity.

Cognitive Impairment

Interindividual differences in learning styles exist among all counselees, but these become most apparent when working with individuals with cognitive impairments. Finucane (1998) identifies several challenges to "traditional" genetic counseling strategies when applied to women with mental retardation; those that involve primarily educational aspects include difficulty understanding abstract concepts such as probability and risk, difficulty using analogies to generalize from one situation to another, limited reading abilities, and, complicating the picture even further, denial of learning problems. In facilitating personal decision making in this population, Finucane thus advocates "shifting the focus from facts to feelings," that is applying a primarily psychosocial rather than informational focus. Technical information can instead be communicated to the individual(s) serving in advocacy and/or custodial roles (Finucane, 1998).

Blindness and Deafness

Visual and auditory impairments present special challenges to carrying out the educational objectives of genetic counseling. Populations with both of these conditions are likely to present for genetic counseling for these and other conditions. Several articles have been published by the Genetics Program at Gallaudet University regarding the special linguistic and cultural needs of the deaf and hearing-impaired population (Arnos et al., 1992a; Arnos et al., 1992b; Arnos et al., 1991a; Arnos et al, 1991b; Arnos 1990). A book, *Signs for Genetic Counseling* (Boughman and Shaver, 1983), describes signs used specifically in genetic counseling. These investigators have emphasized the need for not only interpreters meeting the specific needs of deaf counselees (American Sign Language, signed English, speech reading) but also the use of culturally sensitive educational materials, such as those that replace words such as "affected" and "unaffected" with "deaf" and "hearing" in conjunction with acknowledgment of the view of deafness as a cultural difference rather than a disability to be avoided (Arnos et al., 1992a; Israel et al., 1992).

Visual impairments likely present even greater challenges to the counselee education process given the reliance of genetic counseling on visual tools (e.g., meiosis diagrams, karyotypes) for education. Several organizations provide written information on genetic aspects of visual impairment, including the Foundation Fighting Blindness and the National Eye Institute, which can be made accessible through modern adaptive technologies (low-vision resources).

Scientific Literacy

Educators increasingly are aware of the public's need to have a basic understanding of genetics, disease risk, and health choices within the context of broader scientific and biological literacy. According to the Biological Sciences Curriculum Study (1997), about 95 percent of American high school students take biology in 9th or 10th grade; moreover, human genetics is now included in virtually all high school biology curricula, with the primary focus being Mendelian genetics (BSCS, 1997). Yet despite the increased exposure to human genetics and issues related to genetic testing among high school students, the scientific literacy of the general public lags behind the technological trends and innovations occurring in human biology, genetics, and medicine. Recent estimates suggest that only 20–25% of Americans are scientifically literate (Deane, 2005; Miller, 1998). Civic scientific literacy is conceptualized as a two-dimensional measure that reflects a vocabulary dimension (i.e., the basic scientific constructs needed to read/comprehend competing scientific views in the newspapers or magazines) and the process of inquiry dimension (i.e., understanding of the nature of scientific inquiry) (Miller, 1998). The US 1995 study of civic scientific literacy for these two dimensions found that correct open-ended definitions for the words *DNA* and *molecule* were recorded for 21% and 9% of Americans, respectively (Miller, 1998). The process of scientific inquiry was also understood by 21% of Americans; however, while they had an adequate understanding of the nature of scientific inquiry, Miller and colleagues found substantial misunderstanding about the rationale for choosing a single versus two-group study to evaluate a new drug. For example among the 69% who selected a two-group design, 40% selected this choice believing that if the drug "killed a lot of people" then there would be fewer potential "victims". Such findings have relevance when counseling about participation in cancer/drug treatment trials. Overall, 12% of Americans achieved civic scientific literacy levels of "well-informed" and 25% of "moderately well-informed."

The situation may be improving. A 2003 Harris Poll found that 60% of adults correctly selected "the genetic code for living cells" as the definition of DNA and 67% correctly chose "deoxyribonucleic acid" when asked "What does DNA stand for?" (SERO Corporation, Inc., 2003). Nonetheless, genetic concepts, particularly beyond these basics, are often not well understood, and understanding is influenced by a person's own ethnocultural and educational background as well as his or her life experiences.

A genetic counselor's approach may be influenced by whether a given counselee has any background knowledge on which to build. Many counselees still do not have a frame of reference for standard genetic terminology, such as gene, chromosome, risk, inheritance patterns, and carrier, which represent the basic building blocks for explaining genetic mechanisms. In many instances, the genetic counselor must resort to a mini-course in biology and inheritance before beginning to provide individualized risk assessment information.

A significant disparity exists between literacy skills in the USA and skills required/needed for adequate health literacy (AMA, 1999). *Health literacy*, as defined by the World Health Organization (WHO) in 1998, "represents the cognitive and social skills which determine the motivation and ability of individuals to gain access to, understand, and use information in ways that promote and maintain good health— simply put, the ability to read, understand and act upon health information."

Approximately 27% of the U.S. population (including 22% who are foreign born and 5% of the U.S.-born population) have less than a ninth grade education (National Institute for Literacy, 2000). This very basic level of proficiency has important ramifications with respect to counselees' ability to access genetic information. While the use of written materials such as pamphlets, booklets, etc. can be beneficial for patient education, it is important to evaluate the readability as well as comprehensibility of such materials by the intended audience. Moreover, clients who are unable to read and understand materials may be embarrassed to reveal this limitation; handing them a brochure upside down can provide a quick assessment since readers will automatically right the upside-down material (Scudder, 2006).

Health literacy is critical to deciphering and interpreting health information and resources available via web-based search engines that provide easy access to genetic information for both genetics professionals and the general public. Yet despite the ready Internet/WWW availability, many of the patient education materials on the Internet are not written at an appropriate reading level (8th grade) for the average adult/parent, but have readability levels from 12th grade to college level for pediatric and cancer materials, respectively (D'Alessandro et al., 2001; Friedman et al., 2004).

APPLICATION OF INSTRUCTIONAL AIDS FOR PATIENT EDUCATION

Use of Instructional Aids

The development and use of instructional aids to assist the counselor in explaining concepts is extremely beneficial. The value of colored diagrams, figures, and other materials cannot be overstated. Many graphics already exist, and graphic programs permit the counselor to quickly create useful instructional aids such as ideograms of normal and aberrant chromosomes. Colored markers with interchangeable caps work terrifically to illustrate translocations, deletions, or duplications. Colored pipe cleaners, colored paper clips, and beads on a string are all three-dimensional aids that can provide an easy-to-understand visual analogy of genes as units strung together on the chromosome or of linked DNA bases.

Experience supports the benefit of developing a personal *genetic counseling resource book*. A three-ring binder can be divided into sections, including, for example:

Hospital/center-specific information for easy reference (billing office, major consult contacts, etc.)

Clinical/research protocols in use at your institution for selected conditions

Recurrence risk tables compiled from published data and/or center-specific data

Diagrams illustrating patterns of inheritance (e.g., Mendelian and multifactorial)

Diagrams showing chromosome structure and actual karyotypes (normal and abnormal)

Syndrome-specific information (local support group information, pictures of children and adults with common conditions such as Down syndrome, etc.)

Growth curves (normative and syndrome specific)

Prenatal diagnosis maternal age curves, screening risk tables, etc.

The comprehensive *Genetic Counseling Aids* published by the Greenwood Genetic Center, available in electronic format in both English and Spanish, and/or similar materials developed by the counselor or other groups are an essential part of the counselor's armamentarium of counseling tools. Another full-color genetics flip book, *Genetics Visual Aids for Educators and Health Care Professionals, is* available in Spanish and French versions from CCL Books. It is also extremely helpful to have a series of predrawn tear-off tablets showing two parents, their genotypes, and the four possible genotypes for their offspring. Counselors can also create diagrams that illustrate specific genetic circumstances in front of the client—a skill to be mastered, especially when drawing upside down for the client's benefit. These materials are convenient and can be given to the client to take home.

Patient Letters

The genetic counseling summary letter serves as a valuable and important educational tool for families referred for genetic services. By providing a narrative summary of the information from the genetic visit, the summary letter documents the pertinent aspects of the patient's medical and family history, mechanisms of inheritance, recurrence risks, and recommended follow-up. Moreover, counselees can refer back to the letter for recall of salient points and/or share this with other family members. Diagrams to explain molecular and cytogenetic results can also be included with the letter, along with a copy of the laboratory results.

Audiovisual Materials

Visual aids can further assist the client in understanding genetics information that is often complex. For example, a videotape/digital media reviewing prenatal diagnostic procedures (amniocentesis/CVS) that incorporates the common information to be discussed with all clients provides a means of providing standardized information that is not only time-saving but can be used for quality assurance. Coupled with client-specific individualized counseling, these materials can enhance the process, providing information both visually and in a narrative fashion.

While written or electronic aids can serve to clarify health choices, they cannot replace the human factor in promoting informed choice (Woolf et al., 2005). In a study evaluating the efficacy and utility of a computer-based decision-support aid providing genetic education for breast cancer susceptibility alone or in combination with traditional face-to-face counseling, the computer aid enhanced knowledge in both high-and low-risk women; however, genetic counseling was more effective in facilitating accurate risk perceptions and allaying anxieties in high-risk women (Green et al., 2004). Thus the use of such computer-based decision aids as an adjunct to counseling permits the counselor to shift the focus away from basic education and toward personal risk and decision-making (Green et al., 2005).

Brochures/Pamphlets

Written materials serve as aids to information transfer and are almost universal to health promotion and patient education programs in genetics. They clarify and reinforce the information presented, augmenting the genetic counseling process. Disease-specific brochures are available from individual support groups, many in electronic form.

Designing Informational Materials

In response to the needs of their clients, genetic counselors have always been involved in the development of a variety of educational materials to facilitate the learning process. Writing about genetics often requires the use of technical terminology and concepts that can be confusing. When drafting such materials, consider writing style, vocabulary, layout, typography, graphics, and color. Use the active, not passive voice. Write in short, simple sentences, using one- or two-syllable words. Provide clarification through the use of examples. Avoid the use of jargon, technical terms, abbreviations, and acronyms. In brochures, leave plenty of white space on the printed pages and break up narrative with subheadings, captions, and highlighting of important terms (bold/italic). Important points should be summarized.

Knowledge about the target audience is crucial to producing informational materials on genetic conditions; care should be taken in the development of materials targeting ethnic minorities and patients and their families. Printed materials should be simply written, reinforced with graphics, and pretested with the target audience. Just as language skills differ, people may react differently to graphics, illustrations, and/or analogies. Printed materials should not be simply translated directly from English into other languages.

The importance of formative evaluation in the instructional design of instruments (e. g., questionnaires), media, and both written and visual materials cannot be overstated. To be effective, instructional materials should be developed professionally and undergo systematic pretesting during draft stages. A general three-step review process should include (1) reading level assessment; (2) content analysis; and (3) review by content specialists (US Dept. of Health and Human Services, NIH publication # 92-1493). Readability analysis can be performed with one of many computer software applications. Formal pretesting of materials with the intended audience during development is also beneficial to ensure that the final materials are understandable, relevant, attention-getting, attractive, credible, and/or acceptable to the target audience. Any sensitive and/or controversial elements can be identified and revised as necessary. For additional information on guidelines and resources for developing informational materials, see the Genetic Alliance, Access to Credible Genetics Resources Network (http://geneticalliance.org/atcg).

TENETS OF HEALTH EDUCATION AND PROMOTION: APPLICATION TO GENETIC COUNSELING

As a complement to the tools and techniques used by the genetic counselor *cum* instructor, some discussion of contemporary models of health behavior and their relevance to health promotion programs is warranted. Geneticists and others in medical practice have been rather slow to recognize and utilize the modern principles and practices of learning and behavior theory. However, similar to genetic counseling, health promotion programs seek to improve health, reduce disease risks, and improve the well-being and self-sufficiency of individuals, families, and communities, as well as organizations. Utilizing a multilevel interactive approach, such programs go beyond traditional educational activities by including advocacy, policy development, economic supports, organizational and environmental change efforts, and multimethod programs. Formal awareness and application of the health promotion literature and health behavior models provides genetic counselors with new avenues for clinical practice and research.

Contemporary models of health behavior stem from cognitive-behavioral theories, which are premised on two key concepts: (1) that behavior is mediated through what we know and think (cognition) and (2) that knowledge, while needed, is not alone sufficient to change behavior; factors such as perception, motivation, skills, and personal and social environmental factors also have important roles (Glanz and Rimer, 1995). Behavior is influenced at multiple levels as shown in Table 6-2, including intrapersonal (or individual) factors, interpersonal factors, institutional or organizational factors, community factors, and public policy factors. Several theories describing the interrelationship between these factors and health behaviors have emerged and warrant a brief discussion.

The review of contemporary behavior theories about health promotion that follows is not intended to be exhaustive but rather to heighten awareness of a body of literature of particular relevance to the genetic counseling field. The tenets of health education are certain to have widespread application for genetic counselors involved in the development of patient education materials and service delivery programs. The concepts derived from contemporary behavior theories and health promotion programs are consistent with the underpinnings of the field of genetic

TABLE 6-2. Factors Influencing Health Behavior

Factor Level	Definition
Intrapersonal	Individual characteristics, such as knowledge, attitudes, beliefs, personality traits, self-concept, skills, past experience, motivation, etc.
Interpersonal	Interpersonal processes and primary groups (i.e., family, friends, peers) that provide social identity, support and role definition
Institutional	Rules, regulations, policies, and informal structures, which may constrain or promote recommended behaviors
Community	Social networks and norms, or standards, which exist as formal or informal among individuals, groups, or organizations (e.g., schools, worksites, health care settings)
Public policy	Local, state, federal policies and laws that regulate or support healthy actions and practices for disease prevention, early detection, control, and management

Source: U.S. National Institutes of Health (1995): *Theory At A Glance: A Guide for Health Promotion Practice,* NIH publication 95-3896, p. 16.

counseling that include accessibility of services, attitudes toward health care, perception and beliefs about susceptibility (threat of illness), knowledge about disease, social structure, self-efficacy, decision making, and autonomy. Health education programs improve health, identify and reduce disease risks, manage chronic illness, and improve the well-being and self-sufficiency of individuals, families, organizations, and communities. While it is easy to see the relevance of these concepts to the planning and development of widescale genetic testing and screening efforts (e.g., Tay–Sachs, cystic fibrosis, breast and colon cancer, and newborn screening), these concepts also have applicability to individual genetic counseling encounters, a matter we explore shortly.

Health Belief Model

The first and most widely recognized model that adapts theory from the behavioral sciences to health problems is the health belief model (HBM), which attempts to explain and predict health-related behavior in the context of certain belief patterns. Based on the assumption that the degree of "fear" or "threat" of a disease or condition is a powerful motivating force to behavior, the HBM was first introduced in the 1950s by psychologists in the U.S. to explain the public's use of preventable health services available at that time, such as flu vaccines and chest X-ray screening for tuberculosis (Glanz and Rimer, 1995). The model takes into account a person's perception of the susceptibility and severity of the condition and the practical and psychological costs and inconvenience (perceived barriers) to taking a "health" action. A person's readiness to act (cues to action) reflects the accompanying appraisal of a recommended behavior for preventing or managing the health problem within the context of the perceived threat (Green and Kreuter, 1991; Glanz and Rimer, 1995). The concept of *self-efficacy* was added to the HBM in 1988, to reflect confidence in a person's ability to take action (e.g., change habitual unhealthy behaviors, such as smoking or overeating).

Stages of Change Model

The stages of change model was introduced by Prochaska and DiClemente (Prochaska and Diclemente, 1983; Prochaska et al., 1992) based on work with smoking cessation and drug and alcohol treatment programs. This model views behavior change as a circular process with individuals at varying levels of readiness to change or attempt to change toward healthy behaviors. It is based upon the assumption that people do not change chronic and habitual behaviors all at once, but continuously through a series of stages including the following (Green and Kreuter, 1991; Glanz and Rimer, 1995):

- **Precontemplation stage** (people have no expressed interest in or are not thinking about change)
- **Contemplation stage** (serious thought is given to changing a behavior)
- **Decision stage** (the plan to change is made)
- **Action stage** (the first 6 months after an overt change in behavior has been implemented)
- **Maintenance stage** (the period from 6 months after the behavior change until the behavior is completely terminated)

Consumer Information Processing Theory

Originating from studies of human problem solving and information processing, the consumer information processing theory focuses on the process by which individuals, as consumers, acquire and use information in their decision-making. Although not originally developed for the study of health behaviors, this model can be used to examine why people use or fail to use health information, and hence can be instructional in the design and development of successful informational and intervention strategies. (Glanz and Rimer, 1995). The theory recognizes that there are limitations in the amount of information individuals can acquire, process and remember; hence, choosing the most important and useful points to communicate is critical. Providing information in small, clear, and concise "chunks" that can be handled according to decision rules (heuristics) permits individuals to make choices faster and more easily. The information should be convenient to use and tailored to the audience with respect to amount, format, readability, and processibility. For people to use health information, the material must be available; in addition, it must be viewed as useful or new, and it must be communicated in a "user-friendly" fashion.

The Social Learning Theory

Complex in its design, social learning theory (SLT) incorporates concepts and processes from cognitive, behavioralistic, and emotional models of behavior change. Synonymous with the social-cognitive theory put forth by Bandura in the 1970s, SLT assumes that individuals exist within an environment in which personal factors, environmental influences, and behavior continually interact. The concept of reciprocal determinism is central to SLT, representing a major departure from traditional operant conditioning theory, which tends to view all behavior as a one-way product of the environment. (Green and Kreuter, 1991). In SLT, behavior and environment are "reciprocal" systems. While environment shapes, maintains, and even constrains behavior, the process is bidirectional, with individuals able to create or change (self-regulate) their environment and actions. Learning takes place through direct experience, through indirect or vicarious experience observing others (modeling) or via storing and processing complex information. Self-efficacy, or one's confidence in one's ability to successfully take action, is the most important aspect of sense of self (Bandura, 1986). Not only does self-efficacy influence behavior, but also it may enhance coping and alleviate anxiety.

Theory of Reasoned Action

The concept of *behavioral intention* is central to the theory of reasoned action and represents the final step in the process before any action takes place. Attitudes toward the behavior and perception of social norms favorable to the behavior influence one's behavioral intention. A person's existing skills—skills already possessed, which don't need to be learned—are closely tied to self-efficacy and behavioral intention (Shumaker et al., 1990). For example, a woman who performs regular breast self-exams and obtains regular mammograms before undergoing testing possesses a high self-efficacy about breast cancer screening and the self-confidence and skills necessary to support her behavioral intent to continue or increase her screening behaviors upon learning of the presence of a susceptibility mutation.

Common Sense Model and Transactional Model of Stress and Coping

It has been posited that the health belief model and other decision-making models are limited in their applicability to genetic testing uptake because they account for the cognitive component of decision-making but largely ignore interpersonal and emotional aspects (Gooding et al., 2006; Shiloh et al., 1997), in contrast to the common sense model (CSM) and the transactional model of stress and coping (TMSC). In particular, the CSM (1) acknowledges that an emotional process of "fear control" occurs in parallel to the cognitive process of decision-making and may lead to unconscious responses that run counter to cognitive responses, such as avoiding screening behaviors in order to deny or avoid the health threat, and (2) evaluates the effectiveness of coping strategies in order to allow alternative strategies to be employed (Gooding et al., 2006). The CSM was applied in a study of perceived cancer risk in individuals testing for BRCA1/2 mutations (Kelly et al., 2005) which showed that individuals often have levels of perceived cancer risk that are different from their empiric risk, and these estimates may be resistant to change, often not based on rational factors. For example, contrary to rational expectation, perceived risk of cancer did *not* decrease in individuals who did not have a personal history of cancer and received an informative negative test result. Conversely, perceived cancer risk *did* decrease in individuals with a cancer history and an uninformative negative result, also in contrast to rational expectations. The authors stress that understanding how these estimates form is essential for designing appropriate educational interventions (Kelly et al., 2005).

The transactional model of stress and coping (TMSC) differs from the common sense model in that threats to one's well-being are not appraised but implicit. The individual appraises his/her ability to cope and then implements (1) problem-focused coping strategies (information seeking, lifestyle change) if the stressor is appraised as controllable or (2) emotion-focused coping strategies (seeking social support, avoidance, etc.) if the stressor is appraised as uncontrollable (Gooding et al., 2005). A recent evaluation of the impact of genetic counseling on uncertainty and perceived personal control among parents of children with rare chromosome disorders (Lipinski et al., 2006) employed the TMSC. This study revealed a positive correlation between parents' perceived control of their child's condition and the perception of helpfulness of the genetic counselor. In particular, it was noted that if parents' assessment of their children's condition as serious was accurate, the counselor's promotion of emotion-focused coping strategies was important for adaptation to their children's condition (Lipinski et al., 2006).

FUTURE DIRECTIONS

Many Americans are likely to be faced with difficult and complex decisions about the use of genetic technology to determine personal health risks as well as risks for their unborn offspring. As genetic testing becomes available for more conditions, the traditional format of face-to-face genetic counseling sessions of one to two hours may not be feasible because of time constraints and cost containment pressures arising from managed care. New models to deliver required information to facilitate patient education and informed decision-making must be investigated with attention to quality outcomes and support of patient autonomy.

It is becoming increasingly possible to identify actual gene variants that increase susceptibility to common disease as well as the ability of environmental/lifestyle modification to alter the susceptibility to disease. Of course, the notion of gene/environment interactions in actual practice is not new. For decades we have been preventing mental retardation via dietary modification in individuals with PKU and other inborn errors of metabolism. However, it is now becoming possible to identify variants with a much more modest effect on phenotype and the ability of lifestyle modification to decrease the odds of disease (Florez et al., 2006). It is not yet known whether knowing one's genotype will have a positive, negative, or no effect on motivation to engage in health-promoting behaviors. Education by genetic counselors of counselees and the community on the nature of genetic susceptibility versus genetic determinism is needed in order to enable the type of research that will answer these questions and engage the community in this important endeavor.

SUMMARY

John Naisbett, author of *Megatrends*, cautions that "We are drowning in information but starved for knowledge." Individuals and families affected by genetic disease face a plethora of high-tech information, which they seek to gain true knowledge about their genetic circumstance. *What* is said and *how* information is communicated can have a significant impact on their ability to process the information, and on their understanding. To place more power into the hands of individuals and their families affected by genetic disease is to be sure that they have adequate knowledge—and not just information—about their genetic circumstance. In the role of instructor, the genetic counselor seeks to effectively communicate highly technical genetic information in a way that is compassionate, empathic, and sensitive to the ethnocultural values of the client. In this way, the genetic encounter moves from basic patient education to the multifaceted process of genetic counseling.

REFERENCES

Ad Hoc Committee on Genetic Counseling, American Society of Human Genetics (1975), *Am J Hum Genet* 27:240–242.

Adler NE, Keyes S, Kegeles S, Golbus MN (1990) Psychological responses to prenatal diagnosis: Anxiety in anticipation of amniocentesis (unpublished) cited in Adler NE, Keyes S, Robertson P: *Psychological Issues in New Reproductive Technologies,* Chapter 8.

American Medical Association (1999) Health literacy: Report of the Councel of Scientific Affairs. Ad Hoc Committee on Health Literacy for the Council on Scientific Affairs. *JAMA* 281:552–557.

Andrews LA, Fullarton JE, Holtzman NA, and Motulsky AG (eds) (1994) *Assessing Genetic Risks: Implications for Health and Social Policy.* Washington, DC: National Academy Press.

Arnos KS (1990) Special considerations in genetic counseling with the deaf population. *Birth Defects Orig Art Ser* 26:199–202.

Bandura A (1986) *Social Foundations of Thought and Action.* Englewood Cliffs, NJ: Prentice-Hall.

Beisecker AE, Beisecker TD (1990) Patient information-seeking behaviors when communicating with doctors. *Med Care* 28(1):19–28.

Boud D, Griffin V (eds.) (1987) *Appreciate Adults Learning: From the Learner's Perspective.* London: Kogan Page.

Boughman, JA, Shaver KA (1983) *Signs for Genetic Counseling*, Washington, DC: The National Academy, Division of Public Services, Gallaudet College Press.

BSCS (1997) *Genes, Environment and Human Behavior.* Biological Sciences Curriculum Study, Colorado Springs, CO.

Center for Human & Molecular Genetics (1993) *Catalog of Multilingual Patient Education Materials on Genetic and Related Maternal/Child Health Topics.* Newark; New Jersey Medical School.

Chase GA, Faden RR, Holtzman NA, Chawalow AJ, leonard CO, Lopes C, Quaid K (1986) Assessment of risk by pregnant women: Implications for genetic counseling and education. *Soc Biol* 33(2):57–64.

Collins J (2004) Education techniques for lifelong learning. Principles of adult learning. *RadioGraphics* 24(5):1483–1489.

Cross KP (1981) *Adults as Learners: Increasing Participation and Facilitating Learning.* San Francisco: Jossey-Bass.

Dean C (2005) "Scientific Savvy? In U.S., Not Much". *NY Times,* Aug 30.

Dewhurst ME, Veach PM, Lampman C, Petrtraitis J, Kao J, LeRoy B (2007) Probability biases in genetic problem solving: A comparison of undergraduates, genetic counseling graduate students, and genetic counselors. *J Genet Couns* 16:157–170.

Finucane B (1998) *Working with Women Who Have Mental Retardation: A Genetic Counselor's Guide.* Elwyn, PA: Elwyn, Inc.

Florez JC, Jablonski KA, Bayley N, Pollin TI, de Bakker PI, Shuldiner AR, Knowler WC, Nathan DM, Altshuler D; Diabetes Prevention Program Research Group (2006) TCF7L2 polymorphisms and progression to diabetes in the Diabetes Prevention Program. *N Engl J Med* 355(3):241–250.

Gardiner RJM, Sutherland GR (1989) *Chromosome Abnormalities and Genetic Counseling.* New York: Oxford Univ. Press.

Glanz K, Rimer RK (1995) *Theory at a Glance: A Guide for Health Promotion Practice.* U.S. Dept of Health and Human Services, PHS, NIH95-3896.

Genetic Alliance (2008) Access to Credible Genetics (ATCG) Resources Network. http://geneticalliance.org/atcg.

Gooding HC, Organista K, Burack J, Bieseckcer BB (2006) Genetic susceptibility testing from a stress and coping perspective. *Soc Sci Med* 62:1880–1890.

Green LW, Kreuter MW (eds) (1991) *Health Promotion Planning: An Educational and Environomental Approach* (2nd ed.). Mayfield Publishing.

Green MJ, Peterson SK, Baker MW, Harper GR, Friedman LC, Rubinstein WS, Mauger DT (2004) Effect of a computer-based decision aid on knowledge, perceptions, and intentions about genetic testing for breast cancer susceptibility: a randomized controlled trial. *JAMA* 292(4):442–452.

Green MJ, Peterson SK, Baker MW, Friedman LC, Harper GR, Rubinstein WS, Peters JA, Mauger DT (2005) Use of an educational computer program before genetic counseling for breast cancer susceptibility: effects on duration and content of counseling sessions. *Genet Med* 7(4):221–229.

Harvey EK, Fogel CE, Peyrot M, Christensen KD, Terry SF, McInerney JD. (2007) Providers' knowledge of genetics: A survey of 5915 individuals and families with genetic conditions. *Genet Med* 9(5):259–267.

Holsinger D, Larabell S, Walker AP (1992) History and pedigree obtained during follow-up for abnormal maternal serum alpha fetoprotein identified addition risk in 25% of patients. *Clin Res* 40:28A.

Hsu N, Binns V (2002) Book Review: Genetics Visual Aids for Educators & Health Care Professionals (2nd ed.). *J Genet Couns* 11(1):65–67.

Hyman R, Rossoff B (1984) Matching learning and teaching styles: The jug and what's in it? *Theory Pract* 23:35–43.

Israel J, Cunningham M, Thumann H, Arnos KS (1992) Genetic counseling for deaf adults: Communication/language and cultural considerations. *J Genet Couns* 1:135–153.

Kasper JF, AG Mulley, JE Weenberg (1992) Developing shared decision-making programs to improve the quality of health care. *Quality Rev Bull J Quality Improvement* 18 (6):183–190.

Kelly K, Leventhal H, Andrykowski M, Toppmeyer D, Much J, Dermody J, Marvin M, Baran J, Schwalb M (2005) Using the common sense model to understand perceived cancer risk in individuals testing for BRCA1/2mutations. *Psycho-Oncology* 14:34–48.

Kenen R, ACM Smith (1995) Genetic counseling for the next 25 years: Models for the future. *J Genet Couns* 4(2):115–124.

Knowles M (1973) *The Adult Learner: A Neglected Species* (1st ed). Houston TX: Gulf Publishing.

Knowles MS (1980) *The Modern Practice of Adult Education: From Pedagogy to Andragogy.*

Kumar DD, Ramasamy R, Stefanich GP (2001) Science for students with visual impairments: Teaching suggestions and policy implications for secondary educators. *Electronic J Sci Educ* 5(3), http://unr.edu/homepage/crowther/ejse/kumar2etal.html.

Kupst et al. (1975) Evaluation of methods to improve communication in the physician-patient relationship. *Am J Orthopsychiatry* 45:420.

Kuznar et al. (1991) Learning style preferences: A comparison of younger and older adult females: *J Nutric Elderly* 10(3).

Ley P (1972) Primacy, rated importance and recall of medical information. *J Health Soc Behav* 13:31.

Ley P (1973) A method of increasing patient recall. *Psych Med* 3:217. (refs from Riccardi and Kurtz, 1983 p. 170).

Lipinski SE, Lipinski MJ, Biesecker LJ, Biesecker BB (2006) Uncertainty and perceived personal control among parents of children with rare chromosome conditions: the role of genetic counseling. *Am J Med Genet C Semin Med Genet* 15:232–240.

Magyari T, Smith ACM, Whole K (1994) Effectiveness of multimedia decision-support materials vs. traditional genetic counseling for CF carrier screening. *Am. J. Hum Genet* (abstracts).

Mastropieri MA and Scruggs TE (1992) Science for students with disabilities. *Revi Educ Res* 62:377–411.

Middelton LA, Smith ACM, Irwin A (1996) Consumer expectations and satisfaction with genetic services: Issues to consider in research design and implementation. *J Genet Couns* 5:210.

Miller JD (1998) The measurement of civic scientific literacy. *Public Understan Sci* 7:203–223.

Mittman I (1990) Immigration and the provision of genetic counseling services. *Birth Defects Orig Art Ser* 26:139–146.

Mittman I, Fenolio KR, Lee ES et al (1988) Perinatal genetic services tailored for a multi-ethnic, low Income patient population at a county hospital. *Am J Hum Genet* 43:A241.

Mittman I, (1997) *Genetic Counseling to Communities of Color* (unpublished data).

Mittman, I (1990) A model perinatal genetics program. *Birth Defects Orig Art Ser* 26:93–100.

National Institutes of Health, National Institute on Deafness and Other Communication Disorders (1999) Communicating informed consent to individuals who are deaf or hard-of-hearing. DHHS, NIH Pub. No. 00–4689 (Available online http://www.nidcd.nih.gov/news/releases/99/inform/toc.asp).

O'Connor AM, Stacey D, Entwistle V, Llewellyn-Thomas H, Rovner D, Holmes-Rovner M, Tait V, Tetroe J, Fiset V, Barry M, Jones J. (2003) Decision aids for people facing health treatment or screening decisions. *Cochrane Database Syst Rev* (2):CD001431. Update of *Cochrane Database Syst Rev* (2001)(3):CD001431.

Peters JA, Stopfer JE (1996) Role of the genetic counselor in familial cancer. *Oncology* 10(2):159–166.

Prochaska JO, DiClemente C (1983) Stages and processes of self-change in smoking: Toward an integrative model of change. *J Consult Clin Psychol* 5:390–395.

Prochaska JO, DiClemente CC, Norcross JC (1992) In search of how people change: Applications to addictive behaviors. *Am Psychologist* 47:1102–1114.

Public Education in Genetics (1994) In Andrews LA, Fullarton JE, Holtzman NA, and Motulsky AG (eds) *Assessing Genetic Risks: Implications for Health and Social Policy.* Washington, DC: National Academy Press, pp 185–201.

Riccardi VM, Kurtz SM (1983): *Communication and Counseling in Health Care.* Springfield, IL: CC Thomas.

Ricker KS, and Rodgers NC (1981) Modifying instructional materials for use with visually impaired students. *Am Biol Teacher* 43:490–501.

Schneider KA (1994) *Counseling About Cancer: Strategies for Genetic Counselors.* Boston, Dana Farber Cancer Institute.

Scudder L (2006) Words and well-being: How literacy affect patient health. *J Nurse Practitioners* 2(10):28–34.

SERO Corporation, Inc. (2003) New poll shows dramatic rise in Americans' "DNA I.Q." 27 February. http://www.eurekalert.org/pub_releases/2003-02/kc-nps022603.php. Accessed 7 July 2005 cited in National Science Board. 2006. *Science and Engineering Indicators 2006.* Two volumes. Arlington, VA: National Science Foundation (volume 1, NSB 06-01)

Sharp MC, Strauss RP, Lorch SC (1992) Communicating medical bad news: Parent's experiences and preferences. *J Pediatr* 121:539–546.

Shumaker SA, Schron EB, Ockene JK (1990) *The Handbook of Health Behavior Change.* New York: Springer Publishing.

Smith ACM (1998) Appendix 5.1: Design and Development Model: A Case Example in *A Guide to Genetic Counseling*, (1st ed.). Eds Baker, DL, Schuette JL and Uhlmann WR, Wiley-Liss, Inc.

Tversky, Kahneman (1973) Availability: A heuristic for judging frequency and probability. *Cognitive Psychology* 5: 2-7-232.

U.S. Bureau of Census (1996) *Statistical Abstract of the United States* (116th ed.) In: *The National Data Book.* Washington, DC: Bureau of Census, Dept of Commerce.

U.S. Department of Health and Human Services (1992) Publication 92-1493, *Making Health Communication Programs Work: A Planners Guide.* U.S. National Institutes of Health.

Vermejj GJ (2004) Science, blindness, and evolution: The common theme is opportunity. *J Sci Educ Students Disabil* 10(1):1–3. Reprinted in *the Braille Monitor* 47(3). Available online http://www.nfb.org/Images/nfb/Publications/bm/bm04/bm0403/bm0403tc.htm. Accessed August 28, 2007.

Walker, AP (1996) Historical perspective and philosophical perspective of genetic counseling. in Emory and D Rimoin (eds). *Principles and Practice of Medical Genetics* (3rd ed.).

Wang V (1993) *Handbook of Cross-Cultural Genetic Counseling*, Published by NSGC Special Projects Award. National Society of Genetic Counselors.

Wiel, Mittman (1993) A teaching framework for cross-cultural genetic counselling, *J Gene Couns* 2(3):159–169.

Wlodkowski RJ (1993) *Enhancing Adult Motivation to Learn*. New York: Jossey-Bass, Inc.

Woolf SH, Chan EC, Harris R, Sheridan SL, Braddock CH 3rd, Kaplan RM, Krist A, O'Connor AM, Tunis S (2005) Promoting informed choice: transforming health care to dispense knowledge for decision making. *Ann Intern Med* 143(4):293–300.

World Health Organization, Division of Health Promotion, Education, and Communications, Health Education and Health Promotion Unit (1998) *Health Promotion Glossary*, Geneva, Switzerland: WHO.

7

Risk Communication and Decision-Making

Bonnie Jeanne Baty, M.S., C.G.C., L.G.C.

In all major areas of genetic counseling clinical practice, a central genetic counseling role is to analyze clinical data and calculate risks. Although this is important, the roles of risk communication and aid with decision-making are equally critical in helping clients to incorporate genetic information and use it to improve their quality of life. This is reflected in the large number of studies being published that address these topics. This chapter does not deal with the science of risk calculation or with informed consent (see Trepanier et al., 2004; Berliner and Fay, 2007), but rather with the science and art of risk communication and aid with decision-making. It discusses the literature surrounding these issues, clinical practice considerations, and tools to aid clients in making life-altering decisions and aid counselors in communicating with clients. It is encouraging to note many examples of novel research techniques being used to provide an evidence base for this topic.

Weil identifies risk perception and decision-making as topics that are fundamental to genetic counseling (Weil, 2000, p. 117). The psychological process of risk perception transforms risk information into individualized perceptions influenced by the counselee's life experiences and other sources of information. The calculation, presentation, and discussion of risk figures are central to genetic counseling, and Weil enumerates many domains in which the calculation and discussion of risk are important. Great effort has gone into the generation of accurate risk figures, and these are then used in the service of informed consent and informed decision-making

A Guide to Genetic Counseling, Second Edition, Edited by Wendy Uhlmann, Jane Schuette, and Beverly Yashar
Copyright © 2009 by John Wiley & Sons, Inc.

(Weil, 2000, p. 125). The literature related to risk communication and decision-making is overlapping, as much risk communication leads to some type of medical or personal decision and, conversely, many decisions are informed by risk information.

The phrase "risk communication" consists of both the "communication" aspect and the "risk" aspect. Regarding the communication aspect, effective strategies for good communication in general are equally important in risk communication. This includes the cognitive aspect of communication (e.g., critical thinking, clarity, logic, prioritizing important information, cultural and personal tailoring of information, avoidance of jargon), the psychosocial aspect (e.g., establishing rapport and trust, unconditional positive regard, attention to emotional components, congruence of verbal and nonverbal components, counselor genuineness, shared control of the session between counselor and counselee), and the environment (e.g., privacy, comfortable seating, orientation of counselor to counselee(s), adequate time). Assessing the needs of counselees is critical and should occur early in the session. An interactive style of communication will aid in assessing the counselee's understanding and integration of the information, making sure the counselee's needs are met, encouraging counselee investment in the counseling process, and encouraging shared decision making.

RISK COMMUNICATION

> *Celeste is a 34-year-old woman who comes for genetic counseling to discuss Huntington disease (HD) testing. Her father recently died of HD at the age of 61. The autosomal dominant mode of inheritance seems straightforward: Celeste has a 50% chance of inheriting HD. However, her risk can be altered based on the age of penetrance for HD. Since she is age 34 and has no symptoms, her chance for having inherited HD is 40%. Age of onset is related to CAG repeat size in a group of at-risk individuals, but is not predictive for individuals within that group. Her father's CAG repeat size was 40. CAG repeat size is more unstable when inherited from the father. Results of HD testing can fall into a "gray zone," in which people have intermediate CAG repeat size and may or may not develop the condition. How can you best help Celeste to understand relevant risk information? (Langbehn et al., 2004; Brinkman et al., 1997).*

For purposes of this discussion, risk communication can be defined as a discussion between the genetic counselor and patient and/or family about risks associated with genetic conditions. These may be risks of occurrence or recurrence of the condition; risks, benefits, and limitations of genetic testing; risks of treatment or nontreatment; and related psychological risks associated with these topics.

Factors Impacting Risk Communication

Communication of risk is complex and is subject to internal and external factors, some of which are described below.

Internalization and Retention of Information There is a substantial body of literature suggesting that counselees do not internalize and retain the risk figures that are presented by counselors (Lerman et al., 2002; Julian-Reynier et al., 2003). Accuracy of perceived risk was found to be improved after genetic counseling in some studies, but not altered in meta-analyses of controlled trials (Meiser and Halliday, 2002; Braithwaite et al., 2006).

Overestimation of Risk In cancer genetics studies, there is a tendency for individuals to overestimate their personal risks (Evans et al., 1993; Croyle and Lerman, 1999; Lerman et al., 2002; Matloff et al., 2006; Bjorvatn et al., 2007), and patients and practitioners often do not agree on the patients' risks (Bjorvatn et al., 2007).

Perceptions of Risk This may be a more important determinant of test uptake than actual risk (Lerman et al., 2002). Because of this, researchers have investigated the counselee factors that contribute to their understanding of risk. These may include counselee attributes, interactions with family and others in their social network, and experiences in the professional setting. For example, several studies found that women rely more on their personal experience in interpreting genetic information and understanding cancer risk than they do on professional risk estimates (Kenen et al., 2002, McAllister, 2003, Hopwood et al., 2001, d'Agincourt-Canning, 2005). In a process study that documented actual risk communication in a series of counseling visits, counselors regularly helped counselees to understand the information, but seldom built on counselees' preexisting perspective (Pieterse et al., 2006). (Process studies examine what transpires in actual genetic counseling sessions.) Counselees' risk perception after counseling was unrelated to whether this risk had been explicitly stated.

Risk perceptions are influenced by the following factors (Pearn, 1973; Wertz et al., 1986; Esplen et al., 1998; Van Dijk et al., 2004):

- Seriousness of the disorder
- Personal attributes such as age, education, gender, coping style, risk tolerance, optimism, having a living affected child, desire for children
- Beliefs about etiology, prognosis, and risk management options
- Stress and perceptions of vulnerability
- Familial experience with the condition
- Sense of "likeness" with the affected family member
- Level and accuracy of knowledge
- Heightened media attention
- Discussions in counseling (e.g., whether to have a child, the effects of an affected child on relationships)

There is an excellent review of research findings about risk perception and interpretation by Weil (Weil, 2000, pp. 125–134). He discusses early ideas about the importance of the balance of numerical risk versus burden of the disorder in making a "rational" reproductive decision and notes that this formulation is simplistic. Weil summarizes that reproductive decisions are often influenced more by other factors such as risk perceptions, personal experience, and moral concerns, and there is often poor correspondence between objective and subjective estimates of risk. He suggests that a subjective estimate of risk by the counselor may stifle the client's own exploration of the meaning of risk information to himself. Weil (Weil, 2000, pp. 131–133) also reviews some of the factors influencing the perception of risk figures that have been identified from the behavioral science literature (Table 7-1). Understanding these factors can help the counselor to understand client attitudes and behaviors in relation to risk communication.

Preference for Risk Information   Another area that has been examined is the preference for risk information. Fransen et al. (2006) developed a checklist to assess risk communication in genetic counseling, with the goal of identifying the relationship between aspects of risk communication and outcomes such as risk perception and decision-making. In testing the checklist, they found that counselors often presented the risks of genetic disorders only in proportions and framed the risk in negative terms.

Several studies have documented a preference for receiving probability information in numerical terms (Shaw and Dear, 1990; Julian-Reynier et al., 2003). However, other studies have found that patients differ in their preference for numerical versus qualitative terms (Mazur and Hickam, 1991). In a study of the presentation of risk information during genetic counseling for breast and ovarian cancer, there was little difference in the number of women who stated a preference for percentages, proportions, or population comparisons. In over 40% of cases, risk information was not presented in the counselees' preferred quantitative format (Hallowell et al., 1997). Risk communication using "gambling" odds (1 chance in x) resulted in the most accurate estimate of risk and was the format most preferred by women with an increased risk for breast cancer (Hopwood et al., 2003).

Fear, Anxiety, Uncertainty   In an examination of genetic testing for breast cancer, Press et al. (2000) discuss the adoption of a "risk paradigm" caused by a focus on cancer fear, the risk of developing breast cancer, and the necessity of early screening and testing. They state that epidemiological risks are inappropriately applied to individual women, and these women are pushed into choosing tests and surveillance that do not provide cures or prevention of cancer. The information is presented as tailored for individual women, and the inherent uncertainties are not emphasized. The process also implies blame for illness in women who do not choose testing. They view this emphasis on risk and the possibility of disease as endangering women's sense of well-being. The authors suggest that practitioners (they specifically address nurses) need to help women cope with the anxiety, uncertainty, and fear of breast cancer risk, and carefully examine both the positive and negative aspects of genetic testing.

TABLE 7-1. Factors Influencing Perception of Risk Figures (Weil, 2000)

Factor	Description	Counseling Example
Anchoring	Bias introduced by first concept or risk figure introduced	Counselor: The risk of having another child with Down syndrome is low. Client: So it won't happen again? Counselor: The risk is only about 1%. How does that sound to you? Client: Well..low....I guess. [This client might have been better served if the counselor had avoided the qualitative risk description.]
Cognitive and emotional factors	Individual factors such as optimism vs. pessimism, attitudes toward taking risks, preference for numerical format	Client: I'm not too worried about the result. I doubt that I have it. Conselor: You sound optimistic. Have you thought about how you *would* react if the test showed that you inherited the mutation that your mother has?
Prior beliefs	Client beliefs about level of risk	Counselor: Now that we have a diagnosis, we can tell you that the chance of Jamie's condition happening again is 25%. Client: Wow, you're kidding! Counselor: It sounds like that surprised you. Is 25% lower or higher than you were thinking? Client: Well, my family doctor told me it's one in a million! I think it's probably lower than 25% and I'm not that worried.
Availability	Prior experiences of client	Client: What if I have a miscarriage? My neighbor had an amnio, and she miscarried one week later. Counselor: It can really hit you hard when you know somebody that had a complication. Let's talk a little about our overall experience at St. Mary's.
Representativeness	Inference from small sample to larger group	Client: I don't see how the risk can be 50%. In my family everybody has it! Counselor: Let's take a closer look. We know that 4 of the women in your parents' generation had breast cancer, but we don't really know about the men because they are unlikely to develop cancer if they inherit the mutation. One of your aunts died at a young age, so we also don't know if she had the mutation. Since the women in your generation are young, we don't yet know their experience. When we look at a whole group of families, we see that about 50% of people inherit *BRCA* mutations when their parent has a mutation. We think that having more than 50% in one family is just random chance. That's why I think your chance is still 50%. I can see why you *feel* that the risk is higher. If your test results come back negative, do you think you'll believe the result? Client: I...don't know.

(continued)

TABLE 7-1. (*Continued*)

Factor	Description	Counseling Example
Complexity	Complexity of risk figures	Counselor: We may want to talk more about how you can feel safe if your test result is negative.
		Client: I'm confused. You said that my risk is 50% to have the mutation and 30% to develop cancer if I have it? How much should I worry about it?
		Counselor: Let's take a look at it using some pictures. It may help you to visualize it better.
Uncertainty	Uncertainty associated with the risk figure	Client: You mean I could get Mom's mutation and never even have cancer!
Math ability	Ability to understand numerical values and probability	Client: Since I have two children with it already, that means I should have two without it, right?
Competing values	Competing values and responsibilities	Client: I don't feel like I could lose another baby like that again, but I've always wanted to have a big family.
Consequences	Range of consequences for a specific client	Counselor: We talked about the full range of fragile X syndrome and that it is hard to predict the symptoms for another baby.
		Client: That's what's so hard about this decision. We know we don't want to bring a boy into the world with problems like my nephew, but we wouldn't be sure how bad it would be.
Binarization	Tendency to view risk in two categories (event will occur or not occur)	Counselor: The risk of having another child with OI is 5%. How does that number sound to you?
		Client: Well, it happened before and my risk was much lower. To me it seems like 50–50. Either you have it or you don't.
Need for uncertainty reduction	Emotional need to reduce uncertainty	Client: I just want to know. I'm so sick of wondering, will I have it or not? Nothing could be worse than that!
		Counselor: If you were to test positive, what do you think would change for you?
Risk vs. burden	Concept of risk vs. burden in light of the concepts of uncertainty and undesirability	Counselor: It sounds like you don't know what to do. How do you think your life would change if you had a child with hemophilia?
		Client: Well, I know the risk is pretty high. But I've seen how my mom handled it, and I think our family did pretty well.

Models of Risk Communication: What Conceptual Frameworks are Relevant to Genetic Counseling?

Theoretical models endeavor to provide a framework to explain observed phenomena. Models specific to genetic counseling and risk communication are listed in Table 7-2. If the model fits well with observed data, it can be used to understand the world of the counselee (and sometimes the counselor), design effective interventions, and guide research. These are beginning attempts at understanding the delivery of risk information. The following counseling recommendations were made by the authors of these risk communication models.

o Figure out which facts have the greatest value to the audience. Adapt the message to the cognitive processes of its recipients (Fischhoff, 1999).

o Accept and validate clients' experiences (embodied knowledge) to help increase their self-knowledge, autonomy, and decision-making capacity (Lippman, 1999).

o Explore and challenge personal beliefs before genetic test results in order to improve adjustment in the posttest period (McAllister, 2003).

o Explore counselee's experiences in depth and develop strategies that aid a patient to think through and reflect on those experiences in light of the new information (d'Agincourt-Canning, 2005)

o Focus on variables that can be modified to encourage systematic, deliberate processing of genetic risk information and disable heuristic strategies (Etchegary and Perrier, 2007).

  – Decrease time pressure.

  – Explore client's desired confidence in her decision.

  – Decrease ambiguity of information by clear communication. Definitions should include both what a term means and what it does not mean.

  – Explore *personal* relevance and implications of information before making a decision.

  – Use self-affirmation techniques (e.g., reflecting on important values) to reduce defensive processing of health risk information.

  – Increase client's engagement with risk information.

  – When communicating about risks, include information about managing risks.

  – Present risk information in multiple ways to avoid framing bias and directiveness (e.g., 5% chance of birth defect; 95% change of healthy baby).

Aspects of Risk Communication to Clients

Genetic counselors increasingly recognize the importance of engaging with clients in discussions of risk and decision-making and helping them to incorporate the increasing amount of information and difficult choices into their lives.

TABLE 7-2. Models of Risk Communication

Model	Population	Features	Authors
Riskiness of the gamble	Parents at ↑ risk for affected child	○ The risk of having a child is a gamble. ○ Risk is a combination of probability (uncertainty) and adversity. ○ Riskiness of the gamble is determined by magnitude of probability and level of adversity. ○ Factors influence judgment of adversity (e.g., likelihood of complications, restrictions on parents). ○ Amount, consistency, and clarity of information about factors will influence judgment of adversity.	Palmer and Sainfort, 1993
Embodied knowledge	Prenatal diagnosis clients	○ Women create embodied knowledge by negotiating with biomedical information, transforming it through identifiable processes, and integrating it with their personal beliefs and experiences. ○ Decisions are based on embodied knowledge.	Lippman, 1999
Adapting the message	Individuals at ↑ risk for cancer	○ Formulating an effective risk message begins by characterizing the information needs of the intended audience and what the recipients currently believe. ○ The message should focus on the critical facts that are worth knowing. Those facts need to be transmitted in a credible, comprehensive way. ○ The resulting communication should be tested and the process continued until the audience members experience no more than the acceptable level of misunderstanding.	Fischhoff, 1999
Engagement	Counselees having genetic testing for hereditary nonpolyposis colon cancer	○ Engagement reflects the cognitive and emotional involvement with cancer risk shown by counselees. ○ Counselees demonstrate a gradient from engagement to disengagement that can explain variations in approaches and reactions to predictive genetic testing.	McAllister, 2002, 2003

		o The degree of engagement predicts risk perception. Degree of engagement is influenced by social factors and psychological factors that either facilitate or block the process of engaging with cancer risk.	
		o Engagement fluctuates with time for the same client.	
		o Clients who are intensely engaged with their risk of developing cancer adjust better to a positive test result than clients who are partially (intellectually but not emotionally) engaged.	
Experiential knowledge	Individuals having genetic testing for hereditary breast and ovarian cancer	o Experiential knowledge is composed of empathetic knowledge, derived from connectedness to and knowledge of other family members' experiences, and embodied knowledge, which refers to subjective knowledge derived from bodily experience. o Experiential knowledge is integral to participants' understanding and perception of their cancer risk.	d'Agincourt-Canning, 2005
Heuristic-systematic model	Not applicable	o Effortful, systematic information processing (as opposed to superficial heuristic information processing) is conducive to informed decision-making and improved understanding of risk information. o People who process information systematically form attitudes that are relatively stable over time and resistant to change, and they are more likely to engage in protective health behaviors and make informed decisions. o Variables thought to promote systematic processing include personal relevance, lack of time pressure, perceived need to be accountable for one's judgments, high perceived amount of information needed for the judgment, self-affirmation opportunities, answering reflective questions, entering risk information on a graphical display, and using persolalized expressions of risk information.	Etchegary and Perrier, 2007

215

Practical Aspects Veach et al. (2003) have discussed practical guidelines for presenting risk information. For example, they discuss useful strategies for ensuring that you know your clients' prior beliefs, needs, and ways of processing information; techniques for compensating for counselors' personal biases; strategies that aid clear communication; and strategies to help clients process information. They stress the need to address client emotions during the risk discussion. They also discuss common mistakes when giving information, along with suggestions for counteracting these mistakes. The mistakes include lack of organization and preparation, inflexibility, overload of information and technical jargon, rushing the session, lack of dialog with clients, inappropriate use of close-ended questions, failing to address client emotions and defenses, lack of attention to cultural factors, and inability to admit a lack of knowledge (Veach et al., 2003).

Discourse analysis analyzing use of language and how this might influence decisions showed that counselors used indirect speech, marked by the use of hints, hedges, and other politeness strategies (e.g., use of the phrases "some people" and "most people") to facilitate rapport and to preserve client autonomy (Benkendorf et al., 2001). However, this indirectness may obstruct direct explorations of client needs. Counselors should examine this strategy and consider whether it keeps them from engaging in a client-centered exploration of personal goals and values.

O'Doherty and Suthers (2007) recommended clinical tactics for risk communication in a cancer genetic counseling situation:

1. Encourage clients to use estimates of risk to assist with decision-making rather than as meaningful predictors of future events.
2. Frame the information to clients in multiple ways (e.g., 60% risk of developing cancer and 40% risk of not developing cancer).
3. Provide risk information in terms of absolute probabilities rather than relative risks.
4. Encourage the client to reflect on their professed preferences from different perspectives and over a relatively long period of time (years to decades).
5. Use numerical probabilities as the basis for risk information but include verbal qualifiers to set the numerical risk in the context of other life events.
6. Encourage the client to place the risk of cancer in context by outlining what the diagnosis, risks, and interventions might entail and not entail from the client's point of view.

The CRISCOM Working Group (a European Project on risk communication), published an excellent review of literature regarding risk communication strategies and risk perception in the context of cancer genetic services (Julian-Reynier et al., 2003). Their objectives of risk communication were to modify health behaviors and to facilitate informed decision-making. They discussed the multiple types of risks that must be communicated and two complementary types of risk communication, the probability-based approach and the contextualized approach (personalized information). Examples of the contextualized approach include using the counselee's personal family history, using stories from others, or using culturally tailored messages to illustrate risk information and options. Other contextualized strategies are to elicit and utilize the counselee's views, concerns, and experiences with coping to discuss a plan of action, to tailor messages to the counselee, and to use complementary information tools such as decision aids, leaflets, or videos. The probability-based approach may utilize multiple formats for presenting risk information, including multiple types of numbers, verbal labels, or visual displays. The majority of women express a preference for numerical risk figures, although people often transform these figures into discrete categories. Individual risk estimates, especially short-term risk estimates, are more likely to change behavior than population estimates. Combining visual representations of risk with numerical and written information improves the perceived helpfulness of the information and the accuracy of perceived risk. Gain-framed (positive) messages were more effective in promoting desirable health outcomes than loss-framed (negative) messages. Tailoring risk information and medical recommendations to the individual client may be effective in changing risk perception or screening behavior, and is also sensitive to the cognitive processing style, readiness for behavior change, and confidence in behavior change of the clients. Decision aids appear to be most helpful to clients who are undecided at the time of the intervention. The authors conclude by offering three principles of risk communication: (1) **Assess** a priori beliefs, knowledge, preferences, expectations, anxiety and coping styles of the recipients before formulating a risk communication plan. (2) **Prioritize** information to be given. Put the information in context and use multiple communication strategies and formats. (3) **Follow up** with materials such as leaflets, videos, CD-ROM, personal letters. Consider more than one meeting.

Psychosocial Aspects   Many genetic counselors have noted that attending to the psychosocial aspects of counseling impacts counselees' understanding of risk (d'ydewalle and Evers-Kiebooms, 1987; Lerman et al., 1995, 1997; Soldan et al., 2000; Trepanier et al., 2004; Hopwood, 2005; Berliner and Fay, 2007). Lippman (1999) specifically stresses listening and validating "women's complementary ways of knowing." This has also been expressed in the terminology of listening to patients' narratives (Kenen and Smith, 1995). Using the life history narrative model, counselors invite clients to speak in their own voices, control the introduction and flow of topics, and extend their stories. The counselor is interested in thematic coherence—how utterances express a speaker's recurrent assumptions, beliefs, and goals or cognitive world. This technique has the advantage of including the family and sociocultural perspective and is a useful technique in the initial stages of a risk communication and/or decision-making encounter. Esplen et al. (1998) present a group therapy approach to facilitate integration of risk information for women at risk for breast cancer. They note that most previous attempts to improve communication of risk information focused on the content of specific information and on improving knowledge about risk factors and genetic information, rather than on the emotional impact of being at risk. Their approach incorporates principles of supportive-expressive therapy to address the emotional impact of being at risk for breast cancer in order to promote accuracy of perceived risk. In evaluating the intervention, they found that risk comprehension was improved by 70%, and there were improvements in measures of psychosocial functioning such as cancer-related distress, depression, anxiety and unresolved grief (Esplen et al., 2000). Hopwood (2005) recommends that counselors explore idiosyncratic risk beliefs, personal theories of inheritance, and personal or social resources that underpin coping.

Weil (2000, pp. 134–137) also presents techniques for presenting risk information. These include balanced presentation of risk figures, exploration of the *meaning* of risk figures for the counselee, ensuring that counselees understand the statistical independence of each conception, correcting misunderstanding with a psycho-dynamic origin, resisting excessive reassurance, care in explaining multiple or complex risk figures, and tailoring risk information to clients.

Social Aspects   Another perspective is represented by the work of Bryant et al. (2006). They investigated viewpoints of a variety of people (with and without significant prior experience with Down syndrome) regarding Down syndrome's impact on the affected persons, their families, and society. They found that whether or not participants saw people with Down syndrome within 'a continuum of normality' relates to their views of prenatal testing and termination of pregnancy. Some people focused on the impairment and how this would impact quality of life for families, affected individuals, or both (individual models of disability). Others focused more on social models of disability that identify the role of material and cultural barriers to good quality of life. The authors argue that information available to parents within the prenatal testing context should not perpetuate stereotypes that reinforce a perception of people with a disability as "other," and that materials must be developed with those who have practical experience of living with the relevant condition. This suggests that it is not enough to counsel nondirectively, but that counselors have an obligation to educate people about these viewpoints in order to enable counselees to make truly informed decisions.

Spiritual Aspects   One other important aspect of risk communication in the context of genetic testing is the spiritual aspect. In a study of pastoral counseling in relation to genetic testing, genetic counselors seldom referred clients for pastoral counseling and, in fact, seldom inquired about patients' religious or spiritual values (White, 2006). It is important for genetic counselors to recognize the diversity of spiritual and religious beliefs and to be aware that religious identification does not necessarily indicate a person's beliefs or preferences. Patients may find that their religious beliefs offer hope and strength, or compound their suffering. Questions of "playing God" often surface with new technologies such as genetic testing, including issues of controlling human life, disease, death, and the genome. One point of view is that human beings are part of God's creation and thus part of the natural world and subject to its laws. Another is that by virtue of our God-given reflective capacities and intelligence we are empowered to manipulate nature, and all medical treatments and reproductive technologies harness natural biological systems. Pastoral counselors can provide counseling, and in addition can conduct religious assessments and rituals, help people draw on their religious beliefs to make sense of their circumstances, interpret and affirm patients' decisions in view of their religious background, and help cope with tragedy and loss.

Risk Communication in the Family

Although a discussion of risk communication in the family may or may not emerge in the genetic counseling discussion, family influences play an important role in risk awareness, genetic testing decisions, and outcomes (Croyle and Lerman, 1999; Daly et al., 2001). For this reason, risk communication should include an assessment of the impact of family members who are not present on adjustment to genetic risk and genetic testing decisions, as well as the counselee's beliefs about the effect of their adaptation and decisions on other family members.

In a study of the influence of **significant others** on communication and interactions between healthy women from families with a history of breast/ovarian cancer, social structure affected the meaning and use of genetic information and services (Kenen et al., 2004a). They found that women had strong support from women friends; close communication with sisters, but often limited because of strongly ambivalent feelings; support from partners, but often only under conditions that the partners found comfortable; and more distant communication with brothers. They also discuss gender differences in the use of social support during illness, with women more effectively utilizing the support of family and friends than men.

When **family systems theory** was used to investigate the impact of HD pre-symptomatic testing on families, at least half of families interviewed identified changes in the following areas of family functioning: family membership, family patterns of communication, and future care giving concerns as they influenced current relationships (Sobel and Cowan, 2000). The authors conclude that genetic testing is a family, as opposed to an individual, matter and that family involvement in the decision-making process should be strongly encouraged in order to help families adjust. Families will benefit in pretest sessions from an examination of their patterns of dealing with illness issues, both past and present.

In a study of males at risk for *BRCA1/2* mutations, the principal motivation for seeking genetic testing was **concern for children** (Hallowell et al., 2005). The authors suggest that when it comes to genetic testing the patient/counselee really is the family. Counselors can help the family to acknowledge and weigh the implications for the health of other family members into their decisions about testing. They also suggest that counselors warn parents that their adult children may not support testing, and therefore it may be beneficial to discuss testing with adult children before the testing decision is made.

Another reason that communication about other family members is important is the obligation for counselors to inform **at-risk family members** of their risks.

This need for indirect communication may pose another layer of complexity for the task of risk communication. In a qualitative study to evaluate family communication and family dynamics regarding HNPCC, family members who were persuaded to seek counseling/testing services by the proband were more likely to have counseling/testing and were more likely to seek those services sooner (Peterson et al., 2003). Genetic counselors should attempt to identify existing communication norms within families and ways that family members can take an active role in encouraging others to learn about their cancer risk and options for testing. This may be especially important for more distantly related at-risk relatives. Koehly et al. (2003) stress the importance of a family systems approach to understand how health-related information is diffused through the family and the family members most likely to influence the client's decisions about genetic counseling/testing. They also warn that kinship alone does not sufficiently explain family communication. Characteristics of dyadic relationships such as general communication patterns, support patterns, leadership relations, and lack of conflict are also important. They recommend that practitioners (1) allow clients to define who is family, to capture all persons who may play a role in the process, (2) use a team approach to encourage the use of genetic services, identifying a family leader in the process, and (3) assess and use relational information to identify family members who may be particularly influential and supportive with regard to counseling and testing decisions, as well as persons who may be barriers to the diffusion of information.

In a study of **barriers and facilitators in family communication** about genetic risk for hereditary breast/ovarian cancer and Huntington disease, telling family members about risk was generally seen as a family responsibility, and family structures, dynamics, and "rules" influenced disclosure decisions (Forrest et al., 2003). However, many participants felt that help was needed from the genetics clinic practitioners. This came in the form of holding a group counseling session, writing family letters, and legitimizing the information. Family members also felt a responsibility toward younger generations. Barriers to informing family members of risk included relatives refusing access to at-risk family members (e.g., aunt refusing to tell niece), gender patterns (e.g., women were seen as gatekeepers of important family information), procrastination, reluctance to give information to younger family members, closed family styles of communication, needing time to process one's own risk status or genetic test results, uncertainty about the level of risk, lack of testing in the proband, desire to protect relatives from painful knowledge, preexisting family conflicts and rifts, distant relationships due to deaths in the family, the belief that others did not need to know, prior negative experiences with risk communication, and differences of opinion about who should give information, as well as how and when it should be given.

In a qualitative interview study of people at risk for HNPCC, risk disclosure was stimulated if people felt morally obliged to do so, when they anticipated regret if something preventable happened, if there were, especially fatal, cases in the family, and if professionals recommended disclosure (Mesters et al., 2005). Barriers to disclosure were disrupted and tense family relations, young age of the message recipients, and negative experiences at first attempt to disclose. Gaff et al. (2007) reviewed the process and outcomes of communication of genetic information within families. They discuss a process of (1) making sense of personal risk, (2) assessing the vulnerability and receptivity of the family member, and (3) making a decision about what will be conveyed and selecting the right time for the discussion. Understanding the possible barriers may help genetic counselors to devise effective counseling strategies to aid families with risk communication.

There are several adaptations of pedigree-taking techniques that incorporate exploration of family interactions. These may be used for exploring risk communication in the family as well as factors that are likely to impact on adaptation to and decisions about risk. The social work field has a long tradition of using genograms, which are family histories focusing on intra-familial relationships. Kenen and Peters have extended this technique and developed the CEGRM (Colored Eco-Genetic Relationship Map) and tested its use in breast/ovarian cancer families (Kenen and Peters, 2001; Peters et al., 2004). Engaging in the interactive, insight-promoting CEGRM process provided a tool both for assessing the social context of genetic counseling and helping high-risk women better understand and integrate genetic information into their personal and family identities, health beliefs, and decisions (Peters et al., 2006).

A summary of literature findings about risk communication is presented in Table 7-3. The following counseling recommendations were made by the authors of these studies.

1. Assess the impact of family members who are not present on adjustment to genetic risk and genetic testing decisions, as well as the counselee's beliefs about the effect of their adaptation and decisions on other family members (Croyle and Lerman, 1999; Daly et al., 2001).
2. Encourage family involvement in the decision-making process in order to help families adjust. In pretest sessions, help families examine their patterns of dealing with past and present illness issues (Sobel and Cowan, 2000).
3. Help the family to acknowledge and weigh the implications for the health of other family members into their decisions about testing. Warn parents that their adult children may not support testing, and it may be beneficial to discuss testing with adult children before the testing decision is made (Hallowell et al., 2005).
4. Attempt to identify existing communication norms within families and ways that family members can take an active role in encouraging others to learn about their cancer risk and options for testing (Peterson et al., 2003).
5. Use a family systems approach to understand how health-related information is diffused through the family and the family members most likely to influence the client's decisions about genetic counseling/testing. Allow clients to define who is family, to capture all persons who may play a role in the process. Use a team approach to encourage the use of genetic services, identifying a family leader in the process. Assess and use relational information to identify family members

TABLE 7-3. Risk Communication in the Family: Literature Findings

Authors	Findings
Kenen et al., 2004a,2004b	o Support from close friends and family members is limited by ambivalent feelings and uncomfortable issues. o Women more effectively utilize the support of family and friends than men. o When discussion of breast/ovarian cancer violates the family script, some women try to renegotiate their family script.
Sobel and Cowan, 2000	o Testing causes changes in family membership, family patterns of communication, and future care giving concerns. o Spouses are more depressed by a positive result for their partners than are their partners. o Individuals testing negative may lose membership in the family or be burdened by current or future caretaking responsibilities.
Hallowell et al., 2005	o For men, the principal motivation for seeking genetic testing may be concern for children. o Men generally make the testing decision with other family members, usually their spouse. o Adult children are generally not informed about their father's testing and sometimes resent the secrecy and/or the testing.
Peterson et al., 2003	o Family members who are persuaded to seek counseling/testing by the proband are more likely to have counseling/testing and seek services sooner.
Koehly et al., 2003	o Family members are more likely to discuss genetic counseling/testing if either one carries a HNPCC mutation, if either one is a spouse or a first-degree relative of the other, or if the relationship is defined by positive cohesion, communication, or lack of conflict.
Forrest et al., 2003	o Telling family members about risk is seen as a family responsibility, and family structures, dynamics and "rules" influenced disclosure decisions. o Family members felt a responsibility toward younger generations. o Barriers to informing family members of risk included relatives refusing access to at-risk family members, gender patterns, procrastination, reluctance to give information to younger family members, closed family styles of communication, needing time to process one's own risk status or genetic test results, uncertainty about level of risk, lack of testing in the proband, desire to protect relatives from painful knowledge, preexisting family conflicts and rifts, distant relationships due to deaths in the family, the belief that others did not need to know, prior negative experiences with risk communication, and differences of opinion about who should give information, as well as how and when it should be given.

Mesters et al., 2005	o Risk disclosure was stimulated if people felt morally obliged to do so, when they anticipated regret if something preventable happened, if there were, especially fatal, cases in the family, and if professionals recommended disclosure.
	o Barriers to disclosure were tense and disrupted family relations, young age of the message recipients, and negative experiences at first attempt to disclose.
Gaff et al., 2007	o Communication of genetic information within families includes (1) making sense of personal risk, (2) assessing vulnerability and receptivity of the family member, (3) making a decision about what will be conveyed, and selecting the right time for the discussion.
Kenen and Peters, 2001; Peters et al., 2004,2006	o Adaptations of pedigree-taking techniques (e.g., CEGRM) can explore factors likely to impact adaptation to and decisions about risk, as well as help high-risk women understand and integrate genetic information into their personal and family identities, health beliefs, and decisions.

who may be particularly influential and supportive with regard to counseling and testing decisions, as well as persons who may be barriers to the diffusion of information (Koehly et al., 2003).

6. Help family communication by holding a group counseling session, writing family letters, and legitimizing the information (Forrest et al., 2003).

7. Understand possible barriers and help devise effective counseling strategies to aid families with risk communication. When writing family letters, compromise between providing enough indirect information to maximize the likelihood that relatives will be able to make an informed decision about pursuing counseling, evaluation and/or testing, and overwhelming the relative with information s/he did not request (Gaff et al., 2007).

As Celeste considers testing, you would like her to have accurate information about the scientific facts and a good understanding of possible outcomes for her and her family. You will need to explain not only autosomal dominant inheritance, but also the complications of age penetrance, variation due to differences in CAG repeat size and other causes as yet unidentified, differences in the possibility of expansion from mothers vs. fathers, and the possibility of uncertain results due to intermediate repeat size. If you use an interactive style of counseling, you may be able to assess her level and accuracy of knowledge, and build her trust in your information and ability to help her. It will also be important to understand the issues in her life that relate to the risk of HD. For example, you might explore her relationship to her father and her fears about developing HD, her partner's reactions to the possibility of genetic testing, siblings' risk and the potential for caregiving, and her concerns about children inheriting HD.

DECISION-MAKING

Decision-making will be discussed here in relation to reaching a decision about having genetic testing, management of genetic conditions/birth defects, and reproductive-related decisions, tests, and procedures, as well as the ramifications surrounding these decisions on the counselee and his or her family. Many observers comment on the difference between health services in which the benefits of procedures or tests clearly outweigh the risks and the activity is said to have medical benefit versus "preference-sensitive" health services, in which the ratios of benefit to harm are either uncertain or dependent on patient values (for example, O'Connor et al., 2003). We are mainly discussing situations that fall in the latter category.

You have now had a discussion with Celeste about risk information and family dynamics. How can you help her make an informed decision about having testing? How will your approach change if she is requesting help with the decision vs. appearing to have made up her mind vs. indicating that she will decide in the future?

Factors Impacting Decision Making

Counselees' decisions about testing and risk-reducing treatments are influenced less by their actual risk status than by subjective interpretations of risk and emotional factors (Pearn, 1973; Shiloh and Saxe, 1989; Lerman et al., 2002; van Dijk et al., 2003). The decision of whether or not to test is associated with salient test features such as:

1. The possibility of effective prevention, treatment or screening
2. Health beliefs (e.g., perceived risks, beliefs about etiology)
3. Characteristics of the counselees (e.g., age, family cohesiveness, gender, insurance status, knowledge, levels of pretest worry, need for certainty, personal and family history of the disorder, pessimism, pretest distress, religiosity, desire for children, attitudes toward reproductive alternatives, coping mechanisms, sources of support)
4. Concerns about potential risks (Shiloh et al., 1995; Biesecker et al., 2000; Schwartz et al., 2000; Weil, 2000; Lerman et al., 2002; Ropka et al., 2006)

Genetic counseling does not influence the intention to test or actual test uptake (Lerman et al., 1997; Kaiser et al., 2004; Matloff et al., 2006, Sankar et al., 2006), but it has helped women make decisions about genetic testing (Clark et al., 2000).

In one of the earliest qualitative studies of genetic counseling, Lippman-Hand and Fraser (1979a) performed a qualitative analysis of interviews with 53 parents who had had genetic counseling to characterize the process by which childbearing decisions were made and to determine how counselees resolved the problems created by being at risk. Previously it had been assumed that counselees make informed and rational decisions based on precise, unambiguous recurrence risk information. By examining the actual behaviors of counselees, they observed that counselees viewed widely differing recurrence risks in binary form. The event would either happen or not happen. Although some counselees expressed a desire for advice, they sometimes wanted it as a background against which to view their own choices. The uncertainties inherent in risk information necessitated further processing of factual information to make it relevant. This processing includes the interaction of risk and consequences, the search for socially acceptable alternatives, and integration of the information into the counselee's life circumstances. They found that counselees attempted to limit uncertainties and neutralize problematic consequences by inferring from factual information and their own experiences how they could manage the possible consequences of taking a chance. They identified factors influencing a parent's ability to make a clear decision: presence of a previous normal child, diffusion of decision-making responsibility to others, and recognition that one had already managed the worst. When parents could not develop a sense of coping with another pregnancy, they either decided against reproduction or made a "nondecision" about reproduction by leaving conception to chance ("reproductive roulette"), which served to diffuse responsibility for the decision.

Medical Management Decisions related to treatment and medical management are complex. In women at risk for familial breast cancer, the impact of objective risk information on the intention for prophylactic mastectomy was limited and was mediated by perceived risk (van Dijk et al., 2003). Important determinants of the intention for prophylactic mastectomy in this group were precounseling levels of breast cancer worry and perceived risk, suggesting that genetic counseling is only one event in the entire process of decision-making. One of the factors impacting decision-making is that the results of genetic tests may influence management of a disorder or condition. For example, in *BRCA1/2* testing there was an increase in intentions for surgery or actual surgery in women who tested positive for *BRCA1/2* compared to women who tested negative. Some women choose not to undergo prophylactic mastectomy or oophorectomy before genetic counseling and do not change their decisions after genetic counseling (Miron et al., 2000). The factors most important in influencing risk-reduction surgery decisions were genetic test results, concerns about surgery, timing in life, and early menopause. Intention to undergo prophylactic oophorectomy in women at high risk for ovarian cancer was correlated with perceived risk of developing ovarian cancer and greater perceived benefits of surgery (Fang et al., 2003).

Anxiety and Worry There are several studies that looked at counselee factors that predict interest in testing or specific decisions. In a retrospective survey of genetic counselors, patient **anxiety level** predicted pregnancy management decisions (Wallerstein et al., 2006). Ultrasound findings and actual risks for abnormal outcome, although significantly associated with anxiety, were not the sole predictors of the final decision made. Counselors also reported discussions with patients about history of infertility, whether this was a first and/or a much-wanted pregnancy, whether this was an age-related "last chance" pregnancy, religious views, impact on other family members, and the presence of a previous child with a disability. **Worry** was the most important variable influencing prenatal decision-making (Kenen et al., 2000b). Women at risk because of age assigned the risk to their age category, whereas women at risk because of an abnormal test personalized the risk. Individuals choosing to undergo *BRCA1/2* testing were more likely to be older ($\geq$40 years), to have lower levels of optimism, and to report higher levels of family cohesiveness (Biesecker et al., 2000).

Family In a study of male partners' involvement in reproductive decision-making, male partners seemed to view prenatal diagnosis as either an *information* decision or an *action* decision and appeared to take a more active role in decision making when the decision was viewed as an *action* decision (Kenen et al., 2000a). Regarding *who* influences women's decisions to have prenatal diagnosis, women felt strongly that they themselves were responsible for their decision, although most were also strongly influenced by their partner (Jaques et al., 2004).

In a questionnaire study of men's decision-making about *BRCA1/2* testing (Hallowell et al., 2005), all of the men described their decision to have genetic testing as influenced by their obligations to other family members, primarily their children. For a minority of men, genetic testing presented them with a conflict of duties—their duty to warn their children of their risks versus their duty not to harm them by causing emotional distress. Adult children were often excluded from the decision-making, and some expressed resentment about this. Mothers of potential mutation carriers perceive themselves as having a right to be involved in the decision-making about their at-risk partner's genetic testing.

Social Relationships Many women would have liked to discuss the decision to test with women who had previously had testing (Jaques et al., 2004). Face-to-face counseling was the preferred source of professional information. d'Agincourt-Canning (2006) makes the case that cancer genetic decision-making must be viewed in the context of social relationships. A relational concept of self (rather than an individualistic model of autonomy) provides a better framework for understanding genetic testing decisions; medical choices are made in relation to a continuum of responsibilities toward ourselves and others. She recommends that counselors discussing genetic testing focus not only on the autonomous chooser but also on the broader social circumstances, responsibilities, and commitments of counselees. One example of this concept is a study of consanguineous couples in Israel (Shiloh et al., 1995). The authors found that consanguineous couples' reproductive decisions were influenced by genetic counseling 86% of the time. In many cases, the "influence" was not in changing the reproductive decision, but in providing the couple with information that strengthened their original decision. They recommend that genetic counseling for consanguinity offer help in dealing with the confusion and distress caused by uncertainty, and that it incorporate psychological and decision-making support. They also recommend that health care services should not attempt to disrupt deep-rooted traditional marriage patterns.

DECISION SCALES

There are some useful scales that have been developed to aid with the measurement of decision-making. One widely used scale is the decisional conflict scale (DCS) (O'Connor, 1995), which was designed to measure the level of decisional conflict experienced by patients making health care decisions. The DCS discriminated between those who had strong intentions either to accept or to decline breast cancer screening and those whose intentions were uncertain. There was an inverse correlation between the DCS and knowledge test scores. An informed choice scale that contains measures of knowledge, attitudes, and uptake related to a screening test in pregnancy was developed (Marteau et al., 2001). With this scale, 43% of women were classified as having made an informed choice about the screening test and 57% an uninformed choice.

Two scales were developed that measure satisfaction with a health care decision (Holmes-Rovner et al., 1996; Sainfort and Booske, 2000). Sainfort and Booske discuss the quality of the decision-making process, the quality of the choice, and the confidence in one's decision as important factors is assessing decisions. Elwyn et al. (2003) developed the OPTION scale for measuring patient involvement in shared decision-making. This scale, developed in a primary care setting, showed that practitioners' scores were low on the scale of possible involvement. It would be interesting to see whether results are similar in genetic counseling settings. In developing a decision evaluation scale to evaluate decision aids, Stalmeier et al. (2005) identified three important factors: satisfaction-uncertainty, informed choice, and decision control. The process of shared decision-making, in which the practitioner and the counselee form an alliance in reaching a health care decision, has become an important concept in the health care literature.

Models of Decision-Making: What Conceptual Frameworks Are Relevant to Genetic Counseling?

In a qualitative, descriptive study, clinicians and patients had different goals, purposes, and values regarding prenatal testing (Hunt et al., 2005). The information the clinicians provided patients reflected their clinical interest in identifying and controlling pathophysiology, while patients were most concerned with protecting and nurturing their pregnancy. Patients were not very engaged with relative risks and a utilitarian assessment of the expected value of the knowledge the test could produce. They were primarily interested in promoting the welfare of their baby and managing the sense of vulnerability the screening test itself had provoked. The authors recommend a shared decision-making approach, in which both clinicians and patients bring information and values to the discussion.

Models specific to genetic counseling and decision-making are listed in Table 7-4. The following counseling recommendations were made by the authors of these risk communication models.

1. Parents can use scenarios (series of consequences the parent imagines as outcomes of an event) to evaluate consequences of various decisions and choose the course of action that appears to provide the least loss vs. one whose maximum loss would be acceptable. Part of the development of scenarios involves the parents' perceptions of their ability to cope (Lippman-Hand and Fraser, 1979a, 1979b).

2. Brainstorm alternatives and relevant factors; bring irrational factors to the surface; evaluate alternatives; choose the most important factors and best alternatives; and review and revise the decision (Danish and D'Augelli, 1983; adapted by Veach et al., 2003, pp. 136–139).

3. Using crisis intervention, counselors can be directive in structuring a process to aid the patient in making a decision, while being nondirective about the content of the process and the outcome of the decision (O'Daniel and Wells, 2002). O'Daniel and Wells describe three common phases of crisis intervention:
   a. Beginning phase
      i. Build relationship and join with patient.
      ii. Define and assess the crisis situation.
      iii. Develop goals and an action plan to meet those goals.
   b. Action phase
      i. Collect additional information needed to inform actions.

TABLE 7-4. Models of Decision-Making

Model	Population	Features	Authors
Decision-making under uncertainty	Not applicable	o To assess the probability of an uncertain event or the value of an uncertain quantity, people rely on a limited number of heuristic principles that reduce the complex tasks of assessing probabilities and predicting values to simpler judgmental operations. Sometimes these heuristics lead to severe and systematic errors. o *Representativeness* is the process of assigning attributes based on similarities to another group. *Availability* refers to the process of assessing the probability of an event by the ease with which instances or occurrences can be brought to mind. *Anchoring* refers to the process of making estimates by starting from an initial value that is adjusted to yield the final answer. o A better understanding of these heuristics and of the biases to which they lead could improve judgments and decisions in situations of uncertainty.	Tversky and Kahneman, 1974; discussed in Weil, 2000.
Risk management by neutralization of consequences	Parents making reproductive decisions	o Logic does not drive reproductive decision-making. The subjective factors important in clients' decision-making are not inferior to objective factors, but merely different. o Aid with decision-making needs to account for a lack of purely cognitive factors in decision-making by addressing the processes that counselees actually do use. o Women make child-bearing decisions by attempting to limit the uncertainties they face and by neutralizing problematic consequences by planning how to manage the possible consequences of taking a chance.	Lippman-Hand and Fraser, 1979a,1979b

(continued)

TABLE 7-4. (*Continued*)

Model	Population	Features	Authors
		o Factors that influence a parent's ability to make a decision include the presence of a previous normal child showing previous "success," diffusion of decision-making responsibility to others (e.g., a living child needs a brother or sister), and recognition that they have already managed the worst.	
		o Parents view risk in a binary fashion, thus negating the usefulness of risk estimates. "...No matter the size of the recurrence rate, something can happen—a one in the numerator never disappears no matter the size of the denominator, and this 'one' could be the counselee's child."	
		o Given this binary formulation of risk, the ability to cope with a negative outcome becomes more important than the risk estimate in the decision to have a child.	
Decision analysis	Prenatal diagnosis	o The counselee provides relative values to the potential outcomes of the pregnancy, and the counselor combines those values with the risks to produce a consistent, logical decision.	Pauker and Pauker, 1979
		o Couples' actual decisions differed from the decisions that this logical decision-making tool would predict.	
Rational decision-making	Not applicable	o It is useful to break decisions down, and a systematic model decreases anxiety.	Veach et al. (2003, pp. 136–139); adapted from Danish and D'Augelli (1983)
		o Dealing with emotions is an important component to making a decision.	
Decision-making in natural risky situations	Parents making reproductive decisions	o Individuals in risky situations are interested mainly in information about risk-defusing operators, actions expected to decrease and control the risk. They are less interested in probability information.	Shiloh et al., 2006a; adapted from Huber, 1997

		o Information about consequences of options and about possible controlling actions were evaluated as most helpful.	
		o Decision difficulty was unrelated to counselees' evaluations of the helpfulness of the information but was related to the objective controllability of the information.	
Self-regulatory theory	Not applicable	o Clients are active information processors rather than passive receivers of information.	Leventhal, 1970; Leventhal et al., 1997; adapted by Shiloh, 2006
		o People's perceptions of and beliefs about an illness (illness representations) are important mediating links between health threats and reactions to them.	
		o Cognitive information is integrated into a preexisting framework of life experiences.	
		o Personal experience is unique and can lead to different representations among people with seemingly similar experiences. Thus learning about clients' experience with a genetic condition is not enough to reveal their representations.	
		o In general, a condition is seen as less preventable when a genetic cause is emphasized, thus jeopardizing patients' motivation to change behavior and reduce risks.	
		o Self-perceptions also influence how a client will view genetic information. For example, higher levels of self-reported optimism and perceiving oneself as maintaining a healthy lifestyle may affect genetic risk perceptions.	
Crisis intervention	Prenatal diagnosis for HD	o Practitioners can use a crisis intervention model to enhance autonomy and informed decision-making for patients in crisis.	O'Daniel and Wells, 2002
		o Counselors can be directive in structuring a process to aid in decision-making, while being nondirective about the content of the process and the outcome of the decision.	
Responsibility model	Reproductive decision-making in families at risk for HD	o Regardless of the decision, people present themselves as acting responsibly.	Downing, 2005; Klitzman et al., 2007

(continued)

TABLE 7-4. (*Continued*)

Model	Population	Features	Authors
		○ Decisions are the result of the interpretation and negotiation of responsibility in the family context. How responsibility is configured depends on which relationships are prioritized and may change over time. ○ Responsibilities in counselee, spouse, and children may conflict, and many decisions are dyadic in nature (i.e., they are made by a couple).	
Empowerment model based on transactional theory of stress and coping	Not applicable	○ Genetic counseling process promotes the autonomy of the individual by providing him or her with the tools required to make his/her own decisions and enhances coping and adjustment to the outcome of those decisions through control and mastery. ○ Empowerment is the ability to affect control and positive life changes within a personal context.	McConkie-Rosell and Sullivan, 1999, based on Lazarus and Folkman, 1984

        ii. Address potential barriers to implementation.

        iii. Draw on all strengths that can help patient implement the plan.

        iv. Implement the plan.

    c. Termination phase

        i. Review actions taken and evaluate their success.

        ii. Counselor anticipatory guidance (help patient think about potential future crises, how they might be addressed, and where future support might be found if needed).

        iii. Process client feelings around ending the counseling relationship.

4. It is important for counselors to understand the various factors operating in a family that shape the patient's/client's views of responsibility, explore these factors in the counseling session, identify how clients making different choices can view their choices as responsible, and understand the roles that counselors themselves may play in the narratives that families construct about genetic responsibility (Downing, 2005).

5. Practitioners should tend to the information preferences of their clients, which reflect clients' preferred, implicit decision-making models. Let clients express their questions before providing planned or standard information. Use a shared decision-making approach with psychological counseling support (Shiloh et al., 2006a).

6. Using the self regulatory theory as a framework, Shiloh et al. (2006b) recommend that genetic counselors:

    a. Examine understanding of genetics and heredity in general before any educational attempt is initiated.

    b. Explore specific representations that clients have about particular genetic conditions before predicting or trying to modify their knowledge and reactions.

    c. Investigate clients' prior experiences with genetic conditions, using a personalized approach that would disclose individual meaning of the experience.

    d. Clarify the role of self-representations, types of threat to self-concept and coping behaviors activated in response to these threats, and direct counseling to deal with these issues.

    e. Evaluate the costs and benefits of clients' misconceptions before trying to change them.

    f. Consider interactions and compromises between cognitive and emotional motivations as predictors of counselees' action plans for coping with genetic conditions and risks.

Practical Aspects: Methods for Helping Clients with Decision-Making

The promotion of counselee self-awareness is key to assisting clients who are faced with difficult decisions. Counselees need a conscious awareness of factors that influence their decisions, obstacles to decision-making, and their decision-making style. Veach et al. present suggestions for assisting clients with decision making (Veach et al., 2003, pp. 139–141). These include:

1. Build client self-esteem and competence.
2. Assess prior experience with decision-making.
3. Help client structure and understand the decision-making process.
4. Explore reasons for decision-making.
5. Explore differences among stakeholders in the decision.
6. Recognize cultural influences.
7. Aid with feelings of guilt.
8. Help client obtain support and guidance from significant others and professionals
9. Help client engage in anticipatory activities.

Decision Difficulty   In a field study of counselees seeking genetic counseling to arrive at a reproduction decision, counselees' evaluations of decision difficulty were unrelated to their evaluations of the helpfulness of the information they received in genetic counseling (Shiloh et al., 2006b). Decision difficulty is most likely related primarily to the diagnosis of a genetic condition itself, to limitations in genetic knowledge, to uncertainties inherent in genetic risks, and to moral dilemmas involved in some of the decisions. Lower external locus of control and stronger desire for involvement in medical decisions were associated with more favorable evaluations of information given. Counseling providing more control to clients was associated with higher information helpfulness and lower decision difficulty. The clients most susceptible to decision difficulties were older clients, those with an affected child, and those making decisions involving a moral dilemma or invoking a strong sense of loss (pregnancy continuation/termination and having more children). The information most helpful in making a decision related to potential consequences of choices and possible controlling actions (prevention and treatment). Information about identity of the genetic problem (diagnosis, cause, and prevalence) and probability were most helpful among those considering having more children. This information can be useful to identify clients for whom reproductive decisions will be difficult and for tailoring information that will help such clients reach a decision.

Structured Scenarios   Arnold and Winsor (1984) reported one of the early attempts to use and construct structured scenarios for genetic counseling for a group of women at increased risk to have a child with either muscular dystrophy or a neural tube defect. Study participants found the scenarios generally useful to generate discussion, ideas, and alternatives; to confirm a previous decision; and to facilitate storytelling and emotional processing. A minority found the scenarios biased or unrealistic, or could not imagine themselves in the scenarios. The authors suggest that counselee-generated scenarios may also be a useful technique.

Reflection In a process study of genetic counseling sessions for Huntington disease using discourse analysis, genetic counselors used "reflective frames" (reflective questions to encourage counselees to adopt introspective and self-reflective stances toward their own experience) to aid with decision-making about potential testing, support nondirective counseling, and promote clients' psychological adjustment. Counselors expect clients having genetic testing to be appropriately engaged with the decision-making process and need to ensure that clients have made decisions with sufficient consideration of all possible consequences and free from external pressures. However, clients may resist this counselor agenda, resulting in lack of adequate evidence of reflection. Misalignment between counselors and counselees can lead to client behaviors for the purpose of displaying readiness for HD testing (Sarangi et al., 2004, 2005).

Weil (2000, pp. 145–152) lists 3 goals of the genetic counselor's involvement with decision-making: (1) the decision should be based on adequate assessment of options and consequences and be consistent with counselee values; (2) the counselee should feel that they made the best decision that could have been made at the time, and (3) the process should support and facilitate implementation of the decision. He gives examples of dialog in counseling sessions that illustrate good practice. Suggestions for facilitating decision-making include:

1. Assess and address sources of difficulty.
2. Address the meaning of risk information.
3. Address the counselee's emotions.
4. Provide clear information and guidance.
5. Use scenarios.
6. Explore possible outcomes and the resources for coping with them.
7. Explore the role of others in the decision.
8. Identify areas of agreement and disagreement between spouses.
9. If a counselee requests advice, identify the nature of the issue or impasse and discuss it to help the counselee resolve the problem.

Nondirectiveness and Decision-Making

In many cases, health care professionals have different attitudes toward disability and moral issues such as pregnancy termination compared to lay people (Drake et al., 1996). This makes it important for professionals to examine their role in patients' decision-making and to understand issues of countertransference. Genetic counselors generally have been found to utilize a more nondirective approach to risk communication and decision-making compared to clinical geneticists (Pencarinha et al., 1992). The use of nondirective techniques in facilitating a patient's decision has been in and out of vogue. In the early days of genetic counseling, two opposite stances were used. On one hand, many geneticists distanced themselves from the eugenics movements of the past by adopting a nondirective stance, especially in regard to reproductive decision-making. On the other hand, it was common to explain risks in a way that included an overlay of the opinion of the counselor, who suggested that a rational human being would act in a way that was "socially responsible." With the rise of a more patient-centered ethic of care in the 1980s along with the development of master's-level genetic counselors, practitioners adopted a more functionally nondirective style. More recently there has been a strong movement toward a more nuanced consideration of nondirectiveness in genetic counseling, including the area of decision-making. Emery (2001) discusses the notion of shared decision-making between counselors and counselees as a useful strategy. He notes that medicine in general is gravitating toward this model from the history of a more practitioner-driven model, while genetic counseling is coming from a more consumer-driven model.

Kessler (1997) defined nondirectiveness as involving procedures promoting the autonomy and self-directedness of the client. Nondirectiveness is a way of inter-acting and working with clients that aims to raise their self-esteem and leaves them with greater control over their lives and decisions. Nondirectiveness is an *active* strategy requiring quality counseling skills. Hodgson and Spriggs (2005) made the argument that purposeful dialog promotes client autonomy rather than nondirective counseling. They provide an ethical and practical analysis of a case to further illustrate how this might play out in a counseling setting. They state that there is little evidence to show that nondirective counseling is what clients want, that it is useful in meeting clients' needs, that it is achievable in practice, or that it is a means to respecting autonomy. The person acting in an autonomous manner engages in critical reflection, has understanding, and acts in accordance with his or her values. This concept of autonomy is compatible with values such as obligation and commitment. Genetic counselors can assess the following attributes of an auton-omous choice: whether the client engages in critical reflection, has a fundamental idea of how he or she wants to live, has awareness of influences on deliberation, and is deciding rationally. Genetic counselors should facilitate clients' engagement with the situation, provide support, and encourage active reflection and deliberation, rather than focusing on information, reassurance, and reduction of stress per se. Hodgson and Spriggs' emphasis is on the importance of ***purposeful dialog*** to make an autonomous choice, while Kessler's emphasis is on ***promoting the autonomy of the client*** over their lives and decisions.

Use of Aids for Risk Communication and Decision-Making

Another area of much attention is the use of formal decision aids. In a general review of the evidence base for shared decision-making in health care by the International Cochrane Collaboration Review Group on Decision Aids, randomized trials indicate that patient decision aids improve decision quality and prevent overuse of options that informed patients do not value. (O'Connor et al., 2003, 2004) They define shared decision-making as the process of interacting with patients who wish to be involved in arriving at an informed, values-based choice among two or more medically reasonable alternatives. Patient decision aids are standardized, evidence-based tools intended to facilitate that process in the context of patient-practitioner interactions. They note that decision aids may:

1. Provide information about the options and their relevant outcomes.
2. Help patients personalize this information.
3. Create the understanding that they can participate in decision-making.
4. Promote appreciation of the scientific uncertainties inherent in their choices.
5. Clarify the personal value or desirability of potential benefits relative to potential harms.
6. Help patients communicate their values to their practitioners.
7. Increase skills in collaborative decision-making.

The delivery mode may be print, video, or audio media or Internet-based. They may be self-administered or practitioner-administered. When decision aids were used as adjuncts to counseling they increased knowledge, improved patients' realistic perceptions of the chances of benefits and harms, lowered decisional conflict, reduced passive decision-making, reduced indecisiveness, and improved agreement between patients' values and choices, while maintaining the same level of patient satisfaction and anxiety and demonstrating cost-effectiveness.

These studies suggest that the use of decision aids can be a promising tool to enhance the quality of client satisfaction with the decision and the decision-making process, and in some circumstances may change the actual decision made by the client.

Celeste is considering a test that has life-altering implications and unique personal aspects in terms of optimal timing and whether the information improves her quality of life. There are many possible strategies you could use to help her make a quality decision. For example, she may respond to open-ended questions and an invitation to reflect on her personal experiences, role playing, discussion of practical and coping resources, or use of a decision aid. You can express your belief that she can make a good decision. You can ensure that she has fully explored the option of not testing. Examples of helpful questions include:

o *What made you decide to pursue testing now?*
o *Do you think you are likely to have a positive or negative test result? What brought you to that conclusion?*
o *In the context of HD, how do you think about your responsibilities to your family?*
o *Who else in your family will be affected by your decision? How will it affect them?*
o *What does your partner think about the possibility of testing?*
o *Do you think that testing will relieve uncertainty in your life? Are there things that might still be uncertain?*

- o *How does HD affect your reproductive plans? Would testing change that?*
- o *How does your experience with HD affect your decision about testing? Does it make your decision easier or harder?*
- o *Describe how you imagine things playing out if you test positive.*
- o *Are there things that would be hard if you test negative?*
- o *How will testing improve your quality of life?*
- o *What are the things that would help you in adjusting to your test results?*

Dealing with Children and Young Adults

Risk communication and decision-making discussions with children magnify the complexity of genetic counseling. Significant adults may coerce children into testing because of adult needs rather than appropriateness of testing for the child. Discussion of the ethics of childhood testing are beyond the scope of this chapter, but counselors providing risk information, counseling, and decision-making aid to children and young adults need to establish rapport with the child counselee, ensure that their communication is clear and at an age-appropriate level, and communicate in an interactive manner so they can assess the level of understanding, emotional impact, and, when appropriate, readiness for decision-making. Sarangi and Clarke (2002) state that professionals should be concerned about three sets of consequences regarding genetic testing of a young child for a late-onset [untreatable] disorder or carrier status of a recessive or chromosomal disorder: (1) the child loses their future autonomy as an adult to make their own informed decision, (2) the child loses the right to confidentiality that would be enjoyed by an adult undergoing the same test, and (3) there is potential negative impact of testing and the test result on the child's upbringing. They suggest not adopting blanket policies against testing children without immediate medical necessity, but rather engaging in a counseling process that introduces other "voices" into the discussion (e.g., voice of the child, other families in comparable situations, or policy guidance from relevant professional organizations). Interestingly, they still recommend that the outcome preserve future autonomy by denying childhood testing, but the process is intended to give the parents an opportunity to explore alternatives and reach that conclusion themselves. Some of the counseling challenges in providing predictive testing to 18-year-olds for HNPCC include limited self-awareness and ability to think abstractly, avoidance of difficult issues, and limited life experiences (Gaff et al., 2006). The genetic counselor working with young adults has the challenges of engaging their clients in a reflective process and responding to family dynamics and the different needs of close family members.

Cultural Tailoring

In any discussion of genetic counseling, it is important to consider cultural issues. The research that addresses cultural factors in risk communication and decision-making includes studies with study participants from underserved populations, studies that stratify participants based on ethnic and cultural factors, studies that engage in dialog with underserved clients, and studies that evaluate educational materials designed for culturally diverse populations. For example, in an ethnographic study of 102 amniocentesis genetic counseling sessions with Latina clients, Hunt and de Voogd (2005) found that practitioner and client impressions of decision-making were quite different. Most clinicians said Latinas are likely to decline amniocentesis because they are religious, fatalistic, male-dominated, family-centered, and superstitious. However, patients' discussion of their decision-making and researchers' observations of their counseling sessions were not consistent with these characterizations. Clinicians reported providing less complete information to Latina patients. In an effort to be culturally competent, but lacking a patient-centered approach, practitioners were stereotyping Latina patients and negatively affecting care. The authors suggest that cultural competency training that discourages stereotyping and instead emphasizes open communication and negotiation with individual patients is a better approach.

In a questionnaire study of women who experienced advanced maternal age counseling by counselors practicing culturally sensitive techniques (Eichmeyer et al., 2005), there were large differences in understanding of risk information between Hispanic and Caucasian clients. Overall, 59% of participants had an adequate understanding of risk; however, 71% of Hispanics and 8% of non-Hispanic Caucasians could not demonstrate sufficient understanding of risk. Differences were found when using fractions, percentages, odds, and words, but not when using pictures. The best format for all participants was fractions and the worst format was percentages. Qualitative word descriptions of risk were least understood by Hispanics. The authors suggest that using pictures or pictorial diagrams may be helpful, since they were equally well understood by the two groups.

In an observational study of 28 African American women at high risk for breast/ovarian cancer, cultural beliefs and values influenced genetic testing decisions (Hughes et al., 2003). Test acceptors had higher mean levels of fatalistic beliefs about cancer, higher future temporal orientation, and lower perceptions of familial interdependence than nonacceptors. Using adult learning theory, African Americans' perceived barriers to cancer genetic risk assessment included lack of knowledge; concerns about privacy, discrimination, and eugenics; cultural and religious beliefs (e.g., medical care occurs *after* an illness, genetic testing interferes with God's plan); economic barriers; connection of the term "genetic" with studies attempting to prove racial inferiority; emotional barriers (fear, distress, and stigma); and medical mistrust (Kendall et al., 2007). They suggest strategies for community-based cancer genetics educational programs for African Americans: (1) develop an atmosphere of trust, (2) promote an egalitarian relationship between the expert and the participant, (3) stimulate recall of prior learning, (4) develop an interaction with the participants during the presentation, (5) foster cooperative learning, (6) connect to lived experience, (7) provide feedback to participants, (8) assess achievement of the learning objectives, and (9) use strategies to enhance retention.

In a project designed to tailor communication aids for *BRCA1* counseling for African American study participants, African American focus group participants recommended both ethnic-specific and non-ethnic-specific alterations, resulting in much clearer communication aids (Baty et al., 2003). Important themes included a substantial reduction in technical detail, personalized information made relevant to the lives of the target population, the importance of building trust in the medical system and researchers, avoiding words and images with strong negative associations in the African American community, use of nontechnical images to explain genetic concepts, use of images to energize and personalize word slides, vibrant color, identifiably African American figures, and the use of themes relevant to many African Americans (e.g., religion). Table 7-5 provides examples of these techniques.

Lubitz et al. (2007) used models from educational theories of adult learning and targeted an underserved, ethnically diverse population with low health literacy to develop and assess culturally tailored risk communication. Using focus groups, they compared a "conventional" version that used genes, pedigrees, and quantitative representations of risk with a "colloquial" pictorial version that used analogy, family stories and vignettes, and visual representations of risk, without using scientific words. The colloquial version was easier to understand and conveyed more of a sense of comfort and hope. They concluded that simplicity, analogies, and familiarity support comprehension, while vignettes, family stories, and photos of real people provide comfort and hope. These elements may promote understanding of complex topics in health care, particularly when communicating with people from disadvantaged backgrounds.

Using the example of screening for carrier status for recessive disorders, Atkin (2003) discussed the tension between informed decision-making and prevention. The goal of carrier screening should be informed choice for patients; however, policy in this area also has the goal of the reduction of affected births. He notes that there is an additional overlay when you consider race, ethnicity, and service delivery for underserved populations. Identification of genetic conditions cannot be divorced from previous racist practices, or the widespread discrimination and disadvantage experienced by minority groups. Much of the empirical evidence on people's response to genetic screening and counseling is based on "white" populations. Communication problems are found regardless of the ethnicity of the provider and consumer, but gaps in understanding between professionals and patients are likely to be greater when information exchange takes place across cultural and linguistic divides and when power differences between professionals and clients reflect historical relations of racial exploitation and subordination.

SUMMARY

Risk communication and facilitation of decision-making are core genetic counseling competencies. Genetic counselors will be more effective at these competencies if they (1) understand the needs of counselees in making decisions; (2) explore, respect, and incorporate counselees' personal experiences, beliefs, and attitudes; (3) engage with counselees in the decision-making process; (4) develop effective methods of presenting risk information; (5) utilize an interactive style of counseling; (6) utilize research findings and available training to improve their skills in this area; and (7) develop a coherent, yet flexible set of strategies to work with counselees in

TABLE 7-5. Strategies to Culturally Target Genetic Educational Information (Baty et al., 2003)

Themes	Technique	Examples
Reduce technical detail	o Reduce number and complexity of words o Eliminate jargon and substitute common terms o Break up complex information into components o Eliminate unnecessary detail and keep it in reserve for specific interested clients o Reduce clutter around important messages	o Use of pictures from genetic counseling session with simple text rather than patient letter o Use of "race" rather than "ethnic background"; use of "sex" rather than "gender" o Use of billboard-style messages
Personalize information	o Incorporate human figures in place of or in addition to abstract figures o Include all categories of people you are trying to reach o Exlain why information is important to recipient near beginning rather than end o Use risk figures from the target population	o Superimposition of 2 DNA helices on human figure o Use of picture of woman having mammogram next to picture of average size of lump detected by different screening methods. o Inclusion of working-class men in visual aids used for *BRCA* testing
Build trust	o Identify historic issues that eroded trust of the target population o Use positive rather than negative phrasing	o Use of circular drawing of woman talking with health care provider and friends about her concerns o Use of "choose low-fat foods" rather than "cut back on fat"
Use nontechnical images	o Substitute analogies of common things for technical things	o Use of recipe or instruction manual analogy to describe genetic code
Use images and vibrant color to energize and personalize	o Identify favored (and nonfavored) colors in the target population o Avoid lifeless colors o Find images to reinforce the message	o Use of clay color against blue background for African American visual aids o Use of clip art to energize word messages o Use of study logo based on artwork characteristic of the target population

(continued)

TABLE 7-5. (*Continued*)

Themes	Technique	Examples
Use figures from the target population	o Use cultural consultant to identify features to use in drawing people from the target population o Use photos from the target population	o Use of drawings that use clothing and hair styles rather than skin color to indicate ethnicity
Use themes specific to the target population	o Use literature, cultural consultants, or conversations with people from the target population about your topic	o Use of images from the common religious faiths of the target population o Inclusion of family issues
Avoid negative words and images	o Use literature, cultural consultants, or conversations with people from the target population about your topic	o Use of "gene changes" rather than "mutation" o Avoidance of unnecessary use of the word "aunt" in the African American community

communicating about risk and facilitating informed decision-making. Engaging in effective risk communication and facilitation of decision-making can be one of the most satisfying roles for genetic counselors.

REFERENCES

Arnold JR, Winsor EJT (1984) The use of structured scenarios in genetic counseling. *Clin Genet* 25:485–490.

Atkin K (2003) Ethnicity and the politics of the new genetics: Principles and engagement. *Ethn Health* 8(2):91–109.

Baty BJ, Kinney AY, Ellis SM (2003) Developing culturally sensitive cancer genetics communication aids for African Americans. *Am J Med Genet A* 118(2):146–155.

Benkendorf JL, Prince MB, Rose MA, de Fina A, Hamilton HE (2001) Does indirect speech promote nondirective genetic counseling? Results of a sociolinguistic investigation. *Am J Med Genet (Semin Med Genet)* 106:199–207.

Berliner JL, Fay JM (2007) Risk assessment and genetic counseling for hereditary breast and ovarian cancer: Recommendations of the National Society of Genetic Counselors. *J Genet Couns* 16:241–260.

Biesecker BB, Ishibe N, Hadley DW, Giambarresi TR, Kase RG, Lerman C, Struewing JP (2000) Psychosocial factors predicting *BRCA1/BRCA2* testing decisions in members of hereditary breast and ovarian cancer families. *Am J Med Genet* 93(4):257–263.

Binetti G, Benussi L, Roberts S, Villa A, Pasqualetti P, Sheu CF, Gigola L, Lussignoli G, Gal Forno G, Barbiero L, Corbellini G, Green RC, Rossini PM, Ghidoni R (2006) Areas of intervention for genetic counseling of dementia: Cross-cultural comparison between Italians and Americans. *Patient Educ Couns* 64(1–3):285–293.

Bjorvatn C, Eide GE, Hanestad BR, Oyen N, Havik OE, Carlsson A, Berglund G (2007) Risk perception, worry and satisfaction related to genetic counseling for hereditary cancer. *J Genet Couns* 16(2):211–222.

Braithwaite D, Emery J, Walter F, Prevost AT, Sutton S (2006) Psychological impact of genetic counseling for familial cancer: A systematic review and meta-analysis. *Fam Cancer* 5(1):62–75.

Brinkman RR, Mezei MM, Theilmann J, Almqvist E, Hayden MR (1997) The likelihood of being *affected* with Huntington disease by a particular age, for a specific CAG size. *Am J Hum Genet* 60:1202–1210.

Bryant LD, Green JM, Hewison J (2006) Understandings of Down's syndrome: A Q methodological investigation. *Soc Sci Med* 63(5):1188–1200.

Clark S, Bluman LG, Borstelmann N, Regan K, Winer EP, Rimer BK, Skinner CS (2000) Patient motivation, satisfaction, and coping in genetic counseling and testing for *BRCA1* and *BRCA2*. *J Genet Couns* 9(3):219–235.

Croyle RT, Lerman C (1999) Risk communication in genetic testing for cancer susceptibility. *J Natl Cancer Inst Monogr* 25:59–66.

d'Agincourt- Canning L (2005) The effect of experiential knowledge on construction of risk perception in hereditary breast/ovarian cancer. *J Genet Couns* 14(1):55–69.

d'Agincourt-Canning L (2006) Genetic testing for hereditary breast and ovarian cancer: Responsibility and choice. *Qualitative Health Res* 16(1):97–118.

Daly MB, Barsevick A, Miller SM, Buckman R, Costalas J, Montgomery S, Bingler R (2001) Communicating genetic test results to the famiy: A six-step, skills-building strategy. *Fam Community Health* 24(3):13–26.

Danish SJ, D'Augelli AR (1983) *Helping Skills. II: Life Development Intervention.* New York: Human Sciences Press.

Dolan JG, Frisina S (2002) Randomized controlled trial of a patient decision aid for colorectal cancer screening. *Med Decis Making* 22(2):125–139.

Downing C (2005) Negotiating responsibility: Case studies of reproductive decision-making and prenatal genetic testing in families facing Huntington disease. *J Genet Couns* 14(3):219–234.

Drake H, Reid M, Marteau T (1996) Attitudes towards termination for fetal abnormality: Comparisons in three European countries. *Clin Genet* 49(3):134–140.

d'ydewalle G, Evers-Kiebooms G (1987) Experiments on genetic risk perception and decision making: Explorative studies. *Birth Defects Orig Artic Ser* 23(2):209–225.

Eichmeyer JN, Northrup H, Assel MA, Goka TJ, Johnston DA, Williams AT (2005) An assessment of risk understanding in Hispanic genetic counseling patients. *J Genet Couns* 14(4):319–328.

Elwyn G, Edwards A, Wensing M, Hood K Atwell C, Grol R (2003) Shared decision making: Developing the OPTION scale for measuring patient involvement. *Qual Saf Health Care* 12:93–99.

Emery J (2001) Is informed choice in genetic testing a different breed of informed decision-making? A discussion paper. *Health Expect* 4(2):81–86.

Esplen MJ, Toner B, Hunter J, Glendon G, Butler K, Field B (1998) A group therapy approach to facilitate integration of risk information for women at risk for breast cancer. *Can J Psychiatry* 43:375–380.

Esplen MJ, Toner B, Hunter J, Glendon G, Liede A, Narod S, Stuckless N, Butler K, Field B (2000) A supportive-expressive group intervention for women with a family history of breast cancer: Results of a phase II study. *Psycho-Oncology* 9:243–252.

Etchegary H, Perrier C (2007) Information processing in the context of genetic risk: Implications for genetic-risk communication. *J Genet Couns* 16(4):419–432.

Evans DGR, Burnell LD, Hopwood P, Howell A (1993) Perception of risk in women with a family history of breast cancer. *Br J Cancer* 67:612–614.

Fang CY, Miller SM, Malick J, Babb J, Hurley KE, Engstrom PF, Daly MB (2003) Psychosocial correlates of intention to undergo prophylactic oophorectomy among women with a family history of ovarian cancer. *Prev Med* 37(5):424–431. Erratum in: *Prev Med* 2004 39(1):222.

Fischhoff B (1999) Why (cancer) risk communication can be hard. *J Natl Cancer Inst Monogr* 25:7–13.

Forrest K, Simpson SA, Wilson BJ, van Teijlingen ER, McKee L, Haites N, Matthews E (2003) To tell or not to tell: Barriers and facilitators in family communication about genetic risk. *Clin Genet* 64(4):317–326.

Fransen M, Meertens R, Schrander-Stumpel C (2006) Communication and risk presentation in genetic counseling. Development of a checklist. *Patient Educ Couns* 61(1):126–133.

Gaff CL, Clarke AJ, Atkinson P, Sivell S, Elwyn G, Iredale R, Thornton H, Dundon J, Shaw C, Edwards A (2007) Process and outcome in communication of genetic information within families: A systematic review. *Eur J Hum Genet* 5(10):999–1011.

Gaff CL, Lynch E, Spencer L (2006) Predictive testing of eighteen year olds: Counseling challenges. *J Genet Couns* 15(4):245–251.

Green MJ, Peterson SK, Baker MW, Friedman LC, Harper GR, Rubinstein WS, Peters JA, Mauger DT (2005) Use of an educational computer program before genetic counseling for breast cancer susceptibility: Effects on duration and content of counseling sessions. *Genet Med* 7(4):221–229.

Green MJ, Peterson KL, Baker MW, Harper GR, Friedman LC, Rubinstein WS, Mauger DT (2004) Effect of a computer-based decision aid on knowledge, perceptions, and intentions about genetic testing for breast cancer susceptibility. A randomized controlled trial. *JAMA* 292(4):442–452.

Hall S, Chitty L, Dormancy E, Hollywood A, Wildschut HI, Fortuny A, Masturzo B, Santavy J, Kabra M, Ma R, Marteau TM (2007) Undergoing prenatal screening for Down's syndrome: Presentation of choice and information in Europe and Asia. *Eur J Hum Genet* 15 (5):563–569.

Hallowell N, Ardern-Jones A, Eeles R, Foster C, Lucassen A, Moynihan C, Watson M (2005) Men's decision-making about predictive *BRCA1/2* testing: The role of family. *J Genet Couns* 14(3):207–217.

Hallowell N, Statham H, Murton F, Green J, Richards M (1997) "Talking about chance": The presentation of risk information during genetic counseling for breast and ovarian cancer. *J Genet Couns* 6(3):269–286.

Hodgson J, Spriggs M (2005) A practical account of autonomy: Why genetic counseling is especially well suited to the facilitation of informed autonomous decision making. *J Genet Couns* 14(2):89–97.

Holmes-Rovner M, Knoll J, Schmitt N et al. (1996) Patient satisfaction with health care decisions: The satisfaction with decision scale. *Med Decis Making* 16:58–64.

Hopwood P (2005) Psychosocial aspects of risk communication and mutation testing in familial breast-ovarian cancer. *Curr Opin Oncol* 17(4):340–344.

Hopwood P, Howell A, Lalloo F, Evans G (2003) Do women understand the odds? Risk perceptions and recall of risk information in women with a family history of breast cancer. *Community Genet* 6(4):214–223.

Hopwood P, Shenton A, Lalloo F, Evans DGR, Howell A (2001) Risk perception and cancer worry: An explanatory study of the impact of genetic risk counseling in women with a family history of breast cancer. *J Med Genet* 38:139–142.

Huber O, Wider R, Huber OW (1997) Active information search and complete information presentation in naturalistic risky decision tasks. *Acta Psychol* 95:15–29.

Hughes C, Fasaye GA, LaSalle VH, Finch C (2003) Sociocultural influences on participation in genetic risk assessment and testing among African American women. *Patient Educ Couns* 51(2):107–114.

Hunt LM, de Voogd KB (2005) Clinical myths of the cultural "other": implications for Latino patient care. *Acad Med* 80(10):918–924.

Hunt LM, de Voogd KB, Castaneda H (2005) The routine and the traumatic in prenatal genetic diagnosis: Does clinical information inform patient decision-making? *Patient Educ Couns* 56(3):302–312.

Jaques AM, Bell RJ, Watson L, Halliday JL (2004) People who influence women's decisions and preferred sources of information about prenatal testing for birth defects. *Aust NZ J Obstet Gynaecol* 44(3):233–238.

Julian-Reynier C, Welkenhuysen M, Hagoel L, Decruyenaere M, Hopwood Pon behalf of the CRISCOM Working Group (2003) Risk communication strategies: State of the art and effectiveness in the context of cancer genetic services. *Eur J Hum Genet* 11:725–736.

Kaiser AS, Ferris LE, Katz R, Pastuszak A, Llewellyn-Thomas H, Johnson JA, Shaw BF (2004) Psychological responses to prenatal NTS counseling and the uptake of invasive testing in women of advanced maternal age. *Patient Educ Couns* 54(1):45–53.

Kendall J, Kendall C, Catts, ZA-K, Radford C, Dasch K (2007) Using adult learning theory concepts to address barriers to cancer genetic risk assessment in the African American community. *J Genet Couns* 16(3):279–288.

Kenen R, Arden-Jones A, Eeles R (2004a) Healthy women from suspected hereditary breast and ovarian cancer families: The significant others in their lives. *Eur J Cancer Care* 13:169–179.

Kenen R, Arden-Jones A Eeles R (2004b) We are talking, but are they listening? Communication patterns in families with a history of breast/ovarian cancer (HBOC). *Psycho-Oncology* 13(5):335–345.

Kenen R, Peters J (2001) The colored, eco-genetic relationship map (CEGRM): A conceptual approach and tool for genetic counseling research. *J Genet Couns* 10(4):289–309.

Kenen RH, Smith ACM (1995) Genetic counseling for the next 25 years: Models for the future. *J Genet Couns* 4(2):155–124.

Kenen R, Smith ACM, Watkins C, Zuber-Pittore C (2000a) To use or not to use: Male partners' perspectives on decision making about prenatal diagnosis. *J Genet Couns* 9(1):33–45.

Kenen R, Smith ACM, Watkins C, Zuber-Pittore C (2000b) To use or not to use: The prenatal genetic technology/worry conundrum. *J Genet Couns* 9(3):203–217.

Kenen R, Audern-Jones A, Eeles R (2002). Family stories and the use of heuristics: Woman from suspected hereditary breast and ovarian cancer families. *Soc Health Illn* (25):838–865.

Kessler S (1997) Psychological aspects of genetic counseling. XI. Nondirectiveness revisited. *Am J Med Genet* 72:164–171.

Klitzman R, Thorne D, Williamson J, Chung W, Marder K (2007) Decision-making about reproductive choices among individuals at-risk for Huntington's disease. *J Genet Couns* 16(3):347–362.

Koehly LM, Peterson SK, Watts BG, Kempf KKG, Vernon SW, Gritz ER (2003) A social network analysis of communication about hereditary nonpolyposis colorectal cancer genetic testing and family functioning. *Cancer Epidemiol Biomark Prev* 12:304–313.

Langbehn DR, Brinkman RR, Falush D, Paulsen JS, Hayden MR (2004) A new model for prediction of the age of onset and penetrance for Huntington's disease based on CAG length. *Clin Genet* 65:267–277.

Lazarus RS, Folkman S (1984) *Stress, Appraisal, and Coping.* New York: Springer.

Lerman C, Biesecker B, Bendendorf, JL, Kerner J, Gomez-Caminero A, Hughes C, Reed MM (1997) Controlled trial of pretest education approaches to enhance informed decision-making for *BRCA1* gene testing. *J Natl Cancer Inst* 89(2):148–157.

Lerman C, Croyle RT, Tercyak KP, Hamann H (2002) Genetic testing: Psychological aspects and implications. *J Counsel Clin Psychol* 70(3):784–797.

Lerman C, Lustbader E, Rimer B, Daly M, Miller S, Sands C, Balshem A (1995) Effects of individualized breast cancer risk counseling: A randomized trial. *J Natl Cancer Inst* 87(4):286–292.

Leventhal H (1970) Findings and theory in the study of fear communications. *Adv Exp Soc Psychol* 5:119–186.

Leventhal H, Benyamini Y, Brownlee S, Diefenbach M, Leventhal EA, Patrick-Miller L, Robitaille C (1997) Illness representations: theoretical foundations. In. Petri KJ, Weinman JA (eds.) *Perceptions of Health and Illness.* Australia: Harwood Academic Publishers, pp. 19–46.

Lippman A (1999) Embodied knowledge and making sense of prenatal diagnosis. *J Genet Couns* 8(5):255–274.

Lippman-Hand A, Fraser FC (1979a) Genetic counseling—the postcounseling period: II. Making reproductive choices. *Am J Med Genet* 4:73–87.

Lippman-Hand A, Fraser FC (1979b) Genetic counseling: Parents' responses to uncertainty. *Birth Defects Orig Art Ser* 15(5C):325–339.

Lobb EA, Butow PN, Moore A, Barratt A, Tucker K, Gaff C, Kirk J, Dudding T, Butt D (2006) Development of a communication aid to facilitate risk communication in consultations with unaffected women from high risk breast cancer families: A pilot study. *J Genet Couns* 15(5):393–405.

Lubitz JL, Komaromy M, Crawford B, Beattie M, Lee R, Luce J, Ziegler J (2007) Development and pilot evaluation of novel genetic educational materials designed for an underserved patient population. *Genet Testing* 11(3):276–290.

Marteau TM, Dormandy E, Michie S (2001) A measure of informed choice. *Health Expect* 4:99–108.

Matloff ET, Moyer A, Shannon KM, Neindorf KB, Col NF (2006) Healthy women with a family history of breast cancer: Impact of a tailored genetic counseling intervention on risk perception, knowledge, and menopausal therapy decision making. *J Womens Health (Larchmt)* 5(7):843–856.

Mazur DJ, Hickam DH (1991) Patients' interpretations of probability terms. *J Gen Intern Med* 6(3):237–240.

McAllister M (2002) Predictive genetic testing and beyond: A theory of engagement. *J Health Psychol* 7(5):491–508.

McAllister M (2003) Personal theories of inheritance, coping strategies, risk perception and engagement in hereditary non-polyposis colon cancer families offered genetic testing. *Clin Genet* 64:179–189.

McConkie-Rosell A, Sullivan, JA (1999) Genetic counseling—stress, coping, and the empowerment perspective. *J Genet Couns* 8(6):345–357.

McInerney- Leo A, Biesecker BB, Hadley DW, Kase RG, Giambarresi TR, Johnson E, Lerman C, Struewing JP (2004) *BRCA1/2* testing in hereditary breast and ovarian cancer families: effectiveness of problem-solving training as a counseling intervention. *Am J Med Genet A* 130(3):221–227.

Meiser B, Halliday JL (2002) What is the impact of genetic counselling in women at increased risk of developing hereditary breast cancer? A meta-analytic review. *Soc Sci Med* 54(10):1463–1470.

Mesters I, Ausems M, Eichhorn S, Vasen H (2005) Informing one's family about genetic testing for hereditary non-polyposis colorectal cancer (HNPCC): A retrospective exploratory study. *Fam Cancer* 4(2):163–167.

Michie S. Marteau TM (1999) The choice to have a disabled child. *Am J Hum Genet* 65:1195–1197.

Miller SM, Fleisher L, Roussi P, Buzaglo JS, Schnoll R, Slater E, Raysor S, Popa- Mabe M (2005a) Facilitating informed decision making about breast cancer risk and genetic counseling among women calling the NCI's Cancer Information Service. *J Health Commun* 10 Suppl 1:119–136.

Miron A, Schildkraut JM, Rimer BK, Winer EP, Sugg Skinner C, Futreal PA, Culler D, Calingaert B, Clark S, Kelly Marcom P, Iglehart JD (2000) Testing for hereditary breast and ovarian cancer in the southeastern United States. *Ann Surg* 231(5):624–634.

O'Connor AM (1995) Validation of a decisional conflict scale. *Med Decis Making* 15:25–30.

O'Connor AM, Legare F, Stacey D (2003) Risk communication in practice: the contribution of decision aids. *BMJ* 327:736–740.

O'Connor AM, Llewellyn-Thomas HA, Flood AB (2004) Modifying unwarranted variations in health care: Shared decision making using patient decision aids. *Health Affairs*, 7 October 2004, content.healthaffairs.org/cgi/content/full/hlthaff.var.128/DC1.

O'Daniel JM, Wells D (2002) Approaching complex cases with a crisis intervention model and teamwork. *J Genet Couns* 11(5):369–376.

O'Doherty K, Suthers GK (2007) Risky communictaion: Pitfalls in counseling about risk, and how to avoid them. *J Genet Couns*, May 1, 2007, Epub ahead of print.

Palmer CGS, Sainfort F (1993) Toward a new conceptualization and operationalization of risk perception within the genetic counseling domain. *J Genet Couns* 2(4):275–294.

Pauker SP, Pauker SG (1979) The amniocentesis decision: An explicit guide for parents. *Birth defects: Original article series* 15(5C):289–324.

Pearn JH (1973) Patients' subjective interpretation of risks offered in genetic counselling. *J Med Genet* 10:129–134.

Pencarinha DF, Bell NK, Edwards JG, Best RG (1992) Ethical issues in genetic counseling: A comparison of M.S. counselor and medical geneticist perspectives. *J Genet Couns* 1(1):19–30.

Peters JA, Hoskins L, Prindiville S, Kenen R, Greene MH (2006) Evolution of the Colored Eco-Genetic Relationship Map (CEGRM) for Assessing Social Functioning in Women in Hereditary Breast-Ovarian (HBOC) Families. *J Genet Couns* 15(6):477–489.

Peters JA, Kenen R, Giusti R, Loud J, Weissman N, Greene MH (2004) Exploratory study of the feasibility and utility of the colored eco-genetic relationship map (CEGRM) in women at high genetic risk of developing breast cancer. *Am J Med Genet* 130A:258–264.

Peterson SK, Pentz RD, Blanco AM, Ward PA, Watts BG, Marani SK, James LC, Strong LC (2006) Evaluation of a decision aid for families considering p53 genetic counseling and testing. *Genet Med* 8(4):226–33.

Peterson SK, Watts BG, Koehly LM, Vernon SW, Baile WF, Kohlmann WK, Critz ER (2003) How families communicate about HNPCC genetic testing: Findings from a qualitative study. *Am J Med Genet* 119C:78–86.

Pieterse AH, van Dulmen S, van Dijk S, Bensing JM, Ausems MG (2006) Risk communication in completed series of breast cancer genetic counseling visits. *Genet Med* 8(11):688–696.

Press N, Fishman JR, Koenig BA (2000) Collective fear, individualized risk: The social and cultural context of genetic testing for breast cancer. *Nursing Ethics* 7(3):237–249.

Ray JA, Loescher LJ, Brewer M (2005) Risk-reduction surgery decisions in high-risk women seen for genetic counseling. *J Genet Couns* 14(6):473–484.

Ropka ME, Wenzel J, Phillips EK, Siadaty M, Philbrick JT (2006) Uptake rates for breast cancer genetic testing: A systematic review. *Cancer Epidemiol Biomarkers Prev* 15(5):840–855.

Sainfort F, Booske BC (2000) Measuring post-decision satisfaction. *Med Decis Making* 20:51–61.

Sankar P, Wolpe PR, Jones NL, Cho M (2006) How do women decide? Accepting or declining BRCA1/2 testing in a nationwide clinical sample in the United States. *Community Genet* 9(2):78–86.

Sarangi S, Bennert K, Howell L, Clarke A, Harper P, Gray J (2004) Initiation of reflective frames in counseling for Huntingtons Disease predictive testing. *J Genet Couns* 3(2): 135–55.

Sarangi S, Bennert K, Howell L, Clarke A, Harper P, Gray J (2005) (Mis)alignments in counseling for Huntington's Disease predictive testing: clients' responses to reflective frames. *J Genet Couns* 14(1):29–42.

Sarangi S, Clarke A (2002) Constructing an account by contrast in counselling for childhood genetic testing. *Soc Sci Med* 54:295–308.

Schwartz MD, Benkendorf J, Lerman C, Isaacs C, Ryan-Robertson A, Johnson L (2001) Impact of educational print materials on knowledge, attitudes, and interest in BRCA1/BRCA2: Testing among Ashkenazi Jewish women. *Cancer* 92(4):932–940.

Schwartz MD, Hughes C, Roth J, Main D, Peshkin BN, Isaacs D, Kavanagh C, Lerman C (2000) Spiritual faith and genetic testing decisions among high-risk breast cancer probands. *Cancer Epidemiol Biomarkers Prev* 9(4):381–385.

Schwartz MD, Lerman C, Brogan B, Peshkin BN, Halbert CH, DeMarco T, Lawrence W, Main D, Finch C, Magnant C, Pennanen M, Tsangaris T, Willey S, Isaacs C (2004) Impact of *BRCA1/BRCA2* counseling and testing on newly diagnosed breast cancer patients. *J Clin Oncol* 22(10):1823–9.

Shaw NJ, Dear PR (1990) How do parents of babies interpret qualitative expressions of probability? *Arch Dis Child* 65(5):520–523.

Shiloh S (2006) Illness representations, self-regulation, and genetic counseling. *J Genet Counsel* 15(5):325–337.

Shiloh S, Gerad L, Goldman B (2006a) Patients' information needs and decision-making processes: what can be learned from genetic counselees? *Health Psychol* 25(2):211–9.

Shiloh S, Gerad L, Goldman B (2006b) The facilitating role of information provided in genetic counseling for counselees' decisions. *Genet Med* 8(2):116–24.

Shiloh S, Reznik H, Bat-Mirian- Katznelson M, Goldman B (1995) Pre-marital genetic counselling to consanguineous couples: Attitudes, beliefs and decisions among counselled, noncounselled and unrelated couples in Israel. *Soc Sci Med* 41(9):1301–1310.

Shiloh S, Saxe L (1989) Perception of recurrence risks by genetic counselees. *Psychol Health* 3:45–61.

Sobel SK, Cowan DB (2000) Impact of genetic testing for Huntington's disease on the family system. *Am J Med Genet* 90:49–59.

Soldan J, Street E, Gray J, Binedell J, Harper PS (2000) Psychological model for presymptomatic test interviews: Lessons learned from Huntington disease. *J Genet Couns* 9(1):15–31.

Stalmeier PFM, Roosmalen MS, Verhoef LCG, Hoekstra-Weebers JEHM, Oosterwijk JC, Moog U, Hooderbrugge N, van Daal WAJ (2005) The decision evaluation scales. *Pat Ed Counsel* 57(3):286–293.

Trepanier A, Ahrens M, McKinnon W, Peters J, Stopfer J, Grumet SC, Manley S, Culver JO, Acton R, Larsen-Haidle J, Correia LA, Bennett R, Pettersen B, Ferlita TD, Costalas JW, Hunt K, Donlon S, Skrzynia C, Farrell C, Callif-Daley F, Vockley CW;National Society of Genetic Counselors (2004) Genetic cancer risk assessment and counseling: Recommendations of the National Society of Genetic Counselors. *J Genet Couns* 13(2):83–114.

Tversky A, Kahneman D (1974) Judgment under uncertainty: Heuristics and biases. *Science* 185(4157):1124–1131.

van Dijk S, Otten W, van Asperen CJ, Timmermans DR, Tibben A, Zoeteweij MW, Silberg S, Breuning MH, Kievit J (2004) Feeling at risk: how women interpret their familial breast cancer risk. *Am J Med Genet A* 131(1):42–9.

van Dijk S, Otten W, Zoeteweij MW, Timmermans DR, van Asperen CJ, Breuning MH, Tollenaar RA, Kievit J (2003) Genetic counselling and the intention to undergo prophylactic mastectomy: effects of a breast cancer risk assessment. *Br J Cancer* 88(11):1675–81.

van Roosmalen MS, Stalmeier PF, Verhoef LC, Hoekstra-Weebers JE, Oosterwijk JC, Hoogerbrugge N, Moog U, van Daal WA (2004) Randomised trial of a decision aid and its timing for women being tested for a BRCA1/2 mutation. *Br J Cancer* 90(2):333–42.

Veach PM, LeRoy BS, Bartels DM (2003) *Facilitating the Genetic Counseling Process. A Practice Manual.* New York: Springer.

Wakefield CE, Meiser B, Homewood J, Peate M, Kirk J, Warner B, Lobb E, Gaff C, Tucker K (2007) Development and pilot testing of two decision aids for individuals considering genetic testing for cancer risk. *J Genet Couns* 16(3):325–339.

Wallerstein R, Strmen V, Durcan J, White S, Bar-Lev A, Pruski-Clark J, Wallerstein D, McCarrier J, Twersky S (2006) Factors in decision making following genetic counseling for pre-natal diagnosis of *de novo* chromosomal rearrangements. *Clin Genet* 69(6):497–503.

Weil J (2000) Nondirective counseling, risk perception, and decision making. In Weil J. *Psychosocial Genetic Counseling.* New York: Oxford University Press, Inc. pp. 117–152.

Wertz DC, Sorenson JR, Heeren TC (1986) Clients' interpretation of risks provided in genetic counseling. *Am J Hum Genet* 39(2):253–264.

White MT (2006) Religious and spiritual concerns in genetic testing and decision making: An introduction for pastoral and genetic counselors. *J Clin Ethics* 17(2):158–167.

8

The Medical Genetics Evaluation

Elizabeth M. Petty, M.D.

INTRODUCTION

A comprehensive medical genetics evaluation is the undisputable foundation for an effective clinical genetics visit. Appropriate medical management and accurate genetic counseling are dependent on recognizing the full spectrum of specific symptoms and problems that an individual is experiencing and, ideally, understanding the correct underlying diagnosis. During a medical genetics evaluation, important clinical evidence, reflecting medical concerns and psychosocial issues, and diagnostic clues are meticulously gathered that provide the genetics team with critical information and insights essential for the appropriate management, risk assessment, genetic testing, counseling, and education of an individual or family. Sometimes, all of the needed information can be easily gathered and appropriately considered with one visit to the genetics clinic. Oftentimes, however, because of many factors—such as the later age of onset of many genetic conditions, the overlapping symptoms and signs of some genetic conditions, the rarity of other syndromes, and the natural evolution of some disorders—genetics evaluations over multiple clinic visits, spanning months to years, may be needed before a specific diagnosis can be reached. Careful consideration of all of the information gathered during the medical genetics evaluation(s)

A Guide to Genetic Counseling, Second Edition, Edited by Wendy Uhlmann, Jane Schuette, and Beverly Yashar
Copyright © 2009 by John Wiley & Sons, Inc.

allows the team to provide the best care possible and, importantly, reduces the risk of making mistakes or providing misleading information that could have an adverse impact or negative outcome.

The medical genetics evaluation has evolved over time and encompasses a broad range of clinical activities—from gathering medical and family history information to arranging appropriate genetic testing and follow-up evaluations. Today's medical genetics evaluation encompasses standard elements that are used by physicians across many disciplines, including a full medical history, social history, and review of systems, as well as elements that are unique to clinical genetics, such as a detailed pedigree analysis with risk assessment and a specialized dysmorphology examination to help recognize clinical signs that are diagnostic of specific genetic syndromes (Barness-Gilbert et al., 1989; Cohen, 1989; Saksena et al., 1989; Cohen, 1990; Friedman, 1990; Friedman, 1992; Hall, 1993; Epstein, 1995; Winter, 1995). Some elements of the medical evaluation are comprehensively addressed elsewhere in this textbook, such as family history taking (see Chapter 2) and genetic testing (see Chapter 9), and therefore are not discussed at length here. This chapter specifically focuses on six other key elements of the medical genetics evaluation including (1) the chief complaint or reason for the visit, (2) the history of present illness or relevant medical history, (3) the past medical history, (4) the review of systems, (5) the physical examination, with special attention to specialized examinations for genetic syndromes including the dysmorpholgy examination, and (6) the utility of diagnostic studies and ancillary medical tests in genetics evaluations. Before discussing these elements in more detail, it is useful to understand historical perspectives that illustrate the evolution of clinical genetics and provide a foundation for today's medical genetics evaluation.

Historical Perspectives

Although hereditary diseases and genetic disorders have been described since biblical times and depicted in art throughout the ages, it was not until the last half of the twentieth century that the field of clinical or medical genetics really blossomed into a readily available and widely recognized clinical specialty. During the latter half of the nineteenth century and the majority of the twentieth century, many genetic syndromes and metabolic conditions were first being recognized, defined, delineated, and often named by a wide variety of medical specialists. Many syndromes continue to bear the name(s) of their original describers. In the latter half of the twentieth century, genetics clinic visits and medical genetics literature were largely focused on identifying the cardinal or characteristic features of particular syndromes, describing new syndromes, and determining the inheritance pattern of these syndromes. Some of the syndromes that were first described decades ago have been further characterized or reclassified during the past decade as we learn more about molecular genetics. Bannayan–Rilely–Ruvalcaba syndrome and Cowden syndrome are now recognized as allelic disorders within the spectrum of the PTEN harmartoma syndrome. New syndromes have also continued to be recognized, such as the Loeys–Dietz syndrome, an autosomal dominant connective tissue disorder with some features overlapping with Marfan syndrome.

While new syndromes are still being reported and characterized today, the medical genetics evaluation has become much broader to address not only the diagnosis but, increasingly, preventative strategies, medical or surgical management alternatives, genetic testing considerations, ancillary support options, and psychosocial counseling as well. Clinical genetics services are now well established throughout the developed world. These services have grown and developed over a historical period in which tremendous new knowledge in medical genetics and related biotechnology has been actively sought and rapidly acquired.

The rapid acquisition of new knowledge in genetics and biotechnology has caused a natural evolution of the medical genetics evaluation and shaped the focus of today's genetics clinic visit. After the discovery of chromosome disorders in the late 1950s, cytogenetic testing became available to diagnose particular syndromes. In the early 1960s, growing knowledge about metabolic diseases and employment of screening assays sparked the development of newborn screening programs and biochemical genetics clinics. A new era of molecular genetics began in the 1970s, and by the late1980s DNA diagnostics became increasingly available to geneticists and enabled DNA-based prenatal diagnostic testing. The advent of the polymerase chain reaction (PCR) in 1985 and the birth of the Human Genome Project in 1990 have unquestionably revolutionized the field of molecular genetics and significantly impacted on the medical genetics evaluation. The rapid growth of DNA-based diagnostic tests for monogenic disorders skyrocketed during the 1990s, and the use of DNA-based diagnostic testing for more complex traits became a reality around the turn of the twenty-first century. Clinical applications of molecular genetic testing for many common conditions are predicted to increase in the future. The ongoing development of specialized techniques including oligonucleotide, cDNA, large genomic clone [i.e., bacterial artificial chromosome (BAC)], and single nucleotide polymorphism (SNP) array technology, as well as the increasing automatization and dramatic cost reductions for high-throughput DNA sequencing, will continue to impact the evolution of genetic services. The clinical geneticist today has a wide variety of auxiliary tests readily available to help confirm diagnoses, make predictive diagnoses in asymptomatic individuals, and provide prenatal or preimplantation diagnoses for interested individuals. These rapid advances in genetic discoveries, related technology, and the subsequent media explosion about genetics have also changed, and likely will continue to change, the character of, public desire for, and services provided by genetics clinics.

Surprisingly, despite the extensive growth of clinical genetic services over the latter half of the twentieth century, it wasn't until 1991 that medical genetics was actually recognized as a bona fide medical specialty by the American Board of Medical Specialists. The American College of Medical Genetics (ACMG, http://www.acmg.net/) was also established in 1991 and was formally recognized by the American Medical Association (AMA) five years later in 1996, when it was admitted to their house of delegates. Before formal medical recognition, clinical geneticists, however, have always believed in the importance and uniqueness of the specialty. They see their roles as not only providing patients and their families with the most accurate diagnostic and prognostic information available but also offering them the most up-to-date strategies for management. The expanding scope of available medial genetics services is demonstrated by the fact that clinical genetics services are provided through many different disciplines at academic medical centers including genetics, pediatrics, internal medicine, cardiology, obstetrics and gynecology, neurology, ophthalmology, otolaryngology, oncology, and pathology, as well as multiple disease-focused interdisciplinary clinical services.

The Making of a Clinical Medical Geneticist

To provide accurate, up-to-date information to patients, families, and other healthcare providers about genetic disorders, it is absolutely essential that a thoughtful and comprehensive medical genetics evaluation is performed by a trained clinician. Most often, a medical genetics evaluation is performed by a formally trained clinical geneticist. Practicing clinical geneticists are, for the most part, physicians who have had their initial primary medical training in another area of medicine (such as pediatrics, internal medicine, obstetrics and gynecology, pathology, neurology, or other specialties) and who subsequently obtain at least two years of additional formal subspecialty training in clinical genetics. Traditionally, formal clinical genetics training was available through specialized fellowship training programs, accredited by the American Board of Medical Genetics (ABMG, http://www.abmg.org/), for M.D.s and D.O.s (osteopathic physicians). The ABMG began certifying medical geneticists and genetic counselors in 1981, two years after the creation of the board. Beginning in 1997, accreditation for M.D. and D.O. clinical genetics training programs was granted by the Accreditation Counsel for Graduate Medical Education (ACGME), rather than the ABMG. In rare instances, other professionals (including formally trained Ph.D. geneticists and dentists with interests in genetic syndromes) have assumed active primary roles as clinical geneticists. After completion of a formal training program physicians are eligible to sit for formal board examinations in clinical genetics, and must be renewed on a regular basis through maintenance of certification examinations. Thus Board Certified Clinical Geneticists are individuals who, after completing specialized training, have passed ABMG Clinical Genetics board certification requirements and examinations.

The Role of the Clinical Geneticist

Depending on the individual clinical geneticist's interests, as well as previous medical training, a clinical geneticist may focus his or her practice on specific types of genetic disorders or specific age groups. For example, a board-certified clinical geneticist with a background in obstetrics and gynecology may limit his or her practice entirely to prenatal and perinatal genetics, whereas a geneticist with a background in internal medicine may limit her or his practice to adult-onset disorders. There are many other subspecializations within the broader realm of clinical genetics including neurogenetics, biochemical genetics, and cancer genetics. There are also geneticists who study dysmorphology (literally meaning the study of abnormal forms) and syndrome delineation. These individuals may further specialize in particular kinds of diseases or syndromes, where they rapidly become the "world's expert" on diagnosing and managing a particular condition.

Most clinical geneticists work very closely with genetic counselors and laboratory-based geneticists in providing and delivering comprehensive clinical genetic services. In fact, during a clinic visit the roles of the counselor and the clinical geneticist are often closely intertwined to fully optimize care for patients and their families. The medical genetics evaluation is intimately connected to, and reliant upon, genetic counseling services. The genetic counselor and geneticist often form a healthcare team whose tasks can include:

- Case preparation, including a detailed review of family history and accurate risk assessment
- Genetic counseling and education
- Relevant follow-up, including the accurate interpretation and implication of any genetic or other diagnostic tests

Thus the formal elements of the genetics evaluation provided by the medical geneticists, while essential, are only part of a comprehensive clinical genetics visit where the genetic counselor, clinic staff, and clinical geneticist work closely together to optimally serve the many unique needs of individuals and families seen in a genetics clinic.

Purposes of the Medical Genetic Evaluation

There are several purposes of a medical genetics evaluation (Table 8-1), which may vary considerably depending on the particular disorder or the unique concerns of

TABLE 8-1. Purposes of a Medical Genetics Evaluation

New Patients:
1. Establish or confirm a specific diagnosis
2. Obtain necessary diagnostic tests
3. Provide specific education and support
4. Initiate appropriate referrals
5. Arrange focused medical management and follow-up
6. Determine recurrence risk for patient
7. Assess risk to other family members
8. Provide accurate, individualized counseling

Established Patients (follow-up care):
1. Assess new medical problems and related concerns
2. Determine compliance with recommended management
3. Keep patients informed about new diagnostic and management strategies
4. Provide ongoing age-appropriate education
5. Help coordinate necessary referrals and evaluations
6. Evaluate other at-risk family members

the individual patient or their family. Most often, a complete medical history and physical examination are used to help establish or confirm a particular diagnosis for an individual or for several individuals within a family.

An *accurate diagnosis* remains one of the main goals of the medical genetics evaluation. For a new patient this facilitates appropriate genetic counseling, optimizes medical management, and allows for informative patient education. Specifically, recurrence risks can be most accurately provided when a specific diagnosis is confirmed. In addition, patients and their primary healthcare providers can be correctly educated regarding a particular diagnosis and provided with helpful anticipatory guidance regarding potential problems as well as information about state-of-the-art preventive, therapeutic, educational or vocational, and management options to reduce disease-related morbidity and mortality and, ultimately, optimize the well-being of the individual.

Once a diagnosis is formally established in a patient (including new patients and those with a standing diagnosis), a comprehensive medical genetics evaluation is essential to *help determine the extent of systemic involvement* and to provide *focused medical management* for the patient's unique disease-related problems. This can include both providing anticipatory guidance and addressing new issues. Given that no two individuals with the same condition will have exactly the same medical concerns, social situations, or psychological responses, a comprehensive evaluation of every patient allows medical care and genetic counseling that is specifically tailored to the unique needs of the individual. Referrals to subspecialists and other healthcare providers essential for ongoing care can be tailored to address individual needs and concerns based on medical history information and physical findings. Individualized genetic counseling can be directed to focus on particular patient concerns, and the dissemination of educational information can be targeted to both the individual's desire for information and his or her ability to process and understand the information. On follow-up visits for individuals with a genetic condition who have a particular complaint, a focused but thorough medical genetics evaluation is critically important to address their concerns and questions as well as identify any other new issues that may have been missed by the patient or the primary heath care provider, who may not be as familiar with the condition.

Another important goal of the comprehensive medical genetics evaluation is to *assess other family members* for the condition identified in the proband. There are often medical, surgical, or lifestyle management strategies that can markedly improve an individual's condition, daily well-being, and disease-free longevity. In addition, appropriate anticipation and watchful evaluation for potential problems will enable early detection, improve medical management, decrease morbidity, and, in some cases, reduce early disease-associated mortality. *Appropriate psychosocial support,* occupational or physical therapy, educational opportunities, and vocational resources may allow affected individuals to manage their lives more effectively and productively despite the physical, cognitive, or psychological symptoms associated with the condition. The ability to recognize a specific genetic disorder segregating in a family followed by counseling may provide interested individuals with an opportunity for specific family planning including the use of reproductive technology options, from preimplantation diagnosis to prenatal testing, to avoid the birth of, or plan for the birth of, an affected child as they desire.

A skillful clinical geneticist will take the time to perform a thoughtful and comprehensive evaluation of an individual, even when a particular diagnosis seems quite likely at first glance. Sometimes this evaluation can be accomplished in one visit, while other times it may require a series of visits in a tiered fashion, gathering more information, utilizing additional genetic tests, and employing specialized examinations. As important as it is to give an individual or family a precise specific diagnosis, it is even more important not to mislabel an individual with an incorrect diagnosis based on a hasty evaluation or incomplete review of the patient's medical history, family history, and medical records. It is far better to err on the side of being inconclusive about a specific diagnosis when in doubt than it is to give somebody a wrong diagnosis that could have a significant impact on various aspects of their lives including, but not limited to, their continued healthcare management, sense of self and well-being, and impact on other family members. It is estimated that approximately one-third of patients presenting to a genetics clinic for a diagnosis leave the clinic without a specific diagnosis. It is a common and important practice in medical genetics clinic to continually reevaluate these "undiagnosed" individuals on a regular basis, some syndromes or conditions become more easily recognizable with age and, additionally, the rapid growth of genetic knowledge and resulting diagnostic technology may facilitate making a diagnosis in some individuals over time.

The medical genetics evaluation is clearly rooted in, and has evolved from, the basic and important general components of physical examinations and diagnostic evaluations that are utilized in all areas of medical practice. Importantly, the past and present medical history of an individual, his/her family history, and the physical examination remain critical components of a medical genetics evaluation just as they are in any medical diagnostic evaluation. By the completion of the evaluation the following questions should be addressed and answered:

- What are the medical problems?
- When did the problems arise?
- What other tests or studies would be helpful in this case?
- Why did these problems arise?
- What is the disorder or syndrome?
- Who else may experience similar medical problems?
- What are the chances it might occur again in this family?
- What future problems should be anticipated?
- How can we avoid or minimize these problems?
- How can we optimize the individual's health and psychological well-being?
- Who else should be involved in the care and management?
- How do these problems impact the individual and family?
- Where can the individual and family find more help and information?
- When should we see this person back in the genetics clinic?

THE COMPONENTS OF A MEDICAL GENETICS EVALUATION

The Basic Medical History

One sign of a good medical history of an individual is that it, along with information from a focused, detailed, and accurate family history, will often provide key clues that clearly point to diagnostic possibilities underlying the problems of an individual before there is any information from the individual's physical examination or review of his or her medical records. In fact, it is absolutely essential to obtain a good medical history. The patient's own medical history is critically important in helping to identify particular problems and unique concerns as well as identifying valuable clues to the individual's diagnosis.

The sources of information for the medical history may come directly from the individual, relatives, or a legal guardian. When obtaining a medical history, it is important to consider the individual's cognitive ability and overall reliability regarding the accuracy of the individual's knowledge about specific diagnoses and medical problems. Often, portions of the medical history are provided by the referring physician or other healthcare provider. While these healthcare providers may provide accurate detailed medical information and pose specific questions for the genetics team to address, they may miss or minimize symptoms or issues that are most important to the affected individual. For this reason it is important to take both the individual patient's concerns and the healthcare professional's information into account. In addition to these sources, it is important to review all pertinent available medical records on the patient and other individuals in the family who have similar symptoms or medical problems. This review will be focused on verifying the histories that were provided by the patient, other family members, or healthcare providers. Failure to verify this information with objective data when possible could lead to an unintentionally erroneous diagnosis, despite the best intentions and most accurate recollections of all parties involved. In all cases, it is critical that appropriate permission to communicate with these individuals be obtained.

The medical history is often obtained at the time of the clinic visit. However, for a diagnostic medical genetics evaluation, it is often extremely helpful to have some medical history information from the patient, the patient's family, and the patient's healthcare team before the clinic visit so that appropriate educational materials, specific diagnostic test requisition forms, and appropriate background research on rare conditions can be conducted before seeing the patient. In addition, it is absolutely essential to obtain pertinent medical records before the clinic visit for careful review. Obtaining some of this background information before the clinic visit as part of case preparation (described in Chapter 4) will enable a more focused and more clinically relevant diagnostic evaluation for the patient and the patient's family.

During the clinic visit, sufficient time should be allowed to gather detailed information from the patient or his/her guardian and to explore any areas of particular concern. There are several general components to the medical history that are widely utilized in virtually all medical practices (Tables 8-2A and 8-2B) that are addressed below.

TABLE 8-2A. Basic Components of a Medical History*

Identify the "Chief Complaint" (CC) or "Reason for Visit"	
Determine main questions and concerns of patient, family members, and health care providers when possible.	Important questions can include:
Record the patient's own words when possible.	• "What is your primary reason for this visit?" • "What do you hope to learn or receive from this visit?"

Ascertain the "History of Present Illness" (HPI) or "Relevant Medical History"
Describe patient's problems related to visit.
Identify nature of problems, onset of problems, duration of symptoms, changes in quality of symptoms, previous medical or surgical management; problem-oriented approach

Obtain the "Past Medical History" *Some elements may be included in the Relevant Medical History depending on the age of patient and Reason for Visit.* *Some elements (i.e., prenatal and neonatal history) may be excluded in adult patients who do not have a history of birth defects or cognitive problems.*	

Important elements in a *prenatal* history can include:	• Parents' ages
	• Prenatal exposures (timing important)
	  o Maternal illnesses
	    ■ Fevers, rashes
	    ■ Systemic disorders (lupus, hyperglycemia)
	  o Medications
	    • Prescribed and over the counter
	  o Alcohol, tobacco, recreational drugs
	  o Other environmental
	  o Maternal immunizations
	  o Maternal complications (i.e., major trauma)

Important elements in a *neonatal* history can include:	• Birth history
	  o Delivery—type, complications
	  o Gestational age, size
	• Initial newborn examination
	  o Apgar scores
	  o Length, weight, head circumference,
	• Nursery course
	  o ICU stay, treatments

Important elements in an *infancy* and *childhood* history can include:	• Development history: social, motor, adaptive milestones
	  o Hearing and speech assessments
	  o Vision assessments
	• Childhood illnesses
	  o Type and age of onset

Chronic or major medical problems	• List and indicate age of onset
Surgeries	• Indication, type of surgery, date
Major trauma	• Resulting complications
Hospitalization	• Reason and date
Current medications	• Type and dose • Other nontraditional treatments
Medication allergies	• Type and reaction

(*continued*)

TABLE 8-2A. (*Continued*)

Document the "Family History" *Key elements may be included in the "Relevant Medical History" for inherited conditions*

Describe the "Social History"

Habits	• Tobacco, alcohol, and drugs use
Diet and exercise	
Education	• Highest grade level
	• Academic strengths and weaknesses
	• Special programs/classes
Living situation	• People in home—caretakers and dependents
	• Socioeconomic status
Employment	• Occupation, unemployment, disability
Religious beliefs	
Support systems	

Document a "Review of Systems" (see Table 8-2B)

*Note the sources of the information and reliability of these sources. These can include: patients and/or family member and/or legal guardian; health care provider; medical records.

The "Chief Complaint" or Reason for Visit The first part of the medical history is related to the determination and documentation of what is most commonly referred to in medicine as the individual patient's (or patient's parent or legal guardian if the patient is a child or is unable to express his/her concerns) "chief complaint" or "CC." This identifies and records the major concern(s) or question(s) that initiated the genetics clinic evaluation and need to be addressed. In my own notes, I refer to this as the "Reason for Visit" rather than "Chief Complaint," given that I do not view my patients as complainers and want to start off my notes with a less negative tone, especially since I send copies of my full notes to patients. The referring physician or healthcare provider may have a specific indication or reason as to why a particular patient is being referred for a genetics evaluation; however, it is extremely important to understand and record in the patient's own words his/her own sense of his/her problems and his/her understanding as to why s/he is at the clinic. Failure to do this may leave patients disappointed if, after a lengthy examination and subsequent significant medical bill, they feel their concerns were never fully addressed, even if the geneticist made the correct diagnosis and initiated appropriate management. It is often useful to understand other family members concerns as well. Sometimes an individual will not understand why s/he was referred to a genetics clinic and note that s/he is there only because his/her physician referred his/her for a visit. In this instance, the "Reason for Visit" from the healthcare professional is appropriate to document. Thus the "Chief Complaint" or "Reason for Visit" is most often recorded in the patient's or guardian's own words and elaborated upon as needed by describing referring physician concerns or other family member concerns.

TABLE 8-2B. Review of Systems: A Checklist Looking for Any Symptoms or Problems Not Already Covered

General	Fatigue, weight changes, fever, chills, night sweats, sleep problems
Head	Headaches, trauma
Eyes/vision	Vision changes, glasses, double vision, dryness, pain, discharge
Ears/hearing	Hearing changes, pain, discharge, ringing or buzzing, vertigo
Nose/sinuses	Bleeding, stuffiness, sinus problems, obstruction, smelling problems, postnasal drip
Mouth/throat	Teeth-dental care, sores, bleeding, taste, hoarseness, gagging, choking
Neck	Pain, stiffness, swelling, masses
Lungs/breathing	Shortness of breath, chronic cough, sputum production, wheezing, snoring, apnea, supplemental oxygen use, coughing up blood, chest pain
Breasts	Masses, pain, discharge, exams, mammograms
Cardiovascular	Palpitations, pain, edema, cyanosis, murmur, hypertension, high cholesterol, orthopnea
Gastrointestinal	Appetite, trouble swallowing, jaundice, diarrhea, constipation, stool incontinence, bleeding, vomiting, hemorrhoids, anal pain, bowel movements, indigestion, eating disorders
Genitourinary	Problems with urination, blood in urine, urinary tract infections, kidney stones, nocturia, incontinence, burning
	Women: Pap smears, menstrual history, vaginal discharge, pain, itching
	Men: Testicular exams, testicular pain/swelling/lumps, prostate enlargement, itching, discharge
Sexual	Pain on intercourse, infections, impotence, libido, contraception, sexual preference, sexual activity, pregnancies including live births, terminations, and stillbirths
Endocrine	Thyroid problems, blood sugar problems, diabetes, heat/cold intolerance, growth problems, hormone therapies
Allergic	Seasonal, animals, environmental, eczema (medication allergies go under past medical history)
Musculoskeletal	Fracture history, osteoporosis, scoliosis, joint dislocations, joint contractures, swelling, pain, redness
Hematological	Anemia, transfusions, bleeding problems, bruising
Lymphatic	Lymph node enlargement
Neurological	Fainting, seizures, loss of consciousness, dizziness, weakness, numbness, memory problems, tremors, coordination problems, changes in gait, movement problems, sensory changes
Psychological	Mood changes, anxiety, depression, psychosis, phobias, substance abuse problems, therapy, concentration problems, attention problems, learning disorders
Skin	Itching, rashes, birthmarks, dryness, fragility, healing/scarring, changes in nails or skin

Many clinics will have a check-list review of symptoms. The above list includes a common review of systems. It is not fully comprehensive. You do not need to ask every patient everything on the list.

In addition to formally documenting the main "Reason for Visit," it is important to understand from the patient what questions s/he has regarding his/her health that s/he hopes will be answered at the clinic visit. It is helpful to ask individuals to prioritize their concerns, as sometimes there may be several unrelated issues that s/he hope will be addressed. Often, an individual patient's concerns may be somewhat different than the referring healthcare provider's concerns. Other times, an individual will have a list of issues that s/he would like addressed. There have been more than a handful of patients each year who come to see me in the genetics clinic with multiple pages of typed questions that they want addressed. In this instance, acknowledging their many issues, asking them to prioritize, and explaining the time frame for the first visit can facilitate in making the visit as productive and helpful as possible. Sometimes, an individual's hopes for the visit are beyond the scope of what is possible within a genetics clinic visit. For instance, I have had patients come to my genetics clinic hoping to have "hip surgery" or to "get a new hearing aid." In this instance, it is important to let the patients know the kinds of issues that can be addressed in a genetics clinic, assure them that appropriate referrals will be made, and explain the kinds of outcomes that might arise from the genetics clinic visit. It is therefore critical to know what expectations individuals bring with them to clinic early on in the visit so that it can be as productive and helpful to the patient as possible.

The "History of Present Illness" or "Relevant Medical History" After identifying the "Reason for Visit" it is necessary to describe in detail, as precisely and concisely as possible, what is commonly referred to in medicine as the "History of Present Illness" or "HPI," which is a summary of the individual's present problems related to the "CC" or "Reason for Visit." Since I do not view genetic conditions as an acute "illness" per se, I identify this portion of the medical evaluation as the "Relevant Medical History" in my own notes. When obtaining an individual's "Relevant Medical History," it is often necessary to blend information obtained from the patient, the patient's family members who are present, and healthcare professionals, with objective information as presented in the medical record, including any previous studies or laboratory tests that have been conducted to evaluate the patient's problems, in order to get a full and accurate sense of the constellation of problems.

The "Relevant Medical History" should focus on medical information relevant (or pertinent) to the "Reason for Visit." In this section, it is particularly important to define the nature, onset, and duration of particular problems, understand what has already been done to help diagnose and manage these problems—both within and outside of the medical community—and understand how these problems impact on the individual not only in a medical sense, but also in a psychosocial sense. It is important to ask about and document pertinent positive as well as negative findings. For instance, if an adult is in the genetics clinic for evaluation of possible Marfan syndrome because of a dilated aortic root and tall stature, it would be important to ask about and document other cardinal features, or lack thereof, that can be seen in Marfan syndrome, including eye findings and musculoskeletal features. In this case, it would also be helpful to ask about and document other symptoms seen in related connective tissue disorders. Similarly, if a child with a cleft palate is being seen in clinic, it would be important to ask about features that could be seen in various genetic syndromes associated with clefting, including but not limited to cardiac defects, development, digital anomalies, other birth defects, and family history of clefting. While the "Relevant Medical History" should be concise and focused, it should include enough key information to provide an accurate working differential diagnosis for the patient before the physical examination.

The specific details included in the "Relevant Medical History" will vary from patient to patient depending on age, relevant family history, and types of problems. For example, in a 15-month-old boy presenting with motor and cognitive developmental delays, failure to thrive, and no family history of similar problems, the prenatal, neonatal, immunization, and developmental history of the child is highly relevant; while in a child presenting with short stature, it is critically important to determine whether the growth retardation is of prenatal or postnatal origin as this information will help point the clinician down different diagnostic paths. It may also be important to fully delineate and assess a child's development from the neonatal period onward. Although many children seen for evaluation in a genetics clinic will ultimately require formal developmental testing, including vision and hearing tests, to document the level, extent, and causes of delay as precisely as possible, oftentimes, the key questions and answers obtained in the history can provide a general sense of a child's developmental progress over time. Abbreviated general guides to average milestones in childhood development are presented in several general pediatric textbooks; however, the geneticist should ask more detailed specific questions or refer to a developmental specialist when there are any concerns. It is also important to determine whether the child's development shows continued progress or is static, or if there is a regression with loss of developmental or cognitive skills. A child with Down syndrome will generally make slow and steady developmental progress on a time course lagging behind average children, whereas a child with delays associated with a metabolic disorder, such as X-linked childhood adrenoleukodystrophy, may have early normal developmental followed by a devastating and unexpected period of regression. In addition to standard questions regarding development, it is worthwhile to ask about any unusual behaviors or special talents. The hand-wringing behavior of developmentally delayed girls with Rett syndrome is a very helpful observation. A history of hypotonia and failure to thrive in a neonate who then had a rapid onset of abnormal weight gain in early childhood years would lead a geneticist to consider Prader–Willi syndrome in the differential diagnosis. Before the physical exam, asking specific questions that explore the child's interest and talent in putting jigsaw puzzles together along with his or her unusual behaviors and eating habits surrounding food could appropriately reinforce the suspicion of Prader–Willi syndrome. Thus important clues leading to a differential diagnosis or overall etiology for a patient's problems, and ultimately a diagnosis, may be gained through answers to specific and thoughtful questions about the past medical history and prenatal history.

For a healthy 12-year-old girl with a family history of familial adenomatous polyposis (FAP), it would be essential to include information about which family members have FAP—for instance it is highly relevant to know if the affected family member is a parent or a third cousin—but it would not be essential to include detailed information about her birth history and developmental history in this section. Similarly, for a 45-year-old asymptomatic woman being seen for predictive testing for Huntington disease, key elements of the family history should be included but not early prenatal, development, or childhood history information. For an adult with profound mental retardation, dysmorphic features, and seizures, however, all of those elements should be included. In short, it is essential to include any of the key information that is highly relevant to the reason the individual is being seen in the genetics clinic as this information will be helpful in considering diagnostic, management, and counseling options.

It is very important to assess at the onset how much the patient knows or perceives about her symptoms or condition. Often before reaching a genetics clinic, individuals have been given a tentative diagnosis by their local healthcare provider without much further education or information. Other times, individuals may have made a "self-diagnosis" based on their family history, medical problems of other people they know, or something they have seen on television or read in a magazine, newspaper, or web site. Some patients come to clinic after having gone to libraries or the Internet to read about the condition. It is important to ascertain what preconceived notions and what resources they already have regarding their possible diagnosis. They also may have learned about their condition from other family members if it runs in their family and may not understand the variability of the disease that can exist between family members. It is likewise important to know whether the patient has already initiated contact with national organizations or support groups regarding the diagnosis to determine what connections have already been made and what materials and resources the patient has available.

Individuals coming to clinic may have false hopes or expectations regarding their condition or as to what may happen at the genetics clinic. They may have misunderstandings or may have inaccurate preconceived ideas about their future health based on the limited amount of information they have read. The old saying that a little knowledge is more dangerous than no knowledge at all can sometimes accurately reflect an individual's unrealistic expectations or unwarranted anxieties. Therefore, it is essential to determine the patient's own sense of his/her symptoms and knowledge about his/her condition, as the information that s/he provides for the history will be colored by his/her experiences with, knowledge about, expectations for, and anxieties regarding the condition or problems for which s/he is being evaluated.

The "Past Medical History"   The "Past Medical History" of an individual is also critically important in understanding his/her condition and medical problems. The past medical history for adults and children should describe major or chronic medical illnesses, previous surgeries, any previous hospitalizations, current medications with accurate doses, and medical allergies with the nature of reaction. It is important to understand the various medications, both prescribed and over the counter (including vitamins and herbal supplements), that patients are taking to help alleviate the symptoms they are having. In addition, it is critically important to know of any specific drug allergies that a patient has in the event that it is necessary to prescribe a particular medication for his/her. When possible, it is best to list "Past Medical History" information in chronological order. While specific dates are usually not needed, the years or approximate ages when events occurred are helpful to include. Answers to further questions about injuries, major trauma, and frequencies and types of different chronic illnesses are also important to document.

For neonates, infants, and children, it is essential that a detailed history regarding their mother's pregnancy and prenatal concerns is clearly elicited and well-documented. If this was not included in the "Relevant Medical History," then it should be obtained as part of the "Past Medical History." The child's neonatal and newborn course as well as developmental and immunization history should also be fully explored and well-documented. In the pediatric genetics clinic, it is not uncommon for an individual parent to suspect that something she did or did not do during the pregnancy or before the pregnancy caused the specific problems or condition that their child has. By asking questions about the prenatal history including exposures to any environmental, ingested, or inhaled substances as well as medication use and maternal illness, one can often determine whether or not a parent of an affected child assigns blame to herself, a partner, or perhaps the obstetrician for her child's condition. It is also appropriate and worthwhile to directly ask parents or family members what they feel has caused the problems they or their children have. It is important to ask these questions in a manner that does not suggest blame and is reassuring.

It is useful to determine and document the compliance of individuals with past medical recommendations if possible. Through specific questioning, it is possible to determine an individual's active participation in routine healthcare and preventive medicine strategies (i.e., screening mammography, Pap smears), which may be useful in providing future recommendations for continued care. In addition to asking patients and family members about traditional medical hospitalizations, surgical procedures, and medical management, it is also important to explore whether or not they have sought alternative types of healthcare treatment. It is not uncommon for individuals who have rare syndromes or disorders to find that their primary physicians know very little about their condition, and they may therefore explore alternative healthcare options in seeking answers and treatments for their conditions. In addition, individuals from different cultural backgrounds may seek alternative medical care that difers from standard Western medical care practiced in the United States. Therefore, it is especially important to ask about this. The past medical history should also explore overall general health patterns including diet and exercise.

The "Social History"   The "Social History" of an individual is critically important to elicit, as an individual's social support system may have a significant influence on his/her overall well-being and resources for healthcare management. In addition, an exploration of social history may help identify specific concerns about environmental exposures in the work setting, reveal cognitive or developmental problems during an exploration of the patient's educational history, and provide insights into an individual's physical problems in the work environment due to a disability. In the social history it is important to document an individual's living situation, support system, key relationships, education, employment, exercise patterns, hobbies, and religious beliefs.

This section is where important information about health habits, such as tobacco use, alcohol use, and illicit substance use, is recorded if not directly related to the "Relevant Medical History." When asking about substance use, it is often most helpful to ask questions that specifically document the extent of usage, such as "How many alcoholic beverages do you drink in a typical week?" or, in patients with a known history, "How often do you drink more than three beers per day?" For tobacco use, it is helpful to document when they started smoking and how many packs per day they currently smoke and smoked in the past. If they currently do not use any substances, it is useful to document if they were a former tobacco user, drug user, or significant alcohol user, as this information is relevant to their ongoing healthcare.

Finally, this section can be used to document some unique personal information about the individual that you may draw upon to establish rapport at an annual follow-up visit. For instance, when an individual tells you that art is his favorite subject in grade school, that he just got a new horse, or that he plays on the Special Olympics basketball team, if you document this and ask him about it when you next see him in clinic, it can help establish a good relationship, especially with children.

The "Family History"   As noted above, the family history is a critical component of a medical history. In genetics, this is especially important and therefore has an entire chapter devoted to it in this book (Chapter 2).

The "Review of Systems"   Generally the last, albeit extremely important, component of a medical history is known as the "Review of Systems" or "ROS" (Table 8-2B), where the physician or healthcare provider will ask specific questions about all parts of the body and its functions to determine, in an organized head-to-toe fashion, whether or not there may be other related symptoms that were not brought up in either the "Relevant Medical History" or the "Past Medical History." In addition, a detailed review of systems helps to determine other interrelated illness or problems that may influence the patient's sense of well-being. A detailed review of systems as part of the genetics evaluation may also provide additional clues to an underlying genetic diagnosis. Generally, the review of systems is a series of questions in which the physician will ask about everything from eyesight, dental care, and hearing problems, to problems associated with bowel and bladder function and to problems and concerns related to sexual function. Specific questions related to men's and women's health issues are included in this section. In addition, it is also an excellent time to specifically ask the patient about his/her own sense of their health, whether or not s/he feels s/he is generally in excellent, good, fair, or poor health, and how s/he would describe his/her mood.

For some areas addressed in the "ROS," such as psychiatric problems or sexual dysfunction, individuals may be reluctant to talk about problems in these areas during other parts of the history because of their lack of comfort in raising the topic, embarrassment in talking about such issues, or the private nature of the subject matter. However, when asked specifically about these important aspects of health among a series of other questions, patients may feel more comfortable sharing information about problems that they are experiencing. In my own experience in an adult medical genetics clinic, it is not uncommon for adults to have problems with sexual intimacy or bowel or bladder control stemming from physical, emotional, or cognitive problems related to having a genetic condition that they have not addressed with other healthcare providers. It is therefore helpful to include questions about this in the "ROS" so that opportunities for assistance can be offered to patients who are suffering in silence.

Special Considerations in the Medical History for Geneticists From the medical history the physician obtains significant information about the patient and the patient's concerns about his/her disease or condition and develops a differential diagnosis as to the possible underlying diagnoses that the patient may have. This enables the physician to then provide a well thought out and careful physical examination with a special focus and emphasis on the particular concerns that the patient has, as well as the particular areas of concern that have been addressed through the medical history.

As noted above, the elements in the medical history and their order of presentation will often vary and are somewhat dependent on the particular case. For example, evaluation of a newborn with multiple congenital anomalies would necessitate that information about the pregnancy history, prenatal history, and neonatal history is part of the history of present illness rather than buried in the past medical history. Similarly, evaluation of a child with an inborn error of metabolism or problems with regression of cognitive or motor skills would necessitate that information about childhood development as well as neonatal and prenatal histories are included in the "Relevant Medical History." In genetics clinics, many individuals present to clinic with symptoms of a disease that runs in their family. Clearly in this situation, the family history is a critical part of the history of present illness. Therefore, although the basic components of a medical history always should be included, the order in which they are included may vary depending on the case.

In medical genetics evaluations, a critical component often involves reviewing medical charts carefully. This may include reviewing records of other family members including pertinent pathology reports for any biopsies and autopsy reports of deceased family members who reportedly had similar conditions or features. This is especially important in cases where the patients presenting to clinic are asymptomatic themselves but have a family history of a particular condition. For example, if the patient reports a family history of gynecological tumors it is important to review medical records of affected individuals to determine whether the tumors were ovarian in origin, because the patient could be at increased risk of carrying a *BRCA 1* mutation. However, if the gynecological tumors were cervical or uterine cancer, it is unlikely that a *BRCA 1* mutation is associated Similarly, for asymptomatic adults who are at a 50 percent risk of having inherited a mutated gene causing Huntington disease from a deceased affected parent, it is worthwhile to try to obtain as much information about the affected individual as possible before undertaking genetic counseling and/or genetic testing. This will help to determine whether or not Huntington disease is the correct diagnosis to be considering, since several other neurological conditions can have symptoms that may overlap or mimic Huntington disease. Therefore, in order to provide the most accurate and precise genetic counseling and most appropriate evaluations for a patient, it is important to critically evaluate medical records, not only of the patient but often of additional family members.

The Physical Examination

The General Examination The physical examination in the medical genetics evaluation is based on a standard physical examination (Table 8-3) but contains additional elements that may or may not be routinely done, depending on the particular individual and the specific conditions under consideration. The basic components of a physical examination include an ascertainment of an individual's vital signs, which include heart rate, blood pressure, and respiratory rate, and an overall assessment of the individual's general health, state of mind, and nutritional status. It is important to record parameters of growth including height, weight, and head circumference and to evaluate an individual's general body habitus.

The physical examination is then often done in a systematic fashion, examining the head and neck, thorax, heart, lungs, abdomen, breasts, genitals, musculoskeletal system, neurological system including mental status, and the skin. The order of the examination may vary depending on the patient's chief complaint and age. In pediatric examinations, it is often best to do the most "threatening" parts of the examination (often in children this includes looking in the ears and throat) near the end of the examination and to begin examining the child by observing them and then engaging them playfully in parts of the examination. Most clinical geneticists who examine children have also been subjected to undergoing parts of the examination themselves conducted by children playing doctor. There are several special components of a physical examination in genetics that are utilized in specific situations (Table 8-4).

Cutaneous Examination One critical component in the genetics evaluation is a detailed cutaneous or skin examination to look for any characteristic skin lesions that are associated with neurocutaneous disorders or other syndromes (Spitz, 1996;

TABLE 8-3. Basic Components of a Complete General Physical Examination

Overall general health
Vital signs
Assessment of growth, body habitus, general proportions
Examination by system or structure as appropriate
        Head
        Neck
        Thorax
        Cardiac
        Pulmonary
        Breast
        Abdomen
        Genitourinary
        Pelvic
        Rectal
        Musculoskeletal
        Neurological
        Mental status
        Developmental
        Cutaneous

TABLE 8-4. Special Components of Focused Genetics Examinations

Dysmorphology examination

Describe major anomalies, minor anomalies, and normal variants.
Include key measurements and dermatoglyphics when appropriate.
Assess the pattern of observed features to identify a syndrome.
Obtain photographic/video documentation.

Assessment for specific conditions (examples):

Neurocutaneous disorders
    Careful cutaneous examination for specific signs of syndromes
    Detailed neurological examination
    Ophthalmology examination
    Audiology evaluation when appropriate
    Specialized neuroimaging studies when appropriate
    Specialized examinations of other organs (e.g., kidneys)

Connective tissue disorders
    Detailed examination of joints for contractures or hypermobility
    Examination of body proportions using measurements
    Careful cutaneous examination
    Specialized examinations of other organs (e.g., eyes, ears, heart)
    Specialized imaging studies (e.g., MRI of lower spine)

Sybert, 1997). For example, in Gorlin syndrome, a syndrome characterized by multiple basal cell carcinomas as well as other birth defects, individuals will have a pattern of pitting (small pits), in the palms of their hands and soles of their feet. These pits may be routinely missed unless they are specifically looked for when that syndrome is being considered. Similarly, in a condition such as tuberous sclerosis there are specific characteristic cutaneous lesions such as the shagreen patches, ash leaf spots, and hypopigmented confetti lesions that may be missed if not specifically looked for (often with the aid of a special UV light known as a wood lamp) in addition to angiofibromas of the face.

Body Proportion Measurements Another component of the physical examination that is uniquely important in a medical genetics evaluation is the measurement of body proportions in terms of the length of extremities as compared to the length of the trunk, especially in connective tissue disorders (Pope and Smith, 1995). This assessment can help in the diagnosis of Marfan syndrome, where long arms and long legs with arachnodactyly (long fingers and toes) are associated with having an arm span significantly greater than one's height and having a longer lower portion of the body compared to an upper portion of the body. Therefore, measurements looking at upper to lower segment ratios, arm span, length of fingers compared to the length of the palm, and total hand length are all important diagnostic evaluations in the consideration of Marfan syndrome. Proportional measurements are also important when considering various short stature syndromes to determine whether or not there is proportional short stature or disproportionate short stature. Many of the skeletal dysplasias are classified based on the area of shortened bone growth. Therefore, careful measurements of body proportions can help the clinician develop a differential diagnosis, ultimately leading to appropriate diagnostic studies and a definitive diagnosis. In considering skeletal disorders and connective disorders it is also important to carefully evaluate joints for either contractures or increased laxity, as this may provide important clues to the diagnosis.

Using Photographs   A unique and very important part of the clinical genetics evaluation is viewing photographs of the patient at various ages (Hall, 1996). Some syndromes will typically evolve or change with aging, and therefore it may be useful diagnostically to review photographs of older patients with dysmorphic features at a younger age. For example, as individuals with Williams syndrome age their features often appear more coarse, and when seen as adults they may not present with the widely recognized "elfin" facial appearance of early childhood. Adults with Stickler syndrome, on the other hand, have facial features that may normalize with aging, but their early childhood photos reveal the characteristic facial appearance associated with the condition. In addition, it is often critically important to physically evaluate other affected family members. If this is not possible, sometimes reviewing photographs of these other family members can be of great utility.

The Dysmorphology Examination   In an individual who presents with major or minor congenital anomalies a dysmorphology examination should be conducted in which key measurements are taken and compared to published normalized standards to determine aberrant size, shape, or placement or structural anomalies of certain features such as the eyes and ears. It is important to specifically look for, characterize, and precisely describe and document any major or minor anomalies that may be present.

Major anomalies are often defined as anomalies or malformations that create significant medical problems for the patient or that require specific surgical or medical management. Major anomalies or malformations generally are not considered a variation of the normal spectrum.

Minor anomalies are often described as features that vary from those most commonly seen in the normal population but that, in and of themselves, do not cause increased morbidity.

Describing all major and minor anomalies in great detail as precisely as possible is essential in arriving at the correct diagnosis (Barness-Gilbert et al., 1989; Cohen, 1989; Saksena et al., 1989; Cohen, 1990; Friedman, 1990; Friedman, 1992; Hall, 1993; Winter, 1995; Epstein, 1995). Most often, it is not just one major anomaly or one minor anomaly that makes a diagnosis but rather a constellation of major and minor anomalies that point to a specific syndrome diagnosis or known association.

The presence of a single isolated major anomaly, such as a unilateral cleft lip, has drastically different implications as to etiology, diagnosis, and prognosis than it would for an individual with a median cleft lip and palate associated with polydactyly (extra digits), a congenital heart defect, and low-set ears. To simply say that an individual has polydactyly without defining the number of extra digits, the extent of extra digits (a small nubbin versus an additional well-formed finger), and the precise location (pre- or postaxial referring to the radial/thumb or ulnar/little finger) of the extra finger is of little help in narrowing down the differential diagnosis. When assessing an individual's physical features, it is also critically important to consider race, ethnicity, and familial features. All of these factors will certainly influence the way an individual appears.

Evaluating Dermatoglyphics   Another component of the classic genetics dysmorpholgy examination that is not often conducted any more but can be quite useful in certain situations, is dermatoglyphics. Dermatoglyphics refers to the analysis of finger skin patterns or finger prints. It literally means "skin carvings" in Greek and was coined by the anatomist Harold Cummins in 1926. Given the availability of more sophisticated genetic testing, dermatoglyphics is rarely utilized as a specific diagnostic tool. However, there still are some advantages to looking at dermatoglyphic patterns in clinical patients before diagnostic testing. They are very easy to evaluate, readily available, noninvasive for the patient, relatively inexpensive, and quick. There is a wealth of older genetics literature describing the dermatoglyphic patterns in various conditions. In the diagnosis of trisomy 21, a specific diagnostic index was reported by Rex and Preus in 1982 (Rex and Preus, 1982). They found that examining the hallucal region of the foot (just beneath the big toe on the bottom of the foot) for a pattern known as the tibial arch dermatoglyphic, the fingers for a dermatoglyphic pattern known as ulnar loops, and the palm for a displaced palmar triradius pattern provided quite useful criteria along with other diagnostic features in predicting whether or not a newborn baby had Down syndrome (Winter, 1995). In addition, individuals with sex chromosome abnormalities have characteristic dermatoglyphics. Essentially, the more X chromosomes an individual has, the lower the number of ridges on the fingers. Therefore, an individual with a sex chromosome abnormality such as a man with Kleinfelter syndrome, 47 XXY, will have a lower ridge count on the fingers than a male who is 46 XY.

Classification of Morphogenic Abnormalities   When considering dysmorphic features, it is important to keep in mind how the various abnormalities identified are related to one another.

A **syndrome** is generally recognized and defined when a well-characterized constellation of major and minor anomalies occur together in a predictable fashion, presumably due to a single complex underlying etiology that may be monogenic, chromosomal, mitochondrial, or teratogenic in origin. For instance trisomy 21 (Down syndrome—a numeric chromosome disorder: 47 XX or XY, +21) is a syndrome associated with a predictable constellation of major and minor anomalies that create a recognizable phenotype that allows people who have seen other individuals with trisomy 21 to immediately suspect the diagnosis when they see an individual with the same condition, even though all of the characteristic anomalies are generally not present in any one affected individual. It is relatively common for patients with a specific syndrome to exclaim "I saw pictures of people who look like me!" when they first see or read patient newsletters or educational brochures about their particular diagnosis. When one mother I worked with saw a textbook photograph of a baby with Carpenter syndrome (acrocephalopolysyndactyly type II—a craniosynostosis syndrome) during counseling about her 31-year-old son's recent diagnosis of the syndrome, she remarked that this was the first time in her life she had ever seen "a baby's picture that looked exactly like my son's newborn baby picture."

An **association** is a group of anomalies that occur more frequently together than would be expected by chance alone but that lack a predictable pattern of recognition or suspected unified underlying etiology.

A **sequence** is a group of related anomalies that generally stem from a single initial major anomaly that affects the development of other tissues or structures. Potter sequence is recognized by a constellation of physical findings in which the outward appearance of the newborn is often characterized by flattened abnormal facial features and deformations of the hands and feet. These features, along with poor lung development, are secondary to decreased amounts of amniotic fluid (oligohydramnios), which is most often due to major renal (kidney) abnormalities associated with decreased fetal urine output. The term **field defect** is often used to describe related malformations in a particular region and sometimes is used interchangeably with sequence. The Pierre Robin sequence is, in fact, sometimes referred to as a field defect where the small jaw and posterior displacement of the tongue causing a cleft palate are related to one another in a temporal sense, limited to that field or area of the head. This field defect, however, can be associated with other anomalies in a syndrome such as velocardiofacial syndrome, where affected individuals often have a characteristic facial appearance associated with their cleft palate and cardiac defects. This illustrates the importance of a comprehensive examination in reaching the correct diagnosis for an individual.

When considering dysmorphic features, it is also important to keep in mind the various ways in which structures and tissues can become abnormal. For instance, a structure may be visibly abnormal because of a deformation, disruption, malformation, or dysplasia (Fig. 8-1).

A **deformation** is caused by an abnormal external force acting on the fetus during in utero development that results in abnormal growth or formation of the fetal structure. For instance, fetuses that grow in a uterine environment where not enough amniotic fluid is present (oligohydramnios), as described above in Potter sequence, may have a flattened face due to compression of the face against the uterine wall, resulting in a situation in which there was not enough room for significant movement and full development of the face or facial features.

Another type of abnormality is known as a **disruption,** where normal growth of a fetal structure is halted prematurely. This is seen in the condition known as amniotic bands, where the normal growth of digit or extremity is disrupted or discontinued because of the development of an amniotic band(s) at the end of that extremity. This may result in missing fingers, toes, or hands and feet. Often, disruptions and deformations are relatively isolated and not associated with multiple congenital anomalies.

A **malformation** signifies that fetal growth and development did not proceed normally because of underlying genetic, epigenetic, or environmental factors that altered the development.

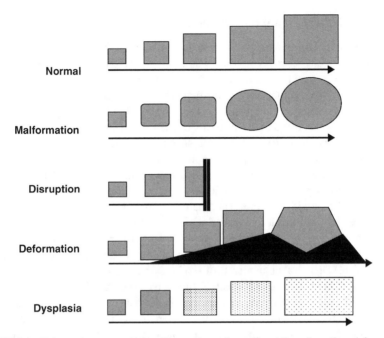

FIGURE 8-1. *Schematic representation of normal growth, malformation, disruption, deformation, and dysplasia of a structure (small square) during the development of the embryo and fetus*

Another type of generalized anomaly is due to **dysplasia** (Fig. 8-1), where the intrinsic cellular architecture of a tissue is not normally maintained throughout growth and development. Many of the skeletal syndromes of short stature are due to dysplasia in the developing bone and cartilage.

It is important for the clinician to use the physical examination to help determine the type of abnormality that exists, as this has quite significant implications for the diagnosis and management of the condition. A relatively common congenital anomaly, unilateral cleft lip and cleft palate, is most often due to an isolated malformation in the structural development of those tissues forming the lip and palate. However, it is important to remember that a cleft lip and palate or other facial clefts may be caused by amniotic bands, in which case the clefting would be considered a disruption of normal growth due to the bands. These two different types of facial clefts are important to differentiate, as they are associated with different recurrence risks for the individual and the individual's family. When evaluating these malformations, deformations, disruptions, and dysplasias, it is extremely useful and important to keep in mind the timing of development of particular organs, tissues, and fetal structures, as this may help determine the time and etiology of the particular abnormality. Basic charts of fetal development can be found in standard medical genetics textbooks and are worth having readily available in the genetics clinic. A general rule of thumb is that most internal organs are formed during the first four to six weeks of fetal development, whereas digits and facial features are defined within the first eight to twelve weeks, and neurological development occurs throughout gestation.

Types of Medical Genetics Evaluations

There are many different types of medical genetics evaluations; they will vary depending on the types of symptoms that a patient presents with as well as the age of presentation. Prenatal evaluation, which is not dealt with at any length in this chapter, is clearly an important diagnostic component of genetics and really its own special field. Prenatal evaluations, however, are rooted in the same general concepts as medical genetics evaluations in terms of the critical importance of good family histories, medical histories, and detailed specialized diagnostic testing.

Another group of individuals commonly referred to medical genetics clinics is infants and children with developmental delays who may or may not have congenital anomalies or other neurological features. Obviously, it is critically important to evaluate newborns with congenital anomalies, birth defects, and ambiguous genitalia in a timely fashion in order to provide specific information and counseling to the often surprised and very distraught family as well as to provide specific information regarding prognosis and medical management for the healthcare team caring for the newborn. The area of inborn errors of metabolism or biochemical disease is a specialized field in medical genetics that looks specifically at metabolism and biochemical problems. Genetic centers may have their own biochemical geneticist experts who specifically focus on diagnosing and managing these types of disorders. A handful of these conditions including phenylketonuria (PKU), galactosemia, homocystinuria, and maple syrup urine disease are screened for in many states during the newborn period so that appropriate management can be immediately initiated. It is important to know what type of biochemical newborn screening, as well as other genetic screening, is standard in the state in which you practice. It is also important to know which state your patient was born in, as this may have implications as to what testing has already been done. The child with learning problems by early school age is also a common cause for concern for families, teachers, and healthcare workers, often resulting in a referral to a clinical geneticist to look for syndromes associated with learning problems and minimal dysmorphic features, such as fragile X syndrome, which generally presents with developmental problems in young boys.

Neurocutaneous disorders, or germatodermatoses, are conditions that are often associated with a variety of features involving the neurological system, skin, skeletal system, and potentially other organ systems (Spitz, 1996; Sybert, 1997). Individuals having one of these syndromes, such as neurofibromatosis or tuberous sclerosis, are often referred to a medical genetics clinic not only for initial evaluation but for continued management and follow-up, as these multisystemic disorders are relatively rare in our population and many primary healthcare physicians may not have the expertise, time, or specialized educational background to fully manage affected individuals in their own practices. Similarly, individuals with connective tissue disorders such as skeletal dysplasias, Marfan syndrome, or one of the many forms of Ehlers–Danlos syndrome are often evaluated and referred to genetics clinics for continued management and follow-up (Pope and Smith, 1995).

There is an increasing and anticipated growing field of adult medical genetics in which individuals with adult-onset disorders including cancer predisposition syndromes and neurodegenerative, psychiatric, cardiovascular, and perhaps, in the future, more complex conditions are referred to medical genetics clinics for evaluation and diagnosis. With the advent and increasing utility of DNA diagnostics for many of these conditions, the area of presymptomatic or predictive genetic testing is a widely growing field that deserves special attention in terms of genetic counseling, consideration of genetic testing, and appropriate cost-effective application of available genetic tests. Presymptomatic and predictive genetic testing for adult-onset disorders is anticipated to be a growing field in medical genetics as more genes are discovered and genetic tests are developed. Thus there are many different indications for individuals to be seen in medical genetics clinics, which necessitate the use of specialized evaluations and approaches as appropriate to the specific situation. For instance, a detailed body proportion examination in a patient referred for Huntington disease would not be indicated, but such an examination would be absolutely necessary in a patient referred for an evaluation of short stature.

Documentation of the Medical Genetics Evaluation

As with any medical evaluation, detailed, precise, and concise documentation of relevant findings, including both the presence of specific findings and the lack of key findings, is extremely important in conveying accurate information to other healthcare providers. A detailed pedigree, which can be facilitated by the use of a computerized pedigree drawing program, is obviously one special documentation service that the medical genetics team can provide to other healthcare providers. Detailed documentation of the medical history and record review also should be clearly presented. The physical findings should be very well documented, and this is often facilitated by the use of specific forms (Fig. 8-2) designed to help rapidly record specific measurements as well as to diagram specific features or cutaneous lesions. In the medical genetics clinic, photographs and videotapes of patients may provide a wealth of information that is ultimately too time consuming or too cumbersome and difficult to convey concisely and accurately in words (Hall, 1996).

There are a plethora of various names for the hundreds of different relatively rare genetic syndromes and disorders; however, these labels often give absolutely no clue to the noninitiated as to what the condition is. Fortunately, the clinical geneticist is well equipped with a special vocabulary of words and terms, often based in Greek and Latin roots, that allow him or her to accurately describe the specific nuances and physical findings of a genetics examination in a relatively concise and precise fashion. However, for genetic counselors just entering the field as well as for many physicians in other specialties, the words sometimes seem more confusing than useful. As is the case in any medical specialty, it is important for all individuals providing clinical genetics services to make a concentrated effort to fully familiarize themselves with the "language of the specialty" in order to effectively communicate with other geneticists and to absorb and appreciate the medical genetics literature. It is equally important for clinical geneticists to communicate information to patients and

NAME: _____ DATE: ____
REG #: _____
DOB: _____ AGE: ____

| VITAL SIGNS |
BP: RA_____ LA_____
    RL_____ LL_____
HR:_____ RR:_____
HEIGHT: ____in _____cm (%)
WEIGHT: ____lbs _____kg (%)

| HEAD - NECK λ |
General description:

HEAD CIRCUM.: _____cm (%)
Cranium/Sutures:
Hair:

Eyes:
    IC: _____cm (%)
    OC: _____cm (%)
    IP: _____cm (%)
    RPF: _____cm (%)
    LPF: _____cm (%)
Ears:
    R: _____cm (%)
    L: _____cm (%)
Philtrum: _____cm (%)
Lips:
Palate and mouth:
Teeth:
Chin:
Neck:

| TRUNK - ABDOMEN |
General description:
    sternum:
    spine:
Breast: Tanner stage: _____
Heart:
Lungs:
    Chest circumference: _____cm
    Inter nipple distance: _____cm
IND_____/ CC_____= _____ (%)
Abdomen:
Umbilicus:
Genitalia:
    penile length: _____cm (%)
    testicular vol.: _____cm (%)
        Tanner stage: _____

| SKIN |
General description:

Freckles - iris:_____ axillary:_____ inguinal:_____
Cafe au lait spots: #_____ size range: _____cm
Neurofibromas: #_____ size range: _____cm
Hypopigmented lesions:
Other lesions:

| EXTREMITIES - PROPORTIONS |
General description:

    laxity:
    contractures:
    digital abnormalities:
LOWER segment: _____cm
UPPER segment: _____cm (HT-LS)
US/LS ratio: ____/____= % (SD)
ARM SPAN: _____cm
WRIST SIGN: ____ THUMB SIGN: ____
HAND: R_____cm (%)
               L_____cm (%)
MIDDLE FINGER: R_____cm (%)
               L_____cm (%)
PALM: R_____cm (%)
               L_____cm (%)
FOOT: R_____cm (%)
               L_____cm (%)
Finger to Hand: _____/_____ (%)
Hand to Height _____/_____ (%)
Foot to Height _____/_____ (%)

| NERVOUS SYSTEM |
Mental status:

Cranial nerves:

Muscle bulk and tone:
Sensation:
Motor strength: Deep tendon reflexes:

| DIAGRAM TO DOCUMENT FINDINGS |
| R   front   L | R   back   L |

| Right hand | Left hand |

FIGURE 8-2. *Example of a form that may be utilized to facilitate documentation of the medical genetics examination*

referring physicians by using terminology that they can readily understand. A physician or counselor who speaks eloquently in unfamiliar terminology to a patient may initially impress the patient but will ultimately provide a disservice to the patient by not providing the patient with adequate information.

DIAGNOSTIC STUDIES

Utility of Diagnostic Studies in the Medical Genetics Evaluation

A variety of diagnostic studies may be required in concert with a clinical evaluation and medical history in order to reach a particular diagnosis for a patient or to provide information about prognosis and medical management for a patient. These tests will include specific genetics-based testing but are not limited only to those genetic tests. For example, in a newborn boy who has excessive bleeding after a circumcision, a DNA-based mutation analysis could both reveal the molecular basis for his bleeding disorder and confirm his diagnosis of hemophilia A, while more routine hematology laboratory tests, such as clotting factor studies, would be most useful in making the initial medical assessment critical to the patient's immediate medical management.

Application of Diagnostic Genetic Tests

Diagnostic genetic tests can be broken down into three large and sometimes overlapping categories including:

- Cytogenetic studies, which may include routine karyotypes, high-resolution karyotypes, molecular fluorescent in situ hybridization (FISH) studies, and chromosome microarray studies
- Biochemical tests, which may include screening urine or plasma samples for the recognition of specific classes of metabolic diseases or specialized quantitative tests to look precisely at specific enzymatic function
- DNA-based diagnostic tests.

These tests, including their clinical utility and limitations, are addressed in detail in Chapter 9.

Other routine laboratory studies may be required in the medical genetics evaluation to help reach a diagnosis or manage patient symptoms. Blood counts, clotting factors, liver and kidney function tests, hormone levels, thyroid studies, acid-base status, and measurements of other breakdown products of metabolism may be useful. None of these laboratory studies is considered routine in the medical genetics evaluation, but they are utilized as necessary depending on the circumstances of individual cases.

Various diagnostic imaging studies are often of great importance and help in the medical genetics evaluation. Specialized imaging studies in the prenatal period are routinely used to look for congenital anomalies, such as detailed ultrasounds and fetal echocardiography. In addition to still photography and video imaging, various types of X-ray studies including skeletal surveys may be of help in determining various genetic conditions including skeletal dysplasias and recognizing bony congenital anomalies that may point to a specific syndromic diagnosis. Specialized imaging studies such as CT scans, MRI scans, and echocardiograms may be required in the evaluation of certain conditions or to help make a specific diagnosis. For example, in Marfan syndrome, where aortic root dilatation and aortic rupture may occur, an echocardiogram documenting aortic root size may confirm the diagnosis. Once the diagnosis of Marfan syndrome is made, routine echocardiograms or, in some cases, other imaging studies such as transesophageal echocardiograms or spiral CT scans of the aorta, will need to be done on a regular basis to monitor the patient for any signs of aortic root problems necessitating more aggressive medical management. Therefore, diagnostic imaging studies in clinical patients can be quite useful not only in initial diagnosis but also in routine follow-up and management.

TOOLS AND RESOURCES OF THE CLINICAL GENETICIST

The clinical geneticist relies on the usual "tools" of the physician, including the stethoscope, reflex hammer, otoscope, ophthalmoscope, and tuning fork. In addition these are supplemented by a variety of measuring devices. The utility of the tools varies depending on the type of examination, but a few basic additional pieces of equipment such as a precisely marked, long (2.5 meter), flexible measuring tape for measuring arm spans and other extremity proportions; a short, clear ruler for accurately measuring proportions and sizes of facial structures such as the palpebral fissure length (PFL), and inner canthi (IC) distance, outer canthi (OC) distance, and inter pupil (IP) distance (Fig. 8-3); a jointed ruler with degree markings to measure the angles of either contracted or hyperextended joints; and large-and small-sized blunt calipers to measure distances and irregular body parts such as various proportions of the calvarium or skull. For measuring the sizes of long bones, especially in squirming children, it is helpful to have a long, durable piece of string that can be marked and later measured. A calculator is helpful in quickly determining ratios between body proportions. In addition to measuring devices, it is sometimes helpful to have a magnifying lens available to closely examine cutaneous lesions. A special ultraviolet

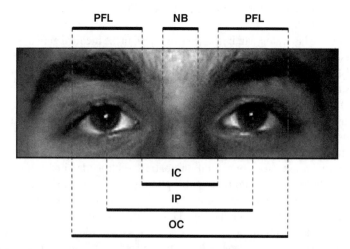

FIGURE 8-3. *Photograph showing the palpebral fissure length (PFL), nasal bridge (NB), inner canthi (IC) distance, inter pupillary (IP) distance, and outer canthi (OC) distance commonly measured in dysmorphology examinations*

light, known as a Wood lamp, can be very useful in examining fair-skinned individuals for hypopigmented lesions such as the ash leaf spots associated with tuberous sclerosis. Still and video cameras are also essential tools to have in the genetics clinic.

A high-resolution digital camera will allow the clinician to directly document specific findings for the medical record as needed. This photographic documentation can be very useful in helping consider diagnostic possibilities at a later date or through consultation with other clinicians (Hall, 1996). It also enables the clinician to share a souvenir photograph with the camera-shy young patient if desired. Other tools or aids may be useful in certain cases. For instance, the use of red disclosing tablets (the type dentists sometimes use to demonstrate food particles between the teeth in proper tooth brushing education sessions) can be useful in the genetics clinic to clearly demonstrate the enamel pits in the teeth of patients with tuberous sclerosis. Clinical geneticists may need to perform a skin biopsy for specialized diagnostic studies and will need 3- to 4-mm punch biopsy kits and local anesthesia readily available in the clinic.

Resources for the clinical geneticist include several very well-written textbooks regarding syndromes and metabolic disorders, a handful of which are listed at the end of this chapter (Gorlin et al., 1990; Beighton, 1993; Pope and Smith, 1995; Baraitser and Winter, 1996; Spitz, 1996; Sybert, 1997; Jones, 1997; Scriver et al., 2001; Nyhan et al., 2005; Emery et al., 2006). Guides to normal measurements are also found in many of the texts but are also specifically well-addressed in a small pocket-sized *Handbook of Normal Physical Measurements* that should be readily available to any geneticist (Hall et al., 2003). Computerized dysmorphology and skeletal dysplasia databases are available and can help clinical geneticists to explore differential diagnoses but should never be relied on as a peripheral diagnostician (OMIM, 2008; Evans, 1995; Winter and Baraitser, 1987; Stromme, 1991; GeneTests, 1993–2008). Online databases and clinical syndrome databases such as POSSUM, OSSUM, and the London Dysmorphology Database can be employed in the evaluation of patients with genetic conditions and may be quite useful in certain cases. The regularly updated Online Mendelian Inheritance In Man (OMIM) can help generate differential diagnoses and has been widely employed by many clinical geneticists as an important initial resource to learn more about the various syndromes they are considering. This database is directly connected through the National Center for Biotechnology Information (NBCI) to other useful genetic databases and Medline searches. The GeneTests database, which identifies DNA diagnostic testing laboratories for various conditions, is also an extremely useful resource that all geneticists should be familiar with. There are many other websites on the Internet that contain useful genetics information or links to useful genetic sites that are too numerous to mention here, including various support group sites for genetic conditions.

UTILITY OF CLINICAL CASE CONFERENCES AND OUTSIDE EXPERT CONSULTANTS

As in any medical specialty where a wide variety of relatively rare conditions are diagnosed and managed, there is great utility and benefit in having clinical diagnostic conferences to discuss cases. These conferences may be utilized to review cases before and after clinic visits to help make a diagnosis and discuss appropriate management. In addition, such conferences are increasingly important, given the ever-changing available genetic technology, as they keep the community abreast of the most current diagnostic options and management strategies for patients. Some conditions are rare enough that any one clinical geneticist may only see this condition once in his or her lifetime, if at all, and therefore may have a difficult time recognizing the condition when first meeting a patient with it. Fortunately, the clinical genetics community is peppered with resident experts for virtually every disease, who are generally very open and willing to provide curbside consultations and expert advice. Sometimes formal consultation with an outside expert is required and always should be actively sought when needed.

Other medical specialists that may be utilized for appropriate medical genetics evaluations include neurologists, cardiologists, oncologists, orthopedists and other surgery subspecialists, ophthalmologists, otolaryngologists, developmental pediatricians, physical medicine and rehabilitation specialists, pain management physicians, audiologists, speech therapists, plastic surgeons, psychiatrists and psychologists, social workers, pathologists, dermatologists, and radiologists. The interaction of all of these healthcare professionals together with the genetics team is often necessary to provide patients with the most appropriate management for their multisystemic disorders.

SUMMARY

The medical genetics evaluation is a critical part of the clinical genetics service for individuals and families with concerns about familial genetic conditions, birth defects, genetic risk for adult-onset conditions, or issues regarding abnormal development. The field of medical genetics is a rapidly evolving and changing field reflecting our ever-increasing knowledge about the human genome. Even within the specialty of medical genetics there are further specializations, with clinical geneticists having expertise in a relatively focused and narrow area of medical genetics. The broad and complex scope of disorders seen in a medical genetics clinic necessitates that the clinician possess an extensive expertise so that s/he can provide appropriate diagnosis and management for patients. Therefore, the genetics clinic is best served by a true team approach in which genetic counselors, medical geneticists, laboratory geneticists, and other healthcare providers interact with the patient and the family to provide appropriate evaluations and comprehensive care. Because of the relative rarity of many genetic conditions, it is important to have access to current medical journals, access to computerized databases, and availability of other medical specialists in order to fully evaluate patients.

In summary, the medical genetics evaluation is a critically important part of a genetics clinic visit. While genetic counselors are not often called upon to conduct a physical examination of a patient independently, a counselor's expert impressions of the patient's features and their assistance with the examination, as well as their often significant involvement in gathering and analyzing medical history information, are highly valued within a genetics team. Importantly, counselors' understanding of and working expertise with the medical examination of their patients will optimize the care of individuals and families who present to medical genetics clinics for evaluation. Thus it is important for counselors who are active in clinical practice to understand all of the elements of the medical genetics evaluation.

REFERENCES

Baraitser M, Winter RM (1996) *Color Atlas of Congenital Malformation Syndromes*, London: Mosby-Wolfe.

Barness-Gilbert E, Opitz E, Barness LA, (1989) The pathologist's perspective of genetic disease. Malformations and dysmorphology. *Pediatr Clin North Am* 36(1):163–187.

Beighton P (1993) *McKusick's Heritable Disorders of Connective Tissue* (5th ed.), St. Louis, MO:Mosby).

Cohen MM Jr. (1989) Syndromology: an updated conceptual overview. VI. Molecular and biochemical aspects of dysmorphology. *Int J Oral Maxillofacial Surg* 18(6):339–346.

Cohen MM Jr. (1990) Syndromology: an updated conceptual overview IX. Facial dysmorphology. *Int J Oral Maxillofacial Surg* 19(2):81–88.

Emery AEH, Rimoin DL, Connor JM, Pyeritz RE, Korf BR (2006) *Principles and Practice of Medical Genetics* (5th ed.), New York:Churchill Livingston.

Epstein CJ (1995) The new dysmorphology: application of insights from basic developmental biology to the understanding of the of human birth defects. *Proc Nat Acad Sci USA* **92**(19):8566–8573.

Evans CD (1995) Computer systems in dysmorphology. *Clin Dysmorphology* 4(3):185–201.

Friedman JM (1990) A practical approach to dysmorphology. *Pediatr Ann* 19(2):95–101.

Friedman JM, (1992) The use of dysmorphology in birth defects epidemiology. *Teratology* 45(2):187–193.

GeneTests: Medical Genetics Information Resource (database online). Copyright, University of Washington, Seattle. (1993–2008) . Available athttp://www.genetests.org. Accessed 12/11/08.

Gorlin RJ, Cohen MM, Levin LS (1990) *Oxford Monographs on Medical Genetics No. 19 Syndromes of the Head and Neck* (3rd ed.), New York: Oxford University Press.

Hall BD (1993) The state of the art of dysmorphology. *Am J Dis Children* 147(11):1184–1189.

Hall, BD (1996) Photographic analysis: a quantitative approach to the evaluation of dysmorophology*J Pediatr* 129(1):3–4.

Hall JD, Froster-Iskenius UG, Allanson JE (2003) *Handbook of Normal Physical Measurements*, New York:Oxford Medical Publications.

Jones KL (1997) *Smith's Recognizable Patterns of Human Malformation* (5th ed.), Philadelphia:W.B. Saunders Company.

Nyhan WL, Barshop BA, Ozand PT (2005) *Atlas of Metabolic Diseases* (2nd ed.), New York: Hodder Arnold Publication, Oxford University Press.

Online Mendelian Inheritance in Man, OMIM (TM). McKusick-Nathans Institute of Genetic Medicine, Johns Hopkins University (Baltimore, MD) and National Center for

Biotechnology Information, National Library of Medicine (Bethesda, MD), 12/11/2008. World Wide Web URL: http://www.ncbi.nlm.nih.gov/omim/.

Pope FM, Smith R, (1995) *Color Atlas of Inherited Connective Tissue Disorders*, London: Mosby-Wolfe.

Rex AP, Preus M, (1982) A diagnostic index for Down syndrome. *J Pediatr* 100(6):903–906.

Saksena SS, Bader P, Bixler D, (1989) Facial dysmorphology, roentgenographic measurements, and clinical genetics. *J Craniofacial Genet Dev Biol* 9(1):29–43.

Scriver CR, Beaudet AL, Sly WS, Valle D, Childs B, Kinzler KW, Vogelstein B (2001) *The Metabolic and Molecular Bases of Inherited Disease* (8th ed). New York:McGraw-Hill online edition: http://www.ommbid.com/.

Spitz JL (1996) *Genodermatoses*, New York:Williams & Wilkins.

Stromme P (1991) The diagnosis of syndromes by use of a dysmorphology database. *Acta Paediatr Scand* 80(1):106–109.

Sybert VP (1997) *Genetic Skin Disorders*, New York:Oxford Universty Press.

Winter RM (1995) Recent molecular advances in dysmorphology. *Hum Mol Genet* 4 Spec No:1699–1704.

Winter RM, Baraitser M (1987) The London Dysmorphology Database (letter). *J Med Genet* 24(8):509–510.

9

Understanding Genetic Testing

W. Andrew Faucett, M.S., C.G.C. and Patricia A. Ward, M.S., C.G.C.

INTRODUCTION

The completion of the Human Genome Project was a phenomenal accomplishment, providing researchers with the reference sequence of the human genome, which has subsequently led to the identification of many genes associated with human disease. Development of new technologies has made it possible to study these genes, search for disease-causing mutations, and develop genetic tests. Genetic testing has the potential to offer dramatic benefits, both clinically and psychologically, for patients and their families. The array of benefits begins with the clarification of diagnosis and prognosis, which assists in decision-making about clinical care. Testing for familial mutations makes available predictive, carrier, and prenatal testing, all of which provide risk assessment for family members of an affected patient to assist them in making complex personal, medical, and reproductive decisions. In addition, there are a multitude of genetic tests available to those with no family history of genetic disease that can provide information about potential reproductive or future health risks.

The process of ordering genetic testing can be a complex and often bewildering process for healthcare professionals. There are challenges related to test selection, laboratory choice, standards of practice, and ethical issues. Commonly, genetic counselors receive requests for genetic testing for disorders for which gene

A Guide to Genetic Counseling, Second Edition, Edited by Wendy Uhlmann, Jane Schuette, and Beverly Yashar
Copyright © 2009 by John Wiley & Sons, Inc.

identification has only recently been reported in the scientific literature. Often these requests come from primary care providers (Whittaker, 1996), but increasingly they come from families who follow the research on the particular genetic disease which has been diagnosed in their family. The immediacy with which peer-reviewed research findings are available on publicly available Internet sites speeds this process.

It is critical that genetic counselors have an understanding of the multitude of factors necessary to evaluate a clinical genetic test. For most tests, no government agency is currently assessing whether the test provides clinically relevant information. In April 2008 the Secretary's Advisory Committee on Genetics, Health and Society (SACGHS), at the request of the Secretary of Health and Human Services (HHS), issued a comprehensive report that proposed a system for oversight of genetic testing in the United States (SACGHS, 2008). This effort and those of other health policy groups will impact the development and utilization of genetic testing in the years ahead.

Currently, genetic counselors must be highly educated consumers as they select a laboratory for genetic testing, a task that calls for an understanding of the types of genetic tests, the mechanics of testing and the specifics of laboratory quality control, qualifications of laboratory personnel, and oversight procedures and practices. Many of these important topics are also addressed in the SACGHS report on the "U.S. System of Oversight of Genetic Testing" (SACGHS, 2008). This chapter focuses on test parameters and the process of identifying a patient-specific "ideal" genetic test, the translation of genetic testing from the research laboratory to the clinical laboratory, and oversight of genetic testing. The role of the genetic counselor is discussed, and clinical cases are used to illustrate the complexities of genetic testing in the counseling setting.

DEFINING GENETIC TESTING

Defining what constitutes a genetic test is not straightforward, and many groups have deliberated on the topic. The EuroGentest Project developed a document outlining definitions from multiple groups (Varga and Sequeiros, 2008). The definition of genetic testing from the Secretary's Advisory Committee on Genetics, Health and Society is as follows:

> A genetic or genomic test involves an analysis of human chromosomes, deoxyribonu-
> cleic acid, ribonucleic acid, genes, and/or gene products (e.g., enzymes and other types of
> proteins), which is predominately used to detect heritable or somatic mutations,
> genotypes, or phenotypes related to disease and health. The purpose of genetic tests
> includes predicting risk of disease, screening newborns, directing clinical management,
> identifying carriers, and establishing prenatal or clinical diagnoses or prognosis in
> individuals, families or populations. Excluded from the definition are tests conducted
> exclusively for forensic and identity purposes as well as tests conducted purely for
> research. Also excluded are tests that are used primarily for other purposes but that may
> contribute to diagnosing a genetic disease or disorder (e.g., blood smears, certain serum

chemistries). For example, cholesterol screening in the general population is not considered a genetic test, but it may reveal a genetic disorder such as an inherited form of hypercholesterolemia.

— SACGHS 2008, U.S. System of Oversight of Genetic Testing:
A Response to the Charge of the Secretary of Health and Human Services, p. 17.

Historically the broad categories of genetic tests were **(1) cytogenetic tests** (chromosome analysis), **(2) molecular tests** (DNA analysis), and **(3) biochemical tests** (enzyme assays, metabolites, protein analysis). Globally, cytogenetic tests detect changes in chromosome number, structure, and arrangement. Molecular tests look for changes in the DNA sequence, methylation, deletions, and duplications, and biochemical tests detect changes in the gene products, such as changes in levels of enzymes and proteins. Evolving technologies have led to considerable overlap between these categories of genetic tests as there are cytogenetic tests that actually use molecular/DNA methodologies, such as FISH (fluorescent in situ hybridization) analysis and chromosomal microarray analysis (CMA). Genetic tests have different clinical applications, and these will influence the specific technology selected (Table 9-1).

In genetic testing, it is often important to take into account both the genotype and the associated phenotype. The genotype is defined as the genetic makeup and the phenotype as the observable traits, characteristics, and symptoms. In an "ideal" genetic test, there is a one-to-one relationship between the genotype and the phenotype. However, as discussed below, it is possible to have a genetic test that can accurately identify changes in genotype but can be quite limited in its ability to predict phenotype, particularly type and severity of symptoms, age of onset, and disease course. This limitation in predicting outcome can be particularly challenging and requires that genetic counselors use a wide variety of critical thinking, educational, and counseling skills in discussing these testing issues with patients.

TEST PARAMETERS

The clinical use of any genetic test should not be initiated until a definite association between mutations in the gene and the disease phenotype has been established. It is important to keep two facts in mind:

- A positive result may be a true positive (individual has inherited the mutation) or a false positive (individual actually has not inherited the mutation).
- A negative result may be a true negative (individual has not inherited the mutation) or a false negative (individual actually has inherited the mutation).

Key test parameters including analytical validity, clinical validity, predictive value, and clinical utility ideally should be reviewed before offering a genetic test; these terms are defined below. For most genetic tests, these parameters vary from lab to lab and are dependent upon the technology utilized, so the genetic counselor should compare these data for each lab being considered. While these descriptive terms are

TABLE 9-1. Uses of Genetic Tests

- Diagnostic/confirmatory
  - Testing designed to confirm or exclude a known or suspected genetic disorder in a symptomatic individual or, prenatally, in a fetus at risk for a certain genetic condition.*
- Predictive
  - Testing offered to asymptomatic individuals with a family history of a genetic disorder and a potential risk of eventually developing the disorder.*
- Presymptomatic
  - Testing of an asymptomatic individual in whom the discovery of a gene mutation indicates certain development of findings related to a specific diagnosis at some future point. A negative result excludes the diagnosis.*
- Carrier risk assessment
  - Testing used to identify usually asymptomatic individuals who have a gene mutation for an autosomal recessive or X-linked disorder.*
- Newborn screening
  - Testing done within days of birth to identify infants at increased risk for a specific genetic disorder so that treatment can begin as soon as possible; when a newborn screening result is positive, further diagnostic testing is usually required to confirm or specify the results and counseling is offered to educate the parents.*
- Prenatal diagnosis
  - Testing performed during pregnancy to determine whether a fetus is affected with a particular disorder.*
- Preimplantation diagnosis
  - A procedure used to decrease the chance of a particular genetic condition for which the fetus is specifically at risk by testing one cell removed from early embryos conceived by in vitro fertilization and transferring to the mother's uterus only those embryos determined not to have inherited the mutation in question.*
- Pharmacogenetic
  - Testing used to identify potential interactions of an individual's genetic makeup with a drug or class of drugs that predict drug effects.
- Prognostic
  - Testing used to predict the probable outcome or clinical course of a disease, or the chance of recovery.

*Definitions abstracted from GeneTests www.genetests.org (section on "About Genetic Services—Uses of Genetic Testing") Accessed December 3, 2008.

familiar to most clinicians and are important for understanding the limitations of any test, they were originally developed for clinical chemistry tests and do not have universally accepted definitions for genetic tests. Where testing for a genetic disease is offered by more than one laboratory, it is often helpful to compare the information from each laboratory and ask the laboratory to explain the discrepancies, if not apparent from the methodologies utilized.

Analytical validity is the ability of a test to accurately measure a given analyte. The analyte is defined as the substance being measured by the test, which can be a specific enzyme, protein, mutation, or genotype of interest. For biochemical genetic testing, the analyte may be easy to define, but molecular test laboratories may define the analyte differently. Using Tay–Sachs disease as an example, in biochemical testing the analyte is the enzyme hexosaminidase. However, considering molecular testing for Tay–Sachs disease, the analyte may be the entire gene, exons, or only specific known mutations. Analytical validity is based on several components:

- *Analytic accuracy* is the degree of agreement of the test result with the "true value" of the analyte. Ideally, this is based on a "gold standard" or reference analyte.
- *Analytic precision* is the agreement between measurements, or the "reproducibility." Ideally, this is known from both an inter-laboratory and an intra-laboratory perspective, for within-run, between-run, and temporal parameters. Since most laboratories develop their own primers for sequence-based tests, the analytic precision of the test can vary if there are mutations in the primer site.
- *Analytic sensitivity* is not only the ability of the test to detect an analyte, but includes a sense of the lower limit of detection of the analyte. Can the test detect levels of 1% or only below 5%? Consider the power of detection of deletions by routine cytogenetic methods versus array CGH (array comparative genomic hybridization) testing.
- *Analytic specificity* is the ability of the test to detect only the analyte of interest, in other words, the proportion of negative results, given that the analyte is not there. In sequence analysis, variants of unknown significance (VOUS) occur often in molecular testing. The presence of VOUS reduces the analytic specificity of the test because without additional testing, the laboratory cannot determine whether the VOUS qualifies as an analyte.
- *Analytical predictive value* is the percentage of all positive results that are true positives.

Clinical validity is the ability of the test to predict the presence of the associated disorder or phenotype. In classical lab practice, it is defined as the percentage of patients who are correctly classified by a test result as having the disease or not. It incorporates clinical sensitivity, clinical specificity, and clinical predictive value. Table 9-2 provides definitions of the test parameters and the formulas used to calculate them.

- *Clinical sensitivity* is the ability to detect disease given that the disease is present, or the frequency of positive tests when the disease is present. The same formulas apply as those used in analytic sensitivity, except that we are referring to the phenotype or presence of the disease. Note that estimations or measurements of clinical sensitivity, although population or epidemiologically based, generally assume a high degree of penetrance. You may have a test that is 100% analytically valid, but with low penetrance the test may have very low clinical sensitivity. If you have a very reliable method for detecting an analyte and the gene is 100% penetrant, with a large enough sample population the estimate of clinical sensitivity may be considered to be close to the analytical sensitivity. Clinical sensitivity/utility and analytic sensitivity are often confused.
- *Clinical specificity* is the ability of the test to discriminate between those with the suspected phenotype or disease and those without it. It is defined in clinical

ical Utility: Test Variable Definitions and Calculations

Disease Phenotype*

Test Result		Present	Absent
	Positive	**A** (True Positives)	**B** (False Positives)
	Negative	**C** (False Negatives)	**D** (True Negatives)

Clinical sensitivity	Probability that person with disease will have positive test result [A/(A+ C)]
Clinical specificity	Probability that person without disease will have negative test result [D/(B+ D)]
Clinical positive predictive value	Probability that person has the disease, given test is positive [A/(A+ B)]
Clinical negative predictive value	Probability that person does not have the disease, given test is negative [D/(C+ D)]
False positive rate	Proportion of all positive test results occurring in individuals who are not affected [1 − specificity] = B/B+ D
False negative rate	Proportion of all negative results occurring in individuals who are affected [1 − sensitivity] = C/A+ C

*Carrier/noncarrier can be used in place of disease phenotype.

Source: Adapted from Holtzman and Watson (1997), p.26; Kroese et al., 2004

chemistry as the frequency of a negative test when the disease is absent. Without a high degree of analytic specificity, a test, by definition, cannot have a high degree of clinical specificity. Some sequence-based tests can only find mutations in 60% of individuals with the disease, and VOUS are frequently found, giving these tests a low clinical specificity (personal communication).

■ *Clinical utility* is the ability of the test to affect positive outcomes, that is, to detect and assist with managing disease, to improve treatment effectiveness, and/or to improve the quality of life (or health) of affected individuals. It refers to the clinical efficacy of using the test. Guidelines for test utilization should be based on clinical utility, and most third-party payers (insurers) require documented clinical utility for test reimbursement. Clinical utility incorporates all of the above parameters, and is based on the presumption of analytical validity. Assessment of clinical utility of a test will generally include and balance clinical, economic, and psychological measures of possible benefit as well as possible harm (Javaher et al., 2008) Evidence of clinical utility is usually not collected during the research or test development phases and may be difficult to document or measure.

Predictive value is the ability of the test to identify the presence of the disease (or absence). This is an important measurement for clinical interpretation and epidemiological studies.

- *Clinical predictive value* (or clinical positive predictive value) is the percentage of positive results given that the disease is present. This does not really refer to the analyte itself, but to the phenotype or disease. It is very important to note that clinical predictive value is a population–based measurement, and the accuracy of measurement is based on the population prevalence of a disease. In this regard, if the disease prevalence in a particular population is high, the predictive value can be very high. However, the results may vary greatly in the general population when the clinical test becomes widely available. If the population prevalence is low, such as in rare diseases, the clinical predictive value is likely to be low also. Estimates of predictive value may be better if the clinical sensitivity is high.

REASONS FOR FALSE POSITIVES AND FALSE NEGATIVES

The genetic counselor or healthcare provider should evaluate each test for the possibility of false positives and false negatives. False positives and false negatives would result in inaccurate information for carrier, diagnostic, predictive, and prenatal testing and have significant implications for healthcare and decision-making. False negatives could lead to false reassurance or a misdiagnosis and additional unnecessary testing. It is important to distinguish clinical false positives and clinical false negatives from analytical false positives and negatives, which refer to the analyte and not the disease (Burtis and Ashwood, 1998). Case #1, presented later in this chapter, illustrates the clinical significance and counseling implications of a false negative result. If the clinical course for a given patient does not match the test results, the counselor should discuss the result with the laboratory and consider either further testing or deferring until better testing becomes available. Case #2, presented later in this chapter, illustrates how important it is to take advantage of evolving technology.

False negative results (individual has disease, but tests negative) can occur as a result of (Kroese, 2004):

- Insufficient analytic sensitivity—the test does not detect the disease-associated genotype
- Untested genes (genetic heterogeneity) are responsible for the disease
- Untested mutations (allelic heterogeneity) are responsible for the disease
- The disease has been misclassified (penetrance or expressivity)
- The genotype is not present in the cell population tested—mosaicism
- Ethnicity-dependent variations in frequency of the genotype

False positives (test positive, but individual does not have the disease) can occur because (Kroese, 2004):

- A lack of perfect analytic specificity
- The test is cross-reacting (testing for polymorphic marker near real disease causing mutation)

- The genotype result is correct, but the phenotype is not visible due to reduced penetrance
- The disease has been clinically misclassified.

COMPLEXITIES OF NEGATIVE TEST RESULTS

It is important that patients understand the meaning of a negative test result. The only true negative result in genetic testing is when a patient tests negative for a known familial mutation. All other negative results could be explained by the limitations of the testing technology, laboratory error, or testing the wrong gene or the wrong mutation(s). A negative result with targeted mutation panel testing is often not a true negative because the patient may have a mutation in an untested part of the gene. Array CGH (array comparative genomic hybridization) tests often have long lists of microdeletion and microduplication disorders that could be detected, but it should be understood that the test only detects a subset of patients with the disease phenotype, correlated with the frequency of copy number mutations seen in the particular disease gene. Sequence-based testing is often described as the "gold standard" in genetic testing, yet most sequence-based tests only evaluate the exons and have limited ability to detect deep intronic mutations or large deletions or duplications of exons in autosomal genes or X-chromosome genes in females.

Often when a clinical genetic test is translated from a research setting to a clinical lab, the full spectrum of disease phenotypes and causative mutations are unknown. The initial test is generally designed to detect a limited number of known mutations associated with the classical phenotype. As additional patients and populations are tested and new mutations are identified, the test may be modified. As an example, copy number changes, such as deletions and duplications, were not initially studied in many conditions because they were predicted to be rare and the technology needed to detect them was complex and expensive. It is now known that these types of mutations are quite common in some disorders and there are many more disorders with such mutations than originally noted. There are likely to be other types of disease-causing mutations that have yet to be identified in the research setting and would therefore not be available in the clinical laboratory.

Genetic counselors should contact the testing lab to verify negative test results in patients who have a strong clinical diagnosis of the suspected disorder. Laboratory errors can explain the negative results, and repeat testing on a new specimen should be considered when the clinical diagnosis is compelling and the clinical predictive value of the test is high. It is also important to evaluate the existing testing methodology and explore alternate methodologies to analyze the same gene for other types of mutations or consider testing other genes that might be causative. These patients should be encouraged to remain in contact with their genetics provider, and the need to consider additional testing in the future as advances are made in testing should be discussed.

VARIANTS OF UNKNOWN SIGNIFICANCE

Before the development of a genetic test, most genes are studied in small populations with precise clinical criteria. Once a test moves to the clinical laboratory, previously unreported gene changes are often identified and their clinical significance is uncertain; these gene changes are known as variants of unknown significance (VOUS). Family studies and functional (gene expression) studies may be available to clarify new variants. Genetic counselors should inquire about the availability of additional studies and the laboratory's policies and costs for such tests. Clinical laboratories formally collaborating with research labs investigating a specific disorder often work with researchers to classify new variants. Patients with a VOUS should also be encouraged to periodically recontact their genetics care provider and/or researcher to determine whether their previously reported VOUS has been reclassified. The American College of Medical Genetics (ACMG) has developed recommendations and a decision tree for interpretation and reporting of sequence variations (Richards et al., 2007).

THE "IDEAL GENETIC TEST"

As illustrated by the preceding discussion, all testing methodologies have limitations and for many genetic conditions, the gene-disease association and clinical spectrum of the condition are not well understood. There may be more than one type of genetic test for a genetic condition, and laboratories may use different testing methodologies, even when testing for the same genetic condition. Therefore, genetic testing may be available utilizing multiple technologies in the same or different laboratories. The "ideal genetic test" has the characteristics listed in Table 9-3, and sometimes providing a patient with the "ideal genetic test" may require the use of a combination of genetic tests. Selection of the "ideal genetic test" requires the use of critical thinking skills to evaluate the genetic testing methodologies and their limitations, determining the testing approach, and considering the indication for testing. The genetic counselor should review the laboratory website or contact the laboratory to ascertain the test parameters described in the sections above and in Tables 9-2 and 9-3 and choose the "ideal" test for each patient based on the individual situation. In selecting an "ideal" genetic test, it is important to also consider cost and test turnaround time, discussed in Chapter 4.

TABLE 9-3. Characteristics of an "Ideal" Genetic Test

- High sensitivity
- High specificity
- Low false positive rate
- Low false negative rate
- High positive predictive value
- High negative predictive value

In 2009, the selection of the "ideal genetic test" for a Caucasian individual without a positive family history of cystic fibrosis would be the American College of Medical Genetics (ACMG)-recommended panel of twenty-three CFTR mutations (Watson et al., 2004). If the patient is of different ethnicity, the "ideal genetic test" may need to include additional CFTR mutations. In a patient who has cystic fibrosis but tests negative for the recommended panel of CFTR mutations, DNA sequencing should be considered. When there is a family history of cystic fibrosis and the familial mutations are known, it is imperative that the relative seeking carrier risk assessment be studied in a lab that specifically tests for the familial mutations. If the familial mutations are unknown, testing should proceed with caution and the residual risk will be unknown. (Watson et al., 2004).

ENSURING QUALITY CLINICAL GENETIC TESTING

Oversight of Genetic Testing Laboratories

Two levels of laboratory standards and guidelines are used in most countries for oversight of laboratories providing genetic testing. In the US, the first level is CLIA (Clinical Laboratory Improvement Amendments) certification, which is government regulated and designed to be a set of minimal laboratory requirements to ensure the safety of the public. CLIA regulations require laboratories to assure that their test results are accurate, reliable, timely, and confidential and do not present risk of harm to patients. All laboratories releasing results to US clinicians or patients require CLIA certification, with the exception of those analyzing patient samples from New York and Washington, where CLIA certification is superseded by state regulatory agencies with additional specific requirements. Verifying that a laboratory has New York state approval for a given test may serve as a surrogate indicator of a quality test. For many genetic tests, such state proficiency programs do not exist and labs must develop internal programs or work with other laboratories offering the same test to organize sample exchanges.

Most quality laboratories follow additional guidelines provided by professional organizations and other certification organizations. In the US, professional guidelines are provided by the American College of Medical Genetics (ACMG), the Association of Molecular Pathologists (AMP), and the College of American Pathologists (CAP). Additionally, laboratories may participate in accreditation programs that meet the CLIA requirements and include additional requirements. Programs are provided by the Joint Commission on Accreditation of Healthcare Organizations (JCAHO), CAP, and other voluntary organizations.

Laboratory accreditation bodies assess factors that are relevant to the laboratory's technical competence, including the

- Qualifications, performance, and technical competency of staff
- Validity and appropriateness of test methods
- Traceability of measurements and calibrations to national standards
- Suitability, calibration, and maintenance of test equipment

- Testing environment
- Sampling, handling, and transportation of test items
- Quality assurance of test and calibration data

[International Laboratory Accreditation Cooperation (ILAC)].

The American College of Medical Genetics has developed "Standards and Guidelines for Clinical Genetics Laboratories," including requirements, considerations, validation, and standards for cytogenetic, biochemical, and molecular genetics tests, accessible at their website.

International Issues

Laboratories outside the US are eligible for CLIA certification, but as of 2009 only a few clinical genetics laboratories in Canada and Germany have applied for this certification. CMS (Centers for Medicare and Medicaid Services), which regulates all clinical laboratory testing through CLIA, currently does not recognize laboratory accreditation programs outside the US. Many laboratories around the world have one or more organizations responsible for the accreditation in their nation. Many of these countries have adopted the International Organization for Standardization (ISO 15189) standards for medical laboratories, have signed a multilateral recognition agreement and participate in the International Laboratory Accreditation Cooperation (ILAC), which accepts laboratory data across the national borders of the participating countries. Javaher et al. (2008) review genetic testing services in European countries, including access to and uptake of genetic testing, regulatory, and financial issues.

Professional Qualifications of Laboratory Personnel

Most countries require that laboratory directors be certified in an appropriate specialty and that laboratory supervisors be certified in laboratory operations and quality control. Certification and educational requirements of other laboratory personnel are quite variable. In the US, genetic testing is considered "high-complexity" testing under the CLIA guidelines and laboratory directors must have a Ph.D. or M.D. degree with board certification in an approved specialty, such as the American Board of Medical Genetics (ABMG), the American Board of Clinical Chemistry (ABCC), and others.

Clinical laboratories must also have a clinical consultant, but the CLIA regulation does not provide specifics regarding training in human genetics. Other laboratory accreditation bodies such as ACMG and CAP do provide guidelines that require genetic expertise and certification. Genetic counselors should check to ensure that the laboratory personnel have appropriate expertise in genetics.

Oversight of Genetic Tests

In the United States, and many European countries, it is the responsibility of the clinical laboratory director to verify the strength of the gene disease association and decide when to make a genetic test clinically available. Clinical lab directors also decide the appropriate testing methodology, and CLIA guidelines require that they provide descriptions of the known and unknown parameters of the test (http://wwwn. cdc.gov/clia/regs/toc.aspx). Most genetic tests are laboratory-developed tests (LDTs) or what were referred to in the past as "home brew tests." The FDA has stated it has oversight authority for LDTs, but this has not been confirmed by the courts, and currently LDTs are not subject to direct government oversight (SACGHS, 2008). The FDA reviews and approves kit-based tests, known as in vitro diagnostic devices (IVDs) and analyte specific reagents (ASRs), which may be used in LDTs. Before a new test can be offered, CLIA requires laboratories to establish and verify the test's analytical performance characteristics but does not review or require outside review of the verification. (Sanderson et al., 2005) The CLIA inspection and laboratory certification process focuses on the analytical validity of the test and does not review clinical validity or clinical utility of a test. Developing an oversight process to decide when a test is ready to move to clinical testing is complex and has been and continues to be discussed by national and international groups.

The Importance and Value of Laboratory Errors and Proficiency Testing

All laboratories make errors, but quality laboratories have multiple processes in place to identify errors and then modify their testing process to reduce the possibility for future errors. Few statistics on laboratory errors are published because most proficiency testing and quality surveillance programs are not punitive but are educational in nature and work to help laboratories continually monitor and improve their testing processes. Research has indicated that most laboratory errors occur in the pre-analytical (sample submission and accessioning) and the postanalytical (reporting) phases and fewer errors occur in the analytical phase of testing (Bonini et al., 2002). Examples of pre-analytical errors include mislabeled samples, testing for the wrong familial mutation, and sample contamination. Post-analytical errors usually involve reporting errors such as typographical errors and sample mix-ups in the reporting process, but they can also occur if reports are confusing and not easily understood by the ordering clinician. Information on the error rate in genetic laboratories is very limited.

Genetic counselors should note that CLIA laboratories are required to have quality assurance programs in place, but at this time are not required to perform proficiency testing (PT) unless they are testing established regulated analytes, which are currently rarely used in genetic tests. Proficiency testing externally validates the laboratory's competence by requiring that a laboratory demonstrate that it can obtain the correct answer when testing samples and is currently considered to be the most rigorous form of performance assessment. Laboratories voluntarily following ACMG or AMP guidelines are required to perform PT. Hudson et al. (2006) surveyed laboratory directors and found that the number of reported deficiencies (defined as the inability to ascertain and report the correct test results in a timely manner) decreased as the percentage of tests that had proficiency testing performed increased. The number of incorrect reports of test results also increased with the number of deficient proficiency tests in the same time period. A laboratory's commitment to proficiency testing is clearly beneficial and worth considering in laboratory selection.

DEVELOPMENT OF A NEW CLINICAL GENETIC TEST

The Research Laboratory–Clinical Laboratory Continuum

New clinical genetic tests are natural outcomes of human genetic research, but defining when a test moves from research to clinical use can be problematic. With completion of the mapping of the human genome, major genetics journals are reporting the discovery of the causative gene or genes for one or more genetic diseases almost weekly. While a lab can set up sequencing or targeted mutation analysis almost overnight, some tests are translated quickly and others are translated slowly to the clinical laboratory setting. Currently, independent assessment of a test is not required, and new tests are offered to the clinical community based on the decision of the laboratory offering the test.

Traditionally in laboratory medicine, new technologies must be tested against the existing technology or "gold standard" (Khoury et al., 2000). Clinical laboratories should perform parallel studies to test samples in both the "old" and "new" technology, and these results should be available for the healthcare provider to review before ordering patient testing using the new technology. Information should also be provided on the limitations of the new technology, including the types of gene changes that may be missed. Unexpected test results should be discussed with the laboratory director to determine whether they might be explained by the technology. New technologies may provide improved detection, faster turnaround times, and lower-cost testing, but they may also increase the frequency of inconclusive results or negatively impact other testing parameters.

A laboratory may decide that a new test is ready to enter clinical practice, but genetic counselors and other healthcare providers must independently decide when to offer new testing and when new technologies should be used instead of existing accepted technologies. Genetic counselors and other healthcare providers must also decide when a patient with strong clinical findings who was not found to have a mutation previously via one technology may benefit from retesting with a new technology.

It is important to evaluate what is known and not known about a test. Often research testing was performed on a tightly controlled patient population; test parameters, including detection rate, types of mutations, and penetrance, will be different in a more diverse patient population. Examples of changes in testing parameters include the predicted penetrance (lifetime cancer risk) of BRCA 1 and BRCA 2 mutations (Khoury et al., 2000; Burke, 2002) and the cystic fibrosis mutation I148T, which was included in the original ACMG panel of recommended mutations but was later found to be a polymorphism in close linkage disequilibrium to 3199del6 sequence change, which was in fact a disease-associated mutation (Watson et al., 2004). Additional factors must be considered when a test moves from diagnostic testing in individuals with clinical symptoms to population-based testing in the public health setting.

In most countries, there is no regulatory agency or professional organization that reviews or approves the introduction of new tests (OECD, 2005). In countries with universal healthcare and/or strong public health systems, reimbursement is limited to tests that have been reviewed by a group of experts appointed by the government or by a governmental healthcare funding agency, and this serves as a de facto test approval system. One model program to review and fund test translation was developed in 2006 in the US, resulting from an international effort to increase the translation of rare genetic tests from research to clinical testing. The Collaboration, Education and Test Translation (CETT) Program, funded by the National Institutes of Health Office of Rare Diseases Research, requires a minimum of one peer-reviewed scientific publication supporting the gene disease association and additional research data to help define the parameters of the test. The CETT Program uses a two-stage review process to evaluate the test, which includes a staff review followed by an expert panel review. The review process considers scientific evidence, proposed testing methodology, laboratory experience with the methodology, potential impact on healthcare, laboratory qualifications and certifications, plan to collect and publicly share mutation and clinical data, plan to provide educational materials, and evidence of a collaboration between the research, clinical, laboratory, and advocacy communities (Faucett et al., 2008).

Many laboratories developing clinical tests have found it necessary and helpful to collaborate with clinical researchers. This relationship provides the clinical laboratory with the researcher's expertise, which can be helpful in determining the significance of an identified gene change and may reduce the number of test results that are labeled as "variants of unknown significance." The researcher can benefit because the clinical laboratory may identify patients that define or expand the clinical spectrum of the condition. Individuals who test "negative" but have a strong clinical diagnosis of a condition may be optimal research candidates to evaluate for other types of mutations or changes in other genes (Chen and Faucett, 2004).

Research Testing Cautions

Chen and Faucett (2004) reported that the pace of clinical test introduction is not keeping up with the pace of test development. In 2004, approximately one-third of tests listed in the GeneTests Internet laboratory directory were only available in research labs. By 2008, this number had dropped to approximately twenty percent.

Appropriately providing research test results to patients raises several difficult issues for genetic counselors. CLIA regulations indicate that provision of individual research results would be non-compliant with federal law. Some Institutional Review Boards (IRBs) have allowed the release of research test results to patients before confirmation by a certified laboratory, although this would appear to be a violation of CLIA regulations. Genetic testing may not be clinically available for all rare conditions, and it may be difficult and expensive for a research laboratory to go through the process of developing a clinical genetic test. It is a reality that some research laboratories are providing genetic test results to patients for clinical use.

Currently in the US, federal legislation states that clinical tests can only be performed by CLIA certified laboratories (Sec. 493; http://wwwn.cdc.gov/clia/regs/toc.aspx) and defines a clinical test as any laboratory data that is communicated to a physician or patient that could be used in diagnosis, management, or patient decision-making (including reproductive planning). Some genetic counselors and researchers are under the false impression that as long as they are not charging for mutation analysis or other molecular genetic or biochemical testing, it would not be considered a clinical test. Federal law does not provide a research exemption or an exemption for "free" testing that provides a patient-specific result. Research results may be released in aggregate (CLIA Sec. 493.3) but individuals should not be told of their status as a mutation carrier or a non-carrier (http://wwwn.cdc.gov/clia/regs/toc.aspx). CLIA regulations apply to all testing that might be used to impact patient care or management, and providing a written report with a research disclaimer does not protect the laboratory or clinician. (Ledbetter and Faucett, 2008).

Researchers, clinical geneticists, and genetic counselors often feel an ethical responsibility to share research results with patients and their families, either out of altruism or a sense of obligation if they provided samples for the gene mapping studies. Researchers and genetic counselors should work to ensure that clinical testing is available for research participants, who should be encouraged to undergo genetic testing in a clinical laboratory. If testing is not available through a clinical laboratory, there are laboratories that are willing to do custom mutation analysis and provide clinical genetic testing in a CLIA certified laboratory for confirmation of a research test result. However, the model of confirming positive research laboratory results through custom mutation analysis in a clinical laboratory (CLIA certified) should be used with caution. This model allows for quality control of the positive test results by the clinical laboratory but does not provide quality control for the negative test results. Laboratory directors surveyed by the CETT Program who provided clinical confirmation of research results reported that they were unable to confirm the research results in at least 5% of cases (personal communication). In the model of "custom mutation analysis," negative research results are not routinely retested in the clinical laboratory and false negative results would go undetected. Additionally, the testing parameters used in a research lab are usually not reported, making it difficult to know when individuals with a "negative" research result should be retested using an improved test that detects additional types of mutations. Case #3, presented later in this chapter, illustrates the clinical implications of disclosing results obtained from a research study.

The reality is that for rare genetic conditions there may be one or just a few laboratories in the world studying the causative gene and the diseases are too rare and test requests too infrequent for test development by a clinical laboratory. Given extremely low prevalence/incidence of a rare genetic disorder and the paucity of data on clinical validity and clinical utility, there are not the same parameters for considering when a test can transition from a research setting to clinical application. As a step toward addressing this complex issue, the American College of Medical Genetics established guidelines for molecular genetic testing for ultra-rare disorders

(2004). Complying with CLIA regulations and providing clinical genetic testing for rare diseases requires the genetic counseling community, research community, and patient advocacy community to work together.

The Role of the Genetic Counselor When Only Research Testing Exists

Genetic counselors should ensure that research testing is being performed under IRB review at the testing institution and that the informed consent process is adequate. The genetic counselor should be aware of his or her own institutional IRB requirements before offering patients and families research testing. Some institutions require that outside research protocols also be approved by their IRB and may not allow genetic counselors to offer research studies and/or research testing without approval. This may make it difficult or impossible for the genetic counselor to facilitate their patient's participation. Genetic counselors in this situation may refer the patient and family to disease-specific advocacy organizations for information about current research studies that may include research testing.

The genetic counselor should make sure the patient understands the difference between research testing and clinical testing. It should be explained that test results for clinical care need to be provided by a CLIA certified laboratory and that most research laboratories do not have this certification. Patients should be informed that research results may be released in aggregate and that the patient and family members will need to confirm any research findings in a clinical laboratory. Clinical laboratories will not accept research results as the basis for prenatal testing and families may not have sufficient time to pursue prenatal testing if research results are not confirmed in a timely manner. Patients and families are often frustrated when clinical testing is not available, and the genetic counselor will need to help the patient and family understand why research testing is not appropriate for clinical use, that genetic testing is not an option at this time, and that the family should contact the clinic on a regular basis to learn about advances in genetic testing. The genetic counselor should not pressure a research (non-CLIA certified) laboratory to perform testing and release results. Instead, genetic counselors should encourage researchers to work with clinical laboratories and patient advocacy organizations to move the test to the clinical laboratory when there are sufficient data to support translation.

Information on a New Clinical Test

In releasing a new clinical laboratory test, the laboratory should define the parameters of the test and provide answers to the questions listed in Table 9-4. Initially, many of the answers may be unknown or may only be known in a controlled population. The genetic counselor should review the information before offering the test to ensure that there are published data to support the test claims. When there are limited or only research population data, this should be clearly indicated in the test description. Limitations of the test and testing technology should be noted. The information should also discuss how new gene changes will be determined to be clinically relevant.

TABLE 9-4. Relevant Factors in Evaluating Genetic Tests

- Detection rate
  - Research population
  - Diagnostic population
  - Carrier testing in general population
- Types of mutations identified to date
- Populations tested to date
- Population specific findings
- Penetrance
  - Research population
  - General population (known or unknown)
- Technology limitations
  - Types of mutations not evaluated by technology (e.g., deletions and duplications)
  - Sample types accepted
- Expected percentage of previously unreported gene changes (variants of unknown significance)
  - How new gene changes will be evaluated
  - When family studies will be needed
  - Charges for evaluation of variants and family studies
- Turnaround time
  - Types of cases in which turnaround time may be extended
- Cost

GLOBAL TESTING ISSUES AND ESTABLISHING POLICY AND PRACTICE GUIDELINES

Numerous elements within clinical practice influence the progression of a new genetic test from a research laboratory environment to acceptance as a clinical standard of care. In determining whether a test is ready to be established as a standard of care, it is necessary to evaluate carefully the outcomes of individual research trials and the comprehensive assessment of outcomes from related research. This evaluation would ideally include a thorough consideration of the medical, psychological, and ethical implications of all potential applications of the clinical test. (Sanderson et al., 2005) Technology assessment conferences and professional organizations' development of practice guidelines are key to establishing and communicating standards of care for use of a genetic test.

Technology Assessment Conferences

One effective format for the evaluation of a new technology or test, or a new or expanded application of an existing technology, used by government agencies in the US as well as many European and Asian countries is a technology assessment conference. These generally include a public session during which presentations are given by experts in the field and an open discussion session is held. This is usually followed by closed sessions in which the members of the expert panel address predefined questions and develop a draft statement regarding the key issues of the specific technology transfer or application. The draft is then critiqued by the panel participants and the statement is finalized.

One early example was the NIH Technology Assessment conference held in 1997, which reconsidered population-based carrier screening for cystic fibrosis (CF). New recommendations were produced based on the results of studies addressing interest in and impact of population-based carrier screening for CF (Kaplan et al., 1991; Williamson, 1993; Bekker et al., 1994; Brock, 1996; Loader et al., 1996). The consensus statement on the topic recommended that CF testing be offered to adults with a positive family history of CF and to couples with no family history who are seeking prenatal care (http://consensus.nih.gov/1997/1997GeneticTestCysticFibrosis106html.htm). Even before publication of the final consensus statement, some genetics centers in the US began offering CF carrier screening to all pregnant patients (personal communication), and one large commercial genetic testing lab began marketing this testing to medical professionals who care for patients of reproductive age.

Practice Guidelines

Perhaps the most powerful influences on professional behavior with respect to genetic testing are practice guidelines from professional organizations or expert opinion statements from recognized entities. It is important to access practice guidelines from both the genetics community and your medical specialty (e.g., American Society of Clinical Oncology genetics guidelines if working in cancer genetics). This is particularly important to do because often practice guidelines are established within individual specialties, making it difficult for practitioners from other disciplines to learn about and apply them. In addition, different professional organizations, even within the same specialty, may endorse practice statements that draw different conclusions.

The guidelines for predictive testing for Huntington disease (HD) are an exemplary example of practice guidelines and effective unified development by different specialists. Initial guidelines for testing using linkage were developed in 1985 by a committee composed of members from the International Huntington Association (IHA) and the World Federation of Neurology (WFN) Research Group on Huntington's Chorea and revised in 1993 when the gene was identified (World Federation of Neurology 1989; International Huntington Association and the World Federation of Neurology Research Group on Huntington's Chorea, 1990, 1994). These guidelines established international standards by which predictive testing for HD continues to be performed. A significant advantage of these guidelines is that they were developed by an interdisciplinary group of professionals, ensuring representation from most groups involved in the care of HD patients and their families. Many of the elements of the HD guidelines have been incorporated into clinical models for predictive genetic testing for other adult-onset diseases, such as spinocerebellar ataxias and hereditary cancer susceptibility syndromes.

When incorporating practice guidelines, genetic counselors should refer to the section in the guidelines that addresses the application of the information. The NSGC, like all professional organizations, suggests that practitioners evaluate the validity of the statement or guideline with regard to the specific circumstances of each patient and use their professional judgment in adhering to or deviating from the recommendations. In addition, it is generally recommended that practitioners who choose not to adhere should carefully document their rationale for this course in the patient's medical record. The NSGC includes a statement of purpose and a disclaimer in each of their published guidelines, as follows:

> Genetic counseling practice recommendations of the National Society of Genetic Counselors (NSGC) are meant to assist practitioners in making decisions about appropriate management of genetic concerns. Each practice recommendation focuses on a clinical or practice issue, and is based on a review and analysis of the professional literature. The information and recommendations reflect scientific and clinical knowledge current as of the submission date, and are subject to change as advances in diagnostic techniques, treatments and psychosocial understanding emerge. In addition, variations in practice, taking into account the needs of the individual patient and the resources and limitations unique to the institution or type of practice, may warrant alternative approaches, treatments or procedures to the recommendations outlined. NSGC genetic counseling practice recommendations should not be construed as dictating an exclusive course of management, nor does use of such recommendation guarantee a particular outcome. Genetic counseling practice recommendations are not intended to supersede a health care provider's best medical judgment.
>
> —Bennett et al., 2003, p. 287–288.

The rapid evolution of new genetic testing has highlighted the need for more practice guidelines to help health care providers make informed decisions about the appropriate use of genetic tests. Given the diversity of factors to be considered in developing practice guidelines for widespread utilization of genetic testing, the need for involvement of governmental agencies including the FDA (Food and Drug Administration), CDC (Centers for Disease Control and Prevention), and CMS (Centers for Medicare and Medicaid Services) has been promoted as one solution. This resulted in a series of appointed committees, including the Secretary's Advisory Committee on Genetic Testing (SACGT) and the Secretary's Advisory Committee on Genetics, Health and Society (SACGHS) (Holtzman and Watson, 1997; Javaher et al., 2008). These efforts have addressed many important issues including oversight of genetic testing, genetic discrimination legislation, gene patents and licensing, coverage and reimbursement for genetic tests and services, and policy issues related to the use and misuse of genetic testing. Other groups, including the Genetics and Public Policy Center (GPPC), Centers for Disease Control and Prevention (CDC) Evaluation of Genomic Applications in Practice and Prevention (EGAPP), the American College of Medical Genetics, and the Clinical Practice Committee of the Association for Molecular Pathology, have also addressed how to keep health care providers informed about how to best use genetic testing.

Given the rapid pace of introduction of genetic tests, frequently genetic tests are available before practice guidelines are developed or technology assessment conferences are held. Often, the decision to offer a patient a genetic test is made on a case-by-case basis. Genetic counselors are encouraged to consult with their team members and other local medical specialists to establish standards of practice for offering genetic tests in the absence of existing professional guidelines or consensus statements. Genetic counselors should be cautious about offering a new genetic test just because it is available–waiting on a test to be reviewed for validity by experts may be safer for a patient or family.

COMPLEXITIES OF NEW TECHNOLOGIES IN THE GENETIC COUNSELING SESSION: ILLUSTRATIVE CASES

As providers of a significant proportion of clinical genetics services in the United States, genetic counselors have played, and will continue to play, a key role in the movement of tests and new testing technologies from research to clinical practice— the technology transfer process. The following cases illustrate this role and stress the importance of thorough counseling of families and ensuring that the informed consent process is followed. The names of the individuals, both professional and clients, and the specific details of these cases have been altered to preserve confidentiality.

Case 1: "Negative" Test Results–Counseling Challenges

Background Sasha Engberg, a healthy 6-year-old female, was seen by her pediatrican, Dr. Dorothy Waxton, for her annual well-child physical examination. During the course of the visit, Sasha's mother, Brynne, told Dr. Waxton that her husband, Donald, currently 28 years old, was recently diagnosed with metastatic colon cancer caused by Familial Adenomatous Polyposis (FAP). The family was devastated and realized that Donald was not likely to survive his cancer. Brynne was understandably worried that Sasha may have inherited this disease, but she didn't want to burden her husband with any additional feelings of guilt. Donald's oncologist had discussed the autosomal dominant inheritance of FAP, and he had given the Engbergs a referral for genetic counseling at the cancer center. However, because of the frequency of medical visits necessary for Donald's surgical follow-up and chemotherapy and his poor stamina, they decided to postpone this visit for a few months. At the pediatric visit, Brynne asked Dr. Waxton if she could order the genetic test for FAP on Sasha, because she would like to learn her daughter's risk status as soon as possible. Dr. Waxton consulted with a pediatric gastroenterologist colleague, who recommended that she submit a blood sample from Sasha to a commercial lab that he had used for sequence analysis of the APC gene. He explained that he had been very pleased with this laboratory because they have simple, easy to read reports and the results are available within 4 weeks. He added that if the child tests positive for a mutation in the gene, it is important to begin surveillance for colon polyps and cancer with annual colonoscopies between 10 and 15 years of age. Dr. Waxton submitted Sasha's blood sample, and within four weeks she received a report from the lab that indicated that no mutation had been identified in the APC gene. She was delighted to be able to share these normal (negative) results with Brynne, who was reassured. Dr. Waxton told Brynne that the genetic lab report still specified that genetic counseling is recommended, and she encouraged Brynne to schedule the appointment at the cancer center.

Two years later, Warren Hargrove, a genetic counselor in the Cancer Risk Assessment Clinic, was scheduled to meet with Brynne. Brynne was not at all happy to be back in the hospital where her husband had recently died after a difficult battle with colon cancer, and she was particularly surprised that Dr. Waxton had continued to recommend that genetic counseling was indicated since Sasha's genetic test for FAP was normal. Warren reviewed the features of FAP, and pointed out that Donald's clinical history was most consistent with this form of polyposis, even his negative family history was consistent since about one-third of patients with FAP are the first in their families to have it. Warren had received the test report of the APC gene sequence analysis performed in Sasha, and he was pleased to see that the laboratory performing the study had done a comprehensive analysis of all 15 exons of the gene in both the forward and reverse directions. Warren asked Brynne what Donald's APC gene sequencing results had identified, as he had not located these results in his hospital chart. Brynne explained that Donald was never studied because Sasha's results were normal and she felt reassured that her daughter was no longer at risk. Warren explained that the test that had been performed on Sasha looked only for the most common types of mutations in the APC gene that cause FAP in about 70–80% of patients, but that these are not the only kind of mutations that can be causative. In fact large deletions and duplications are seen in about 15–25% of patients, and these would not have been detected by the sequence test. Warren recommended that Sasha have another blood test to check for these types of mutations. He also explained that a negative test result for Sasha does not eliminate her risk absolutely in the absence of a known identified APC mutation in Donald, because it is possible that his mutation would not have been identifiable by current technology or that he had a different form of polyposis due to a mutation in a different gene.

Follow-up   Sasha's blood sample was drawn and submitted for analysis of large APC gene deletions and duplications. The test results showed that she was heterozygous for a deletion mutation of exon 15. On the basis of these positive laboratory results, Brynne was counseled that her daughter has a greater than 99% chance of developing features of FAP, particularly adenomatous polyps of the colon and rectum, which have significant malignant potential if not ablated or removed. Based on the natural history of the disorder, it was recommended that annual colonoscopies be performed beginning at 10–15 years of age, with appropriate surgery (colectomy) or polypectomy or ablation (http://www.nccn.org/professionals/physician_gls/PDF/colorectal_screening.pdf).

In addition, it was recommended that Sasha have annual physical exams, including thyroid exam, and a baseline upper endoscopy between 25 and 30 years.

The clinical scenario represented by this case illustrates why all practitioners ordering genetic testing must be aware of the complexities of genetic testing, including the multiple technologies that can be utilized to provide diagnostic information for the same genetic disorder and the limitations of interpretation of test results, particularly in the absence of data on the affected relatives (Giardiello et al., 1997). The differences between laboratories may be extensive with regard to the method used, the level of interpretation involved in reporting results, and the content of the report. Staff members who understand these variables and the indication for the particular analysis should be responsible for choosing the laboratory to be used for genetic testing. To ensure that the most appropriate analysis will be performed for the specific family, the genetics professional should play an active role in selecting the laboratory to perform the study. Additionally, patients and their family members should be fully aware of the limitations of the technology used and the potential need to consider sequential testing to investigate the same diagnosis.

Case 2: Communication about Specificity and Sensitivity of a Genetic Test and the Potential for Improvement as the Technology Evolves

Background   Benjamin Anderson had neonatal hypotonia and mild dysmorphic features noted shortly after birth, which included brachycephaly, flat midface, large ears, and ptosis. During the newborn period, he was evaluated by neonatologist Dr. Jorge Torres, who could not provide a clinical diagnosis to explain Benjamin's constellation of features. The pregnancy had been uneventful, and there were no complications during labor and delivery. The family history was unremarkable and did not include any other relatives with similar features. Dr. Torres ordered a series of genetic tests that were standard of care at that time, including high-resolution chromosome analysis, molecular analyses including *SNRPN* methylation for Prader–Willi syndrome, deletion analyses for *SMN* for spinal muscular atrophy, and evaluation for congenital myotonic dystrophy, as well as metabolic studies and head MRI. An extensive series of blood tests were also performed to check for possible viral and other environmental causes. All test results for Benjamin were normal. Dr. Torres recommended to the family that they schedule an appointment for a complete genetics evaluation. Although Benjamin had hypotonia, he was feeding well and was able to go home at 4 days of age.

During his first year of life, Benjamin continued to have mild hypotonia and had difficulty with recurrent respiratory infections; one bout with pneumonia required hospitalization for two days. While his parents acknowledged that he was developmentally slower than his older sister, they attributed this delay to his recurrent infections and did not feel that a genetics evaluation was needed.

By 2.5 years of age Benjamin had severe developmental delay and had complete absence of speech and in addition had developed autistic behaviors and uncontrolled seizures. His hypotonia had resolved, but he now had mild ataxia. The neurologist taking care of Benjamin recommended that his parents schedule a genetics evaluation in an attempt to gain a better understanding of the cause of his difficulties as well as his prognosis and to make appropriate interventions. The parents expressed concern about the potential risk that their future children might have Benjamin's problems and were now interested in pursuing a genetic evaluation.

Follow-up Deborah Xavier, a genetic counselor coordinating the Pediatric Genetics Clinic at the university-based Children's Hospital, saw Benjamin and his parents in clinic with medical geneticist Dr. Raymond Watts. Before the clinic appointment, all of his previous laboratory test results were reviewed and determined to be up to date and negative. Based on the physical exam and history provided at the genetics clinic, Dr. Watts did not feel that Benjamin's constellation of features suggested any one specific diagnosis but in keeping with various professional practice guidelines (Shaffer et al., 2005; Moeschler et al., 2006; Shevell et al., 2007), he recommended additional genetic testing including subtelomeric FISH, MECP2 gene sequence analysis, UBE3A gene sequence analysis for Angelman syndrome (prior methylation for 15q normal), and fragile X testing. The results of all of these studies were negative. Deborah Xavier contacted Benjamin's mother to review the results, and she was very disappointed that these studies had not helped explain Benjamin's developmental and neurological problems. Deborah explained that we are not able to detect all genetic causes of developmental delays because of limitations in technology. She recommended that Benjamin be seen annually in the genetics clinic, as this follow-up may help determine his specific diagnosis.

Benjamin returned to clinic at 3.5 years of age. On examination Dr. Watts determined that no new problems had developed, but the family was struggling with his significant delays, complete absence of speech, seizures, and recurrent infections. His mother was 8 weeks pregnant, and she and her husband were very concerned about their risk of having another affected child. Deborah Xavier and Dr. Watts met with the parents and discussed a new type of genetic test called array comparative genomic hybridization (aCGH) that had recently been validated and was being used to screen patients like Benjamin for small deletions and duplications of genetic material that would not have been detected by routine chromosome studies (Lu et al., 2007). The use of aCGH tests as an adjunct diagnostic tool with other cytogenetic testing had been recently recommended by the ACMG in a clinical practice guideline (Manning et al., 2007) and a laboratory standards guideline (Shaffer, 2007). Array CGH testing was ordered for Benjamin, and the results identified a duplication of approximately one megabase in Xq28, a region containing the MECP2 gene and flanking regions. A syndrome in which MECP2 is duplicated had been described recently (Del Gaudio et al., 2006), and Benjamin's clinical findings were consistent with most of the patients in that study. The majority of mothers of affected males had been found to be carriers of the duplication with skewed X-inactivation patterns. Benjamin's mother tested positive for the duplication mutation and prenatal diagnosis was offered for her current pregnancy.

This case illustrates the importance of thorough genetic counseling before any genetic testing and clear communication with the client about the current validity and limitations of an earlier test result. In this case, additional genetic testing provided the family with very specific information about the cause of their child's disorder and their risk for having another similarly affected child. As genetic technologies continue to improve, clinical scenarios like this will occur more frequently. Patients seeking genetic testing should be informed about the pace with which these technologies are improving and made aware that our understanding of the validity of testing also changes with research and clinical experience. There are parallel needs to educate the primary care physician referring the family for genetic counseling and the insurance carrier, in the event that additional genetic testing is recommended in the future. Unless insurance carriers understand how rapidly these technologies are evolving, they will deny claims for coverage of additional testing, viewing these as simply repeat analyses. In addition, there is a lag time between implementation of new technologies and development of CPT codings, which is necessary for billing. Depending on the strength of the indication for a genetic test, it may be prudent for some individuals to postpone testing until a better understanding of the technology has been reached and testing is potentially reimbursable.

Case 3: Potential Risks in Clinical Disclosure of Results obtained from Research Studies

Background Amy Shalani has a strong family history of a disease causing severe mental retardation and physical deterioration. Growing up in the early 1980s, she had already lost two of her four affected brothers and seven maternal first cousins, from three different aunts, to this devastating disease. Because of the pattern of occurrence in her family, it was predicted to be an X-linked recessive disease. Amy's mother, maternal aunts, and maternal grandmother, all obligate carriers for the disease, were adamant that the next generation of females in the family be informed about their genetic risks so they could make educated decisions about having children. They sought the assistance of a researcher who was trying to pinpoint the location of the gene on the X chromosome and hoped eventually to study the gene in detail. The researcher was most interested in Amy's family, because it was a large kindred with several living affected males and many obligate carriers to study. He offered to travel over 500 miles to attend Amy's annual family reunion with the intent of gathering detailed clinical information about the entire family and collecting blood samples from as many of the greater than 50 family members as possible. Ultimately, the data obtained from Amy's family, and several other large kindreds with a similar clinical presentation, led to a collaborative effort that resulted in the characterization of the disorder and the identification of the responsible gene. The specific causative mutation in Amy's family was identified. In this case, the researcher was allowed by his IRB to share research results; the researcher was concerned about his ethical duty to the research participants and eventually sent letters to all of the participants to let them know whether or not they were carriers. In Amy's nuclear family, she was reported to be a carrier of the familial mutation and her sister, Jennifer, was reported to be negative for the familial mutation. Amy and Jennifer were told about these test results when they were 12 and 10 years old, respectively.

Follow-up Twenty-five years later, Amy faced decisions about her reproductive options. Based on the information she received from the research, she had decided as a teenager that because she is a carrier she would not ever have children. Now 37 years old and recently married, she and her husband were reconsidering their options. They were seen by Rowena Weinberg, a genetic counselor at the prenatal diagnostic center affiliated with the local Women's Hospital. Amy and her husband, Sean Porter, had done considerable research on the disease on the Internet and had decided that they would like to see whether it was possible to perform preimplantation genetic diagnosis and prenatal diagnosis for the familial mutation causing this X-linked recessive disorder. They provided Rowena with all the documents they had from the research lab that performed the studies, as well as the publications that resulted from these investigations. Rowena contacted a clinical lab that offers testing to confirm results obtained in research labs to determine the feasibility of offering this couple testing. The clinical laboratory found that the results from the researcher were difficult to interpret because of significant changes in genomic databases and nomenclature. After review and discussion with the original research lab, the specific sequence change identified in Amy's family was clarified. The clinical lab required that Amy's testing be repeated in their CLIA certified environment before considering offering prenatal or PGD testing. Amy's blood sample was submitted for confirmatory testing and her studies were normal; thus they did not confirm that she was a carrier of the familial mutation. The lab was concerned that the way in which their sequencing assay was set up might not identify Amy's specific familial mutation. They requested the submission of a sample from Amy's obligate carrier mother to be certain and her testing was positive for the familial mutation. Repeat samples from Amy and her sister (who had two healthy daughters and was 12 weeks pregnant with her third child) were submitted to the clinical lab, and these analyses revealed that Amy was not a carrier for the familial mutation; however, her sister was a carrier.

This case illustrates the significant potential risks of using a research lab for clinical testing. Research labs are not required to follow the same stringent guidelines required by CLIA, such as confirmation of test results, and thus there is a higher risk for inaccurate results from a research lab. All research results should be confirmed in a CLIA approved laboratory. Pre-analytic errors can occur in the sample collection process, particularly in situations where multiple samples are being collected at the same time and location from multiple family members with the same last name. This type of pre-analytical error will impact the validity of results from any lab, clinical or research; thus, sample collection from groups of family members, commonly seen in genetic testing, should be handled with the utmost care to ensure accuracy.

CONCLUSIONS

Genetic testing is now widely available for diagnostic confirmation, predictive testing, carrier, and fetal risk assessment. Genetic counselors have a crucial role in evaluating the clinical usefulness of these tests as they work with patients and their families to assess the medical and personal benefits, as well as the risks, of undergoing testing. Critical thinking and assessment skills are needed to determine whether genetic testing is clinically indicated and in selecting the type of genetic test and the appropriate laboratory. Genetic counselors must be knowledgeable about test validation procedures and laboratory variability. Thorough consideration of the clinical utility of the genetic test and client-focused genetic counseling should precede the use of any genetic test. These considerations are particularly important before the utilization of new technologies, which may have a higher likelihood of inconclusive test results, or use of genetic tests whose outcomes directly influence medical interventions.

To appropriately select a diagnostic laboratory for their clients, genetic counselors must be aware of the rapidly evolving standards by which clinical laboratories are certified and the increasing involvement and oversight of other government agencies and interested entities from the private sector. When a genetic counselor is not familiar with a laboratory, the genetic counselor should inquire about the laboratory's accreditation, the additional voluntary professional guidelines the laboratory follows, and the laboratory's participation in proficiency testing, both external and internal. In addition, it is important to determine the laboratory's experience with the particular test being considered and the specific technology utilized, as well as the training and certification of the laboratory and medical directors and other staff. In general, laboratories that voluntarily participate in multiple certification programs and that adhere to guidelines provided by professional organizations provide testing at a higher standard and should be utilized whenever possible.

Genetic counselors play a critical role in ensuring that their patients receive the "ideal genetic test," one that has optimal parameters for them. Genetic counselors should continue to participate actively in research aimed at evaluating the impact of the genetic testing outcomes and work with other stakeholders in defining enhanced oversight of genetic testing and global practice guidelines for the appropriate use of genetic tests.

REFERENCES

American College of Medical Genetics/American Society of Human Genetics Working Group on ApoE and Alzheimer Disease (1995) Statement on use of apolipoprotein E testing for Alzheimer disease. *JAMA* 274(20):1627–1629.

American College of Medical Genetics (2006) Standards and Guidelines for Clinical Genetics Laboratories. Available at www.acmg.net. Accessed 2007 Dec 4.

Association for Molecular Pathology (2007) Comments to FDA regarding Guidance for Industry and FDA Staff: Pharmacogenetic Tests and Genetic Tests for Heritable Markers. Available at http://www.amp.org/Gov/FDAPGxandGeneticscomments_Final.pdf Accessed 2007 Dec 10.

Bekker H, Denniss G, Modell M, Bobrow M, Marteau T (1994) The impact of population based screening for carriers of cystic fibrosis. *J Med Genet* 31(5):364–368.

Bennett RL, Pettersen BJ, Niendorf KB, Anderson RR. (2003) Developing standard recommendations (guidelines) for genetic counseling practices: A process of the National Society of Genetic Counselors. *J Genet Couns* 12(4):287–295.

Bonini P, Plebani M, Ceriotti F, Rubboli F (2002) Errors in laboratory medicine. *Clin Chem* 48:5:691–698.

Brock DJ (1996) Population screening for cystic fibrosis. *Curr Opin Pediatr* 8(6):635–638.

Burke W, Atkins D, Gwinn M, Guttmacher A, Haddow J, Lau J, Palomaki G, Press N, Richards CS, Wilderoff L, Weisner GL (2002) Genetic test evaluation: Information needs of clinicians, policy makers and the public. *Am J Epidemiol* 156(4):311–318.

Burtis CA, Ashwood ER (ed) (1998) *Tietz Textbook of Clinical Chemistry* (3rd ed.). Philadelphia: WB Saunders.

Caskey CT, Kaback MM, Beaudet AL (1990) The American Society of Human Genetics statement on cystic fibrosis screening. *Am J Hum Genet* 46:393.

Chen B, Faucett A (2004) Overview of Laboratory Testing for Rare Diseases. Available at http://wwwn.cdc.gov/dls/genetics/RareDiseaseConf.aspx Accessed 2008 Dec 4.

CLIA Regulations (including all changes through 1/24/2004). Available at http://wwwn.cdc.gov/clia/regs/toc.aspx. Accessed 2007 Dec 4.

Clinical and Laboratory Standards Institute (formerly National Committee for Clinical Laboratory Standards) Available at http://www.nccls.org/. Accessed 2007 Dec 4.

Collaboration, Education and Test Translation program. Available at http://www.cettprogram.org/. Accessed 2007 Dec 4.

Committee of International Huntington Association and World Federation of Neurology Research Group on Huntington's Chorea (1994) Guidelines for the molecular genetics predictive test in Huntington's disease. *Neurology* 44:1533–1536.

del Gaudio D, Fang P, Scaglia F, Ward PA, Craigen WJ, Glaze DG, Neul JL, Patel A, Lee JA, Irons M, Berry SA, Pursley A, Grebe TA, Freedenberg D, Martin RA, Hsich GE, Khera JR, Friedman NR, Zoghbi, HY, Eng CM, Lupski JR, Beaudet AL, Cheung SW, Roa BB (2006) Increased MECP2 gene copy number as a result of genomic duplication in neurodevelopmentally delayed males. *GIM* 8(12):784–792.

Dequeker E, Cassiman J-J (1998) Evaluation of CFTR gene mutation testing methods in 136 diagnostic laboratories: report of a large European external quality assessment. *Eur J Hum Genet* 6:165–175.

Dequeker E, Cassiman J-J (2002) Genetic testing and quality control in diagnostic laboratories. *Nat Genet* 25:259–260.

Dequeker E, Ramsden S, Grody WW, Stenzel TT, Barton DE (2001) Quality control in molecular genetic testing. *Nat Rev Genet* 2:717–723.

Faucett WA, Hart S, Pagon RA, Neall LF, Spinella G (2008) A model program to increase translation of rare disease genetic tests: collaboration, education, and test translation program. *Genet Med* 10(5):343–348.

Giardiello FM, Brensinger JD, Petersen GM, Luce MC, Hylind LM, Bacon JA, Booker SV, Parker RD, Hamilton SR (1997) The use and interpretation of commercial APC gene testing for familial adenomatous polyposis. *N Engl J Med* 336:823–827.

Holtzman NA, Watson MS (1997) Final Report of the Task Force on Genetic Testing: Promoting safe and effective genetic testing in the United States. Available at http://www.genome.gov/10001733. Accessed 2007 Dec 4.

Holtzman NA, Murphy PD, Watson MS, Barr PA (1997) Predictive genetic testing: From basic research to clinical practice. *Science* 278:602–605.

Hudson KL, Murphy JA, Kaufman DJ, Javitt GH, Katsanis SH, Scott J (2006) Oversight of US genetic testing laboratories. *Nat Biotechnol* 24:1083–1090.

Hyams AL, Brandenburg JA, Lipsitz SR, Shapiro DW, Brannan TA (1995) Practice guidelines and malpractice litigation: A two-way street. *Ann Intern Med* 122(6): 450–455.

International Huntington Association. World Federation of Neurology (1990) Ethical issues policy statement on Huntington's disease molecular genetics predictive test. *J Med Genet* 27(1);34–38.

International Huntington Association (IHA) and the World Fderation of Neurology (WFN) Research Group on Huntington's Chorea (1994) Guidelines for the molecular genetics predictive test in Huntington's disease. *Neurology* 44(9):1533–1536.

International Huntington Association and the World Federation of Neurology Research Group on Huntington's Chorea (1994) Guidelines for the molecular genetics predictive test in Huntington's disease. *J Med Genet* 31(7):555–559.

Javaher P, Kaarlainen H, Kristoffersson U, Nippert I, Sequeiros J, Zimmern R, Schmidtke J. (2008) EuroGentest: DNA-based testing for heritable disorders in Europe. *Community Genetics* 11:75–120.

Kaplan F, Clow C, Scriver CR (1991) Cystic fibrosis carrier screening by DNA analysis: A pilot study of attitudes among participants. *Am J Hum Genet* 49:240–242.

Khoury K, Burke W, Thomson E (2000) *Genetics and Public Health in the 21st Century: Using Genetic Information to Improve Health and Prevent Disease.* New York: Oxford University Press.

Kroese M, Zimmern RL, Sanderson S (2004) Genetic tests and their evaluation: Can we answer the key questions? *GIM* 6(6):475–480.

Ledbetter DH, Faucett WA (2008) Issues in genetic testing for ultra-rare diseases: background and introduction. *Genet Med* 10(5):309–313.

Loader S, Caldwell P, Kozyra A, Levenkron JC, Boehm CD, Kazazian HH Jr, Rowley PT (1996) Cystic fibrosis carrier population screening in the primary care setting. *Am J Hum Genet* 59:234–247.

Lu X, Shaw CA, Patel A, Li J, Cooper ML, Wells WR, Sullivan CM, Sahoo T, Yatsenka SA, Bacino CA, Stankiewicz P, Ou Z, Chinault AC, Beaudet AL, Lupski JR, Ward PA (2007) Clinical implementation of chromosomal microarray analysis: summary of 2513 postnatal cases. *PLoS ONE* (www.plosone.org) 3:e327:1–11.

Manning M, Hudgins L (2007) Use of array-based technology in the practice of medical genetics. *GIM* 9(9):650–653.

Moeschler JB, Shevell M and Committee on Genetics (2006) Clinical genetic evaluation of the child with mental retardation or developmental delays. *Pediatrics* 117:2304–2316.

National Cooperative Cancer Network Clinical Practice Guidelines in Oncology. Colorectal Cancer Screening, v.1.2007. Available at http://www.nccn.org/professionals/physician_gls/PDF/colorectal_screening.pdf. Accessed 2007 Dec 4.

National Institutes of Health Consensus Development Statement on Genetic Testing for Cystic Fibrosis. Available at http://consensus.nih.gov/1997/1997GeneticTestCysticFibrosis106html.htm. Accessed 2007 Dec 4.

National Society of Genetic Counselors. Position Statements. Available at http://www.nsgc.org/about/position.cfm. Accessed 2007 Dec 4.

OECD—Organisation for Economic Co-operation and Development (2005) Quality Assurance and Proficiency Testing for Molecular Genetic Testing: A Summary of A Survey of 18 OECD Member Countries, 2005. www.oecd.org

Pagon R (2007) GeneTests (www.genetests.org), Seattle. Personal communication.

Potter NT, Spector EB, Prior TW (2004) Technical standards and guidelines for Huntington disease testing. *GIM* 6(1):61–65.

Professional Practice Guidelines for Genetic Testing (2006) Conference convened by The Genetics and Public Policy Center; 2006 Feb 1; Bethesda, MD. Available at http://www. dnapolicy.org/resources/Professional_Guidelines_Meeting_Summary.pdf. Accessed 2007 Dec 4.

Richards CS, Bale S, Bellissimo DB, Das, S, Grody WW, Hegde MR, Lyon E, Ward BE, Molecular Subcommittee of ACMG Laboratory Quality Assurance Committee (2008) ACMG recommendations for standards for interpretation and reporting of sequence variations: Revisions 2007. *Genet Med* 10(4):294–300.

Rosoff AJ (2001) Evidence-based medicine and the law: the courts confront clinical practice guidelines. *J Health Polit Policy Law* 26(2):327–368.

Sanderson S, Zimmern R, Kroese M, Higgins J, Patch C, Emery J (2005) How can the evaluation of genetic tests be enhanced? Lessons learned from the ACCE framework and evaluating genetics tests in the United Kingdom. *GIM* 7(7):495–500.

Secretary's Advisory Committee on Genetics, Health and Society. U.S. System of Oversight of Genetic Testing: A Response to the Charge of the Secretary of Health and Human Services. http://www4.od.nih.gov/oba/sacghs/reports/SACGHS_oversight_report.pdf. Accessed October 27, 2009.

Shaffer LG on behalf of ACMG Professional Practice and Guidelines Committee (2005) ACMG guideline on the cytogenetic evaluation of the individual with developmental delay or mental retardation. *GIM* 7(9):650–654.

Shaffer LG, Beaudet AL, Brothman AR, Hirsch B, Levy B, Martin CL, Mascarello JT, Rao KW (2007) Microarray analysis for constitutional cytogenetic abnormalities. *GIM* 9 (9):654–662.

Shevell M, Ashwal S, Donley D, Flint J, Gingold M, Hirtz D, Majnemer A, Noetzel M and Sheth RD (2007) Practice parameter: Evaluation of the child with global developmental delay: Report of the Quality Standards Subcommittee of the American Academy of Neurology and the Practice Committee of the Child Neurology Society. *Am Acad Neur* 60:367–380.

Terry S (2007) Genetic Alliance (http://www.geneticalliance.org/), Washington DC. Personal communication.

Varga O, Sequeiros J (2008) Definitions of Genetic Testing in European and other Legislations. Unit 3 EuroGentest (WP3.4) April 2008. http://www.eurogentest.org/uploads/forms/ form600/option244/BackgroundDocDefinitionsLegislationV1-30April08.pdf

Watson MS, Cutting GR, Desnick RJ, Driscoll DA, Klinger K, Mennuti M, Palomaki GE, Popovich BW, Pratt VM, Rohlfs EM, Strom CM, Richards CS, Witt DR, Grody WM (2004) Cystic fibrosis population carrier screening: 2004 revision of American College of Medical Genetics mutation panel. *GIM* 6(5):387–391.

Whittaker L (1996) Clinical applications of genetic testing: Implications for the family physician. *Am Fam Physician* 53(6):2077–2084.

Williamson R (1993) Universal community carrier screening for cystic fibrosis? *Nat Genet* 1993; 3:195.

World Federation of Neurology Research Group on Huntington's Chorea (1989) Ethical issues policy statement on Huntington's disease molecular genetics predictive test. *J Neurol Sci* 94:327–332.

10

Medical Documentation

Debra Lochner Doyle, M.S., C.G.C.

"Medical documentation, charting, recording"—there are varied names for the activity of making notes that describe the health services rendered to a patient, but all are fairly synonymous. What's perhaps greatly different is the underlying purpose of documenting this information. While *all* practitioners should be motivated, first and foremost, to effectively communicate the clinical events, patient disposition, and plan of action, for practitioners residing in countries without universal healthcare oftentimes the focus is on secondary issues such as mitigating legal liability and/or increasing business efficiencies or reimbursement rates.

The first medical records were journals kept by practitioners to record detailed descriptions of a patient's ailments, treatments, and outcome. Such notes, privy only to clinicians, aided in monitoring the patient's progress after varied treatments, as well as furnished information for ongoing explorations in the field of medicine. Today, medical documentation continues to be an integral part of medical practice, but information obtained through the course of a clinical interaction and transcribed into notes is no longer deemed the sole property of the clinician. While hospitals and healthcare providers are responsible for generating and maintaining medical records, the information contained in the records is increasingly viewed as the property of the patient. Furthermore, many parties such as consulting health and social service practitioners, hospital administrators, peer review organization staff, insurers (third-party payers), self-insured employers, as well as the patient may have access to these records. In addition, medical documentation is often critical to the resolution of disputes that arise over healthcare treatment.

A Guide to Genetic Counseling, Second Edition, Edited by Wendy Uhlmann, Jane Schuette, and Beverly Yashar
Copyright © 2009 by John Wiley & Sons, Inc.

Yet, for all of the importance placed on medical documentation, there is relatively little guidance in the medical literature concerning what to document, when, where, how, and why. These aspects of medical documentation, along with suggestions and examples, are addressed in this chapter. Additionally, some comments regarding disclosure of medical information and medical record retention are provided. While every effort has been made to ensure that the information provided is global in nature, there are several aspects of medical documentation that are unique to practitioners within the U.S, and these areas (e.g., legal, confidentiality, and fiduciary requirements) are delineated as such.

THE IMPORTANCE OF MEDICAL DOCUMENTATION

It is important to recognize that patients' rights are preserved in good medical documentation. It is also worth noting that the best medical documentation cannot and should not replace good communication between healthcare practitioners and their clients (Berry, 1992; Tammelleo, 1995). The most important reasons for recording medical information are as follows:

- To ensure the best possible care for the individual and family
- To document the events of an inpatient or outpatient visit
- To facilitate communication among healthcare providers

Medical documentation is essential for summarizing patient healthcare and communicating the services or treatments provided to or discussed with a client. Healthcare is typically delivered by multiple providers, and the majority of genetic counseling clients are referred by an outside healthcare provider. Therefore, good documentation serves to improve communication between all of the health and social service providers working with a patient (Smith, 1993).

As Mark Twain (1835–1910), the famed American humorist and author, noted— "If you tell the truth, you don't have to remember anything."

The permanent nature of medical records may contribute, now or in the future, to establishing or confirming a diagnosis and to determining an accurate risk assessment. In addition, this documentation can serve to assist genetic counselors in recalling a previous counseling session as they prepare for future consultations with the same client or other family members with appropriate consent. Finally, the institution continues to improve its overall healthcare service when records are selected as part of the hospital or clinic's quality assurance and quality improvement exercises. While the benefits may not be immediately realized by a patient or family, they do hold the promise of long-term improved care for patients in general.

Medical information is also recorded to comply with regulatory requirements and to secure legal protections. Healthcare practitioners have a fiduciary responsibility to compile and maintain accurate medical records. Federal regulations require providers participating in the Medicare program, including hospitals and other institutions, to ensure that medical records are "accurate, promptly completed, filed, retained and are easily accessible" (42 CFR, 428.24) (Stratton, 1994).

Medical documentation is also vital for billing and reimbursement purposes. The regulations pertaining to Medicare are developed by the Centers for Medicare and Medicaid Services (CMS), which also dictates the federal program requirements for Medicaid. The policies developed through CMS have historically been adopted by third-party payers. Therefore, while relatively few genetic patients are recipients of Medicare, regulations or policies pertaining to Medicare are often held as the standard for all healthcare providers and payers. In addition, the Joint Commission on the Accreditation of Health Care Organizations (JCAHCO), the National Commission of Quality Assurance (NCQA), and some state facility licensing statutes require that institutions generate and maintain medical records for licensure, reimbursement, and accreditation purposes.

WHEN SHOULD MEDICAL DOCUMENTATION OCCUR?

Medical documentation should occur with every patient visit and in a timely fashion (George, 1991; Nurses in Independent Practice, 2006). Medical records are typically viewed as accurate and reliable because they are recorded as soon as possible after the clinical encounter. All individuals, including healthcare providers, experience a fading of memory over time. Therefore, it is essential that documentation occur soon after the consultation. In fact, Medicare and the JCAHCO have established standards for record keeping that include specific time limitations for recording or updating medical documentation. For example, Medicare requires that medical documentation must occur within 15 days of hospital discharge (Kapp, 1993).

This is not to say that a genetic counselor is without recourse should additions, clarifications, or corrections to the chart note be desired (Fiesta, 1991). After all, it is critical that the documentation be accurate and truthful. Changes to the medical record, if written, should be obvious and legible. A line is drawn through the entry, making sure that the inaccurate information is still legible. The entry should be initialed and dated, the reason for the error should be stated (i.e., in the margin or above the note if room), and the correct information should be documented. For electronic medical records (EMRs), addendums and/or corrections are feasible, and should follow the same basic principles as for paper. When making a change to an entry in an EMR, the original entry should be viewable, the current date and time should be entered, and the person making the change should be identified as well as the reason for the change. Genetic counselors should explore their institution's policy regarding how corrections and additions should be handled.

EXAMPLE OF ADDENDUM TO LETTER:

Addendum: In further considering Mrs. Jones' reproductive options, it was suggested that artificial insemination might be beneficial. Therefore, Mrs. Jones was contacted and this alternative was reviewed. [date/sign].

WHO RECORDS IN THE CHART?

Every healthcare provider who interacts with a patient has a responsibility to record on the patient's chart the pertinent information concerning the interaction. In some institutions, however, not all categories of healthcare providers are permitted to record in hospital records. In most institutions, authorization is required before a healthcare provider can write in a patient's record. Most genetic counselors who work in hospital settings are able to document in patient's records, but you should inquire within your own institution about the guidelines for recording, signing, and counter-signing patient chart notes. If permitted (see your institution's guidelines), genetic counseling students should have a supervisor countersign their medical documentation. Countersigning an entry implies that another person reviewed the entry and approved the care given; it does not imply that the countersigner performed the service. For this reason, all entries that are countersigned should clearly delineate who performed the services and should be carefully reviewed by the countersigner to ensure the accuracy and completeness of the information presented. It must be emphasized that by providing a signature, the countersigner assumes responsibility for anything written in the notes covered by the signature. For example, if the chart note states that a specified healthcare provider will arrange for a follow-up ultrasound appointment, the countersigner is responsible for ensuring that this appointment is scheduled.

TYPES OF MEDICAL DOCUMENTATION

The term "medical record" typically includes both inpatient hospital-based records as well as outpatient clinic charts, and the guidelines for medical documentation offered here pertain to records of both types whether they are "hardcopy" or electronic. As in other medical specialties, documentation of the genetics evaluation and counseling typically includes the chart note and/or letter to the referring physician. More unique to genetics is a third form of documentation, a letter to the patient or family summarizing the visit.

The chart note and letters of correspondence (letters to the physician and patient) are usually considered "official" documentation, especially if the chart note refers to the correspondence. In addition to the official documentation, records of patients seen in genetics clinics may include standardized forms such as intake forms for collecting demographic information, questionnaires, consent forms, and pedigrees. These forms

TABLE 10-1. Typical Contents of Medical Record for Genetics Encounter

Patient intake form/demographics
Pedigree
Summary chart note, outpatient and/or inpatient consultation
Laboratory report(s): cytogenetics, DNA studies, other labs
Radiology report(s)
Pathology report(s)
Signed consent forms
Photographs
Phone notes
Copies of correspondence: letters to/from referring physician, patient letter
Outside records
Insurance/billing information

help to ensure that pertinent information is collected. Standardized clinical and laboratory record forms also guarantee that desired information is collected and reported in a particular way. Standardized forms are limited, however, in that not every clinical or laboratory circumstance can be anticipated.

A chart note is a summary note that describes a clinical encounter. It includes a statement about the problem (chief complaint) or nature of the referral or visit, history of the present illness, followed by the past medical history (including pregnancy history if appropriate), developmental history, family history, social history, results of the physical examination and review of systems, an assessment or diagnosis, plan, the information or counseling provided, and the recommendations for medical management, treatment, and referral. The chart note is always signed (or electronically signed) and dated (Kettenbach, 1995). There are differing guides and tools for documentation, and as facilities increasingly move to EMRs clinicians may need to use templates that differ from conventions they are accustomed to, but are incorporated into the EMR system their institution is integrating. (Kidneynotes.com, 2005; Richter et al., 2007; Oldfield M, 2007; Swigert, NB, 2006). Electronic record keeping systems offer the advantages of ease of access to information, including chart notes, lab reports, imaged documents, appointment and referral tracking. In addition, EMRs often assist in standardizing vital information regarding the type of visit (new patient referral, established patient visit, etc.) and the duration of the patient encounter, which are required components of medical documentation for purposes of reimbursement (see Medical Documentation for Billing and Reimbursement).

One of the oldest documenting methods is SOAP—an acronym for charting in which each letter stands for a particular section of the chart note. "S" stands for *subjective* and includes the pertinent information that the patient gives the provider (e.g., "The patient reports no leaking of amniotic fluid, bleeding, or illness during her pregnancy"). "O" is for *objective,* which incorporates the measurements and observations of the provider (e.g., "Mrs. Smith walks with a wide-based gait and has difficulties with speech"). "A" stands for *assessment,* a listing of identified risk factors and a review of the information conveyed to the patient concerning each.

"P" refers to the treatment *plan,* which is a description of the recommended treatment or follow-up plan. The SOAP format is described here as it is among the oldest and more commonly used methods; however, it does not include certain information that is critical to medical record documentation within the U.S., namely, the source of the patient referral and the duration of the patient interaction—both governmental and/or fiduciary requirements.

The letter to the referring provider, like the chart note, summarizes the clinical encounter, and sometimes serves the dual purpose of a chart note summary as well as a method of communication between providers. This is a professional standard that facilitates communication between healthcare providers because it serves as written documentation about the genetic counseling session to be included in the patient's medical records maintained by the referring provider. Template letters are used by many clinics and increase efficiency, especially in summarizing patient encounters for common indications and/or procedures, for example, advanced maternal age. The letter can also be a valuable educational tool for the referring physician, since it generally includes information about the diagnosis, its pathology, risks for inheritance, and possible treatment options. Such documentation can be especially useful for rare conditions, since the primary care provider has unlikely encountered similar cases.

The patient letter represents another important form of formal correspondence and has long been regarded as a vital tool of the genetic counseling process. The patient letter, written in comprehensible language, summarizes important information from the genetic visit, the diagnostic issues considered, and the counseling provided. It documents the pertinent aspects of the patient's medical and family history and provides a mechanism for sharing information with family members. Some clinics write a separate patient letter that is copied to the referring physician; others copy the letter to the physician to the family. Many clinics have developed template letters to save time and increase efficiency (see Appendix: Patient Letter Outline).

RECOMMENDATIONS FOR MEDICAL DOCUMENTATION

All documentation should be objective and factual, since the medical record is intended to be a tool for the delivery of healthcare services, documenting clinically relevant information and supporting the assertion that services were performed within the accepted standards of care. The events being depicted are often recorded in chronological order, and the notation should then be dated and signed, or countersigned.

"The length of this document defends it well against the risk of its being read."
Winston Churchill (1874–1965)

As the former English prime minister humorously noted, in general, it is preferable for documentation to be as brief as possible. Only pertinent and relevant information that relates directly to the client's healthcare should be entered. Long narrative paragraphs should be avoided but may be necessary under exceptional circumstances. For example, genetic counseling sessions often include detailed review and assessment of risks associated with multiple factors identified in a family or personal health history. In these circumstances, care should be taken to record all of the pertinent information succinctly. It is imperative, however, that the medical documentation be complete, because there is often a perception that anything not included in the medical documentation didn't happen: "Partial record keeping implies partial healthcare, or 'if it wasn't written it wasn't done'" (Kapp, 1993; Miller http://www.charlydmiller.com/CLASS/document.html last accessed 8-6-07).

If written, records should be neat and legible. Standard medical abbreviations should be used appropriately whether records are written or transcribed. Medical abbreviations help convey complex terms or concepts in a manner that is clear and brief. For example ROM is standard for "range of motion." However, many abbreviations have more than one meaning, depending on context in the medical record. For example, AMA could mean "against medical advice" or "advanced maternal age." If the meaning of an abbreviation is not clear within the context of the note, avoid its use.

All entries in the medical record should be value neutral (Mangels, 1990; Fiesta, 1993). Labels that may be perceived as derogatory should not be used to describe a patient's appearance, condition, or behavior. Some examples of value-neutral terms are compared with connotative terms in Table 10.2. The medical record is not an appropriate forum for airing grievances or differences of opinions. Editorializing about the patient, the family, or other healthcare providers should be avoided.

The source and date of medical information should be documented (e.g., "according to medical records from . . . . Hospital"). If the source of information is not an official document, this should be made clear. Commonly used phrases such as "the patient denied" and "the patient reported" are helpful because they convey both that the patient was asked about an issue and that a specific reply was given.

TABLE 10-2. Examples of Value-Free Language

Connotative	Value Free
The patient's cousin **suffered** from a cleft lip.	The patient's cousin **had** a cleft lip.
Ms. Jones is a 22 yo **unwed** mother of a child with Down syndrome.	Ms. Jones is 22 years old and is a single parent caring for a child with Down syndrome.
Mrs. Smith is a **substance abuser** and is approximately 20 weeks pregnant.	Mrs. Smith admits to continued **use of** alcohol and cocaine during her pregnancy. She is approximately 20 weeks pregnant.

Source: Adapted from Baker et. al., 2002.

Whenever relevant, refer in the medical record to booklets, literature, Internet sites, support groups, or instructional sheets that were used in counseling, or given to the patient. Once referenced, these items also become part of the medical documentation.

Inevitably in the course of a genetic counseling visit, names and other identifying information about the patient's family members will be revealed. It is important to balance the need to document pertinent genetic, medical, and social information about family members with the need to protect the privacy of those family members. If it is determined that the identifying information is relevant to the healthcare of the client and as such must be documented, the record should reflect where the information was obtained and plans for verifying the accuracy of the information.

> For example, "Mr. Barnes reports that his 35-year-old brother was diagnosed earlier this year with hypercholesterolemia after a minor heart attack. Mr. Barnes has indicated that he will speak with his brother, Bernard Barnes, concerning a request to release his medical records to our office."

In the United States, the Health Information, Portability and Accountability Act of 1996 (HIPAA Title II) requires the federal government to develop national standards to protect the privacy of personal health information. These national privacy standards went into effect in April 2003, and all healthcare practitioners are expected to comply with them. These regulations, or how they are interpreted, may impact information genetic counselors often include, particularly on pedigrees. For example, certain aspects of health information are considered "personal" and therefore "protected information." These include full birth dates (month, date and year) of anyone other than the patient. But the age(s) or year of birth only of family members are not viewed as protected. The same is true for dates of death. Full surnames are also protected but can be included if additional information is being sought from the named individual (U.S. Dept. of Health and Human Services, 2007).

If the client is unable or unwilling to assist in the verification of a significant reported history, identifying names may not be useful and should be omitted from the record. The genetic counselor may consider using only initials under these circumstances. Likewise, unrelated individuals (e.g., the friend who accompanies your client to the counseling session) should not be referenced by name in the medical documentation. The genetic counselor should also carefully consider whether information that identifies other family members should be included in the patient/family letter, since these letters are often shared with other family members, friends, and healthcare providers. It is best to discuss with the client in advance what family information will and will not appear in the patient letter.

While the suggestions provided apply to all forms of medical documentation, some additional considerations are worth noting. For instance, in drafting the patient letter, care should be taken to use clear and easily understood language. In addition, medical jargon should be avoided whenever possible and defined when it is used. Explanations of medical terminology should be provided in lay phrases; in some instances parenthetical phrases or notes are sufficient [e.g., "During the examination, Millie was noted to have hypotelorism (closely set eyes)."] (Baker et al., 2002).

DISCLOSURE OF INFORMATION CONTAINED IN MEDICAL RECORDS

> It has been said that the concept of medical confidentiality is as old as the practice of medicine.—Norrie, 1984

The issues of privacy and confidentiality are certainly not new to most genetic counselors. Yet, with all of the discourse surrounding privacy and confidentiality within the field of genetics, few hard and fast recommendations are available. It is worth noting that requests for access to medical records are most frequently initiated from patients themselves as opposed to other family members or third-party payers. By signing a specific form, clients frequently authorize the release of their medical information at the time of applying for insurance or receiving treatment (Smith and Jones, 1991). Nonetheless, when offices receive appropriately authorized requests for medical records, they are required to provide this access in a timely fashion (Fordham, 1993).

Authorization is generally considered adequate when the patient has completed a valid request form that includes the following information:

o The patient's full name and date of birth
o Hospital registration number if available
o Specific information being requested
o Purpose for which the information may be disclosed
o To whom the information is to be sent (name and address)
o Specified authorization expiration date if desired
o The patient's signature (or patient's legal representative's signature accompanied by guardianship papers or power of attorney)
o Date of signature

If the patient is deceased, a letter of authority in addition to the signed request is needed. The letter of authority is given to the executor of a person's estate by the probate court upon their death. Releasing records to anyone other than the executor may be illegal depending on state law. Individual institutions often have guidelines for handling such requests, ensuring that appropriate standards are maintained. On certain occasions it is legally permitted, if not mandated, to divulge medical information without the patient's consent (McCunney, 1996). This circumstance most frequently arises in public health scenarios with respect to duty to report infectious disease or other reportable conditions (e.g., HIV/AIDS, birth defects in newborns, gunshot wounds). In such cases, healthcare practitioners are obligated by state statutes to report the conditions to the appropriate state agencies and do not need to obtain patient or parental permission beforehand.

Perhaps the best guidance for the genetic counselor concerning disclosure of information can be found within the National Society of Genetic Counselors (NSGC) *Code of Ethics*, which explicitly states that "the primary concern of genetic counselors is the interests of their clients. Therefore, genetic counselors strive to ... maintain information received from clients as confidential, unless released by the client or disclosure is required by law" (NSGC, 2006). In fact, many professional societies have formulated guidelines to help healthcare providers make informed decisions about requests for medical information. These professional codes of conduct serve as respected frameworks for healthcare providers in a variety of situations. Again, one's own institution or place of employment is likely to have specific policies in place that should be consulted.

As mentioned previously, HIPAA was enacted in 1996. Section F of HIPAA mandates the establishment of an electronic patient records system, as well as privacy rules for these electronic records. Of particular interest to the genetics community is the Personalized Health Care workgroup, which was tasked with submitting recommendations to the American Health Information Committee that would enhance the integration of interoperable family health history information into EMRs. Since there is not a universally accepted minimum set of family health history data collected, one recommendation made was to develop a core minimum data set with common data definitions to properly collect family health history information. With literally hundreds of EMR vendors and health systems continuing to define their business needs, issues around including genetics information within the EMRs are likely to continue to evolve.

MEDICAL DOCUMENTATION FOR BILLING AND REIMBURSEMENT

The medical record should provide documentation that corroborates the Current Procedural Terminology (CPT®) billing codes used for billing purposes.[1] The CPT® coding system is a mechanism for describing the type and duration of services provided. CPT codes are devised based on the recommendations of a consensus panel of physicians, allied healthcare providers, Medicare carriers, private insurers, consumers, and other interested parties, and are published annually by the American Medical Association. Depending on the CPT® codes used, they may also define levels of complexity and distinguish between new and established patients, whether the patient is self-or physician referred, and inpatient or outpatient consultations. The general rule is that the code that most accurately describes the service rendered is the code that should be used. For most genetic counselors, the code that would reflect the typical patient encounter will be 96040 Medical Genetics and Genetic

---

[1] CPT® is a registered trademark of the American Medical Association.

Counseling Services. However, there are other codes that may be more appropriate under certain circumstances. For example, if the genetic counselor's time is utilized in telephone or online consultations with established patients, there are separate codes for each, depending on the amount of time involved for medical discussion (e.g., 98966–98968 telephone services and 98969 for online medical evaluation). In addition, genetic counselors who serve on multidisciplinary teams may also benefit from billing for their participation in Medical Team Conferences (e.g., 99366–99368). It's important to recognize that CPT® codes are revised annually, and genetic counselors not in private practice should consult with their billing office staff to coordinate billing practices that are acceptable within their facility.

Although the rule is to bill using the codes that most accurately describe the service rendered, the fiscal reality is that some third-party payers recognize certain codes more readily and reimburse those codes at higher levels than other codes. Because of this, billing practices for genetic services are varied across the country. In some areas, genetic counseling is billed as an office visit or consultation using older, more traditional "Evaluation and Management" or E/M codes.

The E/M CPT code components of the patient encounter are as follows:

- Obtaining a history
- Performing an examination
- Facilitating medical decision-making
- Counseling
- Coordinating patient care

Other aspects of the encounter that are considered include the duration (time spent), complexity (high, medium, or low), and level of risk (also ranked as high, medium or low). An institution can use E/M codes even if every component is not a part of an individual case. However, these codes convey the level of complexity and the level of risk associated with a case that the healthcare provider can rightfully claim. E/M codes were designed with physicians in mind, and the financial value associated with the codes was based on physician usage. However, the instructions for use of the CPT® codebook clearly state that, "it is important to recognize that the listing of a service or procedure and its code number in a specific section of this book does not restrict its use to a specific specialty group" (CPT®, 2008). Again, genetics professionals would be well advised to coordinate their billing practices with coding experts such as those found in hospital-based billing offices.

DOCUMENTATION THAT IS SUBJECT TO EXTERNAL REVIEW

What constitutes bona fide medical documentation? The answer to this question varies depending on who is doing the asking. If the question is being asked by a patient, a medical provider, or an attorney, any and all recorded information may be deemed medical documentation. In the broadest sense, virtually all information that is recorded in the regular course of healthcare delivery could be viewed as "medical documentation."

In the strictest sense, however, only the chart note, and in some circumstances the letter to the referring physician (or family), would be considered "medical documentation" and would be requested by a third-party payer in the course of an audit. If, however, other documentation is referenced within the chart note or the letter, it too becomes part of the accepted medical documentation. For example, if a letter is generated to the referring physician in lieu of a clinical chart note, and the letter to the referring physician includes the information that the patient supplied medical records pertaining to her mother's diagnosis of breast cancer that were used for the risk assessment, the letter along with the mother's medical records could be considered the "medical documentation" for this case.

In some circumstances even formal correspondence between physicians is excluded as part of the medical documentation being reviewed. This practice is justified because auditors (known as medical abstractionists), hired by third-party payers or governmental agencies to conduct either a fiscal audit or performance audit find it unrealistic and impractical to hunt through every written document in search of a particular piece of information. For this reason, typically only the chart note, in some cases supplemented by formal correspondence to a referring physician, is reviewed and considered in an audit.

Third-party payers, including Medicare and Medicaid, utilize medical records when they conduct institutional or agency audits. During a fiscal audit, a sample of medical bills will be compiled and the corresponding medical records collected for review. It is less common for nongovernmental agencies to conduct audits; however, as with Medicaid/Medicare audits, the rate of nongovernmental audits has increased in recent years. Healthcare providers and agencies that receive Medicaid or Medicare funds are required to participate in external quality review programs by professional review organizations (PROs), sometimes called peer review organizations or professional standards review organizations. The PROs were created in 1972 by the Social Security Act Amendment specifically for this purpose. The PROs use medical documentation to determine whether appropriate practice parameters were adhered to (e.g., that a pregnant patient was offered maternal serum marker screening or that a pediatric patient received age-appropriate well-child visits). Medical records can also be reviewed by some PROs to investigate for fraudulent or abusive billing practices. For example, a third-party payer such as Blue Cross may question billing patterns of one institution that are not consistent with billing patterns of another comparable institution. To investigate, the payer may hire a PRO to conduct a medical/fiscal audit.

RETENTION OF MEDICAL RECORDS

"Ideally, patient records should be retained forever."—Harris and Thal, 1992

The parameters of record retention have long been debated. There are, of course, numerous practical as well as legal issues in this area. A major issue is that of storage, especially for a large facility that may have many records on clients who have not been seen for many years. Nonetheless, failure to maintain medical records can have serious adverse consequences for patients as well as for the healthcare provider or clinic. Geneticists and their clients know all too well the frustration of not being able to verify a significant medical history in a long-deceased family member whose records are vitally important in accurately assessing a recurrence risk. However, even with the increased use of electronic record keeping as well as microfiche, many institutions find it impractical to maintain records indefinitely.

Many states have statutes that regulate the preservation and retention of medical records. Sometimes these laws also dictate how much can be charged for reproducing a medical record upon request. This is done to prevent institutions from using copying charges to create a barrier to some providers or patients seeking access to the information. There are also federal regulations that concern minimum record retention practices under certain circumstances. For example, the federal patient antidumping law, passed as part of the Consolidated Omnibus Reconciliation Act of 1986, requires all hospitals that participate in Medicare to maintain medical and other records for a minimum of 5 years for individuals transferred to, or from, another hospital (Sickon, 1992). It is generally recommended that medical records containing financial information be retained for a minimum of 3 years for income tax audit purposes.

Genetics record retention policies should be developed with legal advice about federal and state regulations. The American Hospital Association, the American Medical Record Association, and many professional societies recommend retaining original or reproduced (i.e., microfiche or electronic copies) records for a period of 10 years after the most recent adult patient care entry. They recommend retaining pediatric records longer and even advocate that certain portions of the medical record should be retained permanently. Hospitals and other medical facilities should weigh all of these many factors when establishing record retention policies and procedures. Furthermore, there are no published guidelines concerning if, or how, to maintain records of telephone inquiries or patient intake forms for patients who failed to keep or canceled their appointments. Clinics tend to establish individual protocols for dealing with information obtained under these circumstances and are encouraged to seek guidance on the issue from their hospital attorney.

SUMMARY

Medical documentation assists the patient by optimizing patient care and facilitating effective communication between providers. Medical documentation allows providers, institutions, third-party payers, and employers to comply with state and federal regulations. It also assists providers in supporting or defending their practice, should clients initiate legal claims against them or their institution. Understanding the varied uses of the information can be valuable in helping to identify what, where, when, and how to document.

Genetic counselors should consider and periodically reevaluate the various tips recommended for documenting, such as writing brief and succinct notes, keeping comments objective and factual, keeping in mind the necessary CPT® components, and signing and dating all documentation. Furthermore, genetics clinics should develop and implement policies that will confer the greatest degree of privacy and confidentiality to their clients' medical information.

APPENDIX: PATIENT LETTER OUTLINE (adapted from Baker et. al., 2002)

[Genetics Clinic Letterhead]

Date
Patient/Family name
Address

Re: patient name
   Hospital registration number

Dear (Patient, Parent, or Guardian),

I. Introduction (Generally only 1–3 sentences)
   A. Date of visit
   B. Clinic
   C. Reason for referral or visit (include name of referring provider)
   D. Purpose of the letter

II. Body
   A. Description of significant family, medical, pregnancy, and developmental histories and pertinent test results*
   B. Review of physical exam and/or diagnosis*
      a. Findings on physical exam/basis for diagnosis
      b. Interpretation of significant (+) or (−) family history
   C. Natural history of condition
      a. Description of clinical features and prognosis
      b. Incidence of carrier and disease frequency in general population
   D. Explanation of inheritance
      a. Brief description of genes and chromosomes
      b. Suspected or established inheritance pattern(s)
   E. Summary of risk assessment
      a. Recurrence risk
      b. Risks to other family members
      c. Baseline risk of birth defects if relevant
   F. Outline of reproductive options/prenatal diagnosis

---

*Reference the source of this information (i.e., patient/parent report, physical examination, consultation report, medical institution/laboratory from which records were obtained, etc.).

G. Recommendations for medical management, diagnostic workup, carrier testing, etc.
   a. Clear, unambiguous statement of recommendations
   b. Review of referrals made
   c. Laboratory testing undertaken or under consideration
H. Significant psychosocial issues and concerns
 I. Recommendation of nonmedical resources (including contact names, telephone numbers, etc.)
   a. Support services
   b. Patient literature
   c. Educational resources

III. Closing
A. Plan for reporting test results
B. Schedule of return visit to genetics clinic
C. Invitation to recontact genetics clinic
D. Other closing remarks

IV. Signatures
Genetic counselor
Fellow/resident
Attending physician
cc: PCP/others as requested by family

REFERENCES

Baker DL, Eash T, Schuette JL, Uhlmann WR (2002) Guidelines for writing letters to patients. *J Genet Couns* 11:399–418.

Berry R (1992) Patient fights for right to records. *J Am Dent Assoc* 123:238.

Brandt M (1994) New rules for the CPR (computer-based patient record): no more signing on the dotted line. American Health Information Management Association, Chicago. *Healthcare Inform* 11:30–32, 34.

42 Code of Federal Regulations. Sections 482.24. Medicare Conditions of Participation for Hospitals. Condition of participation: medical record services. http://ecfr.gpoaccess.gov

42 Code of Federal Regulations. Sections 415.150-2-8 Teaching Physician Billing Regulations. http://ecfr.gpoaccess.gov

CPT® (2008) http://www.ama-assn.org/ama/pub/category/3113.html

CY 2004 Risk Adjustment Data Validation April 18, 2005 http://library.ahima.or/xpedio/groups/public/documents/ahima/pub_bok1_021587.html

Department of Health and Human Services – The case of Samuel Nigro.M.D., http://www.hhs.gov/dab/macdecision/Nigro.html

DHHS March 12, 2007:HIPAA Title II: Protecting the Privacy of Patient's Health Information, U.S. Dept. of Health & Human Services. http://www.hhs.gov/news/facts/privacy2007.html last accessed 1-7-08

Dollar CJ (1993) Promoting better healthcare: policy arguments for concurrent quality assurance and attorney-client hospital incident report privileges. *Health Matrix* 3:259–308.

Fiesta J (1991) If it wasn't charted, it wasn't done! *Nurs Manage* 22:17.

Fiesta J (1993) Charting-one national standard, one form. *Nurs Manage* 24:22–24.

Fordham H (1993) Judicial commission & risk management: commission routinely receives questions, complaints about access to medical records. *Mich Med* 92:45–48.

George JE (1991) Law and the emergency nurse: poor emergency department record keeping may hamper legal defense. *J Emergency Nurs* 17:167.

Gilbert JL, Whitworth RL, Ollanik SA, Hare FH Jr, James L (1994) Evidence destruction-legal consequences of spoilation of records, Gilbert & Associates, P.C. Arvadea, Colorado. *Leg Med (US)*: 181–200.

Hahn JR (1996) Medical records: information gathering and confidentiality. *Benefits Q*, 4th Quarter 48–56.

Harris MG, Thal, LS (1992) Retention of patient records. *J Am Optom Assoc* 63:430–435.

Hershey N (1994) Evidentiary ruling favorable to physician. *Palinkas v. Bennett. Hosp Law News* 11:4–6.

Hirsh BD (1994) When medical records are altered or missing. *J Cardiovascular Manage* 5:13–14, 16.

Kapp M (1993) *General guidelines for reporting patient care: discharge planning update.* Department of Community Health, Wright State University, Dayton, OH 13:21–22.

Kettenbach G (1995) *Writing Soap Notes* (2nd ed). Philadelphia: F.A. Davis.

Kidneynotes.com April 2005 (http://www./kidneynotes.com/2005/04/tips-for-medical-documentation-and.html)

Mangels L (1990) Chart notes from a malpractice insurer's hell. *Med Econ* Nov 12.

Mark Twain quote: (http://www.brainyquote.com accessed 03/31.08)

McCunney RJ (1996) Preserving confidentiality in occupational medical practice. *Am Fam Physician* 53:160–175.

Medicare Resident and New Physican Guide: www.cms.hhs.gov/medlearn/mmp-guide.pdf

Miller http://www.charlydmiller.com/CLASS/document.html last accessed 8-6-07

Nisonson I (1991) The medical record. *Bull Am Coll Surg* 76:24–26.

Norrie (1984) Medical confidence: conflicts of duties. *Med Sci Law* 24:26.

NSGC Code of Ethics (Adopted 1992, revised 2004, 2006) http://www.nsgc.org/about/co-deEthics.cfm

Nurses in Independent Practice March 2006: (http://dhfs.wisconsin.gov/Medicaid2/hand-books/nip/nip50.htm last access 8/6/2007)

Oldfield, M (2007) Case study: changing behaviour to improve documentation and optimize hospital revenue. *Can J Nurs Leadersh* 20:40–48.

PacifiCare Policy 2005: including references: U.S. Code of Federal Regulations Title 42 Public Health-Conditions for Medicare Payment (http://ecfr.gpoaccess.gov/cgi/text/text-idx?c=ecfr.&sid=1a93322f11eeb69953222561c8bc63d39&rgn=div5&view=text&node=42:2.0.1.2.24&idno=42#42:2.0.1.2.24.2.52.9idx?c=ecfr&sid=1a9322f11eeb699532225611c8b63d39& rgn=div5&view=text&node=42:2.01.2.24&idno=42#42:2.0.1.2.24.2.52.9

Richter E.S, Shelton A, Yu Y. (2007) Best practices for improving revenue capture through documentation. *Healthc Financ Manage* 61:44–7.

Roach WH Jr (1991) Legal review: coping with celebrity patients. *Top Health Rec Manage* 12:67–72.

Sickon AC (1992) Legal review: the medical records implications of state and federal antidumping provisions. *Top Health Rec Manage* 12:83–90.

Smith AW, Jones A (1991) Computerizing medical records: legal and administrative changes necessary. *Healthspan* 8:3–6.

Smith J (1993) Good medical records key to prevention, defense against malpractice claims. *Mich Med* 92:14–15.

Stratton WT (1994) Necesssity of physician's signature on hospital medical records. *Kans Med* 95:57.

Swigert NB (2006) Clinical documentation, coding, and billing. *Semin Speech Lang* 27:101–118.

Tammelleo AD (1995) Good charting-bad communications: recipe for disaster. Case in point: Critchfield V. McNamara 532 N.W.2d287-NE 1005) *Regan Rep Nurs Law* 36:2.

West JC (1995) Punitive damages allowable for record alternation. Moskovitz v Mt. Sinai Medical Center, Sister of Charity Health Care Systems, Inc., Cincinnati. *J Healthcare Risk Manage* 15:43–45.

Winston Churchill (1874–1965) quote: (http://www.brainyquote.com accessed 3/31/08)

11

Multicultural Counseling

Gottfried Oosterwal, Ph.D., Lit. D.

Like many other modern nations, most of them Western, the United States of America has developed into a multicultural society as the result of two main factors: (1) an unabated stream of immigrants and (2) the radical change in the official attitude toward immigration and diversity. The United States has always been a nation of immigrants; until 1965 most of them arrived from Europe, after which time Mexico and Central America were the main sources. Today, however, immigrants come to U.S. shores from areas throughout the world; some 40% are from the continent of Asia, which is home to an immense diversity of values, cultures, and religions (US Census Bureau, 2006). In the past the official approach toward immigrants and diversity was the same as that clearly enunciated by the Founding Fathers: All immigrants were encouraged to abandon their particular culture and values and adopt those of their adopted country, resulting in "assimilation," the "melting pot," and "Americanization" (Oosterwal, 1997). However, since the 1970s the approach has shifted toward **multiculturalism** or **cultural pluralism**. The multicultural approach encourages immigrant groups to keep their traditions, even celebrate them and share them with others as a way of enriching society as a whole.

Although multiculturalism is not without its strong critics (Schlesinger, 1992), the attitude has become commonplace in U.S. society and is applied—sometimes rigorously—to all of its policies, institutions, and organizations. Genetic counseling reflects these developments in society at large. Increasingly, counseling is taking place between people from diverse cultural and religious backgrounds. Multicultural counseling refers to a process whereby a trained professional from one ethnocultural

A Guide to Genetic Counseling, Second Edition, Edited by Wendy Uhlmann, Jane Schuette, and Beverly Yashar
Copyright © 2009 by John Wiley & Sons, Inc.

background interacts with a client from another for the purpose of promoting the client's cognitive, social, emotional, and spiritual health and development. Overall, multiculturally competent counselors are comfortable with differences in values, assumptions, behaviors, and beliefs, and possess the skills to communicate effectively across existing or perceived cultural boundaries.

THE CHALLENGE

At the core of the challenge of genetic counseling across cultural boundaries is diversity. The American population consists of some 175 different ethnocultural groups, each of which is characterized by its own specific **cultural code** (US Census Bureau, 2006), **a set of values and assumptions, notions and beliefs that shape the way people from diverse cultures act and think, relate and communicate; what they consider right or wrong, good or bad, sacred or profane, important or unimportant**. This cultural code shapes the ways that people from diverse cultures interpret disease, death, genetic disorders, and disabilities; perceive of pregnancy and parenting; respond to pain; define family, kinship, and ideal marriage partners; share or conceal information; use or refuse certain foods and medications; and relate to their counselors and care givers.

In Western cultures, illness and disabilities are seen as the result of biophysical or mechanical causes (the **biomedical model**). In many of the cultures of Africa and Asia, disease and disorders are interpreted as the result of divine intervention, which can serve as either a form of punishment or an act of grace, or acts of spiritual powers that seek to do harm (**the magico-religious model**). Genetic disorders are often interpreted as a curse, which often leads to rejection. The experience of and responses to pain, both physical and mental, differ widely, from stoic, private suffering and even denial to dramatic and exuberant public expressions. (See the section on Beliefs about the Causes of Disease and Disorder for further discussion of this topic.)

Although plural marriages are strictly outlawed in Western cultures, some 65–70% of all cultures in the world allow them (Helman, 1994), either as **polygyny** (marriage between one husband and two or more wives) or **polyandry** (marriage between one woman and two or more men) Some cultures of the Middle East and Africa consider the ideal form of marriage to be between cousins, either cross-cousins or parallel cousins. (See the section on Family and Kinship.) In other cultures, such marriages or sexual liaisons are strictly forbidden and considered a negative factor in the development of genetic disorders.

Differences in views about medicine and marriage can have tremendous implications for the process of genetic counseling, especially when discussing family or sexual activity or establishing descent. When people from diverse cultures meet, formally or informally, as neighbors or in a client-counselor relationship, they do so through the lens of their respective cultural codes. An American counselor may interpret an event in a particular way, while her Chinese or Mexican client may perceive the same facts in a completely different way.

MULTICULTURAL COMPETENCY

Competency in multicultural counseling demands four basic skills and attitudes:

1. An understanding of your own cultural code and how it shapes the way you act and think, relate and communicate, perceive reality and judge others. This includes an awareness of the biases and blinders you have developed from your own cultural setting.
2. Knowledge of your clients' ways of perceiving reality: how they interpret illness and disorders, experience and express pain, and view sex, marriage, family, and kinship.
3. An attitude of humility that clearly recognizes and appreciates the diversity of human cultures. No single culture, not even our own, has in and of itself discovered the only way or the best way of being human or of helping people in their pursuit of happiness. We can learn as much from others as they may learn from us.
4. The ability to use other people's cultural codes as a counseling resource. Instead of being viewed as barriers or obstacles, others' values and beliefs should be considered valuable resources, even tools in the process of genetic counseling.

DIVERSITY IS CULTURAL, NOT BIOPHYSICAL

Culture is what sets us apart from the rest of the world. Humans are **cultural beings**, both the creators of culture and a product of it. Although scientists may differ in their opinions of the best definition of culture, over 150 definitions analyzed by Kroeber and Kluckhohn (1952) agree that **culture** refers to a group of people's total way of life: the way they act and think, organize themselves, relate and communicate, make or build things, express feelings and emotions, and respond to the world. It is the manmade part of our environment, the software of our brain, our design for living in realms of life both material and social, mental and spiritual. It is culture that differentiates Mexicans from Koreans, Arabs from Germans, and Russians from Americans. Subcultures within the larger American culture include African Americans, Cuban Americans, European Americans, and Vietnamese Americans. **The core differences among ethnocultural groups are not biophysical, they are**

cultural. They are not external or material; they are rooted in people's cultural codes. They are not determined by skin color or head size or hair texture. Neither are they determined by what we eat or how we dress, walk, and talk. Diversity is rooted in our different value orientations.

The insight that core differences among people from diverse ethnocultural groups are **socially inherited**, not just genetically determined, has a powerful liberating effect. First, it liberates the genetic counselor from the fear of not being able to understand the behavior of clients from diverse cultures. All cultures are **learned behaviors**. With some effort, they can be shared and understood by others. Although it may be difficult, behaviors that are harmful or destructive can also be unlearned. Human behavior is also **logical** when it is interpreted in terms of a person's specific cultural code. What often appears at first as weird or strange or deviant may take on a whole new meaning if interpreted in light of particular values and norms, concepts and beliefs. A person's behavior and ways of thinking can suddenly make sense once you understand what makes them "tick."

Second, the insight that culture is learned and logical liberates the counselor to engage in creative and flexible approaches to genetic counseling. All it takes is a deeper understanding of your clients' particular values, assumptions, and beliefs, and the ability to use them as a resource and a means for more effective results.

Third, the insight liberates the counselor from biases, cultural captivity, and even prejudices. Any culture that shapes us creates biases and blinders. What may at first appear as a deviation or a disorder according to your particular way of thinking may appear to be quite normal in a different setting. For example, a low-income Puerto Rican woman suffers from *ataques de nervios*. These events, which can best be described as epileptic-like seizures, have an emotional base and an important function in Puerto Rican culture. Originally, American psychology either pathologized them as hysteria or considered them to be physical in origin. We now know that such events are a normal part of dealing with trauma and grief in Puerto Rican culture.

Finally, the insight that diversity is cultural rather than biophysical liberates the counselor from the all too facile tendency toward generalizing and stereotyping. There are individual differences in all cultures, even in the most isolated and collectivistic ones. **Cultures are *descriptive* of human behavior, not *prescriptive***. There are many variations among individuals and groups within a single culture.

One of the hallmarks of all cultures is that they are in a constant state of flux, or change. By nature, cultures are **dynamic**; nothing remains the same. These changes constantly demand new and varied approaches, on both an individual level and a collective level. Cultures are also more or less well **integrated**. Each aspect or every element of culture is interrelated with all of the others. Notions of illness, for instance, are interrelated with people's beliefs, social organization, and economic conditions. Because change in notions of time or transportation, family relationships or education, technology or medicine has consequences for all other aspects of a culture, multicultural counseling must be comprehensive. It must include not just evaluation of a person's physical condition but knowledge of his or her entire value orientation.

THE RELIGION FACTOR

People's cultural values and assumptions are universally inextricably intertwined with their religion. The ways people act and think, how they perceive reality and relate to it, are shaped by their view of the existence of a reality other than the physically perceptible one that is believed to interact with our human existence. Religious ideas and expressions are strongly influenced by the culture in which they emerged or developed. This is true not just for American culture, but for cultures everywhere. In the United States and most Western cultures, religion is clearly distinguished and consciously kept separate from the so-called secular aspects of life such as business, education, government, and medicine; in contrast, in most other cultures religion is seen and experienced as the core of life. It shapes the way people view illness and death, and how they relate to and interpret disorders and disabilities. Chronic illness and disorders may be interpreted as a sign of God's displeasure, even punishment, or as a warning to repent and return to the faith of the fathers. In Hinduism and Buddhism, every new birth is considered either a reincarnation or a rebirth of a previously existing being. A disability or genetic disorder may be seen in such cases as direct evidence of a transgression committed in a previous life. Because many cultures interpret disorders and disabilities as the result of curses, spells, punishment for transgressions of a religious or social taboo, or the activities of evil spirits, attitudes toward disabilities and genetic disorders are commonly rather negative and pessimistic. Children affected by chronic disabilities or genetic disorders may be hidden from view, neglected, mistreated, or even abandoned. Their parents may be afraid, both of the symptoms and of the deep sense of shame associated with the disease. Except in emergencies, these families may seldom seek help within the medical system. And when they do, the results are often very poor. Because traditional religious notions and beliefs are deeply ingrained and difficult to change, it may be difficult for them to accept explanations of genetic inheritance or physiological patterns of chronic disease progression. A purely biophysical or medical approach to the problem is therefore of little help in such cases. However, in some cases, the new information received in counseling can be integrated into the traditional belief system. The counselor must not only understand how people from other cultures and religions feel about the problem, but at the same time must develop the ability to use the clients' beliefs, assumptions and even language (such as "grace," "Repentance," "God," "karma," "faith," etc) to explain the situation and help clients to cope.

The counselor should remember that a client's specific beliefs can serve as a great source of strength and comfort, and can be a powerful resource in coping with a disorder or disability. For example, a recent study found that many deeply religious Roman Catholic Mexican Americans believed that they were singled out by God for their roles as parents of a chronically ill or disabled child, partly because of their character and deeds of kindness to others. Many stated that they welcomed the birth of the disabled infant as part of God's plan. Interviews with parents of disabled children in the Latino community often revealed the notion that they had been chosen by God as both a substitute and a model for the suffering of many others (Andrews and Boyle, 1995).

Critical Incident I

Mr Akbar Ali, a 74-year-old Arabic-speaking Muslim gentleman from Algiers in North Africa, was diagnosed with insulin-dependent diabetes and rapidly advancing Alzheimer disease. When the family received the diagnosis, the recommended course of treatment was insulin and a series of family counseling sessions. The family refused both, and seemed quite relaxed. A prayer of thanks was offered to Allah, the Beneficent, the Merciful. The family never returned to the hospital and never came for counseling to deal with the problems associated with Alzheimer disease.

1. How can you explain the family's reaction to the diagnosis?
2. Why did they refuse the insulin and the offer of counseling?
3. Consider the meaning of food and medicines from a religious perspective.
4. How could this issue have been dealt with more effectively?

(For a discussion of this incident, please turn to the Appendix: Responses to Critical Incidents.)

AMERICAN VALUES COMPARED

In our age of multiculturalism, what *is* the American cultural code? America today is a nation in which a host of different streams of culture flow side by side, yet there is a national cultural code. It is rooted in the beliefs of our Founding Fathers and early pioneers, who emigrated primarily from Western Europe. This belief system was then molded and shaped during the settlement of the American frontier. Today, this American code is represented, expressed, and maintained most strongly by the middle class in small-town America.

Is it possible to outline the most obvious and powerful characteristics of this American cultural code? Most social scientists agree that the answer is yes (Stewart and Bennett, 1991). Reflect for a while on the following list of values, which are often expressed in our proverbs and sayings:

- Individualism and egalitarianism
- Action and achievement orientation
- Informality and "fair play"
- Progress and prosperity
- Freedom and democracy
- Privacy and independence
- Risk taking and personal initiative
- Honesty
- Task and time orientation
- Law and justice
- Creativity and innovation

- Efficiency and effort optimism
- Openness and dependability.

Consider also the following culturally loaded terms, which are often used (and abused): victory, success, and youthfulness; mobility, voluntarism, and humanitarianism; competition and confrontation, including the desire to be first (from the First Bank to the First Church); frankness and adversarial relationships; the need to be liked; aggressiveness and violence; racial and religious bigotry. Finally, think of the enormous emphasis in American culture on the notion of self, as in self-awareness and self-reliance; self-esteem and self-worth; self-made and self-realization; self-assertion and self-consciousness; self-help and self-sufficiency; self-satisfaction and self-determination.

Not one of these values is unique to American culture. Australians are at least as individualistic and antiauthoritarian as Americans. But as a whole, this American cultural code shapes the way we act and think, relate and communicate, feel, or even dream. This code also serves as a key to unlocking our understanding of our judgments about others, why "they" are considered "lazy," "deceptive," and "unreliable," "slow," "childish," "authoritarian," "stuffy," etc. Suspending such judgments is essential to unlocking cultural codes.

Not all values shape everyone in the same way or to the same degree. Cultural codes can be viewed as pyramids, with some values at the top and others in the middle or at the bottom. In addition, some values affect us more generally, others more personally. In every culture, persons can be found who in some ways or even many ways do not conform to their cultural code. Moreover, cultures are dynamic; although the core remains basically the same, values do change over time.

FOUR BASIC CORE VALUES

In seminal comparative studies, four core American values have been documented to have the greatest effect on the relationships between health care providers and clients from diverse cultures (Thompson, Ellis & Wildavsky, 1990; Hofstede, 1980) (Table 11-1). These include individualism (in contrast to collectivism), egalitarianism (in contrast to authoritarianism and hierarchical thinking), time and task orientation (in contrast to event and person orientation) and masculinity (in contrast to femininity). Available space does not allow detailed elaboration of the effect of each of these values on the work of genetic counselors in an increasingly multicultural setting. Such insights should come as a result of much personal reflection and meditative

TABLE 11-1. Core Values Compared

American Values	Non-American Values
Individualism	*Collectivism*
Egalitarianism	*Hierarchical Thinking/Authoritarianism*
Time and Task Orientation	*Event & Person Orientation (Building Relationships)*
Masculinity	*Femininity*

study. In what ways, for instance, are you a product of cultural values such as individualism or achievement orientation? How do your views and your client's differ from the American culture's emphasis on task and time orientation?

Individualism versus Collectivism

There is general agreement among social scientists that individualism is the core value with the greatest influence on the American way of life and its national character (Bellah et al., 1986). It shapes the ways we think and feel, and how we relate to others, work, love, experience religion, pursue happiness, organize, engage in politics, and communicate. All happiness or sadness, success or failure, status and position, depends on the individual, which is also the locus of our decision-making and problem solving and where we find our personal identity. Counselors in this value orientation appeal to their clients' own willpower to confront their problem and deal with it. Effective counseling in our American cultural setting means a one-on-one encounter in which an individual communicates with another individual, who is then expected to make a very personal decision. Disabilities and disorders are also experienced and treated as individual problems requiring individual action.

Compare individualism with the core value of collectivism, which is at work in most of the immigrant groups now living and working in the United States: They identify the self not in terms of the individual, but in terms of the group—the (extended) family, the clan, the ethnic group as a whole. In most of these cultures, the locus of decision-making does not lie with the individual but with the group of which he or she is an integral part. In contrast to the United States, where the whole emphasis is on standing out as an individual, in most of the cultures of Africa and Asia the emphasis is on being like the others, thinking like they do. As the Japanese say: "The nail that sticks out is being hammered down." As for Africans the saying "I am what we are" permeates their whole thinking and behavior.

From childhood onward, people in collectivistically organized cultures see themselves first as part of a group, which is the source of their identity and happiness, strength and support. It is also the locus of decision-making and problem solving and determines for them what is right or wrong, good or bad, important or unimportant. Their personhood is experienced and expressed as part of and embedded in their "corporate personality": "When one of us is sick, we all are sick."

Diseases and disorders are indeed personal, but not individual. The self is not shaped by individual thinking and action, as in the Cartesian expression: "I think, therefore I am." It rests instead upon the collective thinking and actions of the group as a whole. A person's status and position, happiness and security, and even his or her future are not based on individual achievements or success, but on the role he or she plays in the group. Group members find strength and support for living and for the pursuit of happiness in this mutual interdependence.

In collectivistically organized cultures, counseling is never an encounter between two individuals, even if the meeting is one-on-one; it always includes a whole family or group of people. The person with the perceived disorder or disability will usually come not alone but accompanied by members of the group: parents and/or siblings, cousins and in-laws. Even in those rare cases when a client comes alone, the counselor must realize that the client does not feel, think, or make decisions as a single individual. He or she is an integral member of a group. The counselor therefore needs to address the "corporate personality" and share with them all the insights, knowledge, and sympathy (or understanding) he or she has to offer.

The counselor should support the development of plans in collaboration with the whole group. In societies based on collectivism, the individual person has never learned to make decisions alone to stand up for him- or herself, or had to "do what is right." If informed about the nature of the disorder or disease, the group will guarantee that the individual client will follow the treatment plan. It is their *plan* and their *responsibility*.

Finally, when it becomes necessary to share bad news, it may be important to first share this information with the closest relatives of the client, who then communicate it to the affected individual. It has been confirmed over and over again that, in a collectivistic culture, sharing bad news directly with the person suffering from the disease may cause great harm. How can we reconcile the diverse expectations created by these two contrasting value orientations? By law, American counselors are required to inform their clients and patients and to insist on "informed consent." Our laws also seek to guarantee privacy and confidentiality and prohibit the counselor from sharing data with others. Privacy and confidentiality, as well as decision-making and problem solving, are rooted in the American value of individualism. To adapt these standards to dealings with clients from collectivistic cultures, it is important to develop a plan with the client and the family early on that addresses how information will be shared. In addition to working more closely with relatives rather than the client, the counselor may want to think carefully about the strength of the language that is used to share "bad news," since cultures rooted in collectivism tend to believe in the idea that as long as there is life there is hope. (See also the section Communicating Across Cultural Boundaries).

Genetic counselors need to be aware that the normative behavior, responses, and expectations of people from diverse cultures toward counseling differ greatly from those of the traditional White-Anglo culture issue when counseling clients from other cultures (McGoldrick, Pearce, and Giordano, 1982). In the United States, patients and clients consider it their right to know the real nature of their condition; however, in most other cultures people do not want to know their real status. Actually, they feel very upset when the counselor or physician tells them "the truth." They consider this rude and intrusive, not respectful of a client's privacy, dignity, and happiness. As part of the process in learning to bridge these differences, consider using the following guidelines:

- Use the client's own culture as a resource: ask about his or her closest relatives and if appropriate request permission to share medical information with them.
- Develop skills to communicate with the client on both relational and cognitive levels. In most cultures, information flows best when it is shared as part of a personal relationship.

- Request guidance from an ethics committee and/or diversity committee regarding the proper approach and language to use when sharing bad news with members of a particular cultural group.

On many occasions specific conflicts emerging from encounters between people from diverse cultures can only be solved through better insights and training, greater creativity and resourcefulness, and using other people's particular values as a resource.

Egalitarianism versus Hierarchical Thinking/Authoritarianism

Most Americans firmly believe that all people are born equal. Therefore, everyone should be treated the same and should have equal opportunities for achievements and success. The fact that we have not always lived up to this core value in no way detracts from its power and importance.

The value of equality, so deeply ingrained in every aspect of American culture, is closely associated with the value of individualism. As a whole, we have no difficulty granting equality to individuals, regardless of ethnic, religious, social, or cultural background. The difficulty arises with regard to granting equality to groups of people.

Most immigrants come into our country from cultures that are hierarchically organized, with clear distinctions between higher and lower classes, between superior and inferior status or position. Ways of thinking and behaving strongly reflect these distinctions. Examples include the following: The male is in many aspects regarded as superior to the female; older persons are more honored than younger ones; children are considered lower than their parents; laypersons are lower than specialists (including counselors); employees and citizens are lower than employers or government officials. Behaviors required by religion often support these distinctions. The caste system in India is a prime example. It is not individual achievement that gives a person his or her identity or status, but his or her position in the caste system.

Many millions of people from (East) Asia (Japan, China, Southeast Asia, India, and others) live by the counsel given by Confucius some 2500 years ago: If you want to find happiness in life, and if you want your society to become a paradise on earth, always obey the five hierarchies: children should always honor and obey and respect their parents, regardless of the circumstances; students and employees should extend this same courtesy to their teachers and employers; citizens should respect their governments; and younger persons should always honor and respect their elders. By extension, this means that the layperson (the patient or client) will show great deference to the expert (the counselor). The attitude of persons from such cultures will be rather formal and respectful, and often conflict with U.S. attitudes of partnership and equal status.

One consequence of the U.S. value of egalitarianism is a preference for simple manners, a high level of informality, and directness. However, clients from authoritarian cultures may feel very uncomfortable with this approach; they may consider American counselors rather disrespectful, even rude, if they interpret behavior in terms of their own cultural code. Respect for the value of hierarchical thinking and authoritarianism that is so prevalent in people from Mexico to Japan demands that American counselors meet certain expectations for their clients: (1) address them formally as Mr. and Mrs. (or at least ask them how they would like to be addressed); (2) treat them perhaps more formally and deferentially than usual; and (3) present yourself at the session well-dressed. In addition, do not be surprised if, when you begin your conversation with one person (usually the one with the symptoms), another person responds. This could be a parent, or a husband, mother-in-law, or elder cousin.

Another aspect of counseling people across the boundary of equality-hierarchical thinking is that a person with authoritarian values will not start a conversation until the counselor speaks. In authoritarian societies, younger people do not speak before older people do, and people of lower status will wait until those of a higher status address them. In addition, people from many Asian cultures hesitate to call attention to themselves. As people in Japan say, "We learn more when we keep our mouths shut." Compare this to the American proverb: "The squeaky wheel gets the grease."

Then there's the issue of trust. Many people from diverse cultures have difficulty sharing their problems with strangers. People from East and Southeast Asia in particular may not feel confident enough to ask questions, even the ones that are uppermost in their minds. As different as they are otherwise, in cultures from Japan to Mexico the attitude is "We don't do business with strangers."

So, how do you cease being strangers and gain the confidence of your clients? First and foremost, you must create an atmosphere of trust; this could involve sharing some snacks or a drink together, demonstrating proper behavior, showing deference, dressing formally, and sharing your own personal issues and experiences with clients. A value characteristic of most people from Africa, Asia, and Latin America, and among Native Americans, is called **reciprocity**. People will respond to intimate questions only when the person asking them first shares some of his or her own experiences. Good relationships in these cultures depend on the level of reciprocity. Clients "give" when we give first. The "giving" of personal data can create a sense of obligation by the client to share relevant clinical information. While such clients will sometimes open up and share intimate data first, this does not let you off the hook, but instead creates the expectation that you will share with them later. Not doing so is considered rude, and often leads to a premature ending of the counseling relationship. Research (Ponterotto et al., 1995) has shown that some 70–75% of counselees from other cultures do not return for another session because of these and other cultural misunderstandings. Of course, the counselor must at all times maintain the appropriate boundaries between the personal and the professional self (McCarthy-Veach et al., 2003).

Helping the client to understand that the counselor sees their professional interaction as building a relationship rather than as a professional contract may bridge this gap. You may want to start your counseling sessions with a brief conversation about your family and your client's family. Icebreakers include questions about how long clients have been in the United States, how we ourselves have struggled with and overcome certain problems, and, if possible, sharing pictures. Often the most effective way of creating a relationship is by offering clients something to eat or drink. Trust is created when people can say: "We have eaten together." Japanese counselors apply this approach with great results. In clinical settings where this type of an interaction is not possible, even offering a glass of water may help to bridge the cultural gap.

Time and Task Orientation versus Event and Person Orientation

Mainstream America sees time like a river flowing in one direction, from its source to its mouth. Time is linear, and can be divided into past, present, and future. In the U.S. the future is the most important of these three. Progress, another key term in the American value system, is geared toward keeping up with the flow of time and shaping its direction. It is viewed as ascending from a primitive past toward a future in which impediments of nature are dominated by human will through science and technology.

From the American perspective, time equals money. It is considered a commodity and is therefore closely associated with work. Because people work for a certain number of hours at a designated rate, we do our best not to "waste time." When meeting with a client, an American counselor comes directly to the point: He or she discusses lab reports, explains the disorder and how it may develop over time, etc. We are extremely task-oriented, and value the efficient use of the limited amount of time we have. We adhere closely to schedules, and feel disappointed when we do not accomplish everything we have set out to do. This sometimes robs us of any joy over what we have accomplished.

Neither this concept of time nor the idea of projecting the future is universal. Many cultures conceive of time as cyclical; the past is seen as a recurring event, not a cause that impacts the future. Time is not a process that can be measured by the clock or the calendar. It is an **event** that combines the present with the past and the future. It can even be envisioned as a space in which things happen.

How do different conceptions of time affect counseling? First, many clients have different attitudes toward punctuality, or "being on time." There is "Filipino time," "hora Mexicana" or "mong lao." "hora Americana," in contrast, is exact; activities are scheduled with a clear beginning and a definite end. Time is apportioned for separate activities: so many minutes are allotted for a prenatal patient and so many for a cancer patient. Such clients may not keep their appointments precisely, and may become annoyed at the resulting irritation exhibited by their mainstream American counselor. "Being late" is a very flexible concept. In Germany or Switzerland not being five minutes early for an appointment is considered late, but in rural Africa or Indonesia an hour or two after the scheduled appointment may be acceptable.

People from areas holding to a non-Western concept of time can feel that a 30- to 45-minute session is not enough time to discuss their problems. People from other cultures may interpret time constraints in one of the following ways: "the counselor is not really interested in us and our problems," or "the counselor is not taking us and our problems seriously." American counselors can come across as uncaring, and always in a hurry, which often prevents clients from asking questions pertinent to their case.

What does this mean for the professional counselor?

- Recognition of differences in time and task orientation demands creativity and flexibility. When it comes to time, suspend judgment and take a "time out."
- Development of the ability to become more culture-sensitive may include considering the way we decorate our offices and arrange our furniture, including the placement of mirrors and plants. This is especially crucial with clients whose thinking is influenced or dominated by **feng shui**. The two cosmic realities of **wind and water** shape every aspect of a person's life, thought, and behavior. The environment where counseling takes place is of crucial importance, because it creates a flow of energy (**chi**), good or bad, that determines a person's health and happiness, feelings and emotions, openness and receptivity.

Gender Roles: Masculinity versus Femininity

The literature on the subject of gender differences across cultural boundaries is vast and continues to grow. The conclusion from current research is that some personality traits occur statistically more often in men, while others occur more often in women. This applies in New York and New Zealand, and even in the primal societies of New Guinea. However, it is culture that determines which traits are considered more favorable than others, and, therefore, which ones should be stimulated and encouraged or downgraded and discouraged. The resulting patterns of masculinity and femininity greatly affect people's identities, attitudes, functions and roles, and physical and mental health.

Traits considered feminine include the following: a greater tendency toward caring and nurturing, more concern about establishing and maintaining social relationships, a preference for group orientation over individual orientation, stronger inclination to help others, and the demonstration of empathy. Feminine traits are further characterized by an inclination toward conformity, a greater sense of responsibility, avoidance of open conflict, and the tendency to use language to resolve conflicts.

Masculine traits include independence, individualism, aggressiveness, self-confidence, and ambition. They are further characterized by a desire to command and control, the expectation that they will be followed, the goals of power, status, and autonomy, self-reliance, action-orientation, an analytical rather than emotional orientation, and an inclination toward competition, programming, and progress. Men panic less and are less frustrated by failure, but they are more interested in pursuing individual interests and personal goals. These traits are also manifested as self-assertion, self-protection, and a tendency toward violence.

In a majority of cultures, masculine traits have been favored over feminine traits, which has often led to considerable differences in status, rights, functions, and positions (Mead, 1935). In other cultures, the differences between masculine and feminine traits are clearly recognized, but seen and treated as complementary. Equality is experienced not in the sameness of tasks or positions, but in recognition of special contributions. There is a clear division of labor, of assignments, and even of positions; for example, politics or governing or going to war is considered a masculine affair, while healing and helping others is valued as a feminine one.

The cultural attitudes and assumptions associated with the differences between the genders greatly affect the process of counseling. They affect the way men and women cope with their problems, listen, accept responsibility, seek social support, and show guilt or shame. Women generally need more time with a counselor than men, as well as more assurances and more comfort. Women who are not assertive and/or see counselors as authority figures may be less likely to ask questions or challenge their directions or conclusions. Women tend to feel more guilt, but men feel more shame, particularly those of Western cultures. Women in male-dominated societies are more inclined to accept the inevitable, while men tend to become confrontational and often distance themselves from the problem. The opposite is true of a client who comes from a culture that favors feminine traits. In such cases, clients will see their counselors more as authority figures. They bond more easily with their counselors, and are less likely to ask questions or challenge the counselors' instructions or advice.

PREGNANCY, BIRTH, AND FAMILY

Pregnancy as Disease

Aside from a few pockets of isolated cultures, the causal relationship between pregnancy and sexual intercourse is now universally understood. The universality of the knowledge about the causal relationship between intercourse and pregnancy does not mean, however, that all people think alike about pregnancy and birth (Oosterwal, 1961). To the contrary, while the physiological processes involved may be basically the same, the cultural responses to these processes differ widely from culture to culture. This has led to a host of different ideas and practices; from the notion of pregnancy itself to the way women should deliver the child, from women's responses to pain and the location where the birth should take place to who the birth attendants should be.

One important difference between Western and most non-Western notions of pregnancy is the idea that pregnancy is a "disease" that needs the attention of a host of specialists. In most cultures, pregnancy is seen as a sign of good health and an event of great vitality worthy of celebration. That view prevents many immigrants from those cultures from participating in prenatal care programs. Often they arrive at the hospital only if an emergency occurs or in an advanced state of labor. In their home countries, deliveries traditionally take place at home or in specially designed places. The woman is surrounded not by medical specialists but by other experienced women, mostly relatives. Men usually are excluded from attending the birth because of the belief that a woman's fluids in childbirth would defile a man, causing weaknesses, ritual uncleanliness, and even severe illnesses. These developments would necessitate special cleansing and rituals of atonement. Most people from other cultures do not share the American expectation that the husband should be present at the birth. It is often wrongly assumed that men from other cultures are less interested or involved in the birth process and bonding with their children. To the contrary, in many cultures, the husband and other male relatives are involved in the process from the moment the pregnancy occurs. The expectant father cannot go out hunting or fishing, must abstain from a host of activities, and is required to avoid certain kinds of food or use others prescribed for the occasion. The pregnant woman is not the only one involved in many rituals and taboos; her husband and immediate family are as well. It takes a whole village, family, or group to have a successful birth and to care for the newborn child.

Another difference between Western and non-Western perceptions is the notion that pregnancy is purely the result of a sexual encounter between a man and a woman. In most cultures, pregnancy is considered a result of both human action and supernatural or divine intervention. Children are seen as a gift from God or the gods, the result of human and divine cooperation. Marriage itself is seen as a symbolic reflection of the sacred marriage between heaven and earth, and pregnancy a result of that divinely instituted supernatural reality. Because pregnancy in most cultures is shrouded in mystery, it is accompanied by a whole set of rituals. The woman, her husband, and her closest relatives are all to follow strictly prescribed behaviors, which may include frequent bathing, avoidance of cold air, continuation of sexual intercourse, exposure to the light of the full moon, avoidance of certain types of food such as pork or chicken or blemished fruits; cessation of hair braiding, etc. Genetic disorders or chronic disabilities are often viewed as the result of breaking taboos; the consequences of actions by a god punishing the woman and her family. In Hinduism and Buddhism, such disorders or disabilities may also be a result of a transgression of divinely instituted taboos committed in a previous life.

Biological Birth vs. Social Birth

One crucial aspect of many non-Western cultures is the clear distinction between "biological birth" and "social birth." To the question "When does a fetus become a person, a social human being?" people from many cultures in Africa and Asia would not give one of the two answers we often use—either at conception or at birth; their answer is at **social birth**. The rituals and stages involved in the process of social birth may vary from culture to culture. At the heart of them all lies the name-giving ceremony. It is only when a child has received a name that he or she becomes a full human being with specific social and legal rights. This explains a host of otherwise misunderstood forms of behavior of non-Western parents. Historically, for example, when a child showed certain genetic deformities or other birth defects, the child was often rejected or even killed. This was not considered murder (infanticide), as the child had not yet received a name. In some cultures, women would not start breast feeding until the child received a name. And parents of premature infants would not visit their child in the hospital until it received a name. In our own culture a person's name is more or less a label, but in many non-Western cultures a name stands for personhood, character, identity, being. In such cultures the importance of asking clients how they would like to be addressed cannot be overstressed.

After birth, people in many cultures observe a special postpartum rest period, during which the mother must follow certain dietary restrictions and avoid taboos and is cared for by other women. This period of rest, the "lying-in" period, lasts from 20 to 40 days. The term used by Mexicans is *quarantena*, indicating 40 days of rest and seclusion. Cultures differ with regard to allowed or proscribed activities and taboos; they range from virtual "house arrest" to the prohibition of sexual contact. For all of these cultures the "lying-in" period serves as a time of companionship with relatives and friends who go out of their way to assist the mother; the result is a strong reduction in or even total avoidance of postpartum (traumatic) stress.

Critical Incident II

Lee Ming is a 26-year-old woman of Chinese ethnic extraction. She and her husband are very concerned about Ming's first pregnancy. Lee Ming grew up in the United States. Against her parents' will, she married an American man she met at college, totally ignoring the feng shui calendar in selecting her wedding day, which indicated that the day she chose was not only totally unsuitable, but outright dangerous. She also paid no attention to her immigrant parents' prescriptive and proscriptive rules regarding pregnancy in Chinese culture. Close to the time of the delivery, Ming became convinced that her first child would be born with a genetic disorder or some other deformity. She recently consulted a Chinese herbalist, who told her to eat more *yang* food to balance the *yin* status of her pregnancy. But she is very afraid of the consequences of not following the Chinese value of "filial piety" (honoring her mother and father's wishes). Although her husband considers it all "weird superstition," Ming has insisted on seeing a genetic counselor.

How might you approach the issue, and counsel Lee Ming and her husband?

(For a discussion of this incident, please turn to the Appendix: Responses to Critical Incidents).

Family and Kinship Relations

There is no other institution in society that has changed so much and so rapidly as the family, which serves as the primary social group in all cultures and societies. This is true worldwide. The issue of family is of immense importance to the genetic counselor because genes are transmitted through families and because genetic conditions are revealed through lines of descent and family history. Therefore, from its very inception genetic counseling has been family-centered and family-oriented.

Complex webs of relationships characterize all human societies; they link people into family groups and regulate sexuality, childbearing, and relationships between group members. The most basic and universal unit is the so-called **nuclear family**, a unit consisting of a husband, a wife, and their natural or adopted offspring. In the United States, Canada, and Europe, such a unit exists *independently* of other such units. In most other cultures, however, the nuclear family was and very much still is part of and embedded in a larger and more extended unit called the **extended family**. Because the nuclear family relies heavily upon the extended family, it is considered a **dependent nuclear family**. It is not the individual but the family that is the main focus of both diagnosis and treatment; thus it is of the utmost importance that counselors become acquainted with the nature of the family, its functions, and the internal relationships among its members.

In the course of a lifetime a person belongs to two nuclear families: the one in which he or she was born and raised as a child, called the **family of orientation**, and the one in which he or she is a parent, called the **family of procreation**. Kinship derives from the existence of one's families. People are said to be **kin** to each other when their relationship can be demonstrated genealogically. From an anthropological perspective, if a relationship can be demonstrated by descent, we speak of a **consanguineal** relationship. If a relationship is based on marriage and/or descent, they are considered **affinal kin**. All societies have clear rules about these relationships; these rules closely regulate how people should behave toward one another, as well as outlining their rights and obligations. Such behavior is expressed in the ways people from diverse cultures refer to their relatives, address them, interrelate with them, or even whether they consider them family. There is a wide gulf between American society and others in this regard. For example, in Western cultures our kinship terminology and the ensuing behavior are strongly determined by generation. We call relatives in our parents' generation uncle or aunt, and members of our own generation are referred to as cousins. Notice that in our parents' generation a clear distinction is made based on the gender of the relative, but no such distinction is made between kin in our own generation. The term "cousin" refers to both male and female relatives.

Given the independent function of the nuclear family in Western culture, the terms father, mother, brother, sister, son, daughter, husband, and wife serve as **descriptive terms**. They apply to one relationship only. In an extended family, the terms father, mother, son, daughter, brother, and sister are classificatory, referring to a whole class of relatives, very much like the Western terms "uncle," "aunt," and "cousin." In most of Africa and Asia, the term "Father" applies to a child's physical and social father, but also to Father's brothers and sometimes to Father's sister's husband and even to Father's father, the men we refer to as uncles and grandfather. The term "Mother" refers also to Mother's sisters, and often to Mother's brother's wife and Father's sisters as well. When a parent dies, or in cases of abandonment or divorce, the child has many other mothers and fathers to watch over him or her. Life in such cultures has much greater stability and continuity, not to mention the deep sense of belonging characteristic of those family constructs and the close involvement of relatives in the growth, care, and development of the child.

American genetic counselors may be confused by the way clients from other cultures characterize their family relationships, often attributing it to a lack of knowledge of the English language. This is not the case; rather, it is rooted in different ways of describing or referring to family relationships. Those kinship relations are of the utmost importance in analyzing a person's family history and genealogy. In addition, kinship relations affect people in every aspect of their daily lives: whom they befriend, whom they trust, with whom they enter into business deals, and even whom they should marry. In many cultures of the Middle East, for instance, there is a preference for a man to marry a "**parallel cousin**," that is, the daughter of Father's brother. In many other cultures of Africa and Asia, the preferred partner is the "**cross-cousin**": the son or daughter of Father's sister or Mother's brother. Therefore, it is important for a genetic counselor to ask pertinent questions about the exact nature of the kinship relations.

People also differ widely with regard to how they trace their descent from a real or assumed ancestor. In most cultures outside the United States, people trace their descent **unilineally**, that is, either through the father or the mother. Descent traced through the father is said to be **patrilineal**. Even our own society is predominantly patrilineal when it comes to family names. In other societies, descent is traced through the mother and is referred to as **matrilineal**. In both cases descent is described as unilineal, since only one parent is regarded as relevant for the purpose of descent. In many cases, a client from such cultures will not even recognize relatives from the other line of descent and will deny that they have any bearing on his or her physical constitution, family history, and genealogy. This is a crucial fact: Many a person considered a relative, even a close one, in our American culture is not considered a relative at all in other cultures and is therefore never mentioned or included in the family history or genealogy. It is a real challenge to work with a person who does not consider his or her patrilineal or matrilineal kinsmen part of the family important to the family history.

Critical Incident III

Sheeba is an 18-year-old female student from Southern Africa who for the last 10 years has been living in the United States with an aunt and uncle, to whom she refers as mother and father. A neurologist suggested genetic counseling because of a suspicion of limb-girdle muscular dystrophy. One of the counselor's first approaches was to obtain a family history. When the counselor tried to establish the number of males in Sheeba's maternal line of descent and the ages of her father and maternal grandmother, confusion arose, because Sheeba is part of a patri-clan that does not include her maternal relatives. Her mother's family was not even considered relatives, and no contact existed. She knew every person in her patri-clan, stayed with her father's brother and his wife, and had intensive contacts with other members of her clan, both in the U.S. and in Africa. Since family history and descent are crucial to an understanding of the possible genetic factors involved, the counselor was at a loss and turned to a colleague for help. What advice might you offer to help her with this situation?

(For a discussion of this incident, please turn to the Appendix: Responses to Critical Incidents.)

BELIEFS ABOUT THE CAUSES OF DISEASE AND DISORDERS

Cultures differ widely with regard to the way people view illness and interpret disorders. In the United States and much of the rest of the Western world, we interpret illness in terms of the scientific paradigm. Disabilities and disorders are caused by biophysical, chemical, and mechanical factors, such as viruses, bacteria, fungi, microbes, and mechanical failures, which can all be studied and manipulated by humans. According to this way of thinking, a clear cause-and-effect relationship exists between all natural phenomena. The processes involved can be observed, measured, and tested. This paradigm is referred to as the **biomedical model**. Although this model has spread around the world with Western culture, most non-Western cultures adhere to other views of illness and disorders, including the **holistic model** and the **magico-religious model**.

In the **holistic model**, people assume and seek to maintain a sense of balance or harmony between human beings and their physical, social, and spiritual environments. Rather than being caused by external physical or chemical agents, illnesses are seen and experienced as a brokenness in the harmony and balance between all things seen and unseen. Because humans are all considered part of and embedded in the totality of the surrounding environment, treatment targets the restoration of harmony. A powerful example of this holistic paradigm is the concept of **yin** and **yang** common in Chinese and other East and Southeast Asian cultures. These two forces are believed to dominate and influence every aspect of life. Illnesses and disorders are the result of too much influence by one or the other of these two forces. If a disease is the result of too much *yin*, it is referred to as a *yin*-disease; a *yang*-disease occurs because of an overabundance of *yang*. Examples of *yin*-diseases include cancer, pregnancy, postpartum depression, PMS, and any other disorder associated with the *yin* organs, such as the heart, the lungs, and the liver. *Yang* diseases are associated with the stomach or the intestines, and range from hypertension and toothache to constipation. The father of modern medicine, Hippocrates, was strongly influenced by this concept. His assistant and later successor, Dr. Galen (Dr. Galenus), adopted this way of perceiving illness and expanded it, using the terms **hot** and **cold** in place of *yin* and *yang*. Hot diseases and disorders included dysentery and sore throat; cold diseases included earache and rheumatism. From the ancient Greeks and Romans, this way of interpreting illness spread to the Arab peninsula. The Arabs carried it with them when they occupied Portugal and Spain. From there, the conquistadores brought the notion to Mexico and all of Inter- and South America. It eventually traveled on to the Philippines and other parts of Asia.

One of the problems encountered in multicultural genetic counseling is that each of the ethnocultural groups affected by this interpretation of illness have conflicting definitions of *hot* and *cold*. Pregnancy and certain genetic disorders may be considered *hot* in one culture but *cold* in another. If a condition is classified as *hot*, then the patient is expected to eat *cold* foods, engage in *cold* activities, and take *cold* medicines. If a condition is instead classified as *cold*, the opposite treatment is required: *warm* foods, treatments, and medication. It is really important for the genetic counselor to be aware of this way of thinking about illness, how it shapes the client's expectations of treatment, and how it affects the way he or she copes with it.

The **magico-religious** model is the most widespread of all paradigms of interpreting illness. In this paradigm, people see themselves and their environment surrounded, even dominated, by supernatural powers on whom they depend for daily life and existence and with whom they may have contact through meditation, prayer, dreams, and visions. As mentioned earlier in the chapter, according to this model diseases, disabilities, and disorders occur as a result of having sinned against God and are interpreted as either punishments or calls to repent and return to "the Straight Path." Illnesses also occur as a result of transgressing certain social and/or religious taboos, breaking of promises, infidelity, dishonesty, or simply having been too harsh toward a spouse or child. Other causes include the casting of spells, curses, or hexes. They can also be the result of the work of evil spirits, which, like the good ones, are all around us. The cause-and-effect relationship in these cases is not organic, but mystical. Keep in mind, however, that to believers it is no less real! Many deeply religious African Americans may be fully convinced that a particular illness or disorder comes as a punishment from God, and that it is He alone who can bring relief, healing, and the power to cope, often through fasting, prayer, sacrifices, and repentance. Many Latino American groups and scores of White-Anglo Christians hold similar views. It is interesting to note here that our English word *pain* is derived from a Greek term meaning *penalty*, a reminder of how for centuries people in the Judaeo-Christian West viewed the relationship between pain and illness and their relationship with God. The magico-religious belief system often coexists in combination with the other models, which may cause some confusion. A counselor may think that the client's responses and understanding are rooted in the biomedical model at the same time that clients are consulting with magico-religious healers: the *curandero* or *curandera* in the Mexican-American community; herbalists and *Suangi*-doctors in the Asian; and the *"Old Lady"* in African American communities.

Each paradigm greatly affects attitudes toward those suffering from certain disabilities and disorders. When birth defects are seen as a result of a curse or spell, caused by hex or witchcraft, or seen as a punishment for transgressions or sins, people tend to hold a very negative view of the affected individuals. In quite a number of cultures outside of North America and Europe it was not uncommon historically for such individuals to be isolated, ignored, or even killed. Even today, in many cultures they are often abandoned, neglected, or kept in extreme isolation. They are often considered a threat to the group and create fear, horror, and revulsion. Because disabilities and disorders in people holding magico-religious views also create a deep sense of *shame* among the relatives, children are often isolated from the rest of the family and hidden from public view. Not until an emergency arises will these disorders be reported to professionals, delaying people from procuring much-needed help, often until it is too late.

To prevent birth defects and disorders from happening, all cultures have developed a host of taboos and an elaborate body of treatment practices and remedies that are handed down from one generation to the next. Many clients from non-Western cultures will first try those practices and remedies before seeking professional advice. Such practices and taboos are especially elaborate for pregnant women and their immediate relatives. Pregnant women cannot go out—or must go out—in the full moon light; they cannot eat certain kinds of food or must eat specially prepared meals. The variations seem endless, and the prescribed or proscribed practices relate to every aspect of life, including bathing, travel, sexual relations, and language. Each of these beliefs in its own way offers comfort, support, and the ability to cope.

Suggested approaches to clients/individuals and families with holistic or magico-religious interpretations of disease include the following:

1. *Recognize* the existence of these models and how they shape the clients' understanding of illness.
2. *Develop* the ability to use these interpretations, including words and concepts, in the process of counseling.
3. *Combine* aspects of these models by stressing the overlap between them, emphasizing their positive and helpful aspects, and considering what each can contribute (synergy) to the solution or the strategy to follow.

Critical Incident IV

Mrs. Lopez, a 34-year-old Mexican-American woman, brings in her 7-year-old daughter, who is suffering from seizures. These are commonly preceded by feelings of confusion, dry mouth, and difficulty in breathing.

The counselor notices that the child is wearing a rather tight red cord around her belly. When asked what it is for, the mother indicates it is to ward off the "Evil Eye," which she suspects is the cause of her daughter's problems. Her *curandera* had suggested her daughter wear this cord, but so far it has provided no relief. What should the counselor do now?

(For a discussion of this incident, please turn to Appendix: Responses to Critical Incidents).

COMMUNICATING ACROSS CULTURAL BOUNDARIES

A common working definition of **communication** in the United States is *the sharing of messages with the least possible distortions.* Such distortions, of course, are inevitable, given certain differences in age and gender, education and socioeconomic background, personal experience, religion, and personality between sender and receiver (Fig. 11-1). In fact, research has confirmed over and over again (Jarndt, 1999) that only about 55–60% of all communication is effective when taking place between

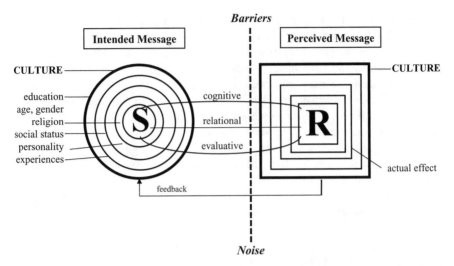

FIGURE 11-1. *Communicating across cultural boundaries. Important factors in cross-cultural communication between a Sender (S) and a Receiver (R) are illustrated. For each party there are multiple layers that impact the ability to both transmit and receive communication messages. These are illustrated by the outer shells and are the same for both parties*

people from the same cultural background. This means that about 40–45% of all communication between counselor and client is unsuccessful. When the client and the counselor come from different cultural backgrounds, that percentage drops to only 20–25%.

In the case of health care and genetic counseling this means that as many as four out of five communications may be unsuccessful, which can be disastrous. The good news is that it is possible to learn to communicate across cultural boundaries and develop skills that can raise this percentage to 60% or even 70%—remember, culture is learned behavior! What is needed to develop such skills are insight into and understanding of the ways people from diverse cultures communicate, recognition of the obstacles, and learning how to overcome them.

A host of factors needs to be considered:

- How do you greet and address each other—formally or informally, by first name or family name, looking each other in the eye or not?
- What kind of relationship is expected between the client and the counselor: paternalistic and hierarchical, or a more equal partnership?
- When listening, is it acceptable to interrupt?
- What types of questions are culturally inappropriate?
- How much time is available for the various activities that make up the process of counseling?

All of these issues are very different from one culture to another. What is appropriate or respectful in one culture may be offensive in another.

In Western culture, eye contact between counselor and client is expected. Avoiding eye contact is not only interpreted as impoliteness or rudeness, but signals distrust or even deception. In many other cultures, however, a woman or a younger person is prohibited from looking a man, older person, or person of authority in the eye. To do so would be highly improper, even insulting. In such cases not looking a counselor in the eye may be considered a sign of respect and recognition of authority. In some cultures, people keep a distance of at least 25–30 inches between them when interacting. In others the distance is even greater. Yet people from many Arab cultures are known to prefer standing toe-to-toe or nose-to-nose, which in the United States is an invasion of privacy and "personal space" that is considered rude and unpleasant. For these and many other reasons, counselors working with clients from diverse cultures need to develop skills in communicating across cultural boundaries.

Three Levels of Communication

Communication takes place on at least three different levels: the **cognitive level**, the **relational level**, and the **evaluative level**. In U.S. culture, most communication takes place on the **cognitive level**. It is primarily verbal, uses rational arguments, is based on facts, and appeals to people's understanding and mental assent (cognition). The *goal* of such communication is "sharing information," "getting the message across," or "making a point." This shapes the whole process of communication throughout American culture, whether it be in education, business, or counseling. In most other cultures, however, especially those of Latin America, Africa, and Asia, communication takes place primarily on the relational and evaluative levels (Fig. 11-1).

The **evaluative level** of communication refers to the way in which clients evaluate the counselor (first impressions): her expertise, trustworthiness, and reliability. They do so based on the way we dress, behave, show deference, and exhibit cultural sensitivity and a sense of humility. Clients may value formal dress and behavior, poise and posture, where we sit or stand, how we arrange our office furniture, and social distance as highly as they value our knowledge and understanding. The *goal* of communication at the **relational level** is not to inform but to establish a communion (from which the English term *communication* is itself derived!). Its purpose is to create or affirm a bond. As many cultures in Africa and Asia put it, the aim of all communication is to create a harmonious relationship between two or more people. Information certainly flows and knowledge is indeed shared in this process, but only as part of and embedded in a harmonious relationship. To create such a personal bond, speaking the truth is avoided or used only in the most euphemistic terms. Because the goal is a warm interpersonal relationship, unpleasant messages are avoided. As American counselors, people using another cultural code can interpret communication that we consider professional and efficient as harsh, cold, and uncaring. Our typical values of information sharing, speaking the truth, individualism, and time and task orientation clash with the Mexican client's values of *personalismo* and **relationship building**, with the Filipino's value of *pakikisama*, and with the Chinese notion of *guanxi*, all of which refer to the building of a warm and personal and harmonious relationship that serves as the very core of all effective communication. That is why even the best traditional American counseling skills and techniques are often ineffective.

How do people cease being strangers so that information may flow leading to understanding? Consider the following:

- Avoid addressing people from the more formally and hierarchically organized cultures by their first names. Address them by their family names, or simply ask them how they would like to be addressed. Remember that in non-Western cultures, names symbolize character, personhood, identity, and personality. Pronouncing names correctly and remembering them from session to session are also of vital importance.

- Before you begin your session, consider sharing some drink or food with your clients. As already discussed, there is no better way in many cultures, whether Mexican, Middle Eastern, African, or Asian, to create or affirm a relationship. As people in Indonesia express it, *"Tidak ada makanan, tidak ada bitjara"* (No food, no talk). When in the more formal institutional setting of a hospital or a medical center, at least offer water or coffee.

- Spend time (perhaps the greatest challenge in our time and task-oriented culture) sharing information about your family, personal interests, issues of concern, etc. The showing of pictures is often appreciated. Ask questions such as, "How long have you been in this country?" "What has been your experience so far?" etc. In American culture counselors often use professional "small talk" as an ice-breaker. The difference is that we consider it "small talk" and an "icebreaker," while others experience this personal sharing as an essential part of effective communication.

Context of Communication

Different **cultural contexts** shape communication modes and styles, forms and patterns. American culture is considered a **low-context culture**. We share this context with the cultures of Northern and Western Europe, Canada, and Australia. However, most immigrant clients come from **high-context cultures**. The use of "high" and "low" does not imply superiority or inferiority. Rather, in low-context cultures, communication is direct and to the point; brief and focused. We use few words, carefully chosen, with definite meanings, and avoid lengthy detours. As the Dutch say, "Anything worth saying can be said short." In contrast, communication in high-context cultures is indirect and implicit. People talk around the subject and embellish the point; this style of communication uses lengthy explanations and employs parables and stories to get the point across. The use of words is an art form aimed at establishing a relationship. It is through parables and stories rather than analysis that they deliver the message. Still, it is not the message itself that is the most important, it is engaging the other person(s) and developing a relationship. Often, therefore, the parables and stories seem on the surface to have little or nothing to do with the topics or issues at hand. A short and pointed question from the counselor on family history or kinship relation may lead to very elaborate stories about events in the lives of the people concerned, and may branch off to include stories about goats or excursions into love affairs. The American counselor needs to resist the idea that the client is "beating around the bush," "stalling," "unwilling to share the truth," "rude," or even engaging in passive resistance. People from high-context cultures who communicate through parables and stories are inclusivistic and holistic, and may therefore come across to the American counselor as "unfocused" and "indirect." The danger is that the American counselor may label this kind of communication "childish" and the behavior associated with it "abnormal." Indeed, the style of communication of people from high-context cultures is very much like the way children in our Western cultures communicate. Other people's use of language may prevent them from being analytical and using abstract reasoning, yet there is nothing about this way of communicating that is childish or abnormal. Such thinking can lead to wrong diagnoses and false interpretations of people's abilities.

One final word about high context and low context: We have used the terms here to refer to cultures as a whole. By extension, they also can be used for individual persons. It is well known that there are high-context *people* in every low-context culture, and vice versa.

Modes of Communication and the Meaning of Words

Every culture has developed its own **mode** of communication: when to listen and when to speak, when to raise your voice (and when not to), when to interrupt, use gestures, show passion, or take sides. In most low-context cultures, people are expected to be low-key, dispassionate, and devoid of affect. They are expected to tell the truth as they see it, no matter what, and to be objective and stay calm, controlled, and nonchallenging. Compare this with the African American mode of communication. In this rather high-context culture within the larger low-context culture of America as a whole, communication is dynamic and dramatic, expressive and self-assertive. People communicate with passion, emotion and affection; show great care and concern; and are person-oriented, spontaneous, and even demonstrative (Kochman, 1981). For a host of historical and cultural reasons, African Americans often find requests for personal information intrusive, considering it an invasion of privacy, excessively personal, and even threatening. Low-context and low-key white Americans, on the other hand, do not experience requests for personal information in this way. They discuss their personal lives and family history freely, and even show a willingness to be vulnerable. In many other cultures, questions about private and personal matters cannot be asked directly. They can be elicited only through story telling, the use of parables, and comparisons with similar family histories. In addition, since many high-context cultures attach great value to reciprocity, counselors should consider the impact on their communication when they share some of their own personal and family issues with disease and disabilities.

Because of their different goal orientations, levels of communication, and use of words, high-context cultures and low-context cultures attach different values and a host of different meanings to individual words. For example, the term "boy" has different meanings to white Americans and African Americans. The same is true for a host of other terms. We have already described cultural differences in the meaning of the words "brother" and "sister." The term "blood" is another example. In some cultures, blood may refer to a reddish substance that circulates through our arteries and veins, as well as to certain relationships between people. In many African and Asian cultures, "blood" represents a person's soul, and denotes character, life, personhood, identity, living being, etc. Blood transfusions and giving blood may be rejected in such cultures because of this association.

These different meanings of words, which make all dictionaries "liars," apply to everyday living: food, clothing, colors, and even numbers. For example, in Chinese culture the number four is associated with death. No counseling or caregiving of a person with this belief should ever take place in a room with the number four or forty-four. In mainstream American culture, the color white stands for purity and cleanliness, innocence, and holiness, but it should be obvious that a white room is not a conducive environment for effective counseling of people from cultures where white is the color of death. In some cultures, the color red is associated with evil, sin, disease, anger, and pain. A number of U.S. hospitals have clearly recognized the significance of these beliefs and are accommodating them by avoiding the use of white personnel coats and by changing bed sheets from white to pastel colors.

No Communication without Identification

There is no better way of developing the personal relationship required for effective communication in cross-cultural counseling than identification. Identification with a client can be defined as the willingness to put yourself in your clients' shoes and walk in them for awhile. This process emphasizes the recognition of underlying common values, is based on empathy and a deep understanding of the client's cultural code, recognizes some clear absolutes, is undertaken for the sake of helping others, and puts the client's needs first. At the same time, the counselor remains true to his or her own cultural and personal values. All of this presupposes the counselor's willingness, as it contradicts the traditional American practice of keeping a certain distance between counselor and client for the sake of professionalism and maintaining a sense of objectivity. The emphasis should still be on "information exchange," communication of professional knowledge, using the right kind of tools and techniques. But in many counseling situations with clients from other cultures, the goals of effective counseling—client satisfaction, level of trust, knowledge, understanding, and effective communication—depend on the counselor's ability to establish a warm and personal relationship.

Many clients from other cultures, confronted with specific disorders and disabilities, suffer from intense feelings of shame and mental anguish for having done something wrong in the eyes of God or the gods or the ancestors, and from being isolated from their own communities. Here, identification means not only empathy and understanding, but the ability to use people's own ways of understanding of the issues to help clarify them and use their own particular methods of dealing and coping with them. All of this requires knowledge about the client's culture, the cultural code that shapes his or her behavior and way of thinking, and a deep sense of humility that recognizes the value of other people's ways. The idea that *there truly is no communication without identification* is an especially powerful sine qua non in the setting of genetic counseling with people from other cultures.

In no way does this mean that counselors must give up their own values, concepts, and ideals, or compromise facts or the truth in any way. What it does mean is that the client can hear the facts, experience the truth, and develop understanding in terms appropriate to his or her own culture.

Great communicators always identify with the needs and interests of others. The most effective approach to genetic counseling across the boundaries of culture is therefore best accomplished through *identification*. Cross-cultural competency in counseling reaches its peak when a counselor knows and understands the client's culture; is able to use his or her cultural values as a resource; and approaches the task with a sense of humility.

CONCLUSION

The purpose of this chapter was to make you more aware of the challenges that increasing ethnicity and cultural and religious diversity present for the profession of genetic counseling. One important consideration is that diversity is not biophysical but cultural. It is not rooted in externals such as skin color or head size or hair texture, but in people's values, assumptions, and beliefs, collectively referred to as the cultural code. Because culture is acquired, other people's cultural values and assumptions can be learned and shared to develop a genuine process of cross-cultural genetic counseling.

There is more than one effective method of cross-cultural genetic counseling. Many of the tools, techniques, modes, and methods used depend on the cultural background of the participants in the process. If different ways of thinking are viewed as complementary rather than contradictory, it leads to greater creativity in professional genetic counseling. Counseling truly becomes "patient-centered," not "disease-centered."

Finally, every culture has its own way of communicating. This is a particular challenge for the professional genetic counselor, whose effectiveness depends largely on the ability to communicate effectively. New skills of communication may need to be developed to enable counselor and patient to communicate on more than one level, in a variety of contexts, and in different modes and styles.

The United States is and will continue to be a multiethnic and multicultural society. This means that the need for multicultural counseling will only increase. Much research still needs to be done with regard to specific populations, both in the area of genetics and multicultural genetic counseling, but great strides have been made in increasing our understanding of and appreciation for different ways of looking at the science of genetic counseling.

APPENDIX: RESPONSES TO CRITICAL INCIDENTS

Critical Incident I

Islam considers the pig an unclean animal. Therefore, Muslims do not eat pork, nor can they use anything made from pigs. In the minds of many Muslims, insulin is still being made from the pancreas of a pig, hence the refusal to take this medication.

Muslims believe that newly born children are the result of a combination of human and divine action. A hundred and twenty days after conception, Allah, the Beneficent, the Merciful, breathes His Spirit—*Ruh Allah*—into the fetus, which thereby becomes a living human being, with specific rights and obligations. At death, the process is reversed. Then Allah sends His angel Israeel to assist the dying person in separating his spirit from the body, which returns to Earth, ashes and dust, waiting for that glorious day of the resurrection and the judgment. Sometimes Allah is believed to take a person's spirit away, but leave the body still alive and well on Earth, resulting in Alzheimer disease, or dementia. This belief is especially powerful in Muslim North Africa. People refer to such a person as *"Baraqa,"* a blessing, or, a "Blessed One." Every one who takes care of such a *"Baraqa"* shares in the blessings that Allah has in store for them. The disease is not seen as a curse, as in our Western culture. It is experienced as a blessing and an honor, and demands respect and rejoicing.

Awareness of this thinking can explain the family's behavior and would result in different ways of approaching them.

Critical Incident II

People in many cultures, including the Chinese, are convinced that intercultural and interracial marriages are wrong, may cause harm, and should be avoided. This is the first rule Ming ignored. In addition, instead of honoring her father and mother (filial piety), she chose her own way, another potential cause of trouble or damage.

The *feng shui* calendar is of great help to the Chinese in their every day decision-making. It spells out clearly which days and hours are good for travel and moving and which are not; which days and hours of the day are good for weddings and sexual relations, to do business and banking, to take care of your health or to make changes in your life. In existence for thousands of years, this calendar still influences the thinking and practices of modern Chinese people. Because Ming had ignored the wisdom of the ages and made her own arrangements, she is very worried about all the potential harm that could have come from it, especially threatening the health of her baby.

Pregnancy and birth are still shrouded in mystery, even among educated Chinese, and therefore involve a host of practices and beliefs. Ming had ignored all of these, giving her another cause for worry.

According to cultural convention, asking forgiveness from and seeking reconciliation with her parents is the first step Ming may have to take. Second, Ming may want to begin to follow traditional Chinese practices to avoid further harm and to give her peace of mind. The counselor should affirm that all things seem well so far, and that, based on physical evidence, no disorders have been detected. Finally, the husband may need to be reminded that one person's superstition is another person's faith.

Critical Incident III

The issue of descent needs to be discussed from both a social and cultural perspective and a biophysical perspective. You might encourage your colleague to first discuss the nature of patrilineal and matrilineal kinship groups, and how people from each relate to other members, perhaps using a pedigree diagram to show patterns of biological inheritance. Once Sheeba sees her relationships in graphic form, she may better understand the issue and be able to supply names and relationships of members of her matri-clan. Then her (classificatory) father and mother will need to be consulted to fill in the gaps so that pertinent family members can be contacted for further information.

Critical Incident IV

The "Evil Eye" is believed to cause considerable harm, primarily among the unborn and younger children, but also among adults. This notion is widespread from Haiti and Mexico throughout Latin America, but is also seen in various forms throughout the cultures of the Mediterranean, Eastern Europe, and Russia, as well as in many parts of Africa and Asia.

The "Evil Eye" is believed to be caused by a hex or spell, created by staring at people and complimenting or flattering them excessively. Symptoms include intestinal problems, aches and pains, fevers, and, in Mexico, *empacho*, the adhesion of food to the stomach wall, which requires surgical removal. The unborn are believed to be threatened by disorders and deformities of a more serious kind. To ward off the effects of the "Evil Eye" pregnant women and younger children will wear protective cords and/or amulets of various kinds.

The counselor may want to start a discussion of the "Evil Eye" to discover the strength of the client's belief, which varies greatly from person to person. Then, with sensitivity and cultural understanding, the counselor may use the synergy of the magico-religious model and the biophysical model to help the client grow in her understanding of the issues involved.

REFERENCES

Andrews MM, Boyle J (1995) *Transcultural Concepts in Nursing Care* (2nd ed.). Philadelphia, PA: J.P. Lippincott.

Bellah R et al. (1986) *Habits of the Heart: Individualism and Commitment in American Life.* New York: Harper and Row.

Bureau of the Census: (2005–2006) *Reports 2005; 2006.* Washington DC: Department of Commerce.

Helman CG (1994) *Culture, Health and Illness* (3rd ed.) Oxford/London: Butterworth Heineman.

Hofstede G (1980) *Culture's Consequences: International Differences in Work Related Values*. Beverly Hills, CA: Sage Publications.

Jarndt FE (1999) *Intercultural Communication: An Introduction*. Thousand Oaks, CA: Sage Publications.

Kochman T (1981) *Black and White Styles in Conflict*. Chicago, IL: University of Chicago Press.

Kroeber AL, Kluckhohn C (1952) *Culture: A Critical Review of Concepts and Definitions*. New York: Random House.

McCarthy Veach Pm, LeRoy BS, Bartels DM (2003) *Facilitating the Genetic Counseling Process: A Practice Manual*. New York: Springer.

McGoldrick M, Pearce JK, Giordano J (eds) (1982) *Ethnicity and Family Therapy*. New York: Guilford.

Mead M (1955) *Sex and Temperament in Three Primitive Societies*. New York: Mentor.

Oosterwal G (1961) *People of the Tor*. Assen: Van Gorcum.

Oosterwal G (1997) *Community in Diversity*. Berrien Springs, MI: Center for Intercultural Relations.

Oosterwal G (2005) *Managing the Multicultural Work Place: the Case of Health Care*. Berrien Springs, MI: Center for Intercultural Relations.

Ponterotto JG et al. (1995) *Handbook of Multicultural Counseling*. Thousand Oaks, CA: SAGE Publications, Inc.

Schlesinger A (1992) *The Disuniting of America: Reflections on a Multicultural Society*. New York: W.W. Norton.

Stewart EC, Bennett MJ (1991) *American Cultural Patterns: A Cross-Cultural Perspective* (rev. ed.). Yarmouth, ME: Intercultural Press.

Thompson M, Ellis R, Wildavsky A (1990) *Cultural Theory*. Boulder, CO: Westview.

FURTHER READING

There are multiple excellent handbooks that address specific issues in varied population groups, cultures and religions. Some are listed below. The *Journal of Multicultural Counseling and Development* is also a useful resource.

DeGenova MK (1996) *Families in Cultural Contexts: Strengths and Challenges in Diversity*. Mountain View, CA: Mayfield Publishing.

Fisher NL (1996) *Cultural and Ethnic Diversity: A Guide for Genetic Professionals*. Baltimore: Johns Hopkins University Press.

Foster GM, Anderson BG (1978) *Medical Anthropology*. New York: John Wiley & Sons.

Galanti GA (1991) *Caring for Patients from Different Cultures: Case Studies from American Hospitals*. Philadelphia, PA: University of Pennsylvania Press.

Gropper, RC (1996) *Culture and the Clinical Encounter: An Intercultural Sensitizer for the Health Professions*. Yarmouth, ME: Intercultural Press.

Hahn RA (1995) *Sickness and Healing: An Anthropological Perspective*. New Haven, CT: Yale University Press.

Kleinman, A. (1980) *Patients and Healers in the Context of Culture*; Berkeley, CA; University of California Press.

Krebs GL, Kunimoto EN (1994) *Effective Communication in Multicultural Health Care Settings.* Thousand Oaks, CA: Sage Publications.

Landy D (1977) *Culture, Disease and Healing.* New York: MacMillan.

Lassiter SM (1995) *Multicultural Clients: A Professional Handbook for Health Care Providers and Social Workers.* Westport, CT: Greenwood Press.

Lipson JC, Dibble SC, Minarik PA (1996) *Culture and Nursing Care.* San Francisco; University of California, School of Nursing Press.

MacCormack CP (1982) *Ethnography of Fertility and Birth.* New York: Academic Press.

Parry JK (1995) *A Cross-Cultural Look at Death, Dying and Religion.* Chicago: Nelson-Hall.

Payer L (1989) *Medicine and Culture.* New York: Henry Holt.

Pedersen P (1994) *A Handbook of Developing Multicultural Awareness* (2nd ed.). Alexandria, VA: American Counseling Association.

Rice PL (1999) *Asian Mothers, Western Births* (new ed.). Melbourne: Ausmed Publications.

Spector RE (1996) *Cultural Diversity in Health and Illness* (4th ed.). Stanford, CT: Appleton and Lange.

Stacey M. (1988) *The Sociology of Health and Healing.* London; Unwin, Hyman.

Sue DW, Sue D (1990) *Counseling the Culturally Different: Theory and Practice* (2nd ed.). New York: John Wiley & Sons.

Wiseman RL, Koester J (eds.) (1993) *Intercultural Communication Competence.* Newbury Park, CA: Sage Publications.

12

Ethical and Legal Issues

Susan Schmerler, M.S., C.G.C., J.D.

Case 1: *When he was about age 32 years, people noticed that Mr. Franks seemed to be short-tempered more often than his usual easy-going self. He was having problems with his short-term memory, and he had problems doing complex tasks. His handwriting deteriorated, he began to drop things, and he frequently tripped while walking. His father was diagnosed with HD on an autopsy. Mrs. Franks, his ex-wife, has an appointment with a genetic counselor to discuss HD in general and the risks for her children (ages 17, 13, and 10) in particular. She is worried about their futures and wants the children tested for HD.*

The issues raised by Mrs. Franks' request are both ethical and legal. They have implications for the children, for Mr. Franks, and for the genetic counselor. For the children, the autonomy of each child, the questions of presymptomatic testing and testing children for adult-onset disorders, the age of consent, and the need for assent are raised. Mr. Franks' privacy, confidentiality, and autonomy are impacted. For the genetic counselor and/or the genetics clinic, defining who is the patient and whether there is a duty to warn are among the questions to be addressed. As we discuss ethical and legal issues for genetic counselors in general, other questions will apply to this case and other genetic counseling situations.

A basic knowledge of ethical theory and principles and an understanding of the law are important in a profession that deals with problems at the cutting edge of science. In this chapter, we look at ethical and legal issues that impact genetic counseling. It is to some extent artificial to address these areas separately, since for

A Guide to Genetic Counseling, Second Edition, Edited by Wendy Uhlmann, Jane Schuette, and Beverly Yashar
Copyright © 2009 by John Wiley & Sons, Inc.

each section of text there is a relationship, a common source, and much overlap with the material in other sections. Because many ethical and legal concepts are complex and easily misunderstood, we will be defining terms throughout this chapter.

It has become tradition in ethics and legal literature to use the feminine pronoun. We continue that tradition here.

ETHICAL ISSUES

Why Study Ethics?

Theoretical ethics does not occupy us on a day-to-day basis. On a personal level, for an individual whose behavior is usually moral, or socially acceptable, the choices she makes are automatic. At times in our personal and professional lives, however, we are unsure how to respond to a situation. There are also situations in which an otherwise moral person may not have the motivation to do the morally right thing. The guidance of rules at these times helps in making the moral choice. An understanding of the source of the rules of conduct may be of value for a more complicated situation.

What Is Moral Behavior?

A society is a community of people that has a common code of conduct, an agreed-upon view of what is acceptable behavior and what behavior is not acceptable. This is what is called morality. There are, for example, certain kinds of behavior that everyone agrees are immoral, and therefore not acceptable, such as killing, imprisoning, and deception. In certain situations, however, society can justify such basically repugnant actions. For example, killing in self-defense is generally deemed justifiable. The sum of this "agreed-upon" conduct makes up a common morality. The goal of moral behavior is to decrease the harms suffered by members of society. Moral convictions, then, provide a standard by which to evaluate our own and other people's conduct and character.

What Is Ethics?

The science of ethics is applied to help us understand the basic themes underlying and governing society's moral behavior. Theories are derived to account for, organize, and explain the themes that are identified, and to place them within a framework that allows rules of conduct to be developed. Ethics, then, is the establishment of a set of guidelines for morally acceptable conduct within a theoretical framework. The particular theory offered usually allows for continuing review of the basis for or justification of any conduct.

Ethical theories use terms that have uniformly accepted definitions. The **principles** offered within a theory are the source of the guidelines for behavior. For example, the principle of nonmaleficence is the source of the guideline "do no harm" among heath care professionals. From principles, values are drawn and rules developed. **Values** are qualities that are considered good or priorities, and are desirable and important. **Rules** are specific guides, and they must be followed at all times. They can be looked at as controls that prohibit or prevent harm. For example, directly causing any of the following harms is prohibited: killing, causing pain, disabling, depriving of freedom, and depriving of pleasure in certain nontrivial situations. To prevent harm, we must follow the rules to keep promises, to obey the law, to do our duty, and to refrain from cheating and practicing other forms of deception. Rules promote and protect basic human interests, both individual and societal. Not obeying a rule usually results in some punishment.

Behaviors that are encouraged by society are said to be the embodiment of **ideals**, or goals to which we should aspire. Not achieving an ideal, or even attempting to achieve it, is not punishable conduct. **Duties** are defined by a person's role in society. They can be, for example, social or professional, and they include behaviors that are required of the person by that role. **Virtues** are characteristics of an individual that are morally desirable (e.g., candor, faithfulness, integrity). **Rights** are justified claims that individuals or groups can make on others or on society. Along with rights must come responsibilities on the part of the individual and obligations on the part of society or other individuals. For example, my right to move about freely obligates you not to unjustifiably block my way. I also have a responsibility to move about only in my own or in public spaces, and to not invade your space.

In summary:

- *Principles* are sources, or guides, for values, rules, duties, and rights.
- *Values* are priorities that are thought to be important and desirable.
- *Rules* are specific guidelines of what should (or should not) be done.
- *Ideals* are goals to which we aspire.
- *Duties* are behaviors that are defined by our professional or social role.
- *Virtues* are morally and socially desirable characteristics.
- *Rights* are justified claims.

Depending on which theory is proposed, the same behavior can be a principle, a value, or an obligation. Trust is a good example. Trust is considered by some to be the overriding principle in medicine. It is also a value derived from the principle of respect for autonomy. Trust is the basis of the provider-patient relation and an obligation derived from the fiduciary (i.e., the confidential or trusting) nature of the doctor-patient relationship.

Ethical dilemmas occur when equally strong arguments exist to justify the application of more than one theory or principle to a situation. To help clarify what appears to be a complicated problem, ethical theories can be applied to organize our thinking about the various choices in a difficult predicament. This is called moral reasoning. Ethical theories provide a structure for case analysis. Disagreements that involve the facts of a case can be separated from those that involve either a difference in the weighting or ranking of the benefits and harms found in the case or an equal weighing of different principles as defined in the case. We will discuss later how the process of moral reasoning can be applied to genetic counseling cases and can be used to derive an ethically justifiable course of action with respect to a particular situation.

Ethical Theories

Theorists have developed many strategies in an attempt to understand moral behavior. Each theory has had its supporters and detractors. There is no one ideal theory. The various theories are not necessarily mutually exclusive. Some modern writers look to more than one theory to provide a comprehensive framework for understanding and directing behavior.

Several theories have had an impact on modern medicine. **Consequence-based utilitarianism** is prominent in medical ethics. The primary focus of this theory is the promotion of happiness. Actions that maximize good and promote the greatest amount of happiness over pain are "right" or acceptable actions. An ethical dilemma is resolved by looking at the consequences of doing or of not doing an action. **Virtue ethics** and **principle-based ethics** have also had a great influence on medicine. The virtue-based theory of ethics focuses on those character traits or virtues a good person should have. Since a person with such traits will naturally act in a morally acceptable way, there should be no need to dictate conduct in a particular situation or to establish general moral rules to determine acceptable conduct. An ethical dilemma is resolved by asking how a virtuous person would act in that situation. Principle-based ethics emphasizes the role of moral reasoning and analysis in ethical decision-making. The core principles of autonomy, beneficence, nonmaleficence, and justice clarify moral duties and obligations. An ethical dilemma is addressed by weighing competing principles, duties, and values. When applied in medicine, these theories are clinician-oriented. A more recent contribution to theoretical ethics is the **ethic of care**. The focus of care ethics is the maintenance and enhancement of caring while conserving the traditional values of other ethical theories. Care ethics is focused on the humanistic virtues, those characteristics that are valued in interactive, intimate relationships. Ethical dilemmas are addressed by promoting respect for equality while at the same time recognizing and valuing differences.

Theoretical Influences on Genetic Counseling

The profession of genetic counseling has developed within the medical model, and has been influenced by the ethical and moral positions of medicine. It has also been shaped by the individuals who have chosen to practice in the field and who view themselves in the context of their relationships. We can gain a greater understanding of the ethical standards that have thus emerged in genetic counseling by more closely examining two theories: the ethic of care and principle-based ethics.

Ethic of Care Humanistic virtues, those that are valued in relationships, are the basis of care ethics. These include in part sympathy, compassion, fidelity, discernment, and love. The source of this ethic comes from natural human caring. The ethic of care is based on interpersonal relations, with mutual interdependence and emotional response emphasized. "Care" in this context is the care for, emotional commitment to, and the willingness to act on behalf of those with whom one has a significant relationship. It involves insight into and understanding of someone else's circumstances, needs and feelings, and a responsiveness to that person's needs as she defines them for herself.

Care ethics is often termed feminine ethics because it emphasizes receptivity, relatedness, and responsiveness, as opposed to logic. The elements of care include relations, attention, compassion, fulfilling the needs of others, and helping others to grow as caring individuals. Attachment is the standard for an ethic of care. Reasoning within the ethic of care framework depends on an understanding as opposed to a knowing, with a focus on relationships. It necessitates attention to context and interrelatedness.

The ethic of care perspective is especially meaningful for the role of a genetic counselor. It is a bilateral theory, involving the relationship of two individuals, with the focus being on the relationship.

Principle-Based Ethics   The study of what is right and what is wrong morally in the practice of medicine has evolved into the field of biomedical ethics. Broadly, this has meant a study of the ethics of the life sciences and healthcare. In a more narrow sense, medical ethics is the code of conduct followed by the medical profession. Beginning with the Hippocratic school, the ethics of medicine has been influenced by virtue- or character-based ethics. In modern times, guidelines derived from principle-based ethics have been used in medical case analysis. The principles of beneficence, nonmaleficence, autonomy, and justice are used to frame the guidelines of this ethical theory.

The role of a healthcare provider (whether a physician or a counselor) defines the duties of that practitioner. The specific duties can come from the employer, the profession, and/or the expectations of society. From these duties are derived the rights of patients and the obligations of the professional. The rules and obligations described below have been organized under one principle only. This is done only for practical purposes. Clearly, the same rules can be supported by different principles, and the same obligations can be derived from more than one principle.

Beneficence   Beneficence is the promotion of personal well-being in others. The type of conduct derived from this principle is positive: We should do good or prevent harm. When benefits are balanced against harms and costs, the outcome should be a net benefit. This principle applies in a society in which one has some discretion in defining one's contribution to the general welfare. It applies specifically in case-related situations, in which the provider and the patient are assumed to have similar values and views of what constitutes a benefit.

Professionally, beneficence requires that the healthcare provider be a trustee of the patient's welfare. The provider-patient relationship is founded on trust or confidence. The provider is an advocate for the patient, acting in good faith for the benefit of that patient. The fiduciary relationship thus constituted requires honesty and fidelity.

Fidelity requires the provider not to withdraw from a patient's care without notice to the patient, to submerge her own self-interests if they are in conflict with the patient's interests, and to put the patient's healthcare interests first. The virtues of candor, loyalty, and integrity are derived from this principle.

Beneficence can sometimes be interpreted as paternalism when, for example, the professional's perception of her duty of beneficence toward the patient and her definition of the limits of the patient's autonomy do not agree with the views of the patient. The refusal by the professional to acquiesce in the patient's wishes, choices, or actions can result in the neglect and violation of the patient's autonomy. In the extreme, paternalism is the opposite of the principle of respect for autonomy. In an emergency situation, however, paternalism is often considered to be justified.

Nonmaleficence   Nonmaleficence, which involves restrictions on behavior as opposed to actions that promote behavior, is framed in negative terms: Do no harm. The rule that we should not inflict harm applies to all the people in our society. "Thou shall not kill" is a moral rule derived from this principle.

Nonmaleficence can be seen as an obligation encompassed by or derived from the principle of beneficence. The ethical issues raised by the use of people as subjects in research or for testing experimental therapies are not uncommon in genetics. Because those issues fall in part under the rules derived from nonmaleficence, it is listed separately here as a principle.

Autonomy   Respect for autonomy is based on the recognition of the intrinsic value of each individual, that person's capacities, and her point of view. It represents the individual's personal rule of self, the need to remain free from controlling interference that may prevent an individual's making of meaningful choices. In medicine, the respect for autonomy is especially evident in the patient's right to decide what will be done to her own body. There are values and obligations derived from this principle, and there are applications of the principle that are relevant both to the healthcare provider and to the patient. We turn now to some of the important obligations derived from the respect for autonomy that are relevant to genetic counseling: truth telling, confidentiality, and informed consent.

TRUTH TELLING   Respect for others requires telling the truth. Both lying and inadequate disclosure show disrespect for other people and threaten any fiduciary relationship. They can add to a patient's reluctance to be honest with the provider or to seek help in the future. Adherence to the rule of veracity is essential for fostering trust in the medical setting. Truth telling is related to the obligations of fidelity and promise keeping that are inherent in the medical relationship. Truth telling also pertains to the management of information that could affect a person's understanding or decision-making. Shielding a patient from the truth is a form of paternalism. Valid consent depends on truthful communication.

The patient also has an obligation to be truthful: She is expected to cooperate in her own care by providing an honest and complete history. She has a duty to inform the healthcare provider of any important issues and to make it known whether she has a clear understanding of the material presented by the provider.

CONFIDENTIALITY   Confidentiality relates not only to the communication between people, but to the fact that a relationship exists between them. In a fiduciary (designating a trust) relationship, any communication that is intended to be kept secret is classified as confidential. A relationship with a genetic counselor or other healthcare provider is a confidential relation. It is dependent on trust. The patient relies on the discretion of the counselor.

It is a goal of society to maintain the public health. It is in the public interest for people to seek and obtain healthcare. Much of medicine involves the individual's having to reveal personal, intimate information. Without access to such information, a provider cannot effectively help the patient. Thus the patient must be able to trust the provider to respect her privacy and the confidentiality of their relationship, which in turn implies the obligation not to share any information without her consent. The patient does not have to ask to have the information kept confidential, because confidentiality is the standard of care. Any breach is a violation of the duty of fidelity. If a practitioner has any standard exceptions to complete confidentiality in her practice, it is her duty to disclose those exceptions to the patient before accepting any confidences.

There is a difference between confidentiality and privacy. Privacy relates to limited or restricted access to an individual. This relates to the person herself, to objects intimately connected with her, and to information about her. A person controls the relationships she has to some extent by controlling what personal information she shares with others. She determines what she wants others to know by allowing them access through a "for your ears only" exchange. The relationship does not have to be professional. Sharing information that has been given in this way, as a secret, without the person's consent is a violation of her privacy.

Confidentiality can be waived by the patient. For example, a waiver has occurred when a patient signs a health insurance form that includes a release for disclosure to that third party. A waiver also is implied when the patient knowingly shares confidences in front of a third party who is not a member of the healthcare team. A patient who contemplates bringing a malpractice suit in which her medical information is an issue will find that she has waived confidentiality in respect to that information.

There are exceptions to the expectation of confidentiality. A state can require by statute that certain information be disclosed. Mandatory reporting usually is restricted to situations in which the value of confidentiality conflicts with the goal of protecting the public health, as in cases of child abuse, or the requirement to report birth defects, specific communicable diseases, or the results of newborn screening. The area of discretionary exception to confidentiality is very controversial. Because of its importance to genetic counseling, we will look closely at the arguments put forward on both sides of the issue in a later section.

INFORMED CONSENT   Informed consent has been obtained when a patient with substantial understanding, and in the absence of control by others, intentionally authorizes a professional to do something. Informed consent is often considered to be the goal of the patient/provider interaction and is an important part of the process of shared healthcare decision-making. A patient's autonomy is manifested in her right to make her own healthcare decisions, including declining treatment and making use of experimental therapies, and in her privacy and bodily integrity. This obligation is especially relevant to research with human subjects.

There are five elements to informed consent that must be met for consent to be truly informed. The threshold element is **competence**, or the capacity to make a rational choice. To be judged capable of making a rational choice, a patient must be rational, as well as able to communicate a choice, to understand the information provided and the consequences of the choices available. A physician is considered to have the ability to make the judgment as to a person's capacity.

"Competency" is a legal term. A person is presumed to be competent to make decisions regarding her healthcare at 18 years of age. Minors can be emancipated as determined by their state statutes to make some or all of their own decisions. A person who is competent to authorize her own treatment is also competent to refuse treatment. A court will determine the competency of an individual if a question of competency is raised. There is a continuum of competency. The criterion that is applied depends on the context of the task. For example, an individual may be considered competent to sign a will while at the same time not competent to make healthcare decisions.

There are two information elements to informed content. The first is the **amount** *and* **accuracy** of the information provided to the patient. Disclosure of the possible benefits and risks of an intervention (e.g., chorionic villus sampling) is an obligation of the professional. Disclosure also includes the obligation to discuss the available alternatives (amniocentesis, maternal serum screening, targeted ultrasound scan). The rule of truth telling, or veracity, is essential to this element of informed consent. The second information element, the **patient's understanding**, presents a myriad of barriers to informed consent. Patients are fearful, sick, or uneducated; they may hold unscientific beliefs; they are in denial; or they may not speak the same language as the provider. It is the obligation of the provider to identify these barriers and endeavor to overcome them.

The consent elements involve **voluntariness** and **authorization** by the patient. As used here, voluntariness means the absence of control by others. The absence of control must be substantial, that is, the patient's authorization has to be an active agreement, an agreement reached not simply by yielding to or complying with a suggestion by the provider.

There are exceptions to the need for informed consent. For more common, low-risk interventions where the risks and benefits are obvious, explicit agreement may not be required, and consent is implied. In emergency situations it is commonly assumed that patients are unable to make decisions about their care or to participate in it because of pain and fear, lack of understanding of the danger to themselves, or an unconscious state. An objective, "reasonable person," standard is applied in these situations. That is, if a reasonable person under the same or similar circumstances would consent to treatment, then consent is presumed.

In summary, the elements of informed consent are:

- Competence
- Information: amount and accuracy
- Understanding
- Consent, including voluntary authorization

Justice   The principle of justice is common to all ethical theories. It can apply at the level of the individual and at the level of society. Individual justice is sometimes explained as giving all people their due, or treating "like" people in a "like" manner. It implies fairness and equitable, appropriate treatment. In healthcare systems, four values are recognized as derived from justice. **Equality** is the provision of equal care for all, while **liberty** is the freedom of choice, for both the provider and the consumer. **Excellence** is the provision of the best possible care for everyone, while **efficiency** is a broad category that includes the containment of healthcare costs, or stewardship.

The application of justice to society involves the intersection of ethics and public policy. This is best illustrated through distributive justice. One level is the distribution of resources. When resources, such as donor organs, are scarce, we want to know who has access to those resources and how qualifications are determined. At this level, justice implies equal access to services. On a second level is the distribution of risks, which is well illustrated by population-based genetic screening tests. The benefits and burdens of false positive and false negative results are considered when establishing cutoffs for distinguishing normal versus abnormal screening results. The sensitivity and specificity of the test are then set to do the least harm and to distribute the benefits and burdens of the testing most equitably.

In the context of genetic counseling practice, the principles we discussed can be thought of as:

- *Beneficence*: We protect and defend the rights of the client; we prevent harm from occurring to the client.
- *Nonmaleficence*: We avoid harming the client or putting her at risk.
- *Autonomy*: We respect the client's right to be self-determining.
- *Justice*: We treat clients fairly, equitably, appropriately.

Ethical Decision-Making

There is no single correct way to approach ethical decision making. We can, however, develop a framework to help bring structure to the facts of a situation and the responses regarding a case by organizing priorities and identifying the underlying principles. Our decisions should be consistent with our profession and personal system of values. An important resource and guide in this endeavor is a code of ethics.

Codes of Ethics

In general, the code of ethics of a profession presents the moral obligations deduced from the kinds of activity in which the members of the profession are engaged. Traditionally a code of ethics consists of a rational and systematic ordering of the principles, rules, duties, and virtues characteristic of the profession and the intrinsic achievement of the ends to which the profession is dedicated. A code can express duties and goals in rules that all members are required to obey. It could also present ideals toward which all members are encouraged to strive. An enforceable code lists those duties that are required, with penalties for failure to perform them. A professional who wants to behave ethically should be able to use the code of ethics of that profession as a guide.

The National Society of Genetic Counselors (NSGC) Code of Ethics (COE) is an important guide for framing the thinking of genetic counselors. Understanding the ethical basis of the COE is one step in the approach to ethical decision making.

The National Society of Genetic Counselors Code of Ethics

The Code of Ethics was written for the members of the NSGC (1992, 2004, 2006) in a format that presents ideals for the profession and practice of genetic counseling. These ideals are goals toward which the practitioner is expected to strive. Such a document does not put forth rules to follow but offers guides for the pursuit of the ideals. As such, it is not an enforceable document.

The NSGC Code of Ethics was written from the ethic of care perspective, which is defined by interpersonal relationships (Benkendorf et al., 1992). The major relationships established by a genetic counselor were used to organize the values, principles, and beliefs that are defined by the profession of genetic counseling. These relationships were identified as being with oneself, the client, colleagues, and society. The following is a closer examination of the elements and values expressed in the NSGC COE.

(1) Section I: Genetic Counselors Themselves

Genetic counselors value competence, integrity, veracity, dignity, and self-respect in themselves as well as each other. Therefore, in order to be the best possible human resource to themselves, their clients, their colleagues, and society, genetic counselors strive to:

1. Seek out and acquire sufficient and relevant information required for any given situation.
2. Continue their education and training.
3. Keep abreast of current standards of practice.
4. Recognize the limits of their own knowledge, expertise, and therefore competence in any given situation.
5. Accurately represent their experience, competence and credentials, including training and academic degrees.

6. Acknowledge and disclose circumstances that may result in a real or perceived conflict of interest.
7. Avoid relationships and activities that interfere with professional judgment or objectivity.
8. Be responsible for their own physical and emotional health as it impacts on their professional performance.

The values enumerated in Section I of the code include competence, integrity, veracity, dignity, and self-respect. The goal for the genetic counselor is identified as being the best resource possible within her relationships. This section is first because within the ethic of care, in order to be open to others, to be receptive and responsive to them, the genetic counselor has to have some degree of self-awareness. She should know what her own system of values includes, have an idea of what her prejudices are, and know how she interprets life experiences. A genetic counselor who cannot or does not hold these values in high regard, in herself as well as in others, will have difficulty achieving the goals and values in the remaining three relationships.

The individual items in this section are guidelines for achieving the goal set forth above. The need to always be prepared (I-1) is emphasized by being placed first. This includes maintaining current knowledge (I-2). Opportunities for continuing education and knowing where to find the necessary resources in order to be prepared are basic to the goal of this section. A standard of practice (I-3) entails more than those specific guidelines written by the profession. It includes what is found in the genetic counseling literature, and what colleagues in similar positions are doing in similar situations. A professional standard serves as a legal guideline for patient expectations. Local genetic associations, such as statewide groups, provide opportunities for comparison and discussion. The ABGC certification examinations also set a professional standard. A license to practice genetic counseling sets a minimum standard for the profession on the state level. Knowledge of and comfort with these standards satisfies the goal of I-3.

Truth telling (veracity) is a fundamental value in healthcare. This starts with the initial encounter with a client or with members of the public. A genetic counselor must accurately represent her training and skills to others (I-5, 6, 7).

In I-8, taking care of oneself is recognized as including not only professional preparation, but also a legitimate self-interest. This involves the duties a person has to herself, such as guarding her own health and life, her material well-being, and the good of her family and friends. To be an effective genetic counselor, to achieve the goal of maximizing the good one can do for others, requires following the above guides.

(2) Section II: Genetic Counselors and Their Clients
The counselor-client relationship is based on values of care and respect for the client's autonomy, individuality, welfare, and freedom. The primary concern of genetic counselors is the interests of their clients. The genetic counselors strive to:
1. Serve those who seek services regardless of personal or external interests or biases.

2. Clarify and define their professional role(s) and relationships with clients, and provide an accurate description of their services.

3. Respect their clients' beliefs, inclinations, circumstances, feelings, family relationships and cultural traditions.

4. Enable their clients to make informed decisions, free of coercion, by providing or illuminating necessary facts, and clarifying the alternatives and anticipated consequences.

5. Refer clients to other qualified professionals when they are unable to support the clients.

6. Maintain information received from clients as confidential, unless released by the client or disclosure is required by law.

7. Avoid the exploitation of their clients for personal advantage, profit, or interest.

The goal of the second section is to provide the best qualitative and quantitative care and services for clients. The recognition that genetic counseling is often provided in the context of a family and in a multicultural community is reflected in the inclusion of "family relationships" in this section. Support of client autonomy in some situations may be an acknowledgment that cultural values in decision-making may include community and family values.

The values that are drawn from this goal also include acceptance, objectivity, veracity, and respect. Items II-1, 2, 3, and 4 address these values. Appropriate, efficient, and prompt services are necessary for the client to be able to exercise her decision-making rights. Item II-5 is an intersection of Sections I and II. The values of honesty and candor necessitate the self-awareness that is one of the goals of Section I. It is not a problem to hold ethical and moral standards that are different from those of your client. It could be a problem if you do not recognize those differences. It could also be a problem if you make a value judgment that in some way influences how that client is treated. The genetic counseling relationship is one of trust and confidence. It is a fiduciary relationship. Because of this, the counselor who cannot support or work with a particular client is required to refer that client to someone who can work with and provide her with the proper services. We cannot, however, decide to stop working with a client without properly notifying her of the situation. Such lack of notice could be interpreted as abandonment. Terminating a relationship also involves the value of fairness.

The value of confidentiality is also drawn from the fiduciary nature of the counselor-client relationship (II-6). Confidentiality not only relates to what is said during the counseling session, but includes the fact that the client sought genetic counseling. It also includes the use of the client's name. This could occur in various circumstances: in front of other clients when on the phone or in the waiting room, for example, during professional presentations that include showing photographs, X-rays, or other client-related documents, when discussing issues related to the client with other professionals during case presentations, in the transmission of client information by fax where errors occur and numbers have not been confirmed, and with the release of client information to anyone when written consent rules apply. Informed consent is one way to ensure that the patient's confidentiality is protected. The laws relating to confidentiality of personal health information are discussed below.

Should a genetic counselor ever release client information without consent? The exceptions to the responsibility of confidentiality are discussed elsewhere in this chapter. Awareness of your own motives and ethical priorities and the repercussions to the counselor-client relationship need to be examined and weighed. Before breaching confidentiality, a genetic counselor should consult with other providers in her institution, if applicable, or with the ethics committee of her professional society. Breach of confidentiality is never to be done lightly.

There are many opportunities to profit from the relationship with the client. If the client's best interests were always placed first, and people were always righteous, then we would not need II-7 (avoid exploitation of clients); it would be moot. However, this is not always the case, as the history of medical research has shown. We need to be reminded that overcharging, providing unnecessary services, and profiting in any way from client information or property is unacceptable. These activities are a misuse of the patient's vulnerability and information.

(3) Section III: Genetic Counselors and Their Colleagues

The genetic counselors' relationships with other genetic counselors, students, and other health professionals are based on mutual respect, caring, cooperation, and support. Therefore genetic counselors strive to:

1. Share their knowledge and provide mentorship and guidance for the professional development of genetic counselors, students and colleagues.

2. Respect and value the knowledge, perspectives, contributions, and areas of competence of colleagues and students, and collaborate with them in providing the highest quality of service.

3. Encourage ethical behavior of colleagues.

4. Assure that individuals under their supervision undertake responsibilities that are commensurate with their knowledge, experience and training.

5. Maintain appropriate limits to avoid the potential for exploitation in their relationships with students and colleagues.

The goal of this section is to maintain and/or improve the quality of genetic services and professional development through the counselor's relationship with colleagues. "Colleagues" include other genetic counselors, healthcare providers, and students. The values that apply to achieving this goal are respect, caring, cooperation, support, and loyalty. Peer support is a valuable vehicle for promoting relationships with others in the profession (III-1). A genetic counselor can advocate for and encourage students through preceptor and mentoring programs. Many students fulfill their Master's requirements by doing questionnaire-based research. Cooperating in such studies not only assists the student but furthers the knowledge base of the profession. There are many local, state, and national forums through which counselors can exchange ideas and resources and provide professional support to others. These would include professional publications. The impact of a peer group of genetic counselors that meets on a regular basis to discuss cases, exchange information, and give one another personal as well as professional support should not be underestimated.

In striving to encourage ethical behavior in colleagues, III-3 is not meant to be interpreted as encouraging watch-dog activity or ethical behavior policing on the part of genetic counselors. An open dialogue with colleagues raises a general awareness of day-to-day ethical issues and can lead to changes in behavior. It is sometimes less threatening to talk about issues on a theoretical level than to address actual events. Opportunities for discussion can be found at regular staff meetings, case conferences, and grand rounds, for example.

There is an overlap in the services provided by genetic counselors and a number of other healthcare providers. Genetic counseling services are also offered in a variety of facilities. Respect for other professionals (III-2) naturally leads to a participation in mutual endeavors that promote the goals of quality services. These can involve educational programs, case conferences, and legislative work. Again, this work can also be in written form in professional publications. The values of cooperation and dedication support an ongoing dialogue with other professionals so that a consensus can be reached in providing the client with the highest quality of care.

Many genetic counselors provide supervision to genetic counseling students. The responsibilities of a trainer include supporting and caring about trainees (III-4). This includes knowing the abilities and limits of the students and not using students for personal gain. Appropriate professional and personal boundaries must be recognized (III-5) in order to meet the goals of this section.

(4) Section IV: Genetic Counselors and Society

The relationships of genetic counselors with society include interest and participation in activities that have the purpose of promoting the well-being of society and access to healthcare. Therefore, genetic counselors individually or through their professional organizations, strive to:

1. Keep abreast of societal developments that may endanger the physical and psychological health of individuals.

2. Promote policies that aim to prevent discrimination.

3. Oppose the use of genetic information as the basis for discrimination.

4. Participate in activities necessary to bring about socially responsible change.

5. Serve as a source of reliable information and expert opinion for policy-makers and public officials.

6. Keep the public informed and educated about the impact on society of new technological and scientific advances and the possible changes in society that may result from the application of these findings.

7. Support policies that assure ethically responsible research.

8. Adhere to laws and regulations of society. However, when such laws are in conflict with the principles of the profession, genetic counselors work toward change that will benefit the public interest.

Genetic counselors have both a personal and professional relationship with society, which are the focus of Section IV of the COE. The goals of these relationships are promoting the well-being of society and access to healthcare. These involve active participation of the individual genetic counselor as a concerned citizen and as a professional. Sections IV-2, 3, 4, and 5 offer ways in which we can be influential. These, as well as IV-1, necessitate keeping up to date with the science of genetics, and with how, when, and where this information is presented to the public. Monitoring legislation that may impact genetic services or testing that is offered to the public is an ongoing challenge. We can provide expert opinions, and we are well positioned to identify instances of misuse of genetic information.

This section also encompasses the principle of justice in the distribution of services and the barriers to services that we work to identify and address. The values and obligations to the client and to society have to be balanced.

In working toward changes in society, a professional works within the laws and regulations of that society (IV-8). This section does not suggest that all counselors should be involved in all activities. The skills and interests of individual counselors should influence those choices. It is an overall important consideration that as professionals we do not compromise our personal and/or professional values when promoting the goals of the Code of Ethics.

Case Analysis

Now that we have a basis for approaching ethical problems and a set of goals to strive toward, we can see how they apply to our practices. This section illustrates how this can be done for a particular situation and could be applied to both clinical and laboratory work.

When a dilemma or an ethical conflict arises in the course of a clinical interaction, it is not always necessary to resolve it immediately. It is helpful to sort out the facts and separate the real dilemmas from disagreements stemming from the use of language or problems with communication. When such issues have been clarified, ethical principles can be applied and an acceptable resolution achieved. The steps listed in this section are a combination of the approaches of several theorists. They are offered as a guide to the process of analyzing a case. The case that follows demonstrates how ethical principles can be used to understand a particular situation.

Case 2: A genetic counselor, Anne, receives a phone call from a friend and colleague, Ben, requesting confirmation of a diagnosis for a young man, Chris. Ben has a client, Diane, who may be related to Chris. If the diagnosis that Diane suggests Chris has is confirmed, she will be at risk for being a mutation carrier for that disorder. Ben has surmised that since Chris lives in Anne's geographical area, it is most likely that he has been seen by Anne. Ben claims that "time is of the essence." Diane has not been able to get a release from her relative, and she is now in her second trimester of pregnancy. The relationship between Diane and Chris is represented in Figure 12-1.

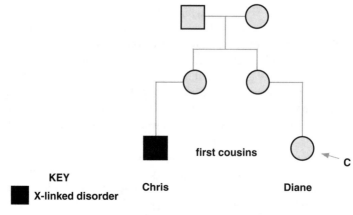

KEY

▪ X-linked disorder

Chris

first cousins

Diane

C

FIGURE 12-1

1. Gathering the Facts   The first step is to gather all the facts, that is, to hear the story of the case. Before beginning the analysis, be sure that there is no other information you want about the case, including social, medical, or genetic facts available to date.

The facts of the case are as follows: Diane was referred to Ben because of her family history (i.e., because of her cousin Chris's problems). Ben has surmised from the description of those problems that Chris has an X-linked recessive disorder. Chris and Diane are first cousins, their mothers being sisters. Anne recognized the description of Chris. Anne does in fact know Chris and his diagnosis. When Anne requested a signed release of information, she was told that Diane had already asked for one but had been refused. Chris's family's reported response was inconsistent with Anne's knowledge of the family, their understanding of his condition, and their concern for other family members. Anne's dilemma: Should she release the diagnosis?

Further information would be helpful in sorting out the issues. For example, how long has Diane been aware of the possible risk? Would knowing her cousin's diagnosis make a difference to Diane's management of her pregnancy? Has the fetal sex been identified on ultrasound scan? We also need to know whether timely, accurately carrier testing and/or prenatal testing is available for Diane, possibly without involving her cousin. These are a sample of the questions that can be asked in this case.

2. Identifying the Parties Involved   The cast of characters of the story has to be defined: Who are the interested parties? Identify the role of each in the case. Who are the decision makers? Who has a stake in the outcome of the case? Who has what information about the case (patient's wishes, family history)? What is the patient's capacity to take part in any decisions that will be made?

The responsibilities of each party should be clear, as should the rights and obligations of each. Any outside influences need to be identified, such as hospital policies or legal implications.

In our scenario the cast includes genetic counselors Anne and Ben and clients Chris and Diane. We should not, however, overlook the interests of the fetus, the father of the fetus, Anne's institution, and society in general. If Chris were a child, his guardian would have to be included in our list. We know, however, that Chris is an adult.

Focusing on the main characters, we can state that Diane has an interest in obtaining the information so that she can make informed decisions after weighing the risks and benefits of testing. She also has a responsibility to bring the family history to the attention of her doctor in a timely fashion, and to pursue a release of information from her family member. Ben has an interest in and a duty to provide the best care for his client, and to use his resources to gain important information for his client. He also has a responsibility to know the standard of practice regarding confidentiality, and a duty to encourage a colleague to act ethically.

Chris has a privacy interest. Not only is his medical information confidential, the fact that he was seen by Anne is confidential. There may be a question of whether he has a duty to his family to share his diagnosis.

Anne has a duty to respect the privacy and confidentiality of Chris. She also has a duty to conform to her profession's code of ethics. If a risk exists, does she have a duty to breach confidentiality and warn Diane? Anne may have a legal duty not to breach confidentiality if her state recognizes a genetic counselor-client privilege, that is, if the confidentiality of the client's information is accorded legal status. The question of a duty to warn is discussed in more detail later in this chapter.

3. Defining the Problem   Asking what decisions are to be made is important for separating the problems of definition or communication from the actual ethical dilemma(s). The way people define a moral problem, the situations they interpret as moral conflicts, and the values they use in their resolution are all functions of social conditioning.

The primary problem in this case is the weighing of the benefits (mainly to Diane) of having medical information against the harms (mainly to Chris) that might be caused by breaching confidentiality. Breaching (or being asked to breach) a professional code is also a harm to the counselor, Anne.

4. Identifying the Principles Involved   Identifying the principles involved in the conflict will help clarify where the various obligations lie. The content of the obligations, and any interobligational conflicts should then become apparent. You can then examine the priorities of the parties involved.

Anne has to weigh the principles of beneficence (helping Diane in the decision-making process and helping Ben fulfill his responsibilities) and nonmaleficence (avoiding unnecessary pregnancy risks and anxiety) against respect for autonomy (Chris's), nonmaleficence (undermining Chris's trust in the profession), and beneficence (helping Ben act in an ethical manner).

5. Resolution   In resolving conflicts, you will find it helpful to use all your available resources, including personnel such as colleagues, religious leaders, hospital or NSGC ethics committees, and an attorney if necessary. In gathering support information, you should also refer to other cases presented in the literature, institutional policies, professional practice guidelines, and the NSGC Code of Ethics.

6. Course of Action   In determining a course of action, apply the principles of the profession in your assessment of the burdens and benefits of all alternatives. Any action you decide to take must be ethically justified on the basis of a good result, primarily for your client and secondarily for any others who may be affected.

7. Evaluation   It is important to evaluate the course of action you pursued. Did it resolve the dilemma presented? Is there any follow-up action necessary? Can another such conflict be avoided in the future? How will the individuals involved deal with the outcome?

Anne's solution to the dilemma will be shaped by how she weighs her various duties. If she feels that Chris's confidentiality should be respected at all costs, she will refuse to provide any information without a signed release. This position can be defended by calculating the theoretical risk of harm to Diane's fetus, and by interpreting Diane's statements as reluctance to pursue the release of information from her cousin. If Anne's goal is to protect Chris's confidentiality while providing some help to Diane, she could contact Chris before responding to Ben. Anne can ask Chris if he would be open to sharing his diagnosis. On the other hand, if Anne has made unsuccessful attempts to obtain consent for releasing the information and believes that the benefits to Diane and the fetus outweigh the harms to Chris, she may elect to provide Chris's diagnosis without a release. This is not a complete list of Anne's options. There are many other issues, such as legal and social implications, in our scenario. Some of these issues are addressed below.

LEGAL ISSUES

The material in the remainder of the chapter is presented to alert you to legal matters of interest to genetic counselors. The discussion is not meant to provide specific legal advice. If such advice becomes necessary, the services of a qualified attorney should be sought. This chapter and the information we are addressing is for educational purposes only.

Relation Between Ethics and Law

As discussed above, moral values result from a combination of cultural factors such as shared values, institutions, and traditions. The rights and obligations derived from this "community conscience" are the moral minimums that are expected of all members of society. Immoral, unacceptable conduct is deterred, prevented, or punished by sanctions imposed by society. Setting boundaries for behavior is the function of the law.

We have already stated that "rights" are justified claims that an individual or a group can make on others or on society. Moral rights, for example, the right to move about freely, are derived from the community conscience. They encompass the right to make and act on one's own choice and to control one's own actions and affairs. They also include the right to certain social benefits and goods, or entitlements. Education is an example of a modern entitlement. Having a right presumes the existence of an obligation on the part of someone else to act in a particular manner. My right to move about freely (e.g., to enter a health facility) obligates others to not unjustifiably restrict my movements (e.g., by blocking the facility entrance).

Rights can be violated or infringed. A violation is unjustified (blocking the entrance to a healthcare facility), while an infringement is a justified overriding of a right (requiring children to be immunized before they enroll in public school).

A legal right is defined by what is legally allowed. Rights are conferred, granted, given, awarded, bestowed, or gained through the law. These rights are not absolute or final. They can be revoked or infringed. An individual has, holds, and owns these rights. A set of rules (that is, our legal system) has been developed so that people can exercise their rights. The legal system has been established as a mechanism for identifying and settling disputes about rights, and enforcing rights by applying those rules. It also allows for judging among claims to rights that may seem to conflict. The rules of law also define the burdens or obligations that are necessary for the exercise of rights.

Sources of Law

The laws that impact healthcare services can be found on the federal and state levels. On the federal level, we have the U.S. Constitution, federal statutes, and case law. The U.S. Constitution is the supreme law of the land. It protects certain individual liberties, such as the freedom of speech, from federal and state government abuses. It limits the actions that the government can take and mandates certain specific governmental obligations (e.g., to convene Congress at least once a year). Any federal or state law that is in conflict with the Constitution is subject to being declared unconstitutional by the U.S. Supreme Court.

Many federal laws have an impact on healthcare in general and genetics in particular. The federal Privacy Act of 1974 limits the disclosure of information obtained by employees of federal services, federal agencies, and government contractors. The Rehabilitation Act of 1973 and the Civil Rights statutes dating from the 1960s prohibit the infringement of a person's rights by private entities involved in employment, housing, or public accommodations on the basis of race or sex, for example. The Americans with Disabilities Act of 1990 adds disabilities to those characteristics covered by the Civil Rights statutes, and extends the Rehabilitation Act to cover private businesses. Employers are prohibited from taking genetic information into account in making job offers.

The Health Insurance Portability and Accountability Act (HIPAA) of 1996 prohibits group health plans from denying individuals coverage on the basis of genetic information, and from using such information to justify charging such persons higher premiums. HIPAA also includes requirements for electronic healthcare transactions for administrative simplification and standardization of protections for the privacy of individually identifiable health information. Genetic counselors are "covered entities" under HIPAA by virtue of either working for a covered entity or being a licensed or certified professional.

Federal laws are enacted by Congress, while the Supreme Court interprets the law through the cases it hears. Supreme Court decisions on issues regarding the federal constitution are binding on all state and federal courts. For example, through a series of cases heard by the Supreme Court regarding a woman's right to make reproductive decisions for herself, the fundamental right to privacy, to make those decisions without undue government interference, has emerged (see e.g., *Roe v. Wade*, 1973). This right is under continuous challenge, the most recent as the federal Partial-Birth Abortion Ban Act of 2003. Challenges to this ban were heard, but not supported, by the Supreme Court in *Gonzalez v. Carhart* (2007).

Within the federal judicial system, a body of case law has developed from the decisions in cases regarding federal law and federal constitutional rights. Once a court decision has been reached, a precedent has been created for future decisions by that court and by lower courts.

For areas regulated by both the federal and state governments, a state may be stricter than the federal government but not more lenient. For example, it is possible to have both federal and state genetic privacy acts. The federal statute may protect genetic information from misuse by public agencies and private enterprises dealing with the public, while the state might elect to expand that protection to cover insurance companies. However, a state could not allow the use of genetic information within the state in a manner proscribed by the federal statute.

States also have constitutions, and the state legislatures enact laws. State court judges look first to the statutes and the case law developed in their respective states. When no state precedents on an issue are found, judges may consider approaches to the issue developed in other states.

Some areas of law, such as public health, insurance, or professional licensing, are left solely to the states to regulate. State laws that infringe on fundamental rights such as reproductive decisions may be upheld only if they are shown to meet a very high standard of importance to that state.

A common problem for professionals is the lack of statutory consistency or uniformity from state to state. A professional can be licensed in one state and not another. Privileges that are recognized in one state may not exist in another, and the limits of confidentiality obligations on healthcare professionals may differ. The federal government does not usually address these areas.

The law is constantly developing and changing, through both the enactment of laws and their interpretation through legal writings and case resolution. A professional should be familiar with the laws in her state that apply to her work and should be aware of changes as they occur.

Medical Decision-Making by Minors

At the age of 18 years, in the absence of cognitive impairment, an individual is considered legally competent. She can make healthcare decisions for herself and enter into contracts. For adults who for whatever reason cannot decide for themselves, family members are the first choice as surrogate decision makers. A court can appoint a surrogate when necessary. For someone who had been competent but is now comatose or mentally ill, a judge may use substituted judgment expressed in advanced directives or past conversations. For the individual who has never been competent (e.g., an infant or intellectually impaired adult), a proxy acts as an advocate and uses her own judgment as to the individual's best interests.

Since parents have direct sovereignty over minor children, they are entitled to make decisions on behalf of their offspring. This right is derived from the notions of family privacy and bonding, parental autonomy, and the legal responsibility of parents for the care and support of their children. Parents are presumed to have the best interests of their child at heart. This presumption can be rebutted by evidence of neglect or abuse. A parent may consent to therapy or decline it, but may not refuse life-saving therapy for a child. Court-ordered blood transfusions are a familiar example.

Most children lack the capacity to make appropriate healthcare decisions for themselves. The participation of a minor in her own healthcare decisions changes with age and circumstances. As the child develops the capacity for moral reasoning and the cognitive skills to recognize cause and effect, and develops a sense of the future, she is entitled to participate more in healthcare decisions. In some states the ages at which a minor may consent to various treatments or procedures are defined by statute. A minor is recognized by most states as emancipated (i.e., accorded adult status) under circumstances such as marriage, pregnancy, or financial independence. The status of "mature minor" is recognized and applied to adolescents who, though not yet 18 years old, are able to demonstrate to a judge that they possess a certain level of maturity and an understanding of the consequences of medical decisions. This status is usually invoked in situations in which the state has an interest in encouraging the adolescent to seek medical care that she might not pursue if her parents were to be informed, as with the treatment of venereal disease. The President's Commission for the Study of Ethical Problems in Medicine and Biomedical and Behavioral Research (1983) recommended that to the extent possible, individuals who are recognized to lack decision-making capacity still be consulted about their preferences, out of respect for them as individuals.

The Law and Genetic Counseling

A medical malpractice suit is a public accusation of wrongdoing that has not yet, and may never, be proven. Usually such an action is brought by an individual against the provider. Malpractice issues for genetic counselors could be expected to be addressed most often in terms of the laws that govern medical malpractice: contract, battery, and negligence.

The nature of the provider-patient relationship is fiduciary and can be considered contractual. All transactions between the parties in the relationship require a high degree of good faith and fairness. One party (the patient) places her confidence and trust in the other (the provider). She incorporates the statements of the provider into her thinking and behavior. Certain conditions (e.g., the maintenance of confidentiality with respect to disclosures made by the patient) are understood or implied. There should be no failure on the part of either party in regard to these understandings. Some rules of law that may apply include:

- Neither party should exert pressure or influence on the other.
- Neither should take selfish advantage of the trust of the other.
- Confidences shared should not be used to benefit one or disadvantage the other without full disclosure and consent.

When a provider agrees to take care of a patient, an obligation to properly attend to the patient is established. This obligation lasts as long as both parties agree to the relationship, or until the relationship is affirmatively terminated by either party. For a specialist, this duty ends when the consultation or testing is completed. A provider who totally neglects a patient or fails to give the patient any care or attention while a need for continuing care exists may be considered to have abandoned that patient. Such abandonment also constitutes negligence. Abandonment can also be a breach of a contract with the patient to provide personal professional services, but is not a common basis for law suits in medicine.

A second basis for malpractice is battery. Battery is an unwanted, unconsented touching. The legal prohibition of this type of behavior is reflected in the necessity for consent. It is not necessary that there be physical injury, financial loss, or an unsuccessful treatment. The injury can be to personal dignity, creating the feeling of having been insulted or violated.

Most malpractice cases are the result of real or perceived negligence. Suits in genetics are usually based on claims of injury to a patient because a provider either did not use or misused certain information or a technique. Examples of misuse of information include the failure to recognize a genetic disorder in a child, a misdiagnosis, the ordering of a wrong test, or the misinterpretation of a laboratory result. Failure to act may also be the basis of negligence. Not taking a family history, not ordering the appropriate tests, and not identifying a high-risk situation are examples of failure to act. Failure to provide complete and accurate counseling has been the basis of negligence claims. The provision of incorrect recurrence risks for hearing loss was the basis of *Turpin v. Sortini* (1981), while *Schroeder v. Perkel* (1981) claimed a failure to diagnose a child's cystic fibrosis.

If a person thinks she has been injured by a battery or by negligence, she can initiate a malpractice suit. Malpractice is a tort action. A tort is an injury or wrong done by a private person, as opposed to one done by the government or a government agent. The injury can be to the person herself or to her property, as the result of a negligent act or intentional misconduct. Only injuries for which compensation in money damages can be recovered are included.

A tort action has four elements that must be proven by the person who brings the suit (the plaintiff):

(1) There was a provider-patient relationship and a **duty** owed by the defendant (the person being sued) to the plaintiff.

(2) The defendant **breached** that duty either by not doing what should have been done (failure to act) or by having done something improper (deviation from the standard of care).
(3) The breach of the duty was the direct **cause** of the harm suffered by the plaintiff.
(4) An actual **injury** (physical, financial, or emotional) resulted, which can be compensated for by the courts.

The first element, *duty*, is shown by looking at the standard of care of the profession. The substance of the duty is established through the practice of the profession. A professional who represents herself as and provides services as a specialist must possess and apply the knowledge and use the skill and care that a reasonable, well-qualified specialist in that field would use in a similar case or circumstance. This may not necessarily be the highest level of practice. An appropriate level of skill and knowledge, good practice, can be defined through national certification requirements, practice guidelines, a scope of practice, and codes of ethics. These provide an objective, uniform measure of the standard of care for that a professional.

The plaintiff then has to show that the provider did not conform to those standards (i.e., she *breached her duty*) either in what she did or what she did not do. The *causation* element is usually most difficult to prove. The birth of a child with defects is often the harm claimed by parents and is said to have resulted in two specific torts, wrongful birth and wrongful life.

The tort of wrongful birth is a specific negligence tort; it can be brought by parents when a child is born with a disorder or a defect. The defendants could be a physician and/or other healthcare providers, the hospital or university that employs them, and/or support services such as a laboratory. The parents must show that if they had known there was an increased risk, they would have avoided the birth of an affected child. The duty that was owed to them comprised accurate genetic counseling and an explanation of risks and available tests. By not providing the plaintiffs with the information that was needed, the defendant breached her duty and deprived this set of parents of their right to make an informed decision. A breach could involve the failure to use due care in performing and interpreting tests, to diagnose a genetic condition or ascertain the genetic nature of a condition, or to inform the plaintiffs of accurate risks and available tests. The parents then claim that the breach of duty they have demonstrated is the cause of the birth of the affected child, since they allege that if they had been properly warned, they would have avoided the child's birth.

A claim can be brought by a child against healthcare providers asserting that the child should not have been born. In such wrongful life suits, an affected child claims there was a duty owed to its parents by the healthcare providers to inform them of possible defects in future children. As in the wrongful birth suit, it is claimed that the failure to meet that duty deprived the parents of the right to make informed decisions, resulting in the birth of the child with defects, and possible pain and suffering. The child has to assert that it would have been better not to have been born at all than to be born with defects and with pain and suffering. These claims are not usually successful. The courts usually do not see life itself as an injury.

Fraud is another example of a tort that may involve genetic counseling. A pattern of unfounded statements of reassurance are fraudulent, as is the making of promises that are known to be false. If a patient claims to have been intentionally misled by the provider, she will further assert that having relied on the provider's false counsel, she was prevented from making an informed decision.

Lawsuits are brought for different reasons. Some are used to punish the wrongdoer, while others are used to challenge existing laws. The remedy sought is a compensation for actual injuries.

The remedies for malpractice depend on the injury claimed. A contract can be enforced by the court. Money damages can be awarded for breach of contract or tort claims. Administrative sanctions can include suspending a license or funding, or assessing fines. For a more detailed discussion of the elements of a law suit as they relate to genetic counseling, see Schmerler (2007).

No one likes to be sued. It is devastating, insulting, embarrassing. It uses up valuable time and resources. You can do everything according to the standards of the profession. You can follow every suggestion you find here and elsewhere. There still is no guarantee that you will never be sued or that you will prevail if you are named in a suit. You can, however, minimize the possibility of finding yourself in court by observing the following recommendations, both with your colleagues as a profession, and as an individual professional.

(1) **What Can Be Done As a Profession?**   As mentioned above, courts look to the standards of the profession to ascertain the duties and obligations of its practitioners. A profession can actively set its own standards by developing practice guidelines and by offering certification and recertification. If the individuals who practice the specialty neglect to act to do these things, standards may be set by legislators and other healthcare providers.

The profession of genetic counseling has taken an initiative to ensure the quality of its practitioners by establishing the American Board of Genetic Counseling (ABGC). The ABGC administers a national certification examination. The profession's national organization, the National Society of Genetic Counselors, Inc. (NSGC), sponsors and supports the development of practice guidelines. It provides the vehicles (*Perspectives in Genetic Counseling* and the *Journal of Genetic Counseling*) for the publication and disbursement of these guidelines. The Code of Ethics, accepted through ratification by the NSGC membership, is another source of the profession's standards.

Licensing of genetic counselors is in the public interest and defines the scope of practice, minimum education requirements, and standards of practice in that state. A counselor-client privilege can be created that would impose confidentiality obligations specifically on genetic counselors. It also provides a means to take action against individuals who practice incompetently despite being able to enter the profession.

(2) What Can Be Done As Individual Professionals?   It is most important to be aware of and comply with the standards of practice of the profession. The ultimate goal is to provide the highest quality of care, not because doing so will keep you out of court, but because it is an ethical principle of the profession. Reasonable errors in judgment should not lead to malpractice claims. Other considerations are examined below.

(a) Effective Communication Is Paramount   Communication, both with the client and with colleagues or team members, should be based on realistic expectations. Informed consent is the goal of the dialogue that involves the disclosure of the information the client needs to make a decision. A signed consent form is a record of that communication process. It does not replace the process but is written evidence that the communication took place. In addition to a formal consent form, it is helpful to include a note in the client chart stating what was said, that the client understood the material, and that all her questions were answered. This may seem obvious, but it cannot be said too often: Open communication is a key element in preventing malpractice claims.

(b) Keep Accurate and Complete Records   The purpose of a chart is to communicate with other healthcare providers and to document what was done and why it was done. Documentation provides a record of the information given to you by the client and by you to the client. If an electronic medical record system is used, such interactions as significant telephone calls, emails, as well as important face-to-face conversations should be included. If a paper chart system is employed, notes should be typed. At a minimum, they should be written in ink. Each page in the chart needs a signature. Knowing what not to write is as important as knowing what to include in the chart. Abbreviations and acronyms that have multiple interpretations should be avoided. For example, AMA stands for "against medical advice" in a hospital context and "advanced maternal age" in the context of genetic counseling. Gratuitous remarks about a client (personality or appearance) are not useful. Open criticism of another professional's judgment should not be included. Careful documentation can be used to support your position that professional standards of care were met. (Please see Chapter 10, Medical Documentation for further information).

(c) Preserve Patient Confidentiality   When you are asked to release information from a client's chart, only information generated by your office should be included. Records you used to form your opinion may be included. Do not provide information on the telephone unless you are absolutely certain the person you are speaking with has the client's permission to hear it. Middle names and social security numbers are good identifiers in this situation. (Consider the position Anne in Case 2 was put in by her colleague Ben's request.)

(d) Do Not Practice Without Malpractice Insurance   Confirm your insurance coverage with your employer. It is not wise to assume that your employer's insurance

policy covers you in all situations. Genetic counselors are often asked to provide services at the private offices of an employer's medical staff or in a testing unit off campus. Several have found out the hard way that neither their employer who originally sent them nor the office they were providing services in included them in their insurance policies. Insurance policies can be purchased through your professional organization if your employer does not provide coverage or if you are in private practice.

(e) Be Prepared to Terminate an Unsatisfactory Relationship Barring any statutory obligations, a professional is free not to enter into a relationship with a particular client. If you need to sever your relationship with a patient, it is prudent to take affirmative action to notify the patient, suggest substitute care, and clearly document why the relationship was ended.

AREAS OF PRACTICE RAISING ETHICAL AND LEGAL QUESTIONS

Genetics is at the cutting edge of science, ethics, and law. The possible applications of genetic information have ramifications that go far beyond medical care. Ethical, legal, and social considerations should be in the forefront of all aspects of genetics, and were incorporated as an essential part of the Human Genome Project (Andrews et al., 1992).

The following topics are a few of the subjects that are not easily settled and have been debated often over the years. They have been selected because they represent some of the ethical dilemmas that arise in genetic counseling, and are used here to stimulate continuing discussion by genetic counselors. The pros and cons published in the literature are presented for each topic. They are offered in no particular order.

Sex Selection

Case 3: Mrs. B was referred for counseling and possible testing because of her age (36 years). She had one child, a girl of 2 years. Mrs. B's dress, her attitude, and her vocabulary made the genetic counselor think of someone much younger. She was most interested in the earliest possible identification of fetal sex. That was the focus of her questions. Relative risks and benefits of the various procedures available were of only passing concern to her. The genetic counselor gave her the benefit of the doubt, although her colleagues agreed that the patient's information may have been falsified.

The desire to have offspring of a chosen gender was not created by the availability of prenatal techniques. Cultural, economic, and political pressures throughout history have resulted in the development of an astonishing array of pre- or periconception techniques used by parents to influence the gender of their offspring (Jones, 1992). Today, medical techniques for the preconception, preimplantation, and postimplantation identification of sex are available. Because the techniques applied after implantation are inevitably associated with abortion, they stimulate the most discussion. The American Society for Reproductive Medicine (2001) relaxed its opposition to sperm-sorting if the technique is used for the purpose of family balancing. It discourages the use of preimplantation genetic diagnosis for sex selection, which some people find less morally objectionable.

Arguments in support of sex selection emphasize social and economic benefits. Besides the identification of a fetus with a sex-linked disorder (e.g., hemophilia, Duchenne muscular dystrophy), positive factors are cited that include benefits to the family by enhancing parent-child compatibility, reducing neglect and abuse based on sex, and reducing the number of unwanted children. Benefits to society include reducing the birth rate and slowing population growth, and secondarily improving parent-child relations (Warren, 1985). In some cultures, the desire of parents for sons is extremely powerful. Sex selection may also enable parents to fulfill religious or cultural expectations. Parents could thus achieve not only individual preferences but also traditional and religious goals.

Legal arguments emphasize the constitutional protection of procreative liberty and privacy (Robertson, 1990). As long as the reason for termination is not questioned in any other context, how can such questioning following prenatal diagnosis be justified?

Those who argue for the prohibition of sex selection find that the harms outweigh the benefits. Deleterious effects on parents, besides the costs in time and money, include the guilt and physical effects of repeated pregnancies and terminations. A failed attempt at gender selection could lead to rejection of the child of the undesired sex and increased burdens on any children of the desired sex. Society is seen to be harmed through the reinforcement of sex stereotypes, and the devaluation of the human worth and contributions of the undesired sex. The ACOG Committee on Ethics (2007) opposes providing sex selection for personal and family reasons because the use could be seen as a form of sexism. A slippery-slope argument suggests that sex selection is a first step toward more intrusive genetic engineering. A shift in the use of technology from a physician-patient model to a service provider-consumer model could lead to market exploitation of the technology (Jones, 1992).

Can we solve this dilemma in a way that does not limit women's rights or involve termination? The request for sex selection is a symptom of a greater social and cultural problem of the unequal value assigned to people on the basis of gender. The suggestions of solutions that address the issue in terms of legal prohibition, professional coercion, or moral sanctions serve to reinforce in part and ignore in part this basic problem. The elimination of the economic and cultural basis of the need for sex selection will make it less attractive and unnecessary.

For genetic counselors, sex selection highlights the necessity of balancing the need to be culturally sensitive with the need to follow our ethical obligations to ourselves. Although Fletcher and Wertz (1987) found that M.D. and Ph.D. geneticists were supportive of prenatal diagnosis for sex selection, only 32% would do the testing in their centers. Because the purpose of prenatal diagnosis for sex identification is to trigger the abortion of the undesired-sex fetus, many institutions do not accept it as an indication for testing. It may, however, be impossible to completely avoid participating in the practice of sex selection, since the client has a right to obtain available information about the sex of her fetus.

Mrs. B of Case 3 decided to have an amniocentesis for advanced maternal age. Fetal sex could not be determined on ultrasound scan. The results of the test revealed a chromosomally normal female. There was disagreement among the medical professionals whether to share with or withhold from the patient the fetal sex.

Presymptomatic Testing in Children

Case 1 revisited: In Case 1, Mrs. Franks had her own reasons for requesting HD testing for her minor children. Would we approach such a request in the same way if the children themselves had asked to be tested to see if they were going to get their father's illness? If the 17-year-old was in a serious relationship that may lead to marriage, and she asked for testing, how would we respond? These issues are not as straightforward as they may first appear.

Advances in molecular genetics have led to presymptomatic and/or predisposition diagnostic testing. They highlight questions regarding intrafamilial relationships and disclosure and confidentiality of personal information. When testing is applied to the care of children, these issues are magnified. Such testing has the potential for great benefits and great harms.

Wertz et al. (1994) assessed the risks and benefits of testing in the process of developing guidelines for the testing of children. They categorized genetic tests in terms of their utility. Testing can offer immediate medical benefits for the child, as in the case of newborn screening for treatable diseases (e.g., phenylketonuria), or it can be of benefit to the older child when making reproductive decisions (e.g., carrier testing for cystic fibrosis). Some testing that does not offer benefits to the child is nevertheless requested by parents or the child, or done to benefit another family member.

Presymptomatic testing for children may be considered beneficial for several reasons. Psychologically, such tests benefit parents by removing worries due to uncertainty, by avoiding resentment from children later in life, and by facilitating the planning necessary to provide support for an affected child. Social benefits include taking advantage of available technology and helping to prepare for the future. Presymptomatic testing offers such medical benefits as encouraging vigilance in healthcare or eliminating the need for intensive medical surveillance. Many parents consider it their role, responsibility, and right to decide whether and when to test children (Mitchie et al., 1996).

The harms that may result when children are tested include disturbance of the parent-child or sibling-sibling relationships, damage to a child's self-esteem, unwarranted anxiety related to the anticipation of symptoms, and the removal of the child's right to decide whether to be tested as an adult. The conflict between the parents' interest in making decisions for the well-being of the child and the interest of the child in self-determination is influenced by the age of the child.

At present, the testing of children cannot be justified for disorders in which symptoms are rare in childhood and for which no treatment is available (e.g., Huntington disease). A committee of the British Clinical Genetics Society

(Working Party, 1994) recommended that there be a general presumption against testing when there is no direct health benefit to the child. The American Society of Human Genetics (ASHG) and the American College of Medical Genetics (ACMG) (1995) presented a joint report suggesting points to consider when parents raise the issue of testing children. The report emphasized the importance of medical, social, and psychological issues. The NSGC, while endorsing the ASHG/ACMG statement, developed its own resolution addressing the issue (1995). The positions of these organizations concurred on, among other things, acknowledged benefits and risks of such testing. They differ in that the NSGC addresses prenatal testing. Some of the discussion on these statements can be found in *Perspectives in Genetic Counseling* (vol. 17, no.4 and vol. 18, no.1). Two committees of the American Academy of Pediatrics addressed this issue. The Committee on Genetics (2000) recommended that testing of children under the age of 18 years be done only if there is immediate medical benefit to the child. The Committee on Bioethics (2001) recommended against predictive testing of minor children for adult-onset disorders. Borry et al. (2006) reviewed international guidelines and position papers concerning presymptomatic testing for children. They found there was a consensus that supported testing only if there is a medical benefit to the child. Although there does not seem to be a consensus regarding the time at which to test children for disorders for which medical intervention is available (e.g., familial polyposis), it is agreed that testing should be considered by the time clinical surveillance would be initiated.

One approach to Mrs. Franks' request could be to discuss testing risks and benefits with the older child, who would soon be approaching the age of majority, and not test the younger children until they were at that same age.

The Use of Genetic Information for Discrimination

Case 4. Sophia was a clerical worker for a small public relations firm. After arranging to take several vacation days to care for her 47-year-old mother as she was being transitioned to a nursing home, she was fired from her job. Sophia was told that her position was being eliminated. She later learned that a co-worker had shared with her employer that Sophia's mother had early-onset Alzheimer disease.

Genetic discrimination occurs when genetic information is used to treat individuals differentially, to deny them normal privileges, or to treat them unfairly. This issue is particularly important in the areas of employment and insurance coverage, when a person's privacy rights are in conflict with the rights of the employer or insurance company to have the information needed for determining the extent of coverage. On May 21, 2008, President George W. Bush signed into law the first civil rights legislation of the new millennium—the Genetic Information Nondiscrimination Act (GINA). GINA provides protections against genetic discrimination in both the health insurance and employment settings. The health insurance provisions of the law take effect in 2009, and the employment protections will take effect approximately 6 months later.

The federal Americans with Disabilities Act of 1990 (ADA) prohibits discrimination in employment on the basis of disability. Disability is broadly defined by the ADA as a physical or mental impairment that substantially limits one or more life activities. A person who has a record of having such an impairment or is regarded in this light is defined by the act as disabled even when there is no apparent incapacity. Included in the definition of disability, then, are people with a genetic predisposition and those who are asymptomatic carriers of a late-onset disorder.

Employers and insurers have been permitted to consider risks in making underwriting decisions and to refuse to cover preexisting conditions. This can lead to a restriction of job mobility for people with genetic conditions. Other questions are raised by the use of predictive tests as well: What is the reliability of genetic tests in predicting future health status? How is "preexisting" to be defined? Who decides which tests are appropriate? Who will pay for them?

Insurance companies are regulated by the states. Until recently, state laws tended to focus on testing rather than on the information itself. Hudson et al. (1995) presented recommendations for the protection of individuals from genetic discrimination. One purpose of HIPAA is to improve the portability and continuity of health insurance. To help achieve this goal, Congress imposed limits on preexisting condition exclusions and prohibited discrimination against individuals and beneficiaries based on health status. These regulations supercede less strict state laws. However, insurance companies have a strong financial incentive to avoid risk. In assessing rates, insurance companies use information on current health status, family history, and medical records. An individual applying for insurance must answer the questions truthfully. Not being truthful about a known future risk is fraud and grounds for denying or canceling coverage.

Duty to Warn Third Parties

Case 5: *Mr. W had a personal and family history of multiple pregnancy losses. Chromosome analysis revealed that he has an apparently balanced translocation. He has two siblings living in another state. They are both of childbearing age.*

The responsibility of healthcare providers to third parties is a continuously developing and controversial area. Genetic information can be relevant to those who are related to a genetic counselor's client. A duty to warn third parties can be derived from the counselor's responsibility to society. Variations of this scenario have been discussed in the genetics and ethics literatures: What if Mr. W's siblings are aware of the family history? What if they are not? What if they are patients in your practice? What if there is an ongoing pregnancy? Any one of these situations could arise in your practice. Considering the pros and cons of the possible professional positions prepares you for addressing them.

It can be argued that the impact a client's genetic information has on the risks for her relatives and their children puts this information into a category that is different from other medical information. This difference is thought to limit the provider's duty of confidentiality. We can consider the issue from the point of view of those third-party relatives who seek the information and of those who may have risks of which they are unaware.

The President's Commission for the Study of Ethical Problems in Medicine and Biomedical Research (1983) supports the position that the duty to prevent harm may at times limit the professional's duty of confidentiality. They outline conditions that should be met before a patient's confidentiality is breached. First, reasonable efforts to convince the patient to consent must have failed. Second, there should be a high probability that the harm (risk of occurrence) will occur if the information is not shared and that the information will actually be used to avert that harm. Third, the risk must be to an identified third party, and the disorder must be a serious one. Finally, only the genetic information needed to prevent that harm (i.e., needed for diagnosis or treatment) should be shared. The commission strongly advised that any professional considering breaching a patient's confidentiality have the circumstances of the case reviewed by an appropriate third party. There is no definition given of "reasonable," "high probability," or "serious" disorder.

In developing a code of ethics for the Council of Regional Networks (CORN), Baumiller et al. (1996) incorporated the commission's recommendations. In their Code of Ethical Principles for Genetics Professionals, they recommended that in the infrequent circumstance that there will be great harm, a provider can override the patient's confidentiality after first informing the patient. Again, "great" harm is not defined, and we do not know how that is related to the seriousness of a disorder. From this point of view, it would not be acceptable for a genetic counselor to contact relatives without consent to inform them they are at risk for an untreatable disorder or for a disorder for which the testing is common, public knowledge. ASHG (1998) concludes that "a healthcare professional has a positive duty to inform a patient about potential genetic risks" to her relatives.

The reasons for *not* sharing a patient's genetic information without consent are well presented by Fost (1992). He points out that genetic counseling situations do not usually involve imminent life-threatening risks to third parties. He also emphasizes that the doctor has a special relationship with the patient but none with her relatives, who are strangers to the provider. Genetic information involves areas of life that are very personal, such as one's identity and reproductive fitness. Privacy concerns should be of essential importance. Fost points out that there are no legal mandates for reporting genetic information to third parties, and telling at-risk relatives is not a recognized obligation or duty. Any harm suffered by that third person was not intentionally inflicted by the patient, but is the result of an act of nature.

The responsibility to a party who is not your client is emphasized in the special situation of monozygotic twins. Heimler and Zanko (1995) confronted this issue when a request for predictive testing for Huntington disease was made by one of a pair of monozygotic twins. The authors required the third party (the other twin) to participate in the testing situation. This position stimulated some debate in the genetic counseling literature (Hodge, 1995; Reich, 1996).

Suter (1993) and Pelias (1991) agree that a genetic professional has the primary duty to respect the privacy, autonomy, and confidentiality of the client with whom she has direct contact. There are few legal cases that support a duty to warn of a risk for genetic disease. In *Schroeder v. Perkel* (1981), the court found that the duty owed by a physician was to provide a diagnosis in a timely fashion to the parents of a child with cystic fibrosis. The duty to warn that was recognized in *Pate v. Threlkel* (1995) was for the physician to take steps to warn the immediate family of the hereditary disease risk. Informing the patient of the inherited nature of her disease and the need to share the information with her relatives was considered to be sufficient to fulfill the duty to warn. The New Jersey Superior Court, in *Safer v. Estate of Pack* (1996), asserted that a physician's duty to warn is not always met by informing the patient of the hereditary nature of the disease. These cases not withstanding, disclosing patient health information is now regulated by the Privacy Rule of HIPAA. Obtaining patient consent for such disclosure is required, with only a very few, specific exceptions. Disclosure can cause financial harm in the form of higher insurance rates, loss of employment opportunities, and possible loss of insurance, as well as emotional harm. The possible consequences of disclosure and nondisclosure should be carefully weighed. Noncompliance with the Privacy Rule could lead to civil or criminal penalties.

Both ASCO (2004) and the AMA (2004) promote the actions of physicians that encourage patients undergoing genetic testing to notify relatives of the information related to the risk of disease. Encouraging open communication among family members can help circumvent conflicts. It is useful to offer some clients a written summary or an article about the condition in question that can be shared with relatives. Some families may benefit from group genetic counseling sessions.

Unexpected Findings

Case 6: Mr. F is the normal healthy father of a child with developmental delays. The child has been found to have a chromosome deletion that may have occurred as the result of a parental chromosome translocation. Studies of the parents reveal that Mr. F has a 47,XXY chromosome complement, which suggests that he is infertile.

The story of finding nonpaternity during family genetic testing is familiar. However, unexpected information can occur in a variety of testing and professional situations. For example, an unexpected chromosome abnormality or variant can be detected, an ambiguous ultrasound scan finding may be observed, or a conflict of interest can come to light. At times, test results are open to interpretation or subject to controversy.

When deciding how to approach the unexpected findings, we have to weigh the benefits and harms of nondisclosure with those of disclosure. The first considerations include the relevance of the information to the client's situation and the consequences of the finding(s).

The arguments for disclosing incidental findings are based on the principle of respect for autonomy. The information belongs to the individual. Duty to the client requires truth telling and full disclosure. The client may learn of the findings in a different context from some other provider. Beneficence would require that we avoid undermining the client's trust in the profession, which could happen if she learns a genetic counselor was not totally honest with her.

The reasons for nondisclosure of an unexpected finding should be compelling. Arguments for *not* disclosing incidental findings include respect for autonomy. A person has a right not to know, and disclosure may violate that right. Because issues such as nonpaternity or gene carrier status can be emotionally charged, the principle of nonmaleficence may prevail in some situations. ASHG 1996 recommended that family members not be informed when nonpaternity is discovered unless paternity was the purpose of the testing. However, facts relevant to medical decision making cannot be justifiably withheld.

The President's Commission 1983 recommends that the client be advised before testing of the possibility that unexpected information may be revealed. Details of your institutional policy on disclosure (if one exists) should be included in any discussion of possible test results.

Duty to Recontact

Case 7: *You had been following a patient with features of Noonan syndrome when the mutations responsible for this condition were identified. At the next scheduled appointment, you discussed this new information and offered testing of the patient. In the back of your mind you remember that there were a number of children you saw over the past years for the same indication, but whom you have not seen on a regular basis. With no electronic medical record system available, you wonder how important it is to dig up the names of the families.*

A major difference between genetic testing and diagnosis and other areas of healthcare is the rapidly increasing volume of information created by new genetic technologies. This creates a continuous need to examine the impact of the rapid advances in genetics on professional practices. New applications for tests and easier access to testing could possibly lead to the recognition of new rights and privileges for clients. We must address the implications of these changes to our duties to clients with whom we once had a professional relationship.

Usually the duty a professional owes a client lasts as long as there is a need for the professional's services, for example, for the duration of an illness. Part of the duty is the full disclosure of known facts and information regarding the genetic condition. For the specialist, the duty to the client usually ends with the consultation.

Pelias (1991) suggests that there may be a continuing obligation to recontact the client when new information becomes available that would have an impact on that client's decision-making. This expanded duty to disclose could be based on the recognized duty of physicians to recontact patients when new information regarding past medication or therapy is discovered. Genetic counselors deal in information. This possible new duty may apply to information regarding changes in diagnostic availability and new implications of prior test results. The Social Ethical and Legal Issues Committee of ACMG examined this issue (1999). They concluded that because the primary care provider has an ongoing relationship with the patient, he should be responsible for reminding the patient to keep in touch with a genetics healthcare provider for changes in the field that may affect his care. A geneticist would be responsible for providing clinical updates only to those patients with whom she has a continuing relationship.

As in all situations, documentation by the consultant that includes a request to the client to keep in touch with the genetic clinic, especially if individual circumstances change or develop, is important. The counselor may also include in client letters statements about the potential future availability of testing and technological dvances and information about genetic support groups, especially those providing members with periodic updates with respect to scientific and medical developments. However, these efforts may not relieve the provider of her duty to recontact that client. A communication in writing by means of a first-class letter to the last known address is evidence of a good-faith effort to notify a former client. It is not clear how far back in time the duty to recontact would apply.

The argument that there is no duty to recontact involves the client's responsibility for herself and her own healthcare. As an adult, she should keep up to date regarding any testing or services available to her. She should contact the healthcare provider on a regular basis if her concerns are ongoing. The administrative nightmare that a duty to recontact may present to some practitioners is often included in the argument. Respect for the client's autonomy can also be invoked. Not every client wants to keep thinking about the reasons that brought her to genetic counseling. Some need to "put the past behind them," while others have preferred to change providers. By initiating contact with the client after a period of time, we may be violating her right to privacy and her right "not to know."

CONCLUSIONS

The goal of this chapter was to introduce you to some of the ethical and legal issues that impact genetic counseling. The subjects addressed were a sampling of those that many practitioners confront at some time. Hopefully, a sense of the depth of these issues will stimulate ongoing discussion, research, and further study.

READING LIST

Aboul-Enen FH, Ahmed F (2006) How language barriers impact patient care: A commentary. *J Cult Diversity* 13(3):168–169.

Americans With Disabilities Act of 1990, 42 U.S.C. S12101, 12201-12213 (Supp. V 1994).

Andrews LB (1992) Torts and the double helix: malpractice liability for failure to warn of genetic risks. *Houston L Rev* 29:149.

ASHG Statement (1998) Professional disclosure of familial genetic information. *Am J Hum Genet* 62:474–483.

ASHG (1996) Statement on informed consent for genetic research. *Am J Hum Genet*, 59:471–474.

ASHG/ACMG Report (1995) Points to consider: ethical, legal and psychological implications of genetic testing in children and adolescents. *Am J Hum Genet* 57:1233–1241.

Baier AC (1986) Extending the limits of moral thinking. *J Philos* 133(10):538–545.

Bartels DM, Leroy BS, Caplan AL (eds) (1993) *Prescribing Our Future: Ethical Challenges in Genetic Counseling*. New York: Aldine DeGruyter.

Baumiller RC, Cunningham G, Fisher N, Fox L, Henderson M, Lebel R, McGrath G, Pelias MZ, Porter I, Seydel F, Willson NR (1996) Code of ethical principles for genetics professionals: an explication. *Am J Med Genet* 65:179–183.

Beauchamp TL, Childress JF (1994) *Principles of Biomedical Ethics* (4th ed.). New York: Oxford University Press.

Benkendorf JL, Callanan NP, Grobstein R, Schmerler S, FitzGerald KT (1992) An explication of the National Society of Genetic Counselors (NSGC) Code of Ethics. *J Genet Couns* 1(1): 31–39.

Borry P et al. (2006) Presymptomatic and predictive genetic testing in minors: a systematic review of guidelines and position papers. *Clin Genet* 70:374–381.

Brody H (1976) The physician-patient contract: legal and ethical aspects. *J Legal Med* (4):25–29.

Capron AM (1979) Tort liability in genetic counseling. *Columb L Rev* 79:619–684.

Committee on Ethics, American College of Obstetricians and Gynecologists (2007) ACOG Committee Opinion No. 360: Sex selection. *Obstet Gynecol* 109(2 Pt 1): 475–478.

Committee on Genetics, American Academy of Pediatrics (2000) Molecular testing in pediatric practice: a subject review. *Pediatrics* 106:1494–1497.

Council on Ethical and Judicial Affairs, AMA (1995) The use of anencephalic neonates as organ donors. *JAMA* 273(20):1614–1618.

Crossley M (1996) Infants with anencephaly, the ADA, and the Child Abuse Amendments. *Iss Law Med* 11(4):379–410.

Elliot C (1992) Where ethics come from and what to do about it. *Hastings Center Report* 22(4):28–35.

Ethics Committee of the American Society for Reproductive Medicine (2001) Preconception gender selection for nonmedical reasons. *Fertil Steril* 75(5):861–864.

Fletcher JC, Wertz DC (1987) Ethical aspects of prenatal diagnosis: views of U.S. medical geneticists. *Clin Perinat* 14(2):293–312.

Fost N (1992) Ethical issues in genetics. *Med Ethics* 39(1):79–89.

Fost N (1993) Genetic diagnosis and treatment. *Am J Dis Child* 147:1190–1195.

Gert B, Berger EM, Cahill GF Jr, Clouser KD, Culver CM, Moeschler JB, Singer GHS (1996) *Morality and the New Genetics*. Boston: Jones and Bartlett.

Gilligan C (1982) *In a Different Voice: Psychological Theory and Women's Development*. Cambridge: Harvard University Press.

Gilligan C (1987) Moral orientation and moral development. In: Kittay EF, Meyers DT (eds) *Women and Moral Theory*. Savage, MD: Rowman and Littlefield Pubs. pp 19–33.

Gonzalez *v.* Carhart (2007) 550 U.S.

Harris *v.* McRae (1980): 448 U.S. 297.

Heimler A, Zanko A (1995) Huntington disease: A case study describing the complexities and nuances of predictive testing of monozygotic twins. *J Genet Couns* 4(2):125–137.

Heyd D (2003) Male or female, we will create them: the ethics of sex selection for non-medical reasons. *Ethical Perspect* 10(3–4):204–214.

Hodge SE (1995) Paternalistic and protective? *J Genet Couns* 4(4):351–352.

Hogben S, Boddington P (2005) Policy recommendations for carrier testing and predictive testing in childhood: A distinction that makes a difference. *J Genet Couns* 14(4):271–281.

Hudson KL, Rothenberg KH, Andrews LB, Kahn MJE, Collins FS (1995) Genetic discrimination and health insurance: an urgent need for reform. *Science* 270:391–393.

In re Baby K (1993): 832 F. Supp. 1022 (E.D. Va.).

In re T.A.C.P. (1992): 609 So. 2d. 588.

Jones OD (1992) Sex selection: regulating technology enabling the predetermination of a child's gender. *Harv J L Tech* 6:1–61.

Karns LB, Roche M, Yashar BM (2005) *An Ethics Casebook for Genetic Counselors. 2nd edition: Ethical Discourse for the Practice of Genetic Counseling.* NSGC.

Kuczewski MG (1996) Reconceiving the family: the process of consent in medical decision making. *Hastings Center Rep* 26(2):30–37.

Maher *v.* Roe (1977): 432 U.S. 464.

Mahowald MB (1993) *Women and Children in Healthcare: An Unequal Majority.* New York: Oxford University Press.

Maley JA (1994) *An Ethics Casebook for Genetic Counselors.* Charlottesville: University of virginia.

Medearis DN Jr, Holmes LB (1989) Th use of anencephalic infants as organ donors. *N Engl J Med* 321(6):391–393.

Mitchie S, McDonald V, Bobrow M, McKeown C, Martequ T (1996) Parents' responses to predictive genetic testing in their children: report of a single case study. *J Med Genet* 33:313–318.

National Commission for the Protection of Human Subjects of Biomedical and Behavioral Research (1983) *The Belmont Report.* Washington DC: US Government Printing Office.

National Society of Genetic Counselors (2006) Code of Ethics. *J Genet Couns* 15(5):309–312.

National Society of Genetic Counselors (1995) Prenatal and childhood testing for adult-onset disorders. *Perspect Genet Couns* 17(3):5.

Natowicz MR, Alper JK, Alper JS (1992) Genetic discrimination and the law. *Am J Hum Genet* 50:465–475.

Nelson RM, Botkin JR, Kodish ED et al. (2001) Ethical issues with genetic testing in pediatrics. *Pediatrics* 107:1451–1455.

Noddings N (1984) *Caring: A Feminine Approach to Ethics and Moral Education.* Berkeley: University of California Press.

Partial-Birth Abortion Ban Act of 2003 (18 U.S.C. 1531).

Pasquerella L, Smith S, Ladd R (2001) Infants, the dead donor rule, and anencephalic organ donation: should the rules be changed? *Med Law* 20(3):417–423.

Pate *v.* Threlkel, 661 So.2d 278 (Fla. 1995).

Pelias MZ (1986) Torts of wrongful birth and wrongful life: a review. *Am J Med Genet* 25:71–80.

Pelias MZ (1991) Duty to disclose in medical genetics: a legal perspective. *Am J Med Genet* 39:347–354.

Pelligrino E (1989) Character, virtue and self-interest in the ethics of the professions. *J Contemp Health Law Pol* 5:53–73.

Pelligrino E (1993) The metamorphosis of medical ethics: a 30 year retrospective. *JAMA* 269 (9):1158–1162.

President's Commission for the Study of Ethical Problems in Medicine and Biomedical and Behavioral Research (1983) *Genetic Screening and Counseling: Ethical and Legal Implications.* Washington DC: US Government Printing Office. pp. 41–88.

President's Council on Bioethics (2003) Beyond Therapy: Biotechnology and the Pursuit of Happiness.

Rehabilitation Act of 1973 (29 U.S.C.A. S791 *et seq*).

Reich E (1996) Testing for HD in twins. *J Genet Couns* 5(1):4749.

Robertson JA (1990) The Randolph W. Thrower Symposium: Genetics and the law, procreative liberty and human genetics. *Emory L J* 39:697–719.

Roe *v.* Wade (1973): 410 U.S. 113.

Safer *v.* Estate of Pack, 677 A.2d 88 (N.J. Super. Ct. App. Div. 1996).

Schmerler S (2007) *Lessions Learned: Risk Management for Genetic Counselors.* New York: Springer.

Schroeder *v.* Perkel (1981): 87 N.J. 53, 432 A.2d 834.

Social Ethical and Legal Issues Committee, ACMG (1999) Duty to re-contact. *Genet Med* 1(4):171–172.

Spital A (1991) The shortage of organs for transplantation: where do we go from here? *N Engl J Med* 325(17):1243–1246.

Suter SM (1993) Whose genes are these anyway: Familial conflicts over access to genetic information. *Mich L Rev* 91:1854–1908.

Troug RD (1997) Is it time to abandon brain death? *Hastings Center Rep* 27(1):29–37.

Turpin *v.* Sortini (1981): 643 P.2d 954 (Cal.).

Warren MA (1985) *Gendercide: The Implications of Sex Selection.* Totowa, New Jersey: Roman and Allanheld.

Wertz DC, Fanos JH, Reilly P (1994) Genetic testing for children and adolescents. *JAMA* 272(11):875–881.

Working Party of the Clinical Genetics Society (UK) (1994) The genetic testing of children. *J Med Genet* 31:785–797.

13

Student Supervision: Strategies for Providing Direction, Guidance, and Support

Patricia McCarthy Veach, Ph.D., L.P. and Bonnie S. LeRoy, M.S., C.G.C.

INTRODUCTION

Supervision is an essential component of genetic counseling education, serving three primary purposes: (1) promoting the professional development of student supervisees who are the genetic counselors of the future, (2) ensuring continued provision of quality patient services, and (3) serving a gate keeping function regarding those individuals who enter the profession (Bernard and Goodyear, 1998). Since supervision typically is done *on top of* other job responsibilities, it pays to be strategic. Therefore this chapter describes the supervision process in a systematic manner and offers practical suggestions for improving the efficiency and effectiveness of supervision activities. The content is geared toward genetic counselors who are new to providing clinical supervision, but the information is also helpful to students who are supervisees. In writing this chapter, we have drawn upon extensive literature from

A Guide to Genetic Counseling, Second Edition, Edited by Wendy Uhlmann, Jane Schuette, and Beverly Yashar
Copyright © 2009 by John Wiley & Sons, Inc.

the mental health counseling and psychotherapy fields, a growing literature on clinical supervision in genetic counseling, and our combined 45 years of experience as counselor educators and clinical supervisors.

The sections that follow define supervision and present goals regarding desired outcomes. Different roles and responsibilities of the supervisor and student are described, and supervision methods and techniques are delineated. Suggestions for assessment and evaluation are provided. Ethical and legal issues are raised, and challenging dynamics inherent to the supervision relationship are also discussed. To illustrate major concepts, examples of critical incidents experienced by genetic counseling supervisors and students are included.

The ultimate outcome of effective supervision is a student who progresses toward becoming a fully competent genetic counseling professional. The American Board of Genetic Counseling (ABGC) has established proficiency criteria by identifying practice-based competencies that an entry-level genetic counseling professional is expected to demonstrate (Fine et al., 1996). Graduate programs that are accredited by the ABGC must provide clinical experiences that ensure that students develop these competencies. Thus it is crucial that supervision goals and student evaluations are tailored to specifically address student progress in the areas of the practice-based competencies.

The ABGC practice-based competencies (Fiddler et al., 1996) consist of four domains, and each encompasses the practice skills necessary for students to demonstrate expertise within the domain. These competencies are presented in an appendix to Chapter 1 of this text. Clinical supervision constitutes an essential vehicle for advancing student development of these practice-based competencies. Assessment of the extent to which student skill development has been achieved needs to occur through the supervision relationship, with the supervisor and student working together as a team. This chapter provides some guidance toward the development of effective relationships in the supervisory setting so that the supervisor and student may learn and grow together.

DEFINITIONS OF SUPERVISION

Various definitions of student supervision exist in the professional literature. Bernard and Goodyear (1998) define supervision as an intervention that promotes the transmittal of skills, knowledge, and attitudes of a particular profession to the next generation in that profession. Supervision also ensures that patients receive a certain minimum quality of care while supervisees work with them to gain their clinical skills. Weil (2000) defines genetic counseling supervision as an activity that helps students develop and gain an increased awareness of ethical issues and their resolution, develop greater awareness of their professional *blind spots*, and become socialized to the profession. According to Weil, clinical supervision includes advice, insight, and support concerning one's cases, clinical skills, and broader aspects of professional development.

Implicit in these definitions are three components: (1) an ongoing relationship between the supervisor and student that consists of guidance and support; (2) activities that promote socialization into one's profession; and (3) a focus on the development of professional behaviors or skills for the benefit of one's clientele. The supervision relationship evolves over time and generally ends after a specified time period. Supervisors and students need to develop trust and rapport, and they must have mutual goals in order to maintain a viable relationship.

Clinical supervision consists of both individual supervision and peer group supervision. Individual supervision typically involves a supervisor who is an experienced genetic counselor and a student with less genetic counseling experience than the supervisor. Peer supervision consists of individuals with comparable levels of experience who participate in ongoing meetings to provide support, guidance, and feedback regarding difficult cases and general professional life and work issues (Zahm et al., 2008). As discussed in more detail in Chapter 5, peer supervision can serve practicing genetic counselors by further enhancing their skills and professional growth.

Individual clinical supervision is the focus of this chapter because it is the primary method of student clinical training in the genetic counseling field. A prevalent method used in individual supervision is *live supervision* (Hendrickson et al., 2002; Lindh et al., 2003), in which a supervisor is present for part or all of a student's genetic counseling sessions. Live supervision is combined with consultations involving a priori review of the student's case preparation, post hoc review of performance with patients and written documentation (letters and clinic notes), discussion of the student's professional growth, and role modeling of behaviors expected of genetic counselors.

GENETIC COUNSELORS AS CLINICAL SUPERVISORS: RESPONSIBILITIES

The genetic counseling supervisor has several responsibilities regarding student clinical practice, including being available to meet with the student, offering support and guidance as needed, providing clear, timely, and balanced feedback, setting expectations for the student, and following up to be sure goals are met (Hendrickson et al., 2002). The supervisor also has a responsibility to employ an approach different from that which would typically occur with patients in genetic counseling encounters. The skills that a genetic counselor uses to counsel patients are distinct from those used to supervise students, and this difference is important for supervisors and students to appreciate because being an effective genetic counselor does not automatically make one an effective supervisor (McCarthy et al., 1988). For instance, the primary theoretical approach to genetic counseling involves nondirectiveness with the intent of facilitating and supporting autonomous patient decision-making (McCarthy Veach et al., 2003). Genetic counselors are careful to assess each patient's perceptions and belief systems and to work within the patient's values framework. In contrast, supervisors in the clinical setting strive to help students practice within the profession's accepted values framework and to separate their own values from those of their patients. Moreover, one of the most frequent interventions that genetic counselors use with their patients is information-giving (Bartels et al., 1997). Yet effective genetic counseling supervisors may provide little or no information; rather, they encourage students to learn how to obtain information on their own, thus increasing their problem-solving skills.

SUPERVISION GOALS AND DISCUSSION TOPICS

Goals

Goals are aims or expectations regarding the skills that a student is expected to achieve, and, as such, they provide a framework for supervision. Broadly conceptualized, clinical training goals reflect one's answers to the following questions: As a result of this rotation, what should students know? What should they be able to do? How will they feel about their professional development? Goals are most effective when they are explicit, specific, measurable, and feasible (i.e., they reflect aims that are within a student's ability range, and there are sufficient opportunities to achieve them). Two distinct models that may be used to establish goals are the Discrimination Model and Bloom's Taxonomy.

The **Discrimination Model** developed by Bernard and Goodyear (1998) classifies student skills into four categories based on whether the skills primarily involve overt behaviors or covert feelings or thoughts. Examples specific to genetic counseling are illustrated:

- **Process Skills:** These are "doing skills" that consist of the actual techniques and strategies used in a genetic counseling session:
  - The student obtains appropriate family, medical, and social histories.
  - The student uses open-ended questions to help patients express concerns.
  - The student is able to manage expressions of strong emotions by patients.
- **Professional Skills:** These are "doing skills" that involve adherence to professional standards of behavior, including adherence to ethical standards of the profession:
  - The student comes to genetic counseling sessions adequately prepared.
  - The student documents genetic counseling session data accurately in patient charts.
  - The student seeks consultative help when needed.
- **Personalization Skills:** These are "feeling skills" that pertain to the internal, subjective reactions students have toward their patients, toward genetic counseling, and toward their supervision relationships:
  - The student recognizes how patient loss triggers the student's own grief reaction.

- The student is able to tolerate ambiguity in sessions.
- The student seeks feedback during supervision in a nondefensive manner.
- **Conceptualization Skills:** These are "thinking skills" that involve cognitive processes such as case analysis and patient conceptualization:
    - The student formulates appropriate and specific plans and strategies for sessions.
    - The student anticipates patient reactions to genetic information.
    - The student is able to interpret patient response/nonresponse accurately.

The second model is **Bloom's Taxonomy** (Bloom et al., 1956), presented in Table 13-1. Developed for use in educational settings, this taxonomy consists of a hierarchy of learning processes from basic memorization of facts to highly sophisticated critical thinking. The novice student is more likely to have memorized basic genetic information but tends to lack skills requiring application, critical analysis, and evaluation of cases. One would expect more skills representative of higher levels of the hierarchy to be demonstrated as a student gains supervised clinical experience.

The Bloom's Taxonomy model can be used by both supervisor and student to assess the student's skill level in various clinical settings and to establish specific goals for attaining or improving upon skills. The following example illustrates how Bloom's Taxonomy Model could be used to assess students' confrontation skills [a *process skill* in the Bernard and Goodyear (1998) Discrimination Model]:

Knowledge Level: Students repeat what they have learned about confrontation from their classes, answering questions such as, What is confrontation? What is an example of a confrontation statement?

Comprehension Level: Students demonstrate their understanding of what confrontation generally is intended to accomplish in a genetic counseling session and why it is important by explaining reasons for pointing out discrepancies to patients.

Application Level: Students identify the type of confrontation that might be appropriate for a particular type of patient and demonstrate in a role play how they would actually confront such a patient.

Analysis Level: Students identify aspects of a patient's situation they would want to challenge (e.g., pointing out inconsistencies between a patient's comments and nonverbal behaviors regarding termination) as well as factors that might promote or hinder their use of confrontation with this patient.

Synthesis Level: Students connect their confrontation responses to patient goals by articulating how confrontation about a particular patient's inconsistent behavior helps the patient make the best decision for herself.

Evaluation Level: Students judge the effectiveness of their confrontation in meeting its intended goal for a given patient and provide evidence to support their assessment.

TABLE 13-1. The Application of Bloom's Taxonomy for Developing Genetic Counseling Goals

Beginning Level Skills

Know
Recall or recognize appropriate facts, concepts, principles. List, repeat, memorize, recall, state.

Examples

1. State the mode of inheritance for neurofibromatosis.
2. List the etiology, symptoms, and prognosis for the major genetic conditions dealt with in the metabolic diseases clinic.

Comprehend
Translate, interpret, extrapolate from data, charts, graphs, etc.

Examples

1. Interpret a pedigree to identify a family at high risk for cancer.
2. Translate information presented in scientific articles into language understandable to the patient.

Intermediate Level Skills

Apply
Use facts, concepts, and principles in a hypothetical or real situation. Illustrate, demonstrate, use, give an example.

Examples

1. Illustrate for a patient the difference between dominant and recessive inheritance in a way that the patient can understand.
2. Provide information about chromosome studies to patients in easy to understand terms.

Analyze
Compare and contrast information, deduce, dissect, break down.

Examples

1. Compare and contrast the possible psychosocial impact of the diagnosis of Down syndrome in a first pregnancy for a 25-year–old versus a 41-year-old woman who comes to clinic with a long history of infertility.
2. Determine from available data the most appropriate follow-up plan for a given case.

Advanced Level Skills

Synthesize
Integrate information, consolidate, build, join

Examples

1. Consolidate data from a patient's family history and from blood test results to identify what information is important to communicate.
2. Integrate and convey information from several sources in the literature that is important for a particular patient.

TABLE 13-1. *(Continued)*

Evaluate
Critique information, assess, judge, debate, determine the worth of...

Examples

1. Assess patient's likely reaction to a proposed counseling plan and modify as needed.
2. Assess the extent to which patients understand the information presented in a genetic counseling session.

Source: Genetic counseling examples based on Bloom, ed. (1956).

Discussion Topics

A variety of topics may be discussed in clinical supervision, and examples are listed in Table 13-2. The primary discussion topics can be categorized as patient-related issues, issues pertaining to the student counselor, and issues pertinent to the supervision relationship (Hendrickson et al., 2002). These topics can be used as a reference when structuring supervision sessions.

TABLE 13-2. Supervision Discussion Topics

Patient-Focused Topics

- Patient diagnosis/symptoms
- Assessment of family and medical history
- Interpretation of risk figures and test results
- Determining genetic counseling approach (e.g., type of information to provide and how to present this information)
- Conceptualizing patient dynamics (e.g., patient indecision)
- Planning student responsibilities for genetic counseling session
- Setting short-term and long-term goals
- Assessing patient progress (e.g., patient decision-making)
- Identifying ethical/legal issues
- Recognizing boundary issues in genetic counseling

Student-Focused Topics

- Genetic counselor/patient dynamics
- Impact of personal perspectives on provision of genetic counseling
- Clinical skills progression
- Professional development

Supervision Relationship Topics

- Relationship between supervisor and student
- Boundary issues in supervision (e.g., confidentiality)
- Administrative issues

Source: Hendrickson et al. (2002).

SUPERVISOR AND STUDENT ROLES

Two processes, *support* and *guidance*, form the basis of all styles of supervision to varying degrees (Hart and Nance, 2003). Support refers to a focus on students' feelings about themselves and their thoughts and feelings when working with patients. Guidance refers to conceptualizing patients' issues and needs and learning about and using specific genetic counseling techniques/interventions. Support and guidance vary along a continuum from low to high. These processes are evident in the various roles adopted by supervisors and students over the course of their relationship.

Bernard (1988) defines four types of supervisor and student roles: consultation, teaching, counseling, and evaluation. Each role has a place within the supervision relationship, and, ideally, supervisors and students are versatile in their use, shifting among roles as needed. It is important to remember that genetic counselor supervisors usually have had little or no formal training in clinical supervision. Most individuals who are not formally trained typically use, and overuse, the role in which they are most comfortable, or they rely on the types of supervision approaches they experienced as students. The following examples demonstrate how supervisors and students can be more versatile in their use of roles and thus enhance the effectiveness of the supervision experience.

Teaching Role

When the supervisor is in the teacher role and the supervisee is in the classical student role, the primary interaction is instruction, with an emphasis on guidance. The teacher is a resource person who shares information, skills, and strategies, which the student is seeking. The focus is on the development of the student's skills as a genetic counselor. Teaching activities include demonstrating, explaining, and interpreting events from genetic counseling sessions, and identifying appropriate interventions. The supervisor exerts a fair amount of power over this interaction, as the "expert" who provides at least some of the answers. Novice supervisees who are eager for models of what to do usually prefer the supervisor to assume the teaching role. Supervisors who adopt a teaching role may vary between directive modes of teaching (e.g., "This is what you should do. . .") and evocative modes (e.g., "What can you think of to do? Here is what I would suggest").

Consultation Role

Consultation is the principal activity through which supervision typically is conducted (Boyd, 1978). When the supervisor is a consultant and the supervisee is a consultee, they interact collaboratively. Objectives are mutually agreed on, the supervisor encourages the student to self-evaluate, and the focus of supervision is on the student's patients. Consulting activities include brainstorming possible strategies and interventions, generating options for the patient, and discussing patient needs.

The consultant (supervisor) acts as a facilitator who works with the consultee (supervisee) to determine effective planning and action. The consultee has a great deal of personal responsibility for goal-setting, evaluation, and problem-solving. Supervisees who are more advanced usually prefer consultation.

Counseling Role

When the supervisor is in a counselor role and the student is in a client role, the primary interaction is one of exploration with the goal of promoting self-awareness and growth. Here the focus is on the student as a person, and thus support is emphasized. The supervisor assists the student to recognize developmental tasks and become aware of personal issues that may affect responses to patients. For example, beginners typically struggle with issues of competence and confidence (Hendrickson et al., 2002; Loganbill et al., 1983). A supervisor in the counselor role can introduce a discussion of these dynamics and help to normalize them (e.g., "Most students feel some anxiety about their skills. Is that what you are feeling?"). The supervisor plays a role in helping the student identify feelings and defenses and understand how these inner experiences affect the genetic counseling relationship. However, the supervisor is *not* responsible for helping the student change these defenses or reactions. This distinction maintains an important boundary in that the supervisor does not provide psychotherapy for the student. If personal counseling or psychotherapy appears to be appropriate, the supervisor should discuss with the student a referral to a therapist. The counselor-client roles tend to be adopted infrequently in the typical genetic counseling supervision relationship.

Evaluation Role

When the supervisor is an evaluator and the student is an evaluatee, the primary interaction is critiquing and feedback giving, and the focus is on accountability. The supervisor acts as a gatekeeper assessing the effectiveness of the student's service provision. In this interaction, elements of administrative supervision often blend with clinical supervision. Evaluation activities include formal and informal assessments, goal-setting, and giving and receiving feedback. Three aspects of the clinical experience are generally included in the evaluation: the student's skills, the genetic counseling services provided, and the supervision relationship itself. The process of evaluation is covered in more depth later in this chapter.

Examples of Supervisor—Student Roles

No single role is the absolute "right" role to assume in clinical supervision. Supervisors and students move in and out of these roles depending on the students' support and guidance needs. The following supervisor-student interactions illustrate how the different roles described above can be applied effectively to the same scenario.

Scenario: *The student has just completed a genetic counseling session in which the patient started to cry as she heard the results of her genetic testing. The student had responded by repeating extremely complicated information about the test results in a rapid, highly technical fashion, at which point the supervisor elected to take over the session. Later, during a supervision discussion, the case was reviewed and the issue was discussed.*

Teaching Role
Student: Is what I did OK? If not, what should I have done instead?
Teacher: This is what I think you should have said to empathize with the patient. . . .

Consultation Role
Consultee: I missed my chance to address her feelings. I'd like to figure out some ways that I could respond when patients cry.
Consultant: Why don't we talk about different strategies? Sometimes I will wait a few moments before saying anything. What sorts of approaches have you thought of trying?

Counseling Role
Client: It's not usually like me to ignore a patient's feelings. I don't know what was going on.
Counselor: Maybe you felt distressed by her reaction?. . . Let's discuss this.

Evaluation Role
Evaluatee: I had to be sure she got all the information she needed, but I think I could have done it better.
Evaluator: I'm glad you realize that. There might have been a better way to present the information. I think your timing was part of the issue.

It is important to note that these roles are not always discrete; elements of more than one role may be evident in any particular supervisor-student interaction. Furthermore, a mix of roles may be optimal. For example, in the preceding scenario, the supervisor might want to use a combination of the four roles to thoroughly process the genetic counseling incident. Finally, both members of the supervision relationship influence the roles that are expressed by the other party (e.g., the student may "pull for" the evaluator role by asking for feedback; the supervisor may encourage the student to act as a client by asking how the student feels about counseling a terminally ill individual).

The following scenario provides another illustration of different supervision roles with the student initiating a specific role.

Scenario: *Your student comes to you and says, "I just saw a couple who were referred for prenatal diagnosis. I went through a detailed explanation of advanced maternal age and the associated risk factors. I also explained the amniocentesis* *procedure, but I just don't know if they 'got it.' I mean, I asked a few times if they had any questions, but they kept saying 'no.' I really don't know if they understood any of the information." The following are examples of the different directions in which the ensuing discussion could proceed.*

Teaching Role

Student: How can I tell if they understood?
Teacher: Next time, after you've given some important information, try asking the patients to summarize what they heard you say.

Consultation Role

Consultee: I would like to figure out a different approach.
Consultant: Let's brainstorm other approaches. What other ways have you tried to find out if patients understand information? What might you do?

Counseling Role

Client: I have no idea if I'm doing any good!
Counselor: This seems to be bothering you. Maybe you're operating from an assumption that when you ask patients if they have any questions, they'll tell you. But your intuition says that's not working.

Evaluation Role

Evaluatee: I really don't think they understood anything.
Evaluator: What cues were you picking up on that suggest they didn't "get it"?

STUDENT RESPONSIBILITIES

Students' responsibilities in clinical supervision include developing versatility in responding to the supervisor's different roles of consultant, teacher, counselor, and evaluator; coming prepared to supervision; being open and responsive to feedback; following through on supervisor assignments and recommendations; disclosing important information; asking for assistance when faced with counseling issues beyond their competencies; and engaging in honest self-evaluation.

Students have the ability to influence the types of roles that their supervisors use in their supervision interactions, and therefore they must do their best to recognize what type of role they need in a given situation and how to ask for it (Bernard, 1988). For instance, if students need support to talk through their emotional reactions to a difficult case, then it may be effective to assume a client role and "ask" their supervisors to adopt a counselor role. If they desire direction with respect to case preparation, then a teaching role may be optimal. If they desire feedback, they can adopt an evaluatee role complementary to the evaluator supervisor. Finally, if they wish to collaboratively "troubleshoot," they should be a consultee and ask their supervisors to be consultants.

Receiving Feedback

Student: My supervisor never provided any clear or specific feedback. At the end of the placement, I received a very negative evaluation. What can I do to keep this from happening in future rotations?

Response: When supervisors are too "laid-back" and not fulfilling their obligation to provide constructive supervision, the student must take a more active role in seeking feedback. The student can request that they schedule a specific time for supervision sessions and then come well prepared. The student can also ask the supervisor to provide feedback on specific behaviors (e.g., "How clearly do you think I explained X-linked inheritance to the patient?"). The student can also request more global feedback ("What skills do you think I am doing fairly well, and which ones do you think I need to work on?").

Just as supervisors have a responsibility to provide feedback appropriately, students have a responsibility to appropriately receive it. We offer several guidelines for receiving feedback that supervisors can recommend to their students at the beginning of a clinical rotation.

Clarify Feedback—Let your supervisor know that you heard and understand the feedback; ask for clarification until you do understand.

Share Your Response—When receiving feedback you will have both cognitive and affective reactions. Let your supervisor know how this feedback makes you feel and what you think about it.

Accept Positive Feedback—Awareness of your strengths is as important as awareness of areas for improvement; do not gloss over positive feedback too quickly. You may want to use this feedback to think of new ways to adapt your strengths to different situations.

Reflect on Feedback—Take time to absorb, synthesize, and reflect on feedback you have received and think about ways to apply feedback in subsequent genetic counseling sessions.

Accept Corrective Feedback—Remember that corrective feedback is necessary for your development as a genetic counselor. Everyone has areas for improvement, so try to welcome this information rather than avoiding it.

Test Validity of Feedback—Although everyone's perceptions are valid in their own worldview, they are not necessarily the absolute "truth." If the feedback does not fit with your perceptions, ask for clarification and check it out with others. Usually you will discover the valid part of the feedback if you persist in trying to understand it.

Exercise Personal Responsibility—As you develop your skills, you will become more aware of your own strengths and weaknesses. Take responsibility by asking for feedback about specific behaviors and issues that are challenging for you.

Avoid Feedback Overload—If you begin to feel overwhelmed with information, let your supervisor know that you have had enough and would like to continue the conversation at a later time. It is important to realize that processing and assimilating feedback can take time.

SUPERVISION METHODS

Supervision relationships may be more likely to start off "on the right foot" and develop into a strong working alliance if supervisors use a variety of methods and strategies to "frame" the relationship. Table 13-3 contains a list of general strategies for structuring positive supervision relationships (Fall and Sutton, 2004).

Supervisors typically use a variety of methods when conducting supervision. Different methods are evident in the various types of verbal responses that supervisors use. Based on a classification system developed by Danish et al. (1980), McCarthy et al. (1994) identified 11 supervisors' verbal responses, which are presented in Table 13-4, along with examples specific to supervision in the genetic counseling setting. These responses cluster into three categories:

- **Continuing responses,** which encourage the student to talk and are particularly useful for initial exploration of a topic.
- **Leading responses,** which are supervisor statements that shape the direction of the conversation. They are particularly helpful once initial exploration of a topic has been completed.

TABLE 13-3. Strategies for Effective Supervision Relationships

- Establish clear written goals or clarify goals written by the students' training programs.
- Discuss the roles of both supervisor and student, including your model of supervision.
- Disclose to students what the process of supervision will be like as well as your expectations.
- Describe the evaluation process, including your expectations, timing, and criteria.
- Establish a process to resolve conflict.
- Establish a process for ongoing feedback apart from any formal evaluation.
- Respect students while offering constructive feedback.
- Maintain professional boundaries.
- Discuss the *double bind* that may occur as a result of encouraging students to disclose their limitations while they simultaneously are being evaluated with respect to their suitability for the profession.
- Acknowledge students' anxiety, and identify its sources.
- Create an atmosphere in which students are both supported and challenged.
- Use communication techniques such as metaphors, analogies, and humor.
- Encourage a more egalitarian relationship through collaboration.
- Monitor the supervision relationship itself by expressing "here-and-now" reactions.
- Be fully present with students.

Source: Adapted from Fall and Sutton (2004).

TABLE 13-4. Supervisor Verbal Techniques

Continuing Responses

Encourage the student to talk

1. *Content responses* to reflect student statements
   Example: "To summarize, you told me that from the family history, you feel the patient's risk for cancer is low."
2. *Affect responses* to reflect student feelings
   Example: "It sounds like you feel uncomfortable when a patient becomes angry."

Leading Responses

Supervisor leads discussion

3. *Open questions* to get at process issues
   Example: "Tell me, how would you approach this issue?"
4. *Closed questions* to get at details
   Example: "What is the recurrence risk for neural tube defects?"
5. *Interpretations* to provide insight
   Example: "When the discussion turns to complicated information, it seems that you start talking really fast to avoid discussing it in any detail."
6. *Confrontations* to point out discrepancies
   Example: "You do a better job than you give yourself credit for. Maybe you're being too hard on yourself."
7. *Advice-giving* to suggest alternative behaviors
   Example: "Next time when a patient appears upset, wait a few moments before jumping in."
8. *Influence responses* to try to alter student views
   Example: "It isn't usually helpful to tell patients that they should not feel bad."
9. *Information-giving* to provide facts, resources, etc.
   Example: "Direct gene analysis for this disorder is available through many commercial and academic labs in the U.S."

Self-Referent Responses

Supervisor self-revelations

10. *Self-disclosure* to reveal supervisor personal information
    Example: "When an adolescent is involved, I find that it works best if I take the time to talk with the teenager alone."
11. *Self-involving* to provide supervisor personal reactions about the student
    Example: "I enjoy working with you because I think our counseling approaches are similar."

Source: Examples based on McCarthy et al. (1994).

- **Self-referent responses,** which involve revelations by the supervisor of autobiographic information or personal reactions to the student. Self-reference is particularly helpful for normalizing student experiences (e.g., "I have difficulty working with angry patients, too."); modeling appropriate interventions (e.g., "This is how I explain a balanced chromosomal translocation to a patient.");

dealing with supervision impasses (e.g., "I get frustrated when you say 'Yes, but...' to my suggestions, because I sense you really don't want to hear my ideas."); and providing feedback (e.g., "I'm very pleased at how thoroughly you prepped your last case.").

In addition to specific verbal responses, supervisors can use different techniques during supervision. These include modeling of counseling interventions (the supervisor demonstrates a skill either through a role play with the student or in an actual genetic counseling session, which the student observes); assigning homework (e.g., "Locate and summarize the research findings regarding Marfan syndrome."); and referring the student to other sources (e.g., "Contact the molecular diagnostics laboratory for more information on testing for myotonic dystrophy.").

Live supervision is a prevalent supervision method (Hendrickson et al., 2002; Lindh et al., 2003) that involves sitting in for part or all of the student's genetic counseling sessions. Within a live supervision model, the supervisor may cocounsel (use a team approach and share counseling responsibility with the student), consult with the student outside the room during sessions, and debrief after sessions. In preparation for live supervision, supervisors provide *anticipatory guidance* by discussing cases before seeing patients, reviewing session outlines, and role playing (Hendrickson et al., 2002). They also assess student readiness, allowing students to take over more elements of the session as they gain skill and confidence. Within genetic counseling sessions, supervisors allow students sufficient time before interjecting comments and they *hand back* the session to students after their interjections. After genetic counseling sessions they encourage students to critique their interactions with patients and they provide specific feedback to their students.

It is extremely important that, from the outset of their relationship, the supervisor and student schedule and faithfully adhere to a regular meeting time; otherwise the student's professional development will not get the time and attention that it deserves. Prepping and debriefing cases "on the fly" will lead to rushed, confused, and incomplete supervision. In addition to establishing a regular schedule for supervision, a comprehensive evaluation of cases can be initiated by having students keep a journal summarizing their impressions of their sessions. When students document their impressions immediately after a session and make more detailed written comments at a later time, both affective and cognitive issues are more likely to be identified. Affective issues typically emerge immediately after a session, and cognitive details develop more fully from later reflection. Before meeting with the supervisor, the student can self-evaluate by reviewing case notes and/or tapes (if sessions are taped) and by identifying particular questions or issues to be discussed.

Students (and supervisors) can also complete a brief genetic counseling session evaluation form, for instance, rating each session on a 10-point scale (1 = my worst session, 10 = my best session) and briefly explaining their ratings. Supervisors can use students' completed rating forms in several ways: reviewing student ratings at the end of each day or each week in order to quickly assess how students believe they are doing, independently completing the forms and comparing their ratings with those of their students, beginning supervision sessions with a discussion of the students' ratings, and watching for general improvement in ratings over the course of the rotation and intervening if this is not happening.

METHODS FOR ASSESSING STUDENT SKILLS

Formal Case Presentations

Formal case presentations provide a vehicle for assessing student counseling skills, providing students with feedback about their genetic counseling behaviors, and generating interventions for working with a particular patient. Although they can be done in individual supervision relationships, the benefits are usually greater when formal case presentations are done in small groups with a designated supervisor acting as facilitator, such as in a class setting. A typical case presentation consists of both a written and a verbal summary of the case, followed by discussion, which includes brainstorming and feedback.

Case presentations are most effective when students are focused in their verbal and written descriptions. However, students often have difficulty "getting to the point." They spend so much time on relatively trivial details that the most important information may be neglected entirely or come up too late to address it adequately. There may be several reasons for students' failure to focus, and these are listed in Table 13-5. To help students focus, the supervisor can assign stimulus questions. Examples of stimulus questions include:

1. What was the reason given for referral?
2. What were the patient's expectations of this session?
3. Summarize the medical and family histories and provide a risk assessment.
4. What were the major medical and genetic issues involved in this case?
5. What were the major psychosocial issues involved in this case?
6. What options did the patient have for decision-making?
7. What is your follow-up plan?
8. What are 1 or 2 questions you have about the case and/or your performance?

Feedback is an essential component of case presentations. One important ground rule for feedback provision during case presentations is that everyone should begin with one positive feedback statement and then one corrective statement. The supervisor should enforce this rule in order to prevent two possible dynamics— either everyone praises the student to the extent that no constructive learning occurs, or everyone "gangs up" and overwhelms the student with corrective feedback. The supervisor should ask group members who raise criticisms to specify what they would have done if it had been their patient. Group members also can be asked to illustrate their suggestions through brief role plays. Because numerous ideas can be generated quickly during case presentations and these ideas vary in their value, the

TABLE 13-5. Reasons for Students' Failure to Focus in Supervision

Fishing—The student does not know how to focus or has not transferred this skill to genetic counseling relationships.

Where's the Road Map?—The student lacks a framework for conceptualizing patients, thus failing to see the bigger picture (e.g., fails to recognize a family history of mental retardation in multiple generations and affecting only males is a possible cue for fragile X syndrome or some other form of X-linked mental retardation). Students often lack a framework when they have limited prior experience with a given genetic condition.

Going with the Flow—The supervisor derails the student's presentation by throwing out several ideas at once, and the student follows along this divergent path.

Birds of a Feather—The student's behaviors mirror patient behaviors (e.g., the patient's descriptions are scattered and the student repeats this pattern in supervision). This dynamic is called "parallel process" by some theorists (Ekstein and Wallerstein, 1972).

Pressure Cooker—The student experiences intense emotion (e.g., anger, frustration, agitation) and deals with it by "blowing off steam" or talking on and on in great detail.

I've Got a Secret—The student withholds certain information because it is anxiety-provoking. For instance, the student feels anxious about the supervisor's reactions to "mistakes", a patient's experiences touch on the student personal issues (e.g., unresolved issues about death), there is a lack of trust in the supervisory relationship, and/or the student wishes to prevent anticipated consequences of telling the supervisor certain information (e.g., if the student does not disclose about failing to confront a prenatal patient's alcohol abuse, the supervisor never figures out and addresses this resistance).

Shot Gun Approach—The student irrationally believes that there is one crucial piece of information that, if the supervisor only knew it, would allow the supervisor to tell the student exactly what to do with a given case or with similar cases in the future. Failing to recognize which pieces of information are the most critical, the student feels compelled to repeat verbatim what transpired in the genetic counseling session.

I'm No Good—The student greatly magnifies mistakes, placing the supervisor in the position of providing reassurance, minimizing the errors that have occurred, and withholding corrective feedback. The student's unconscious agenda (perhaps trying to mask insecurities) prevents a focused discussion of the case.

The Laid-Back Supervisor—The supervisor provides little or no guidance regarding how to present cases, thus putting the onus for deciding what to discuss on the student. This type of "laissez-faire" approach generally is viewed as undesirable by both novice and more experienced students (Allen et al., 1986).

---

supervisor should summarize the most valid points. The supervisor also needs to be sensitive to the emotional state of the student presenter and call a time-out if the student becomes too anxious or discouraged. It is also important that the supervisor monitor the time and the process (e.g., "I see that we have 10 minutes left. How are we doing with the questions that you had about this case?"). This technique actually is similar to what one does in the clinical setting, where patients are informed of time limitations and their responsibility to raise any issues that have not yet been discussed.

Supervision discussions usually are based on a combination of supervisor observations made during live supervision and on indirect data about the student's genetic counseling cases. As students gain clinical experience, more of their supervision discussions are likely to involve indirect data such as information obtained via self-reports and case notes, with the student providing verbal and written summaries of what transpired in a session. Elements of the formal case presentation (e.g., stimulus questions, feedback process, etc.) can be used informally when supervisors and students meet individually to debrief regarding their counseling sessions and when discussing student self-reports and case notes.

Supervisor: My student reported on a counseling session I had not observed. I questioned the way in which some information appeared to have been given to the patient—in a complicated way which I felt the patient probably did not understand. My student's response was "You weren't there—you are only second guessing." How can I better handle case reviews of sessions that I did not directly observe?

Response: A formal case presentation is one way to provide detailed supervision when the supervisor was not present during the session. The student benefits from analyzing the specifics of the case, presenting them chronologically, and identifying aspects of the case that require consultation. A well-conducted case presentation can enhance the student's clinical skills. In addition, because self-report is limited by the student's skills in accurately assessing and explaining what occurred and by the student's comfort with disclosing relevant information (including mistakes), direct data also are desirable. When possible, sessions should be videotaped or audio taped. These methods provide first-hand information that affords a more valid record of what occurred (Hendrickson et al., 2002), and they allow the supervisor and student to more quickly address important issues because they do not need a detailed session summary.

In this situation, we recommend that the supervisor initially adopt a counselor role to address the affect implied by the student's response. For example: "You seem frustrated by my feedback. Do you think I've jumped to the wrong conclusion?" This response invites the student to explore the supervisor-student relationship in the "here and now," and it may open the door for a meaningful discussion. For instance, perhaps the supervisor *does* reach conclusions too quickly, or the student may feel too threatened by corrective feedback to assimilate the supervisor's comments. Once this process issue is explored, discussion can return to identifying aspects of the student's approach that helped and hindered the patient's understanding.

Surveying Patients

Another type of assessment approach based on direct data concerning student performance involves surveying the student's patients. Some would argue that the ultimate test of whether genetic counseling is effective is the extent to which patient expectations are met. Survey results from patients served by the student could be incorporated into the feedback given to the student during supervision. Table 13-6 provides a sample patient survey form.

TABLE 13-6. Examples of Questions to be Used in a Patient Satisfaction Survey

1. How well do you feel your student counselor understood your situation?

1	2	3	4	5
Not at all well				Extremely well

2. How well did your student counselor explain information about your condition, testing options/ results, etc. to you?

1	2	3	4	5
Not at all well				Extremely well

3. How comfortable did you feel with your student counselor?

1	2	3	4	5
Not at all comfortable				Extremely comfortable

4. What is one thing your student counselor did especially well?
5. What is one thing your student counselor could have done better?

Formative and Summative Evaluations

Evaluation is the "hallmark" of supervision (Bernard and Goodyear, 1998), playing a vital role in the development of competent professionals and in assuring quality service provision. There are two major types of evaluation in supervision – formative and summative. Formative evaluation, the most common type, consists of informal feedback that focuses on the student's day to day behaviors with specific cases and patients. We have outlined several suggestions for providing formative evaluations in Table 13-7. These suggestions consist of specific behaviors intended to minimize some of the common difficulties encountered with this type of evaluation.

> **Student:** As a student, I experienced a few sessions in which the genetic counselor/ supervisor jumped in and started speaking with the patients regarding a topic I was just getting to.
>
> **Response:** In providing formative evaluation, timing, privacy, and accuracy are extremely important [see Table 13-7]. Generally students benefit more when they are permitted to complete a session with the supervisor taking note of what to "fill in" at the end. Later, at an appropriate time and place, corrective feedback can be given. This strategy will more likely lead to a change in counseling approach than interrupting the student during a session that is, for the most part, going well.
>
> Certainly there are occasions when it is necessary for the supervisor to step in quickly (e.g., to correct an inaccurate statement that would shut down an important avenue of discussion with the patient). We recommend that at the

beginning of their relationship supervisors discuss with their students when, why, and how they might "step in" during counseling sessions. They should ask their students how they think they will feel when that happens, describe strategies they will use to "hand back" the session to the student after stepping in, and also identify ways that students can let them know if they need assistance at any point in a session.

Summative evaluation is a more formal activity in which supervisors and students look at the "whole package" and make judgments about the student's overall functioning. Because summative evaluation is based on a judgment about how well the student has done so far, it tends to be more comprehensive than formative evaluation. Therefore, summative evaluation should not focus on a single case or behavior but rather on the student's general professional development. Guidelines for conducting summative evaluations are listed in Table 13-8.

Evaluation can be a difficult activity for several reasons (Bernard and Goodyear, 1998). Students usually feel anxious about evaluation because it touches on their personality and intelligence. Supervisors may also feel anxious if they think they will open "Pandora's box" (e.g., Will I have to fix what I call attention to? Is my student's problematic performance due to poor supervision on my part? What if my impressions are wrong?). Both supervisors and students may feel anxiety as they struggle to fully explain and understand judgments about complex human skills (e.g., what does it mean that a student "lacks sensitivity to cultural differences"?).

TABLE 13-7. Suggestions for Providing Formative Evaluation

1. **Timing**—Pick the right time, as soon as appropriately possible after the behavior has occurred.
2. **Private**—Select the right setting; privacy is important.
3. **Balance**—Begin with one or two things the student is doing well before moving to corrective feedback.
4. **Affect**—Recognize the emotional impact your feedback is having on the student.
5. **Warn**—Avoid surprises; it is best to drop a hint of what is to come.
6. **Self -Control**—Keep your own reactions under control and in perspective. It may be a familiar mistake to you, but it's the first time for the student.
7. **Accuracy**—Be sure of all of the facts involved.
8. **Behavioral**—Keep the student's personality out of the discussion. Focus on the precise behavior that the student either is exhibiting or failing to exhibit that requires modification.
9. **Focus**—Keep the conversation on the student; don't compare the student to other supervisees.
10. **Rebuild**—Close with an effort to restore the student's confidence.
11. **Delay**—Think before you speak. Often when we have a strong reaction to an immediate situation, our responses tend to be more emotional and off-putting. With reflection the feedback can be more effectively delivered. Consider telling the student that you would like to discuss the case tomorrow, thus allowing you time to plan your supervision approach.

Source: McCarthy Veach et al. (2008).

TABLE 13-8. Guidelines for Conducting Summative Evaluations

1. Develop minimum evaluation criteria. Articulate the standards against which you are comparing the student. Students often agonize over how much importance to place on the feedback they receive when they lack an awareness of these minimum standards. One approach is to review with the student the practice-based competencies established by the ABGC before the start of the clinical rotation. Another approach involves working with the student to identify goals for developing a set of skills for the particular rotation on which the evaluation will be based.

2. Seek strong administrative support from your employers and the academic program director. Clarify who is the ultimate authority, use agreed-upon evaluation methods, and identify due process procedures for students whose performance is problematic.

3. Follow a standardized procedure. The method and timing of evaluations should be consistent across students and, to the extent possible, across training sites.

4. Hold students to a reasonable number and level of practice-based competencies they are expected to demonstrate.

5. Consider student developmental differences. Different skills are expected from students in their first rotation versus the last rotation.

6. Articulate clear evaluation criteria and methods.

7. Evaluate qualitatively and quantitatively.

8. Obtain input from several sources (other supervisors, the student, patients, etc.).

9. Document evaluations in writing and include examples of student behaviors.

10. Include specific suggestions about what the student can do to improve.

11. Be flexible. Your goals for the student may need to be modified over time.

Source: Bernard and Goodyear (1998)

Evaluations at the Completion of a Rotation

At the end of a clinical rotation, the supervisor should complete an evaluation summarizing the student's overall performance. If, during the rotation, the student worked with other genetic counselors, the supervisor should elicit and incorporate their feedback into the final evaluation. The supervisor and the student should set aside a time to meet and review these evaluations and formally bring the rotation to a close. Completed evaluations should be provided to the student and forwarded to the student's genetic counseling program director.

One strategy for making the final evaluation meeting more interactive is to ask students to "self-evaluate," first completing the evaluation form the way they believe their supervisor will complete it and then completing it a second time to indicate their perceptions of their own performance. Similarities and discrepancies can be discussed at the final meeting. It is also recommended that supervisors and students conduct a "mid-rotation" evaluation meeting at which they complete as much of the form as is relevant at that time and then discuss their ratings. In this way, the student will have time left in the rotation to address any corrective feedback. This strategy can alleviate student anxiety triggered by the question of "What does my supervisor *really* think of me?"

At the end of the clinical rotation, students should complete an evaluation to provide feedback about the supervisor and to communicate overall impressions about the rotation. Although graduate programs usually provide a form and mechanism for this evaluation, the supervisor might consider soliciting additional feedback. For example, one form that provides student feedback about the supervisor's goal setting and feedback skills is the *Evaluation Process Within Supervision Inventory* (Lehrman-Waterman and Ladany, 2001), a 21-item measure with a 7-point rating scale (1, strongly disagree ... 7, strongly agree). Sample items include: "My training objectives were established early in the relationship," "My supervisor and I created goals that were realistic," "My supervisor balanced his or her feedback between positive and negative statements," and "The feedback I received was directly related to the goals we established." This form could be completed midway through the rotation and/or at the end of the rotation.

SUPERVISEE AND SUPERVISOR CHARACTERISTICS

Developmental Considerations: Novice Versus Advanced Supervisees

Student developmental differences constitute an important factor to consider when selecting and implementing supervision interventions and when evaluating student performance. There are several ways in which novices may differ from more advanced students with respect to their competencies and supervision needs. These differences may be viewed on a continuum, rather than as "all or nothing."

Developmental Levels Students vary as they gain counseling experience in areas such as competence, emotional awareness, autonomy, identity, respect for individual differences, purpose and direction, personal motivation, and professional ethics (Borders and Leddick, 1987). As they develop competency in each of these areas, students will fluctuate among stages characterized by some authors as stagnation, confusion, and integration (Borders and Leddick, 1987). This progression is nonlinear and discontinuous and requires supervisors to tailor their responses accordingly.

Dependence on Supervisor/Patient Novices tend to depend on the supervisor for direction, feedback, and validation, whereas advanced students function more independently. Novices are also highly dependent on patient reactions as a basis of validation (e.g., "The patient was angry... that must mean I did a poor job of answering her questions."), while advanced students are more realistic about patient reactions.

Anxiety Novices experience more "global" anxiety about their competencies; they fear that they are "terrible" genetic counselors, while advanced students will usually have more specific anxiety (e.g., "I have difficulty confronting male patients"). Advanced students may also have greater performance anxiety because they feel they have to be expert genetic counselors.

Motivation Although novices may be afraid of supervision, they are also eager for it and usually feel as if they can't get enough. Some authors (e.g., Kadushin, 1968) believe that advanced students may be resentful of supervision, regarding it as one more "burden" in an already overloaded schedule.

Personal Responsibility Novices often suffer from the "Whose problem is it?" phenomenon, feeling overly responsible for all aspects of the genetic counseling relationship (e.g., if a patient is unable to decide whether or not to have an amniocentesis, novices believe the indecision persists because they did not explain risk factors adequately). Novices usually lack a clear understanding of their professional role because they lack genetic counseling experience. Advanced students are usually more realistic about their responsibilities as genetic counselors; when they feel overly responsible, it may be a clue that something in the case touched on a personal issue.

Professional Self-Concept Crystallization Novices typically have poorly defined concepts of themselves as genetic counselors. They have many questions about their strengths and weaknesses, and whether they are capable of being helpful. Their self-concepts are fairly fragile and based primarily on patients' reactions. Advanced students have more stable and accurate self-concepts that are more resistant to idiosyncratic patient reactions and genetic counseling experiences.

Supervision Needs Novices generally are a more homogeneous group with respect to their supervision needs. Typically their concerns include: Can I learn the necessary counseling techniques? How do I meet patient needs? What is my role as a counselor? How adequate am I as a counselor? Do my patients like me? (Littrell, 1978). Advanced students are much more heterogeneous given their varied counseling and supervision experiences.

Clarity of Supervision Goals Novices are more inclined to set goals that are too global and unrealistic (e.g., "I will learn everything there is to know about all metabolic diseases during my 8-week rotation in this specialty clinic."). Advanced students have a more precise understanding of what they need to accomplish, and therefore their goals tend to be more specific, feasible, and individualized. Novices may have inappropriate goals based on their limited understanding of genetic counseling (e.g., "I want to like and be liked by every patient."). In contrast, advanced students have a deeper and fuller appreciation of genetic counseling and therefore can set appropriate goals.

Supervisor: I have a student who is in her final rotation and already has a job in a pediatric setting. This is a prenatal rotation. She was an excellent student throughout her program but seems to be 'blowing off' this clinical experience. One obvious difficulty was motivation, but more difficult for me were the "I know it all" attitude and the disbelief of her previous supervisors that she wasn't doing well. What do I do?

Response: This student needs to be reminded of the original goals of the rotation. Problems like this will be less difficult to deal with if you have written criteria for passing the rotation and a written consent to supervision. Acknowledging that supervision has lost some of its thrill for this advanced student may also be helpful. Ask her to identify supervision activities that would be more challenging and then include some of these in addition to required activities during your time together.

Furthermore, this situation provides an excellent opportunity to discuss how competent professionals must make efforts to prevent themselves from viewing their patients and their clinical work as routine or boring. We recommend that you talk frankly with the student about the risk of "cutting corners" in her clinical work once she graduates. It might also help to discuss how she may hit plateaus where she feels stagnant in her work and to brainstorm with her ways to manage those experiences (e.g., participate in peer group supervision, seek variety in her work, etc.).

It is important to select supervision strategies that are appropriate for students at different skill levels. If possible, the supervisor should assign less complicated cases to novices and save more challenging ones for advanced students. Any case is additive for the novice who has done little or no genetic counseling. The supervisor should be more selective with advanced students, who may need greater depth or breadth of experiences. Initially the supervisor should be more highly structured with novices to diminish their anxiety and to increase productive use of time. The supervisor may also want to take an expert, teacher role with the novice, while primarily using a more collaborative, consultant role with the advanced student. To the extent possible, supervisors should allow advanced students to conduct part or all of their genetic counseling sessions alone in order to approximate the way that they will provide genetic counseling once they graduate.

Supervisors must also monitor their internal reactions to students who are at different levels of training. Common dynamics that may arise include:

Identification—It may be harder to identify with a novice, especially if the supervisor has been a genetic counselor for a long time.

Self-Efficacy—The supervisor may feel superior to a novice, but threatened by the advanced student who has highly developed skills.

Responsibility—The supervisor may feel more responsible for novices and may experience separation issues as they develop skills. The supervisor may feel less responsible for advanced students, believing they can "take care of themselves."

Expectations—The supervisor may mistakenly assume that novices have fewer competencies than they do; conversely, the supervisor may mistakenly assume that advanced students have certain competencies that they do not possess. Discussion of student experience and an assessment of student skills at the beginning of supervision can help to clarify competencies and assist in establishing appropriate goals for skill development.

Novice Supervisors

As they gain supervision experience, supervisors typically encounter developmental issues similar to those of their students. Novice supervisors in particular face challenges as they work to clarify their new role, experiment with different techniques, and gain confidence. Recommendations to help supervisors "grow into" their new role include (Polanski, 2000):

- Examine your own professional development and experiences as a supervisee and draw from those.
- Think about the differences between your clinical practice and your supervision practice.
- Draw upon models of good supervision provided by supervisors in your own training.
- Engage in co-supervision with a colleague, if feasible.
- Participate in a peer supervision group.
- Establish clear boundaries with supervisees.
- Address your novice status directly with supervisees and discuss any reactions they may have.
- Remind yourself that you have more experience than supervisees and more objectivity regarding their clinical situations.
- Don't be afraid to engage in trial and error.
- Don't apologize. You have a great deal to contribute as a novice.

Cultural Considerations

Cultural characteristics are important factors in supervision, just as they are in genetic counseling relationships. Culturally sensitive supervisors assist their students in becoming aware of their own biases, beliefs, and values, they encourage them to learn and understand their patients' worldviews, and they help them develop culturally appropriate clinical interventions (Sue and Sue, 1981). Similarly, supervisors work to recognize their own biases, attempt to understand their students' worldviews, and continually expand and use their repertoire of culturally appropriate supervision methods. Genetic counseling students who are members of groups that are underrepresented in the profession respond well to supervisors who attempt to distinguish between student behaviors that are characteristic of their cultures and those that are unique to them as individuals (Schoonveld et al., 2007).

COMMON SUPERVISION CHALLENGES

Ethical and Legal Issues

A number of ethical issues may arise during the supervision relationship. Two common ethical challenges involve multiple role conflicts and confidentiality limits. These issues should be addressed, especially since supervisors usually work with a "captive audience," that is, students who have no choice about being part of the relationship (Stout, 1987).

Multiple Role Conflicts

Multiple role conflicts within supervision are virtually unavoidable because of the supervisor's triple allegiance to the student, the student's patients, and to the genetic counseling profession. Conflicts that pose the greatest likelihood of problems in supervision involve other relationships the supervisor has or may eventually have with the student (e.g., boss, instructor, research advisor, recent classmate, friend). If possible, the supervisor should suspend other relationships with the student during the period of supervision as this will help to define and maintain appropriate boundaries and reduce the potential for loss of objectivity.

Confidentiality Issues

There are limits to confidentiality within supervision relationships, and students vary in their awareness of these limits. For instance, some students worry excessively about the possible ramifications of their disclosure to supervisors. They struggle with the question of how open to be with the supervisor who ultimately will evaluate them, and they may fear that anything they say is "fair game" for the supervisor to share with others. On the other hand, some students believe that everything they say is completely confidential. The supervisor is responsible for clarifying and upholding confidentiality limits. A supervisor should never promise that everything a student says and does will remain confidential. In some cases, information revealed during the supervision relationship needs to be divulged to the director of the program as it may have negative repercussions for patient services. Confidentiality limits should be discussed at the beginning of the supervision relationship and they should be reviewed before discussing particular issues for which student privacy might not be maintained. In this way, a student may choose not to disclose certain information, and the supervisor should respect this choice. If the information is not crucial to the student's performance with patients, it can remain undisclosed.

Supervisor: I have been working for about 4 months with a student who initially was doing very well. One day she seemed to have uncharacteristically low energy. I asked how she was, and she said "Fine, just fine." Later as her performance declined, I pressed for an explanation, and she stated that she had some personal problems and did not want to discuss it with me. Her academic and clinical work are suffering, and the change in her personality is significant. What should I do if she will not talk to me?

Response: As her supervisor, you have the responsibility to address the unidentified problems because they are affecting the student's ability to learn and to provide adequate genetic counseling. Since the student declined to explain the reasons for the changes in her behavior, you should respect her right to keep personal difficulties confidential. However, you are responsible for ensuring quality patient care. Therefore, if the student's problems continue to affect her ability to provide patient care, it is appropriate for you to acknowledge her right to confidentiality regarding the reasons for her diminished performance, and refer her to a professional who can help. Depending upon the situation, it also may be appropriate to suggest a leave of absence from the clinical rotation. In such situations, it is important to maintain written documentation specifying her clinical performance and to consult with appropriate parties to determine an action plan (e.g., the student's program director) (Forrest et al., 1999).

When a student's behavior indicates a serious problem, it is important that a supervisor maintain clear boundaries, in particular keeping "performance" separate from the "cause" (Forrest et al., 1999). For instance, in this situation, the cause may be that the student is depressed; however, from your perspective as a supervisor, the issue is that she is late to sessions and is unable to concentrate on what patients tell her. You role is not to excuse her performance because of her depression, nor is it to "cure" her depression. You should remind her about confidentiality limits and also state that any actions that you take are intended both to be helpful to her and to ensure that patients receive appropriate care.

Problematic Performance

In clinical supervision there is potential for inappropriate behavior by both supervisors and students. Supervisors may fail to provide timely, accurate feedback, attend superficially to the student's clinical work, distort evaluations, and waste time in supervision gossiping, talking about their own cases, or trying to impress the student. Students, on the other hand, can withhold critical information, waste time in supervision discussing trivial points, and express either so much anxiety or hostility that the supervisor is hesitant to give feedback.

Student problematic characteristics/behaviors may also include lack of technical knowledge, failure to incorporate supervisor feedback, persistent anxiety, lack of interpersonal skills, failure to follow through on responsibilities (e.g., being unprepared), defensiveness, lack of conceptualization skills, overdependence on the supervisor, lack of professionalism, failure to get along with others in the clinic, hostility, disrespecting the supervisor, ethical violations, and disrespecting patients (Lindh et al., 2003). Some students may also seek special or atypical considerations (Lindh et al., 2003).

Supervisor: I have a student who is significantly older than me and came to our clinic with some related experience. However, the student is a novice in the area being supervised and has some difficulty with being a beginner at anything. How do I handle this?

Response: This issue can be addressed concretely by reviewing with the student Bloom's Taxonomy [see Table 13-1] and the practice-based competencies defined by the ABGC. The student's actual skill level can be documented, and specific goals for achieving more advanced skills can be established.

> We also recommend addressing the "white elephant" in the room. For example, "I realize that you are coming to clinic with relevant prior experience. If I were you, I imagine I might find it challenging to take directions and feedback from a younger supervisor." [Supervisor waits for student's reply to this statement and then says . . .] "I wonder how we might recognize and handle any conflict that comes up because of it."

Anxiety

As mentioned above, anxiety comprises one type of challenging student characteristic. Anxiety affects students' clinical performance and their openness to supervision and feedback (Fall and Sutton, 2004). Sources of student anxiety may include being observed and evaluated, being in a new clinical rotation and needing to acclimate, feeling for the first time as if they have to prove they can actually do what they came to graduate school to do, and holding irrational beliefs that when they counsel they must be all-knowing and make a difference in every patient's life. Supervisor strategies for addressing student anxiety include (Fall and Sutton, 2004) encouraging students to talk about their fears, showing that you understand how challenging their situation is and communicating affirmation and support, working collaboratively and in a consultative style, setting clear goals to reduce the magnitude of what they are doing, clearly stating your expectations in order to place limits on what seems like a "limitless" environment, providing clear and relevant feedback, self-disclosing your own feelings of anxiety during your training to normalize their situation, and using occasional humor.

Lack of Preparation

Lack of preparation is another common challenge (e.g., students have not adequately prepped a case, they do not follow through with an approach that you worked out with them before counseling a patient, etc.). Approaches for understanding and addressing lack of preparation include (Fall and Sutton, 2004) the following. First, find out whether the student knows and understands what you mean by "being prepared." You may need to role model how to prep a case. Another reason for lack of preparation is that when supervisees feel unsafe, they will try to hide as much of their skills, work, and themselves as possible. Directly addressing their unsafe feelings usually is helpful. There may be personal issues interfering with a student's preparation, and this deserves careful review as many supervisees will not readily volunteer such information. Finally, lack of preparation may be a result of discouragement, disorganization, or lack of commitment. Explore the student's individual situation and how one or more of these factors may be interfering with adequate preparation.

Unconscious Dynamics

Unconscious dynamics play a large role in the supervision experience for both parties. The supervision relationship can generate strong affective reactions (Stout, 1987). Students may develop intense emotional responses to their supervisors (adulation, resentment), and vice versa. These feelings often are based on transference and countertransference, that is, reactions prompted by one's past history with other significant relationships (McCarthy Veach et al., 2003). Examples include students either greatly admiring authority figures or resenting them, and supervisors losing patience with dependent or rebellious students. Sometimes students act out their patients' emotions on their supervisors (anger, anxiety, etc.). Such acting out can be difficult to detect and manage because it is done unconsciously.

Supervisors may have unconscious or conscious agendas such as wishing to impress their students with how much they know, wanting to prevent students from developing their skills because then the supervisor would not be needed anymore, and avoiding discussion of feelings because they are afraid of developing a close relationship. Additional issues involve gratification of one's own needs (e.g., having rescuer fantasies, wishing to be the ultimate authority), various anxieties (over being evaluated by each other; anxiety about strong patient or student emotions, performance anxiety), imposing one's values on the patient or student (e.g., beliefs about abortion or mental retardation), fear of being disliked, and overidentification (with patients or the student). To the extent that these issues are unrecognized, they can compromise the work of supervision. Supervisors should reflect upon their supervision performance (Stout, 1987) by regularly asking themselves, "Whose needs are primarily being met? Is what I'm doing within the realm of supervision?" Supervisors should avoid irrelevant, excessive self-disclosure and excessive probing into students' personal lives, and they should set and adhere to a regular time and private professional location for supervision (McCarthy et al., 1994). Supervisors may wish to meet periodically in peer supervision groups to consult about their supervision issues, and/or they may prefer to raise certain issues with the student's genetic counseling program director.

SUPERVISION AGREEMENTS FOR CLINICAL SUPERVISION

A written supervision agreement for clinical supervision is one mechanism for helping to set boundaries regarding multiple relationships and for clarifying confidentiality limits. A written agreement facilitates a communication process that involves discussion between the supervisor and student of the basic elements of supervision goals, processes, and outcomes (McCarthy et al., 1995). Such discussions can be facilitated by a written document that formalizes and clarifies the relationship, educates the student about the nature of supervision, and provides the student with a model of the informed consent process for use with patients.

A written supervision agreement may include the following information: purpose of supervision, supervisor credentials, pragmatics of the supervision relationship (e.g., frequency, length, location, missed sessions, contacting in emergencies), description of supervision processes (e.g., the methods that will be used, roles and responsibilities of each party), administrative issues (e.g., description of evaluation procedures, due process procedures), ethical and legal issues (e.g., confidentiality limits, possible multiple relationship conflicts, guidelines for patient treatment), an addendum for clarifying or adding to the statement based on the supervisor and student's discussion, and a statement of agreement (indicates understanding of and adherence to the contract). The Appendix provides a sample of a supervision agreement for use in genetic counseling supervision. This sample can be modified to fit individual supervisor situations.

> **Supervisor:** A student entered into the supervisory setting being defensive and resistant to the process. These reactions, it seemed, stemmed from the student's own uncertainties about herself as a professional (low self-esteem), as well as personal conflicts from her life experiences. How should I deal with her behavior?
>
> **Response:** A supervision agreement for clinical supervision can be helpful in clarifying expectations concerning the student's attitude and handling of personal issues. A written statement allows you to specify your expectations of the student, including the expectation that she will develop awareness of the effects of her personal issues on the quality of her genetic counseling service provision. You should discuss and sign the agreement at the beginning of the clinical rotation and give a copy to the student for reference.
>
> We further recommend that you monitor your reactions for possible counter-transference. For instance, what feelings do her resistance and defensiveness trigger in you—Sympathy? Concern? Frustration? Do you find yourself over-identifying—remembering being really scared when you were a student and therefore feeling reluctant to provide any corrective feedback that might make her feel worse? Try to set aside your countertransference and gently suggest to your student that her reactions are due to her low self-esteem. Ask her what the two of you can do to manage feedback in a way that she can "hear it," and periodically check to see how she is feeling about feedback in subsequent sessions.

CONCLUSIONS

Similar to the practice of genetic counseling, clinical supervision involves many complicated skills that take time and practice to develop. One should not expect to automatically be able to perform the skills necessary to be an effective supervisor or student. Much effort goes into a supervisory relationship, and one's preparation for a role of active responsibility in this relationship, whether supervisor or student, will help ensure a successful experience. It is important to remember that investing time in becoming an effective supervisor is both a personal and a professional responsibility. Effective supervisors positively shape the future of the genetic counseling profession.

APPENDIX: EXAMPLE CLINICAL SUPERVISION AGREEMENT FOR THE GENETIC COUNSELING SETTING*

(Sample Agreement, Each Clinic Individualizes)

AGREEMENT FOR GENETIC COUNSELING CLINICAL SUPERVISION AT THE XXXXX CLINIC

The purpose of this form is to acquaint you with your supervisor, to describe the supervision process and expectations, to involve you in planning your supervision

*Adapted from: McCarthy et al. (1995).

experience, and to give you the opportunity to ask any questions you may have regarding supervision.

Your Supervisor I hold a Master of Science degree specializing in genetic counseling and am certified by the American Board of Genetic Counseling. I have worked in the university setting for approximately 8 years. My clinical work has largely involved patients with general genetics concerns, metabolic diseases, and familial cancers. I have supervised genetic counseling students in these clinical settings since 1989.

Practical Supervision Concerns We will meet weekly for one-hour individual supervision sessions. All these sessions will be held in my office. We will arrange a regular meeting time before your first clinical experience at this setting. Because your placement at this site is a requirement of your genetic counseling program, attendance at all sessions is mandatory. In the event that you are unable to attend a clinic or a supervision session, you are responsible for making alternative arrangements in advance, if possible. I will provide you with my phone and pager numbers.

Practical Clinical Concerns I am ultimately responsible for the genetic counseling services provided in these clinics, including the services provided to any patient seen by students. You are responsible for coming to clinic on time and professionally attired. You are responsible for preparing the cases assigned to you in each of the clinics. This includes coming prepared to discuss the medical, genetic, and psychosocial aspects associated with the specific disorders encountered. We will discuss the cases before each clinic and together, we will decide on the most appropriate counseling approach. You will be expected to write clinic notes and follow-up letters to referring health professionals and the families you have seen in each clinic.

Objectives of this Clinical Experience During your clinical experience at this clinical setting, you are expected to learn the following:

- Take inclusive and appropriate family, medical, and pregnancy histories
- Prepare a case in the appropriate manner to include the most up to date medical and genetic information
- Assess any genetic risk and communicate that risk to the to the patient and family in a way they can understand
- Facilitate patient and family decision-making
- Offer supportive counseling
- Write clinic notes and follow-up letters to patients, families, and referring health professionals
- *Additional objectives appropriate for this particular clinic may be added here.*

Supervision Process Clinical supervision is an interactive process intended to monitor the quality of patient care, improve clinical skills, and facilitate your professional and personal growth. As a student, you have the responsibility of learning and growing professionally through these clinical experiences. This includes coming prepared to supervision, being open and responsive to feedback, following through on all assignments and recommendations, disclosing important information, asking for assistance when you are faced with counseling issues beyond your competence, and engaging in self-evaluation. You can expect to receive timely verbal and written feedback on your clinic assignments and progress with your clinical experiences. You can also expect to have a supportive environment in which to explore patient-related concerns. You will be expected to actively participate in the supervision process.

The possible benefits from this experience include improvement of your genetic counseling skills and an increased sense of your professional identity. The possible risks to you include discomfort arising from challenges to your genetic counseling knowledge, abilities, and/or skills.

Evaluation and Due Process   The clinical settings in which you will be seeing patients are part of an accredited graduate program in genetic counseling, so you may use your clinical experiences here as part of your logbook of cases needed to apply for your board certification. As your supervisor, I will provide you with ongoing written and oral feedback throughout this rotation. A formal written evaluation will be conducted upon completion. Evaluation criteria include your performance in the clinical setting. I will also determine the extent to which you have met the set of objectives for this rotation and assess your progress in attaining the skills necessary to practice as a genetic counselor. A formal written evaluation of my supervision will be solicited from you at the end of the rotation.

If at any time you are dissatisfied with your supervision or the evaluation process, please discuss this with me directly. If we are unable to resolve your concerns, you are urged to discuss them with the director of this genetic counseling graduate program.

Legal/Ethical Issues   Supervision is not intended to provide personal counseling for you. You are strongly encouraged to seek counseling if any personal concerns arise. In general, the content of our supervision sessions is confidential. My evaluations of your development are shared with the director of this program and may be discussed in supervision meetings. The purpose of supervision meetings is to assist clinical supervisors in exploring methods that may improve a student's progress. The formal written evaluations are kept in your file in the program director's office. You can expect that I will not discuss your progress with your fellow students. Limits to confidentiality include, but are not limited to, treatment of a patient that violates the legal or ethical standards established by the institution or the genetic counseling profession.

Addendum   After discussion with your supervisor, please write any statements you would like to add (You may attach additional pages, if necessary):

Statement of Agreement   I have read and understand the information contained in this document.

_____   _____

(Supervisor(s) Signature)   (Date)

_____   _____

(Student Signature)   (Date)

REFERENCES

Allen GJ, Szollos SJ, Williams BE (1986) Doctoral students' comparative evaluations of best and worst psychotherapy supervision. *Res Pract Prof Psychol* 17:91–99.

Bartels DM, LeRoy BS, McCarthy P, Caplan AL (1997) Nondirectiveness in genetic counseling: A survey of practitioners. *Am J Med Genet* 72:172–179.

Bernard JM (1988) Receiving and using supervision. In Hackney H, Cormier LS (eds), *Counseling Strategies and Interventions* (3rd ed.). Englewood Cliffs, NJ: Prentice Hall, pp. 153–169.

Bernard JM, Goodyear RK (1998) *Fundamentals of Clinical Supervision* (2nd ed.). Boston, MA: Simon & Schuster, Inc.

Bloom BS, ed. (1956) *Taxonomy of Educational Objectives, Handbook I: Cognitive Domain*. New York: Longmans, Green.

Borders LD, Leddick GR (1987) *Handbook of Counseling Supervision*. Alexandria, VA: Association of Counselor Education and Supervision.

Boyd J (1978) *Counselor Supervision: Approaches, Preparation, Practices*. Muncie, IN: Accelerated Development, Inc.

Danish SJ, D'Augelli AR, Hauer AL (1980) *Helping Skills: A Basic Training Program* (2nd ed.). New York: Human Sciences Press.

Ekstein R, Wallerstein RS (1972) *The Teaching and Learning of Psychotherapy* (2nd ed.). New York: International Universities Press, Inc.

Fall M, Sutton JM (2004) *Clinical Supervision: A Handbook for Practitioners*. Boston: Allyn and Bacon.

Fiddler MB, Fine BA, Baker DL, ABGC Consensus Development Consortium (1996) A case-based approach to the development of practice-based competencies for accreditation of and training in graduate programs in genetic counseling. *J Genet Couns* 5:105–112.

Fine BA, Baker DL, Fiddler MB, ABGC Consensus Development Consortium (1996) Practice-based competencies for accreditation of and training in graduate programs in genetic counseling. *J Genet Couns* 5:113–121.

Forrest L, Elman N, Gizara S, Vacha-Haase T (1999) Trainee impairment: A review of identification, remediation, dismissal, and legal issues. *Couns Psychol* 27:627–686.

Hart G, Nance D (2003) Styles of counselor supervision as perceived by supervisors and supervisees. *Couns Educ Superv* 43:146–158.

Hendrickson S, McCarthy Veach P, LeRoy BS (2002) A qualitative investigation of student and supervisor perceptions of live supervision in genetic counseling. *J Genet Couns* 11:25–50.

Kadushin A (1968) Games people play in supervision. *Soc Work* 13:23–32.

Lehrman-Waterman D, Ladany N (2001) Development and validation of the Evaluation Process Within Supervision Inventory. *J Couns Psych* 48:168–177.

Lindh H, McCarthy Veach P, Cikanek K, LeRoy BS (2003) A survey of clinical supervision in genetic counseling. *J Genet Couns* 12:23–42.

Littrell JM (1978) Concerns of beginning counselor trainees. *Couns Educ Superv* 18:29–35.

Loganbill C, Hardy E, Delworth U (1983) Supervision: A conceptual model. *Couns Psychol* 10:3–42.

McCarthy P, DeBell C, Kanuha V, McLeod J (1988) Myths of supervision: Identifying the gaps between theory and practice. *Couns Educ Superv* 28:22–28.

McCarthy P, Kulakowski D, Kenfield J (1994) Clinical supervision practices of licensed psychologists. *Prof Psychol Res Prac* 25:177–181.

McCarthy Veach P, LeRoy BS, Willaert R (2008) *Providing and Receiving Feedback in Clinical Supervision: A Supplemental DVD Workbook*. Minneapolis, MN: University of Minnesota.

McCarthy Veach P, LeRoy BS, Bartels DM (2003) *Facilitating the Genetic Counseling Process: A Practice Manual*. New York: Springer.

McCarthy P, Sugden S, Koker M, Lamendola F, Maurer S, Renninger S (1995) A practical guide to informed consent in clinical supervision. *Couns Educ Superv* 35:131–138.

Polanski, P. (2000, Winter). Training supervisors at the master's level: Developmental considerations. *ACES Spectrum Newsletter*, 3–5.

Schoonveld CE, McCarthy Veach P, LeRoy BS (2007). What is it like to be in the minority? Ethnic and gender diversity in the genetic counseling profession. *J Genet Couns* 16:53–70.

Stout CE (1987) The role of ethical standards in the supervision of psychotherapy. *Clin Superv* 5:89–97.

Sue DW, Sue D (1981) *Counseling the Culturally Different*. New York: John Wiley & Sons.

Weil J (2000) Introduction. *J Genet Couns* 9:375–378.

Zahm K, McCarthy Veach P, LeRoy BS (2008). An investigation of genetic counselor experiences in peer group supervision. *J Genet Couns* 17:220–233.

14

Genetic Counseling Research: Understanding the Basics

Beverly M. Yashar, M.S., Ph.D.

Research creates an opportunity to expand our understanding of our world, to shine a light onto an issue that is either open to broader explanation or has not previously been investigated. Designing and successfully implementing an effective research study is filled with numerous opportunities for both success and failure. The process is demanding, time consuming, and stressful. So why embark on this process? Research allows us to discover something novel, not only in our area of interest and but also in ourselves as investigators. Working through a research project creates the opportunity to develop new skills in critical thinking and analysis.

Since research attempts to break new ground, there is no guarantee that it will be successful. While our failures often can tell us as much as our successes, the goal of this chapter is to provide you with guidance that will help you tip the balance toward success. We will be looking at research as a process that has a specific structure composed of discrete steps (Fig. 14-1). Research is a complex process that requires us to use both the left and right sides of our brains and to be simultaneously creative and practical. In the end (or more accurately, from the start) research requires taking a leap of faith into the darkness.

A Guide to Genetic Counseling, Second Edition, Edited by Wendy Uhlmann, Jane Schuette, and Beverly Yashar
Copyright © 2009 by John Wiley & Sons, Inc.

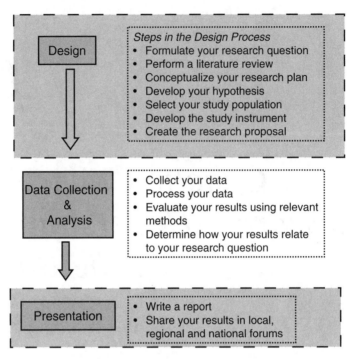

FIGURE 14-1. *The Research Process. The entire process of taking a research project from start to finish is illustrated in this figure. The actual discussion in this chapter is focused on the first and third phases. Many aspects of the analysis portion of the process are project-specific and a full discussion is beyond the scope of this chapter. The reader is encouraged to explore additional texts for guidance on this critically important phase*

This chapter touches on all aspects of the process but focuses on study design and presentation. We will take a step-by-step approach and provide general guidance to help you successfully approach, navigate, and complete these components. While our perspective will be grounded in the social sciences as opposed to laboratory-focused research, many of the concepts are broadly applicable. A number of excellent textbooks (referenced at the end of the chapter) are available that discuss individual topics in more detail.

If we knew what it was we were doing, it would not be called research, would it?
—Albert Einstein (1879–1955).

WHY DO RESEARCH?

The knowledge that is generated by a research study can provide insights and can be used to effect change and improve our work as genetic counselors. This process is driven by a unique way of thinking that is exemplified in the definition of the word itself. The word "research" is derived from the French word *recercher* meaning "to seek out, to search closely" (Harper, 2001). The prefix "re" means anew or over and over again. Consequently, research is an iterative process in which an investigator is able to answer questions that explore the "who, what, when, where, and why" of a phenomenon and develop an understanding of why these answers are true. A research project can help answer questions like:

- How effective are newborn screening programs?
- Why do clients in seemingly identical clinical settings make different decisions?
- What are the best resources and methods for helping my patients understand their risk?
- Which approach to structuring a counseling session is most responsive to the needs of my patients?
- When should genetic research results be transitioned into clinical care?
- How does my client's cultural heritage impact a counseling session?

The iterative component of research refers to the fact that simply asking and answering a question once is insufficient. In the world of research you have proven the truth of your answer when multiple experts reach the same conclusion. While researchers are continually striving for objectivity, the process itself and the resulting outcomes are extremely sensitive to error. Consequently, the process of repetition helps to ensure accuracy and allows a researcher to answer a single research question using a variety of approaches. For example, the question "When should genetic research results be transitioned into clinical care?" might be explored by asking:

- How do patients use risk information to make decision?
- What is the impact of unregulated tests on public health?
- What is the economic impact of new genetic tests?
- What are the psychological implications of false negative test results?

The answers to these questions are complementary and support the development of a more completely nuanced understanding of the original research question. In addition, the varied approaches may reflect the unique interests of the investigator and the available resources.

Genetic counseling research is focused not only on the practice itself but also on the varied clinical, social, legal and ethical issues that inform both our practice and our professional identity. A quick scan of the tables of contents of the *Journal of Genetic Counseling* finds research projects with a variety of perspectives. This variety reflects the diverse interests of individuals within the profession and demonstrates that interested researchers have explored a wide variety of questions, employed varied methodologies and applied novel theoretical lenses to explore and understand our practice (Bedard et al., 2007). Chapter 7 in this book, "Risk Communication and Decision-Making," provides multiple examples of the diverse research interests of our community.

A critical factor unifying these varied approaches is reliance on evidence-based methods. This demands that the researcher forms his or her clinical research question in response to a recognized need for information, searches for the most appropriate evidence, critically appraises it, seeks to incorporate the results into a strategy for action, and finally evaluates the outcomes. Evidence-based medicine is formally defined as an approach to healthcare that promotes the collection, interpretation, and integration of valid, important and applicable patient-reported, clinician-observed, and research-derived evidence (McKibbon, 1995; Sackett et al., 1996). High-quality research allows clinical researchers to evaluate in advance the impact of planned changes to clinical practice and can help us to understand and bring about change to the practice of genetic counseling. As stated in our Code of Ethics, genetic counselors are encouraged to participate in actions that have the purpose of promoting the well-being of society and access to healthcare (Bennett et al., 2006).

DEFINING RESEARCH: A WAY OF THINKING

How do we know what we know? What is true and/or real? There are multiple ways of defining truth. From a nonscientific perspective "truth" is based on agreement between various parties and can be defined by legal precedent, ideology, revelation, formal logic, intuition, or common sense. In research, "truth" is based on the belief that observation and cataloguing of experiences can help us understand what we know. Consequently, defining "truth" in research is dependent on a compilation of methods, tools, and techniques, and it is these methods that set it apart from other means of acquiring knowledge.

Research provides a background against which claims for knowledge can be evaluated, and provides a way for researchers to communicate and compare their findings. However, the results are not absolute. It is important to recognize that while the observations remain constant, our analysis and interpretation may change over time.

WHAT MAKES SCIENTIFIC KNOWLEDGE DIFFERENT?

Research is a unique activity in its insistence on objectivity—holding to this standard can be quite difficult given the nature of being human. Our perspectives on how the world around us works (i.e., the rules that govern our lives) are continually influenced by our personal experiences. It is these anecdotal experiences that are a central part of how we explain and bring order to the world around us. These experiences form the basis of a *subjective* perspective in which one's thinking is conditioned by one's previous experiences, educational background, discipline of study, philosophy, and social heritage. In research, when we strive to attain an *objective* perspective, we are working to understand a topic (explain a phenomenon) in a way that does not introduce the researcher's (i.e., our own) interests and perspectives. Objectivity gives research its special character, as it can help us to identify and develop constant explanations of natural phenomena.

Objectivity should be considered as both a method and a goal. It is easiest to think of objectivity in terms of a controlled experimental situation that produces the same or similar results, that is, the findings are replicable. In a practical sense, a research result is deemed to be objectively "true" when independent researchers arrive at the same conclusion. This insistence on replication helps to protect research from the biases of the researchers. In certain disciplines (i.e., molecular biology, biostatistics, clinical research), the process for obtaining objective results and the reasons why objectivity is so valuable are relatively easy to understand. Even in disciplines that are striving to understand individual motivations and perspectives and are less concerned about the generalizability of their results, pursuing this knowledge in the name of research demands that the researcher strives to remain as objective as possible. No matter what research discipline you ascribe to, the following precepts should be kept in mind:

- Apply a systematic scientific approach to identifying and developing your research question, formulating and testing your hypothesis, and collecting and analyzing your data. This ensures that data are gathered according to a scheme that is ordered and methodical.
- Strive for rigor (accuracy and exactness) in all phases of the project. This is especially true in data analysis, but begins with the design of the project.
- Develop a comprehensive research plan that serves as the blueprint for the actual work.
- Be open to critical inquiry from others and be self-critical.

This mind-set makes it possible to define discrete characteristics of a successful research project and to begin to understand how to approach designing, implementing, and analyzing a research project in which the results are valid and verifiable.

CHOOSING AN EXPERIMENTAL APPROACH

While there are many absolutes about the process of designing and implementing a research project, there are also multiple opportunities for you as a researcher to make decisions that are determined by your unique interests. Selection of your experimental approach (choosing a quantitative or qualitative method of investigation) is one such example. In a *qualitative* study the investigator is focused on describing variation in a phenomenon, situation, or attitude, and working to understand the deeper meaning of individual experience. Often the aim is to produce a complete, detailed description. In a *quantitative* approach, the research is focused on quantifying variation, utilizing precise and generalizable statistical methods, and looking at cause and effect.

In **qualitative studies**, data are generally collected in the form of words as opposed to numbers and the results are evaluated in terms of themes or categories (Creswell, 1998; Greenhlagh and Taylor, 1997; Mason, 2002). The goal is generally discovery, description, understanding, and interpretation. The analysis is interpretive rather than measurable and is highly context dependent. This type of approach often leads toward the development, rather than testing, of a hypothesis and/or theory.

A qualitative study can consider details and nuances of subjects' replies and explore multiple interpretations of answers (Table 14-1). The process is highly dependent on communication and observation, and subjects generally have freedom in their responses,

TABLE 14-1. Features of Qualitative and Quantitative Research (Neill, 2007)

Qualitative	Quantitative
The aim of qualitative analysis is a complete, detailed description.	Quantitative research is focused on classification, counting, and construction of statistical models that explain the observations.
Can be very useful in early phases of a research project.	Recommended during later phases of research projects.
Researcher may only know roughly in advance what he/she is looking for.	Researcher knows clearly in advance what he/she is looking for.
The design emerges as the study unfolds.	All aspects of the study are carefully designed before data are collected.
Researcher is the data-gathering instrument.	Researcher uses tools, such as questionnaires or equipment to collect numerical data.
Data are in the form of words, pictures, or objects.	Data are in the form of numbers and statistics.
Qualitative data are richer, more time consuming, and less generalizable.	Quantitative data are more efficient, able to test hypotheses, and more generalizable. However, these studies may miss contextual details.
Researcher tends to become subjectively immersed in the subject matter.	Researcher tends to remain objectively separated from the subject matter.

that is, they can describe their experiences in their own words. Methods of choice can include individual, in-depth interviews and focus groups. Participants are asked to respond to general questions, and the interviewer or group moderator probes and explores their responses, works to identify and define participants' perceptions, opinions, and feelings about the topic or idea being discussed, and, for a focus group, tries to determine the degree of agreement that exists in the group. This type of research is exploratory and open-ended. Qualitative research is extremely effective in discovering the meaning events have for the individuals who experience them. It is interpretive in character; the analysis is dependent on interpretation by the researcher. Thus the quality of the findings from a qualitative research project is directly dependent upon the skills, experience, and sensitivity of the interviewer or group moderator.

Quantitative studies measure characteristics and experiences with numerical categories that are analyzed statistically. This method generally relies on structured questions in the form of a survey with predetermined response options. It does not restrict the types of research questions that are being explored; rather, it imposes a specific structure on the ways in which the research questions are explored and the results are gathered and evaluated (Table 14-1). In quantitative research, it is the responsibility of the researcher to assess the validity and reliability of the study instrument (i.e., the data collection tool). In this approach it is critical that the researcher develops questions and responses that have the same meaning to all participants and really measure what the researcher intends to measure. The upside of this approach is that it is possible to explore the experiences of greater numbers of individuals and in general it is viewed as more objective.

Qualitative research can generate rich, detailed data that provide an in-depth understanding of a topic. Quantitative research generates reliable, population-based data and is well suited to establishing cause-and-effect relationships. (Table 14-1) The decision of whether to choose a quantitative or a qualitative design is both philosophical and practical (Neill, 2007). Which method you choose will depend on the nature of the project, the type of information needed, the context of the study and the availability of resources (time, money, and human). Are you looking to gain new knowledge or develop new theories or methods to apply to the research process itself? Alternatively, is your research going to be focused on applications in which you are trying to understand an area of practice and working towards improvement or change (also known as clinical or translational research)? It is important to keep in mind that while these are two different philosophies, they are not necessarily contradictory (Glasziou et al., 2004). In fact, elements of both designs can be used together in mixed-methods studies. Combining qualitative and quantitative research is becoming more and more common.

Combining both types of research can result in:

- Better research development—one approach can be used to inform the other, i.e., qualitative research results can be used to develop a quantitative study instrument.
- Increased validity—confirming results from different data sources and different mechanisms
- New ideas, fresh perspectives, and the identification of contradictions

---

Whichever method or methods you use, it is critical that you utilize purposeful, reflective reasoning, and analysis to guide your decision-making. Maintain an open mind, be willing to identify and deal with your biases, and be prudent in your decision-making and willing to reconsider your perspectives, conclusions, and decisions. Achieving this goal demands that you are habitually inquisitive, diligent in seeking out relevant information, and focused and persistent in your inquiries and analysis. At the end of the day, using critical thinking skills will help you to be successful in all phases of your research project.

THE RESEARCH PROCESS

No matter how long or short the time period you have to undertake a research project, it is critical to approach your research in a stepwise manner that breaks it down into a process composed of discrete phases: design, data collection and analysis, and presentation (Fig. 14-1). This approach will help you organize your work and goes a long way toward ensuring the success of your research (Botti and Endacott, 2005; Endacott, 2004a, 2004b, 2005a, 2005b, 2005c; Kumar, 2005). For illustrative purposes, the design process itself has been broken down into seven discrete sequential steps. The order in which these steps are undertaken can vary from project to project and researcher to researcher. To the novice researcher, it is often difficult to envision where your project will lead; however, the more time you can spend anticipating and critically evaluating your end point(s) and how the steps in your research plan will get you there, and anticipating problems that may arise along the way, the higher the likelihood of successfully completing a project that provides answers to your questions. The research plan helps you impose "a method to the madness."

Design Step 1: Formulate Your Research Question

The first phase of designing your research plan is to formulate your research question. Where can you find good research ideas? Curiosity is a critical first step in identifying a potential project. What have you been learning about in class, observed in your clinical rotations, heard discussed in conferences, or presented at seminars? What did you find interesting or intriguing and wanted to know more about? Your daily professional world is a great place to start (Table 14-2).

Reading current literature can also help you identify topics of interest. Look at the table of contents from journals of interest to genetic counselors, including but not limited to the *Journal of Genetic Counseling, Genetics in Medicine,* and the *American Journal of Medical Genetics.* Read abstracts from recent genetics professional meetings or those related to your interests. In addition, exploring the tables of contents and reading articles in journals of interest can help you develop research ideas that refine or extend previous research. What are the existing theories that support your clinical work? Can these be built upon or should they be contested? Look at recent projects that have been funded by relevant agencies like the Jane Engelberg Memorial Followship or the Audrey Heimler Special Projects Award at NSGC. Requests for proposals (RFPs) from funding agencies are another possible starting place. These documents generally describe new questions that need addressing and identify general approaches that thought-leaders in the field see as important. Even if you are not going to be applying to these agencies, evaluating RFPs can be a great way to identify interesting research questions. Let your creative juices flow. Just because the topic you have identified has been previously researched, it does not mean that the specific question that you want to answer has been asked. Your perspectives will be unique—use them.

Give yourself permission to identify new areas for exploration. This can be a very exciting part of the process. Think big—at first nothing should be out of the realm of possibility. You will have plenty of time to determine what is going to be workable and to evolve the project in order to ensure success given the constraints of your environment. This is the point in the process where everything is possible.

Once you have identified your general area(s) of interest, it is important to consider how interested in this topic you really are. Research projects require a lot of time;

TABLE 14-2. Developing Practice-Based Research Questions (Endacott, 2004a)

Identify areas of your clinical practice that:
You "use" but don't work effectively
You "use" but you don't know why they work
You "do" differently from others or from the way that you were taught
We should be doing but we "don't"
Impact how our patients approach improving their health and well-being

make sure that this is something that you really want to do. Is this a topic that you really care about? Ask yourself why you chose this topic and exactly what you want to discover. The steps outlined in Table 14-3 provide a practical approach to developing a research idea that you will enjoy pursuing.

TABLE 14-3. Identifying and Developing a Research Idea (Kumar, 2005)

Step	Guidance	Questions to Ask Yourself
1. Define the purpose of your study and identify a broad area of interest.	Work to be as clear and precise as you can.	Make sure you really care about this topic. Ask yourself why you want to do this research and what you hope to achieve.
2. Dissect the broad idea into subareas.	This is a place to really brainstorm multiple ways of exploring your research interest	Have I explored my research idea from multiple perspectives?
3. Select a subarea.	This should be the idea that you find most interesting.	Do I really "care" about this idea? Ask yourself why this is appealing.
4. Raise a specific research question.	Make sure that it relates to your original research problem	Ask yourself if this question will allow you to really explore your area of interest.
5. Undertake a literature review.	Determine what is already known about your topic. Be sure to consider relevant related areas. This will help you begin deciding if your question is worthy of research.	Has this idea been explored previously? If yes, why is it worthy of replication or follow up? If no, why not?
6. Formulate an objective and specific aims (or subobjectives).	This is derived from your research question and should take the form of action-oriented statements.	Make sure that the specific aim is doable and related to your objective.
7. Assess your specific aim(s) in terms of feasibility.	Ask yourself if it passes the "so what" test—will this analysis make a difference to me—to others? Define the obstacles • Knowledge, available data, time, cost Weigh the benefits against the costs.	How much work is involved? Is the scale of the project • doable? Do you have: • enough time? • enough money? • access to the needed expertise? Are there ethical considerations: • what population will you be studying? • are they accessible?
8. Double-check that you are still interested in your project.	Make sure that the project possess relevance, adds to a body of knowledge, and supports your interests.	Are you still interested? Do you agree with the objectives? Do you have the needed resources?

Design Step 2: Perform a Literature Review

With a good research idea in hand, it is important to explore the existing literature so that you can see what is already known about the topic. This search will help you gain a fuller understanding of the history of explorations in your topic. This analysis helps you to figure out what is really known and what is still unknown and where your research results will fit into the current body of knowledge. This review can also help you identify theories or conceptual frameworks that you can use to support your proposed work.

At first, this search is going to humble you. You may think that all the good ideas have already been asked and answered. However, this is the time to really use your critical thinking skills. Evaluate what has already been accomplished, figure out its strengths and weaknesses, and recognize that there are multiple ways of asking and answering a question, each of which, if rigorously developed and applied, will yield complementary insights. What possible failings or issues are there in the previous research? What is appropriate for future analysis? This review will help you develop objectives (including subobjectives/specific aims) that are grounded in the literature, doable, and relevant to the field.

So How Do You Get Started on Your Review?   Ask your advisor, mentor, supervisors, and senior students what the most credible (usually peer reviewed) and useful journals and conference proceedings are in your field. Also ask for advice on identifying seminal or "classic" papers that you should definitely read. You might also look for a study that resembles your research idea. Ask yourself what the investigators considered relevant in their review of the literature, that is, what information was reviewed in the introduction of the paper? Aside from helping you to figure out the current state of thinking about the topic, this will help identify relevant issues that you need to consider and help you begin to think about how you might measure things and preview common problems. You can use these past experiences to identify and avoid common traps and pitfalls.

You will need to immerse yourself in the literature so that you can become familiar with the field. In the beginning you will be spending the majority of your time reading. It's normal to be overwhelmed by the possibilities. It is impossible to read everything that might be relevant; instead, read selectively. Before bothering to read any paper, make sure it's worth it. Scan the title, then the abstract, and then glance at the introduction and conclusions. Before you try to understand all the nitty-gritty details of the paper, skim the whole thing and try to get a feel for the most important points. If it still seems worthwhile and relevant, go back and read the whole thing. Be sure to pay careful attention to the methods and results and evaluate how well they support the conclusions. You may want to take notes while you read. Even if you don't go back and reread them, this process can help you to focus your attention and forces you to summarize as you read. And if you do need to refresh your memory later, rereading your notes is much easier and faster than rereading the whole paper.

One Last Detail   This is the point in planning your research project when you should start to figure out how you are going to keep track of your references, including not just the citation but relevant information gleaned from the articles. There are a number of excellent online bibliographic management programs, including Citation Manager, EndNote, and RefWorks. Some of these may be available for use through your local library. This is a good point in your research project to learn how to access them and to start using them to keep track of your literature search.

Design Step 3. Conceptualize Your Research Plan

Once you have decided on your research question, it is time to transform it into a format that will drive the next phase of developing your research plan, your *objective(s)* and *subobjective(s)* or *specific aim(s)* (Table 14-3). The **objective** defines the overall thrust of your study. It sets the relationships and associations that you want to establish or discover and summarizes what will be achieved by the study in general terms. The objective is derived from your research question.

The **specific aim(s)** describes the specific aspects of the topic that you will be investigating. It should break down the general objective(s) into smaller, doable pieces and systematically address the various aspects of your research problem. Each specific aim has a single purpose that is clear and nonredundant and is generally specified in terms that rely on action words like determine, compare, verify, calculate, describe, and establish. Avoid the use of vague nonaction verbs such as appreciate, understand, or study.

Specific aims are generally focused on key factors that you believe influence or cause the problem (these are identified from your literature search), and they should specify what you will do in your study, and the order in which they will be performed. Formulating specific aims will help you focus your study and narrow it down to the essentials. If properly formulated, specific aims will facilitate the development of your research methodology and help to orient the collection, analysis, interpretation, and utilization of data. It should help you organize your study into clearly defined parts or phases and help you avoid collecting data that are not strictly necessary for understanding and solving the problem you have identified.

> For example, if your research question is focused on the consequences of gene discovery in common complex diseases, then the general *objective* of your study might be to explore ways in which clinical genetic medicine can accommodate the growth of genomic medicine. A *specific aim* could be to assess public perception of genetic results from association studies or to determine how genetic counselors decide when genetic research results should be transitioned into clinical care.

Take care to make sure that the specific aim(s) of your study:

- Cover the different aspects of the problem and its contributing factors in a coherent manner and in a logical sequence
- Are clearly phrased in operational terms, specifying exactly what you are going to do, where, and for what purpose

- Are realistic considering your resource constraints (especially your own time!)
- Really allow you to test your hypothesis or provide answers to your research question

Finally, remember that research is an iterative process, and that iteration also applies to the design process. Make sure that at each step in conceptualizing your research plan your decisions are logical, doable and support your ultimate goals (Table 14-3). If not, you will need to go back and restart the process from an earlier stage.

Design Step 4 (Optional). Develop Your Hypothesis

Based on your work to this point in developing your research project [your literature review, critical analysis of previous results and supporting theories, and the development of your research objectives and specific aim(s)], you may have discovered that you can postulate testable explanations for the problem. If so, you can formulate a hypothesis(es) in addition to the study objective.

The *hypothesis* takes the form of a prediction about the results of your research; it defines the relationship(s) between one or more factors (variables) and the problem you are planning on studying in a format that can be tested. It describes in concrete terms what you expect to happen in the study and provides an explanation for the expected results (Table 14-4). In doing so it brings direction, specificity, and focus to your research study and becomes the basis for the subsequent design of your project. The hypothesis generally states what the investigator believes to be the most probable explanation for the phenomenon he or she is planning on studying.

Consequently, the hypothesis:

- Represents the best hunch of the researcher and is simple, specific, and conceptually clear
- Is a tentative proposition, but is related to a body of knowledge
- Has unknown validity, but is capable of being tested and measured
- Specifies a relationship between variables that is one-dimensional, i.e., tests one relationship at a time

While generating a hypothesis at the start of a research project has the advantage of helping to guide the research project, not all projects are well suited to the strictures imposed by a hypothesis. If an area of research is novel and truly exploratory, generating a hypothesis can oversimplify the investigation and limit the process. Since a hypothesis defines testable relationships, the existing body of literature (either specific to the topic or related) must be sufficient to define testable components of the hypothesis. If your project is going to be the first to explore a topic, generating a hypothesis will likely not be useful and may need to wait for the generation of appropriate observations.

TABLE 14-4. Issues in Study Design, Implementation and Analysis

Component	Issues to Consider
Hypothesis	Evaluate the validity of your hypothesis. Ask if it is specific enough to be researchable yet still meaningful. How certain are you of the relationship(s) between variables?
Variables	What will you be measuring? What degree of error is acceptable?
Study Population & Sampling	Which individuals or group will you need to work with to answer your research question?
	What are the important characteristics of your entire population? How will you choose your sample? How big is big enough? Does your sample need to be representative? If so, of whom or of what, and what degree of accuracy is acceptable?
Study Instrument	How will you get the data you need to test your hypothesis? What tools or devices will you use to make or record observations? Are valid and reliable instruments available, or do you need to construct your own?
Data Collection— Logistics	What is your timeline? How much leeway do you have? How will you coordinate the various steps? Will interviewers, observers, or analysts need to be trained? What level of interrater reliability will you accept?
Data Processing & Analysis	What analytical and statistical tools will be applied to the data? What results will allow you to accept or reject your hypothesis? Do the findings show numerical differences, and are those differences important?
	What skills do you need to develop or expertise to identify in order to accomplish this?
Ethical Considerations	Can the data be collected and subjects' rights still preserved?
The Research Proposal	Make sure to write for your reader and follow all agency requested requirements in the final document.
Interpretation & Conclusions	Was your initial hypothesis supported? What if your findings are negative? What are the implications of your findings theoretically, how do they change your original assumptions, or your interpretation of the literature? What recommendations can you make for public policies or programs in this area? What suggestions can you make for further research on this topic?

So How Do You Go About Designing Your Hypothesis?   First you need to figure out what concepts you want to understand. These are your variables. They translate your concept into an objective and measurable construct and define the type of data you will be gathering and analyzing. The *hypothesis* states the relationships between variables so that they can be tested experimentally. It may take the form of a cause-effect statement, or an "if X, then Y" statement. Remember that the hypothesis makes **tentative** predictions about how we expect the variables to **covary**. The variable that measures the assumed cause in the relationship is called the **independent** variable (i.e., the variable that is postulated to explain another variable), and the effect or outcome is called the **dependent** variable (i.e., what is affected by the independent variable). While research is inherently reductionist (we are always trying to simplify the issue), it is never so simple as to assume that there are only cause-and-effect relationships. In generating your hypothesis it will be important to take into

account variables that affect, connect, or link the relationship between the independent and dependent variables. *Extraneous* variables can impact the dependent variable but are generally not measured in the study, while the *intervening* variables link the independent and dependent variables and are necessary in order for the independent variable to impact the dependent variable.

A Few Words About Measurement   Since variables provide a way of measuring a concept they can be operationally defined and measured. Attributes are the specific values or characteristics of a variable. This could be accomplished in quantitative research by assigning numbers that are amenable to statistical analysis (age, height, or weight). As an example from the NSGC Professional Status Survey, if the variable were "years employed as genetic counselor," the attributes could be "0–5," "5–10," "10–15," "15–20," and "20+ " years of experience (Parrott and Del Vecchio, 2007). If the variable were degree of job satisfaction, the variables could be "very satisfied," "satisfied," "dissatisfied," or "very dissatisfied." In qualitative research this is accomplished by coding in which the researcher extracts concepts from data, identifies themes, and develops interpretations.

There are varied levels of measurement. These variations determine the type of statistical analysis that can be conducted and, therefore, the type of conclusions that can be drawn from the research. The rules that are used to assign labels to variables (the attributes) are a critical component of measurement. If the rules used to assign the labels are poorly designed the outcome(s) can be meaningless. In all forms of measurement the attributes that are used to categorize your variable should form categories that are both *mutually exclusive* and *exhaustive*. *Exhaustive* means that there must be enough categories so that all the observations will fall into some category. *Mutually exclusive* means that the categories must be distinct enough that no observations will fall into more than one category.

Design Steps 5 and 6. Develop Your Materials and Methods

You have decided on your objectives and specific aim(s) and determined whether it is appropriate to develop a hypothesis (and, if needed, designed one). What to work on next? You will now need to set up the overall strategy for accomplishing your specific aim(s). In this phase you will have to decide what data you need to collect to meet your research objectives, and how you will gather and analyze it. Table 14-4 identifies the topics that you will need to consider. Remember the weeding out and narrowing down that occurred as you moved from identifying your research idea to setting objectives and specific aims? Why did you go through this process? It allowed you to develop an idea for your research project that was valid, verifiable, rigorous, and ultimately doable. Similar critical criteria must be applied to the development of your study design, in which you figure out how you are going to actually explore, test, and hopefully answer the questions you have identified. In this phase of designing your project it will also be important to work on anticipating any roadblocks you may encounter and to make a specific plan for how you will address them.

During this phase of study design, it will be important to consider the feasibility of actually getting the work done. What are the obstacles in terms of knowledge, availability of relevant data, time, and/or resources? Do the benefits outweigh the costs? There is a constant struggle between being as rigorous as possible in your design while considering the practicality of designing a project that can be completed. Think small (the details of the day-to-day) and think big (ask yourself why is this important and why do I care?). Do you have sufficient time to accomplish the work that you are proposing? If you are going to be working with human subjects, are there ethical constraints to the work that you are proposing? Think about whom you will need to identify as collaborators. Will they be able to help you? And finally, figure out what resources you will need. These can include getting access to specific patient populations, the cost of survey design, statistical consultants, research assistants, recording equipment, and office supplies.

Design Step 5. Selecting Your Study Population

Often during the process of identifying and designing your research question you will have also defined exactly who you want to study, that is, the members of your study population. For example, if your research will be focused on understanding the utility of newborn screening in Alaska, then the broad parameters of your study population have been identified. However, there are times when your research question is developed independent of a specific population. If you are interested in exploring the public's attitudes toward genetic testing for bipolar disease, your study population could include anyone in the entire world. In either instance, it will be impossible to interact with every individual relevant to your research question. You will need to determine exactly which individuals you will be studying. Exactly who will you ask to participate in your research? Who in the "public" will you be interviewing or surveying? Sampling provides a means of saving time and minimizing cost. Careful sampling of your population can help ensure that your research provides comprehensive information that is representative of the entire group. However, it is important to be aware that since sampling provides an estimate of your population, it is also subject to "error." Depending on the type of research project and the objectives, an investigator may be more or less concerned about this issue.

Generally in exploratory research or in a project that is based on qualitative methodology, the researcher will use a ***nonrandom sampling method*** that focuses on volunteers and individuals who are easily accessible (i.e., they are in the "right place at the right time"). For these types of studies the parameters of the study population itself are less important than the exploration and the generation of new insights and hypotheses for future research. The advantages of using ***nonrandom selection*** are that the method is minimally expensive, the sampling is easy to obtain, and understanding the characteristics of the population itself is of minimal importance. Consequently, the results can be sensitive to bias (the quality of a measurement or analysis that results in misrepresentation) with regard to the selection of study participants by the researcher.

If a research project is focused on understanding an issue within the context of a specific population (how much do genetic counselors know about direct to consumer genetic testing?), it may be important to develop a sample that is representative of the entire population. Since it is going to be impossible to interact with every genetic counselor, it will be important to apply *random or probability sampling*. This selects a subset of individuals in the population that are representative of the entire population. When appropriately applied, *random sampling* provides a solid estimate of the entire study population. This sampling methodology is more commonly associated with quantitative studies and can be used to test a hypothesis and develop population statistics.

When using random sampling to construct your study population, it is important to work on minimizing bias. Think very carefully about who comprises the entire population and consider any special structures that may exist in the larger study population. These substructures may necessitate employing additional sampling precautions, including systematic random, stratified random, and cluster sampling (Creswell, 2003; Hulley et al., 2001; Kumar, 2005; Marczyk et al., 2005; Rubin and Babbie, 2007). Deciding between these options is dependent on a variety of factors that include the structure of your study population (are there strata or clusters you need to be aware of), your research question, and the available time and money. As you define your actual sample, it is important to evaluate this issue carefully and comprehensively.

How Big a Sample Do You Need?   The size of the sample depends on the type of research design being used; the desired level of confidence in the results; the degree of accuracy desired; and the characteristics of the population of interest. There are a variety of statistical methods to assess whether a sample size is adequate (i.e., power calculations). This topic is beyond the scope of this chapter.

How Good Is Your Sample?   It is important to realize that there will always be a difference between the sample statistics and the true population mean or average. Error is an inherent by-product of sampling. The guiding principles of sampling include working to provide the best approximation of the population and avoiding bias in sample selection. While increasing your sample size will increase the accuracy with which it represents a population, bias can still arise because of either nonrandom selection or incomplete or inaccurate representation of the population, that is, the sampling frame is wrong or important components of your population can't be identified or won't participate.

Finally, take the time to consider your choices about your study population in light of your research objectives. Does your final population still allow you to gain information that is relevant to your research objective? If your research is focused on improving the quality of healthcare in Alaska and you are sampling a population based in Alaska, then you will have likely selected the correct population. However, if the objective of your research is to determine the cost effectiveness of newborn screening in general, then only studying Alaska (with its very low population density) may not be the optimal study population.

A full discussion of the concepts and practice of sampling is beyond the scope of this chapter, and interested readers are encouraged to start with the references in the bibliography and then explore focused texts on this topic.

Design Step 6. Develop the Study Instrument

There are a variety of ways in which you go about collecting the data for your study. The tool that you use to collect your data is known as the study instrument. *Primary data collection* is gathering data directly from those who hold the information. This method often includes using surveys, interviews, focus groups, and clinical trials. Alternatively, you can extract research data from *secondary sources*, like clinic forms, chart notes, clinical records. Each method has it owns benefits and limitations.

All things being equal you should work to ensure that the tool or tools you use to gather your data, that is, your study instrument, provides you with the highest-quality data. There are limitations to both primary and secondary data collection in terms of *accuracy* (how well your methods and results measure the true value) and *reliability* (the consistency and stability of your methods and results). Whether you choose to collect your data face to face, on the telephone, or via the web, before you make your decision consider the strengths and drawbacks of each approach, how much bias is acceptable, and what type of an error rate you can tolerate. It is also important to think about mechanics, available time, money, skills, and other resources. Table 14-5 provides a brief overview of two types of research tools (interviews and question-naires/surveys) and highlights critical factors to consider.

Design Step 7. Create The Research Proposal

Often a necessary step in the development of your plan is finding support and/or funding for your project. Convincing someone to give you these needed resources will usually require that you write a research proposal. This document can be used to convince others (including your research committee) that there is merit to your proposed project (is the question that you are asking worthwhile?) and that it is workable (will you be able to answer your question using the proposed plan?). So while the process of writing a proposal may seem onerous and time consuming, it is also a very important way of ensuring that your research is appropriately organized to effectively answer your proposed question(s) (Locke et al., 2000). If appropriately developed, your research proposal should translate your idea into a work plan that defines what you are going to be doing, how you will be doing it, and when it will happen. It can help you figure out where you may have problems and plan for how you will deal with them. Writing a proposal can help you to establish a timeline for your project. It can also be useful in generating an Institutional Review Board (IRB) application. Often the required components and the level of detail are similar to those of an IRB application (see section *The Human Side of the Equation*). Finally, it can optimize communication with not only a funding agency but also other members of your research committee and working group.

TABLE 14-5. Study Instruments—A Comparison

	Interviews	Questionnaires and Surveys
	This is a useful approach when you want to measure individuals' perceptions or attitudes. This approach can help provide in-depth insights when little prior information exists on a topic. Subjects are allowed to answer questions (Interviewer probes) using their own words, and depending on the type of experimental approach and study design the Interviewer may have flexible or inflexible responses.	This approach is especially helpful when the study population is large and maintaining anonymity is an issue in reporting. It can be useful for measuring behaviors and perceptions.
Data		
Depth of Information	Very High—High	Moderate
Reliability	Can range from Very High to Low. This variation depends on the method of data collection and the skills of the researcher in interpretation.	Very High
Study Population		
Research Setting	Location is constrained	Location is not constrained
Culturally Responsive	Depends on focus and skills of researcher	Depends on focus and skills of researcher
Errors in Data Collection		
Interviewer-Dependent Bias	Sensitive. If interviewer is inflexible in their responses, then this is less sensitive.	Insensitive
Interviewer-Dependent Skill	High—Low	Insensitive
Subject-Dependent Bias	High	Low—Very High. Depends on the quality of the instrument. It is not possible to clarify ambiguities in questions or answers. Also impacted by who chooses to participate in the research
Cost	High	Generally less expensive

A well-organized research proposal focuses on both the big picture and the minutiae. In a research proposal often "the devil is in the details." Consequently the process of developing a research proposal can serve as a highly useful step in the development of your research project. This activity can provide you with the opportunity to really think through your project from start to finish. An effective proposal should delineate the research problem, provide a convincing argument for why it needs to be explored, and demonstrate that your planned approach (i.e., your methodology) is adequate for the task. As noted previously, it is critical to determine what format the funding agency requires and follow its instructions faithfully. If no guidance is provided you can look at the instructions from a similar agency. The web site for the Office of Extramural Research at the National Institutes of Health has a wealth of useful information and guidance about the grant process. While there is no single universally acceptable and correct format, there are a set number of tasks that must be accomplished in a proposal, often in a very condensed format. Generally a research proposal contains sections that include the following information:

- Introduction, which includes:
  o Background
  o Your research question
  o Significance
- Objectives and specific aims
- Study design
- Time line
- References

The *Introduction* section generally serves multiple purposes. In its simplest form it introduces the study and states the research question. In general this section of a proposal answers the question "What is this study all about?" and explains why it is important to find an answer. This section provides the reader with general information about your research purpose and plan.

In addition, the Introduction section answers the question "Why bother to undertake this study?" by providing a justification for your proposed work. This is usually grounded in previous research. To be able to develop this section you will need to identify and discuss related work (provide a relevant literature review) and explore how your research question was previously investigated. As part of this review, you will need to address the shortcomings of existing work in the area, and demonstrate how your approach will differ from and be an improvement over existing work. This section should remind you of the work that you undertook to develop your research idea. In fact, much of the work that you did while developing your research project can be reused to write the Introduction section of your proposal. You may also be asked to include a section that discusses the significance of your research. The focus and content of this section should explore how your research results will add to the existing body of knowledge. In some cases, this section will ask you to explore the broader implications of your research.

The content of the sections of your proposal that present your *objective(s)*, *hypothesis*, and *specific aim(s)* will be derived from the work you did while conceptualizing your research plan. Make sure that the information that is provided in the Introduction section provides adequate justification for these sections of the proposal.

The *study design* provides information on the mechanics of your research. It defines and justifies the methodology that you will be using to accomplish your research. It generally describes where the work is going to be taking place, describes how you will gather information (what your study instrument is), defines your study population (sample size and sampling design), and defines the methods of data analysis. It also generally discusses your budget (including material, people, and equipment support) and defines a time line for accomplishing the proposed work.

This section also generally contains a discussion of the problems or limitations of the proposed work, identifies possible roadblocks, and provides a plan for how you will deal with these potential issues. This section can also include information about relevant resources that you will be utilizing to help you accomplish the proposed work (i.e., additional expertise or collaborators). Finally, it is important to remember to refer to all relevant literature.

It is critical that you present your ideas for investigating your research question in as much detail as possible, and present a reasonably detailed plan for how you will accomplish this work. Generally you will be able to reuse parts of the proposal in the final write-up. This means that a well-written proposal makes for a well-written final report.

Finally, pay close attention to the writing itself. Be sure that your document is logically organized (i.e., do your arguments make sense intellectually and are they presented so that the reader can understand and evaluate them?). If you present your research plan in a strong, error-free manner, your reader is more likely to take the time and effort to really understand it. If your writing is weak, your reader is more likely to become confused and distracted and it is less likely that she or he will be won over by your arguments. Work on making your writing as clear and compelling as possible. To that end, it is worthwhile to consider the importance of striving for simplicity, clarity, and brevity in your writing. No matter your purpose, work to produce a proposal that is accessible. Often this can be accomplished by enlisting the help of others who are working with you on your project. Give them the opportunity to read and critique your document. While it may be painful to imagine receiving this feedback, in the end it will help you produce a stronger final document that will support your goals.

DATA COLLECTION AND ANALYSIS

This topic is beyond the scope of this chapter and is an interesting and exacting discipline in its own right. As you design your research project, this part of the process should also be carefully evaluated (Table 14-4). Often data processing and analysis will require that you develop new knowledge and skills, and depending on your time frame, scope and focus of your project, and your prior expertise you may want to enlist additional expertise to help you complete this phase of your research The following references are a good starting place:- Creswell, 2003; Hulley et al., 2001; Kumar, 2005; Marczyk et al., 2005; Mason, 2002; Rubin and Babbie, 2007. Establishing a plan for data entry and coding will help minimize errors in your data and increase the efficiency of your analysis.

PRESENTATION: PULLING IT ALL TOGETHER

Research in genetic counseling is focused on generating new perspectives on our profession. Its value is maximized when it is shared with the entire community. Making sure that others are aware of the results of your work is a critical end point of the entire research process. Your goal in research presentation is to share your work with a greater audience so that it can be evaluated against the current standards in the field, can be incorporated into the existing body of research, and can become a steppingstone to new ideas. There are multiple opportunities to share your work. These can include your final write-up, peer-reviewed manuscripts, book chapters, and presentations at local, regional and national meetings (including both talks and poster presentations). In each case there will usually be specific requirements and instructions about the format, content, and length. It is essential that you review these guidelines and follow them as precisely as possible. This will ensure that your proposed presentation receives a comprehensive and fair review.

If you are preparing a thesis, your graduate school will have specific requirements for the content and format of this document. If you are preparing a manuscript for submission to a journal, there are usually instructions on the journal's web page or in the paper edition of the journal itself. Be sure to follow these instructions explicitly.

Below are some ideas on how to go about developing a research article. A full discussion of this topic is provided by Bowen (Bowen, 2003).

- The **Abstract/Summary** is designed to tell the reader what your study was about and your conclusions. It should be short (generally a paragraph) and to the point. While it always appears at the start of a paper, it is generally the last thing that you will write since it is based on the content of all the other sections.
- The **Introduction** allows you to state clearly what the research is about and includes the relevant background information (i.e., places your research in context, introduces the reader to the topic, provides important definitions). It should include content that explores your research topic and lays out the central question(s). This section is similar to that contained within the introduction of your proposal but, depending on the actual format of your write-up, may be more detailed (a thesis) or more focused (a manuscript).
- The **Materials and Methods** section describes all aspects of how the study was carried out. It contains information about the study design, participants, procedures for data collection, measures that were used in the data analysis, and the actual process of data analysis.
- The **Results** section is a factual presentation of the findings from your analysis. Use tables, graphs, figures to enhance and clarify the presentation of your information and results.
- The **Discussion/Conclusion** section provides a systematic and thoughtful interpretation of your findings and discuses the implications. Start by restating your topic and briefly summarizing your results. Bring in the main points, but

don't go into too much detail. Your discussion is the place where you go beyond the summary. Work to provide an answer or answers in light of everything that you have done and discussed. Your conclusions must be linked to the evidence provided by your results.

- **References**
- **Figures/Tables/Appendices/Supplementary Materials**

Another important forum for sharing your research can be professional meetings. These are often competitive and require submission of an abstract that describes your work. Like other forms of research writing, there are often specific guidelines on format and word limits. Look carefully for these instructions, as failure to comply can result in your abstract not even getting a review. When your research is accepted for presentation there will also be guidance about the format for your presentation (for both talks and posters). Pay close attention to these instructions; they are very important in ensuring that your presentation goes well.

THE HUMAN SIDE OF THE EQUATION–ETHICAL RESEARCH

Genetic counseling research is often dependent on participation by human subjects. This type of research is subject to review by an Institutional Review Board (IRB) that decides whether human subjects are being treated ethically. The history of regulation around human subjects research is long and checkered. In the U.S., there are multiple branches of the federal government [Office for Human Research Protection, Office for Research Integrity, the FDA (Food and Drug Administration)] that are focused on protecting the rights of human research subjects. The IRB serves as the local face of this regulatory system; its regulations apply to both subjects and researchers. A full discussion of this topic and the basis for the current ethical principles that govern IRB practice is beyond the scope of this chapter and, interested readers are encouraged to review the documentation from the IRB boards at their institutions (Bankert and Amdur, 2006; Human Research Protections Program Operations Manual: University of Michigan, 2008; NCPHS, 1979). Highlighted below are some general principles.

What Defines a Human Subject?

The federal regulation defines a human subject as any living individual or fetus about whom a research investigator obtains data via interaction or intervention (45 CFR 46, 2001). This regulation also includes human tissue, but excludes deceased individuals, and consequently research on them (including their tissue or information) is not protected by IRB regulations. In addition, research that is conducted on individuals participating in public behaviors (i.e., observation of anonymous individuals on the street) is not regulated by the IRB.

The federal regulations defining human subjects also apply to identifiable private information. This requires that researchers carefully consider what constitutes

TABLE 14-6. Critical Elements of an IRB Review

Evaluate and ensure:
Risks to subjects are minimized
The risk/benefit ratio is reasonable
Equitable selection of subjects
Informed consent is appropriately obtained and documented
Safety monitoring of data, where appropriate, is sufficient
Appropriate protection of privacy and confidentiality
Adequate protection of vulnerable subjects

identifiable private information. According to the Health Insurance Portability and Accountability Act of 1996 (HIPAA), private health information is defined as information (including demographic information) about a patient that (1) is created or received by a healthcare provider; (2) relates to the past, present, or future physical or mental health of the patient; provision of healthcare to the patient; or payment for the provision of healthcare to the patient; and (3) identifies the patient or with respect to which there is a reasonable basis to believe it could used to identify the patient (HIPAA, 1996). While HIPAA does not directly govern research, it does regulate holders of medical records (e.g., hospitals, physicians, insurers, and healthcare clearinghouses) that are essential to conducting research.

As a general rule, any research that involves human subjects and relates to private behavior or information is considered human research and subject to protection by an IRB. It is critical that you determine while you are designing your project whether it will be subject to IRB review and contact your local board for discussion. Since genetic counselors often wear both research and clinical "hats" for their patients, it is important to remember that human research is distinguished from medical practice in that:

- The purpose is focused on obtaining general knowledge rather than on improving individual patient health.
- Direct benefit to the participant is possible, but unknown.
- The validity of the method is also unknown.
- The short-term goals are focused on new knowledge that may (or may not) ultimately impact patient care in the long term.

At the end of the day, the IRB and the review process are focused on protecting human subjects from the risks associated with research. It is important to realize that the review process (from the perspective of both the investigator and the subject) is geared toward minimizing potential risks and maximizing benefits. General elements of an IRB review are identified in Table 14-6.

How Do You Approach the Process?

Start by reviewing the IRB website at your institution. If the documentation is limited, look at the sites at other large medical research institutions (The IRBMED at the

University of Michigan Medical School is a good place to start). Familiarize yourself with all the documentation that you will be required to complete and work to understand the purpose of these documents from the perspective of the review process itself. It can also be helpful to figure out how your application will be reviewed and learn what committees will be evaluating it and how long it will take at each step. As with all other phases of your research project, work on learning from others about how to successfully navigate this process. Talk with your colleagues about how to develop the application. If you have done a good job of developing your research plan and your research proposal, the process of creating the application should be relatively straightforward.

The amount of time that it will take to get from start to finish (i.e., approval) will depend on your institution and the type of project that you are undertaking. It can be very helpful to talk with the IRB staff to get some information about how long it will take early in the development of your project so that you will know how it will impact your timeline for starting and completing your project. It is important to recognize that investigations into topics that would be considered sensitive or difficult to address in a clinical setting will also raise red flags in an IRB review. These include sexual attitudes, preferences, or practices; use of alcohol, drugs, or the like; information that could impact financial standing, employability, or reputation; topics and information that could result in social stigmatization or discrimination; psychological or mental health information; and genetic information (Markel and Yashar, 2004; Pelias, 2004). This makes it even more important to ensure that your application and informed consent document (if needed) are carefully and comprehensively drafted so that the IRB reviewer(s) can easily understand what you are intending to do and can evaluate the risks and benefits to the potential participants.

SEEING IT THROUGH TO THE END

It can be very hard to maintain a positive attitude and stay motivated throughout the entire research process. It would not be uncommon at different points in a research project to feel that your project is boring, to worry about how you are going to get it all done, or even to feel insecure about the validity of what you are attempting to study. These are all normal feelings and often arise when you have lost focus about the purpose of your project and the end point(s) that you are working towards. To help you stay focused and motivated, force yourself to manage your research time so that you are working on your project every day. Procrastination is not your friend—try to set up daily, weekly, and monthly goals, make them realistic, and work hard to attain them. In addition, setting up regular meetings with your advisor can help you stay on track. The more opportunities you create to present and talk about your research, the easier it will be to work on—talk to other students and plan regular meetings with your committee members. Not only will this help you keep on track, it will also be helpful when you start to analyze your results or if you run into problems with your project. Of course, a natural consequence of all these conversations is that you will receive criticisms about your research. Learn to deal with it. This is an innate element of the research process and central to the success of most projects. The more you can work on bouncing your ideas off of others and getting regular feedback, the higher your likelihood of success.

CONCLUSION

Research is a complicated process. The topics that have been presented in this chapter are meant to help you understand the big picture; however, to be successful at this endeavor you will need to delve more deeply into each content area. Why make the effort? Undertaking your own research project will provide you with multiple benefits. Working through a research project will allow you to develop a broader perspective of the current clinical practices in genetic counseling. The skills, including critical thinking, creative problem solving, and oral and written communication, that you will need to develop in order to successfully complete your research project will complement your clinical genetic counseling skills. By becoming part of the research community, you will broaden your definition of yourself as a genetic counselor and have the chance to contribute something truly novel to the profession.

REFERENCES

Bankert EA, Amdur RJ (eds.) (2006) *Institutional Review Board: Management and Function* (2nd ed.). Sudbury: Jones and Bartlett.

Bedard AC, Huether CA, Shooner K, Buncher CR, Warren NS (2007) Career research interests and training of genetic counseling students. *J Genet Couns* 16:645–653.

Bennett RL, et al. (2006) Code of Ethics of the National Society of Genetic Counselors. *J Genet Couns* 15(5):313–323.

Botti M, Endacott R (2005) Clinical Research 5: Quantitiative data collection and analysis. *Intensive Crit Care Nurs* 21(3),187–193.

Bowen N (2003) How to write a research article for the *Journal of Genetic Counseling. J Genet Couns* 12(1):5–21.

Code of Federal Regulations. *Title 45, Part 46 (45 CFR 46)* (2001) *DHHS protection of human subjects*. Retrieved December 8, 2008, from http://www.hhs.gov/ohrp/humansubjects/guidance/45cfr46.htm

Creswell JW (1998) *Qualitative Inquiry and Research Design: Choosing Among Five Traditions*. Thousand Oaks, CA: Sage Publications.

Creswell JW (2003) *Research Design: Qualitative, Quantitative and Mixed Methods Approaches* (2nd ed.). Thousand Oaks, CA: Sage Publications.

Endacott R (2004a) Clinical Research 1: Research questions and design. *Intensive Crit Care Nurs* 20(4):232–235.

Endacott R (2004b) Clinical Research 2: Legal and ethical issues in research. *Intensive Crit Care Nurs* 20(5):313–315.

Endacott R (2005a) Clinical Research 3: Sample selection. *Intensive Crit Care Nurs* 21 (1):51–55.

Endacott R (2005b) Clinical Research 4: Qualitative data collection and Analysis. *Intensive Crit Care Nurs* 21(2):123–127.

Endacott R (2005c) Clinical Research 6: Writting and research. *Intensive Crit Care Nurs* 21 (4):258–261.

Glasziou P, Vandenbroucke J, Chalmers I (2004) Assessing the quality of research. *Br Med J* 328:39–41.

Greenhlagh T, Taylor R (1997) How to read a paper: Papers that go beyond the numbers (qualitative research). *Br Med J* 315:740–743.

Harper D (2001) Online Etymology Dictionary. Retrieved December 8, 2008, from http://www.etymonline.com/index.php

Health Insurance Portability and Accountability Act (HIPAA) of 1996, P.L. 104-191, 119 Stat. Retrieved December 10, 2008, from http://www.hhs.gov/ocr/hipaapre.html

Hulley SB, Cummings SR, Browner WS, Grady D, Hearst N, Newman TB (2001) *Designing Clinical Research* ((2nd ed.)). Philadelphia: Lippincott Williams & Wilkins.

Human Research Protections Program Operations Manual: University of Michigan (2008). Retrieved December 5, 2008, from http://www.research.umich.edu/hrpp/om/FullOM.pdf

Kumar R (2005) *Research Methodology* (2nd ed.). Thousand Oaks, CA: Sage Publications.

Locke LF, Spirduso WW, Silverman SJ (2000) *Proposals That Work* (4th ed.). Thousand Oaks, CA: Sage Publications.

Marczyk G, DeMatteo D, Festinger D (2005) *Essentials of Research Design and Methodology*. Hoboken, NJ: John Wiley & Sons, Inc.

Markel DS, Yashar BM (2004) The interface between the practice of medical genetics and human genetic research: What every genetic counselor should know. *J Genet Couns* 13 (5):351–368.

Mason J (2002). *Qualitative Research* (2nd ed.). Thousand Oaks, CA: Sage Publications.

McKibbon MA (1995). *The Medical Literature as a Resource for Evidence Based Care: Working Paper from the Health Information Research Unit*. Ontario: McMaster University.

National Comissions for the Protection of Human Subjects of Biomedical and Behavioral Research (1979) The Belmont Report: Ethical principles and guidelines for the protection of human subjects of research. Retrieved December 5, 2008, from http://ohsr.od.nih.gov/guidelines/belmont.

Neill J (2007) Qualitative versus Quantitative Research: Key Points in a Classic Debate. Retrieved December 5, 2008, from http://wilderdom.com/research/QualitativeVersusQuantitativeResearch.html

Parrott S, Del Vecchio M (2007) Professional Status Survey 2006. Retrieved December 8, 2008, from http://www.nsgc.org/client_files/career/2006_PSS_RESULTS.pdf

Pelias MK (2004) Research in Human Genetics: The tension between doing no harm and personal autonomy. *Clin Genet* 64:1–5.

Rubin A, Babbie E (2007) *Research Methods for Social Work* (3rd ed.). Pacific Grove, CA: Brooks/Cole Publishing Company.

Sackett D, Rosenberg WMC, Muir Gray JA, Haynes RB, Richardson WS (1996) Evidence based medicine: what it is and what it isn't. *Br Med J* 312:71–72.

15

Professional Identity and Development

Elizabeth A. Gettig, M.S., C.G.C. and Karen Greendale, M.A., C.G.C.

INTRODUCTION

The field of genetic counseling has evolved in response to scientific and technological developments in molecular and clinical genetics, along with changes in healthcare delivery and policy. The role of genetic counselors in the delivery of genetic services has expanded to fill niches created by these advances. As we continue to develop as a profession, it is important to remain flexible in articulating our professional identity and committed to professional development, individually and collectively.

In this chapter, we discuss the concept of professional identity and development—enhancing knowledge and skills while growing in our professional abilities and in our individual jobs. We discuss how we move from a student identity to a professional identity, what that transition entails, and how we conduct ourselves professionally. Professional identity can be viewed as the integration of professional roles and experiences into a cohesive self-image. We also address the topics of lifelong learning, certification, and licensure. Professional development activities include continuing education, specialized training, research, moving into a subspecialty of practice, focusing on a specific project/disease group, or simply redefining one's role as a genetic counselor. Professional development can also encompass moving beyond one's job to involvement in institutional, regional and national activities.

A Guide to Genetic Counseling, Second Edition, Edited by Wendy Uhlmann, Jane Schuette, and Beverly Yashar
Copyright © 2009 by John Wiley & Sons, Inc.

THE GENETIC COUNSELING PROFESSION AND ROLE EXPANSION

The genetic counseling profession is relatively new, having had its start in 1969 when the Sarah Lawrence College program accepted its first class of 10 students. As this book goes to press, there are more than 2500 genetic counselors practicing in the United States and Canada and a couple hundred more in countries around the world. New areas of practice have been created as genetic counselors have recognized unmet needs and developed new services in response. Genetic counselors' success in these new roles has often opened new doors for others in the field. These new directions were once referred to as "non-traditional" roles; however, today we can acknowledge the diversity of available roles and recognize that an individual who self-identifies as a "genetic counselor" may in fact not provide genetic counseling!

The National Society of Genetic Counselors (NSGC) has played a critical role in promoting and sustaining role expansion. As individuals have moved into new areas of specialization, groups of genetic counselors interested in a specific area have formed special interest groups (SIGs). Pediatrics, Prenatal, Cancer, Neurogenetics, Cardiovascular, Assisted Reproductive Technologies/Infertility, Industry, and Public Health are just some examples of SIGs that have been established in NSGC. SIGs enable genetic counselors to network with colleagues working in the same area, fostering collaborations and professional development. Most SIGS use Listservs and designated areas of the NSGC website to keep members informed about advances published in the medical literature, to advise each other on difficult cases, and to share information from relevant conferences. Several SIGs have produced materials to introduce their subspecialty to students or to those new to the specialty and have developed and distributed documents for other healthcare providers, insurers, and the public.

Role expansion can be tracked via the NSGC's Professional Status Surveys, which were initiated in 1980. Members are surveyed every two years regarding focus of work, responsibilities, salaries, faculty appointments, professional activities (e.g., presentations, publications, committees), employer support for continuing education and other job benefits, and job satisfaction. A summary of the results is published by the NSGC and may be accessed in the "Career" section of the website. Many genetic counselors have utilized the survey findings to help expand their roles, create new positions, and negotiate increased compensation, autonomy, and benefits. Each survey provides a quantitative and qualitative "snapshot" of the profession, and as a series they demonstrate changes over time in response to economic, social, and other factors.

In summary, genetic counselors have spearheaded efforts to expand their professional roles, enhancing job satisfaction and contributing to the richness of the profession. We predict that the field will continue to move into chronic, common diseases as more interventions become available. We believe that changes in the science and in the healthcare marketplace will lead future generations of genetic counselors to continually reassess and redefine their professional roles and responsibilities. Role expansion of genetic counselors is discussed in greater depth in Chapter 17.

PROFESSIONAL IDENTITY

According to Benveniste 1987, a profession is an occupation that meets the following criteria: application of skills based on technical knowledge, requirements of advanced education and training, formal testing of competence, controlled admission, membership in professional associations, allegiance to a code of conduct, and sense of responsibility to serve the public. In fewer than 30 years, genetic counseling has become a unique and established profession. In 1997, Kenen, a sociologist, noted that the genetic counseling cohort, even at that relatively early stage, fulfilled most of the criteria used to define a profession (Kenen, 1997). These include its own body of knowledge (which combines content from genetics, medicine, ethics, and psychology), dedicated training programs, an accrediting body, a certification process [overseen by the American Board of Genetic Counseling (ABGC)], a professional society [the NSGC], a journal (the *Journal of Genetic Counseling*), a newsletter *(Perspectives in Genetic Counseling),* and a Code of Ethics (adopted by NSGC).

The term "professional" traditionally referred to an individual who was employed in a profession. However, this term is currently applied more broadly, to refer to any individual who is responsible for providing a particular service to internal clients (e.g., co-workers) or external clients (e.g., patients) (Maister, 1997). Professionalism refers to the extent to which one identifies with his/her profession, accepts its values, and acts accordingly (Morrow and Goetz, 1988). Professionalism can be evidenced by an individual's ability to meet normative expectations and effectively provide a given service to clients and colleagues.

Professional identity is also related to finding self-meaning connected with one's work (Olesen, 2000). The most important aspects of a person's professional identity are the ability to self-reflect, master a body of knowledge, practice ethically, display professionalism, and have a lifelong intention to participate in continuing education. This identity connects us and brings a commonality among professional genetic counselors, encompassing genetic counselors working in both clinical and non-clinical roles.

Professional Identity: The Genetic Counseling Student

It is useful to stay in contact with my colleagues/friends from grad school because they are the only ones who truly understand some of the struggles, fascinations and the feeling of not knowing something or doubting our skills. It is also helpful to be able to talk to colleagues in my own clinic, but I don't feel quite as open as I do with my classmates.

I was fortunate in that while I was a student, I developed close relationships with several of my classmates. While we were doing rotations, we frequently discussed interesting cases, and debated different approaches to take with challenging patients. Now, even though we're scattered across North America, we still support each other in these ways. I have really appreciated this because we all "get" things about each other's work that our family and friends do not.

—Quotes from recent graduates

The student usually has begun to develop an emerging professional concept even at the time of interviewing for genetic counseling programs when responding to the frequently asked question, "What do you perceive the role of a genetic counselor to be?" As the student begins training, it is common to find that the initial definition of the practice of the genetic counselor evolves from a concrete definition found in a textbook to a more fluid version based on clinical experiences and interactions with clinical supervisors and instructors in training programs. The genetic counseling student initiates his/her professional development with his/her first graduate courses and continues the learning process throughout his/her life. The student will learn the nuances of practice while in training and will be exposed to the fundamental principles of genetic counseling.

Lavin and Hyllegard's 1996 contention that higher education is an important catalyst to personal development holds true for genetic counseling students. Regardless of professional roles and job descriptions, genetic counselors have similar graduate training that unites all of us. Graduate training fosters the development of professional self-esteem and identification with the profession. Students often begin their studies with a lack of confidence and have concerns about failure or are anxious about their perceived ignorance. The unfamiliar clinical environment may appear threatening, and the student may feel out of place. However, the commitment to academics and the motivation to succeed inevitably result in effective and successful practitioners. The identity changes from a student mindset—with concerns including grades and academic issues—to becoming a professional genetic counselor, with responsibility to clients, colleagues, and employers. The thirst for knowledge and intellectual stimulation results in a sense of changed identity as the individual moves from student to practitioner. This discovery of empowerment through education and the attainment of professional qualifications becomes the foundation of professional identity.

Upon graduation, students usually attain a broader sense of the meaning of genetic counseling and a wider appreciation of what constitutes the field. No longer directly supervised, the new genetic counselor may develop his/her own style of counseling and thereby craft (at least in part) his/her own professional self. The process involves not merely talking with the patient and imparting information—it is much more complex and includes development of a deeper understanding in the domains outlined in the profession's Code of Ethics (e.g., self, patients, colleagues, and society). The former student is now a professional genetic counselor—albeit an inexperienced one—with all the responsibility and values associated with that designation.

As you make the transition from student to genetic counselor, mentors will play an important role. Early mentors likely will be faculty at your training program and clinical supervisors. Later mentors may include colleagues whom you meet through networking, serving on committees and other professional activities in addition to colleagues at your institution. Throughout your career, it is important for your professional development to seek out guidance through mentors.

Professional Identity: The Genetic Counselor

The transition from student to professional was a really good one, because I could finally implement the type of counseling techniques I wanted to use without being supervised and judged in each session by a counselor with a different counseling style from me. I guess what I am trying to say is that it was useful to learn from each counselor's technique, but in the end I was itching to implement my own in freedom.
—Quote from recent graduate

Everyone has their own personal identity, but the collective profession of genetic counseling also has a professional identity, which stems from membership in a socioculturally distinct group (Cox, 1993). Genetic counselors' shared beliefs are easily found in the NSGC Code of Ethics (accessible at NSGC website). Genetic counselors value competence, integrity, dignity, and self-respect in themselves as well as in each other. Genetic counselors' relationships with other genetic counselors, genetic counseling students, and health professionals from other disciplines are based on mutual respect, caring, cooperation, support, and a shared loyalty to their professional goals. The relationship of genetic counselors to segments of society or to society as a whole includes interest and participation in activities with the goal of promoting societal well-being (NSGC Code of Ethics). Professional identity may include physical, biological, and stylistic features or shared worldview, norms, values, goals, or sociocultural heritage (Cox, 1993). Personal identification varies within and between cultural groups, while professional identity is formed by shared experiences in training and practice as noted above. Our cultural identities, which influence our personal and professional identities, may be associated with power, prestige, and status and at times may conflict with our shared identity as genetic counselors (Hogg, 2003; Bell and Nkomo, 2001; Ragins et al., 2000).

Our Code of Ethics has captured many elements that enhance personal and professional growth. As genetic counselors, we must first provide quality services and experiences to clients/populations by engaging in "active listening" and analyzing the content of patient encounters. Second, we must maintain good working relationships with colleagues, staff, clients, and the families or populations with whom we work. Genetic counselors must be lifelong learners because of the ever-changing nature of our profession. Therefore, we must be committed to attaining continuing education, certifications, and licensure. We must keep an open mind with regard to new knowledge, approaches, and techniques and must continually reevaluate what we bring to the therapeutic relationship through self-reflection, peer supervision, journaling, and other means.

From an outsider's point of view, genetics is constantly changing—some might even say that the field has become overwhelmingly complex, even chaotic. Each day or week may bring new gene discoveries, new treatments, or new clinical trials. What once was not possible may become possible. Consider the example of cystic fibrosis. When the genetic counseling profession began in the early 1970s, the gene for cystic fibrosis (CF) had not been discovered. The life expectancy for a child born with CF at that time was not more than 20 years. Now with the discovery of the CF gene, more effective treatments, lung transplants, and earlier diagnosis through newborn screening, it is probably not unreasonable to expect that a child born today with classic CF may live into his 50s and have a relatively typical life experience complete with an education, employment, and a family. In 2006, the predicted median age of survival was 37 years, quite an accomplishment (CF Foundation, 2007; Strausbaugh et al., 2007). With the discovery of the CF gene also came carrier testing, prenatal diagnosis, and attempts at gene therapy. Clearly there have been numerous advances in a short period of time, illustrating the need for genetic counselors to keep their knowledge current in order to provide accurate information.

The practicing genetic counselor who does not continually keep abreast of developments through continuing education, self-study, or other means (especially if practicing in relative isolation) may not be able to offer the patients seeking his/her services the latest information and the most complete array of options.

PROFESSIONAL CONDUCT

My experience may have differed from some of my classmates because I'm the only counselor at my hospital, but I found that I had to really shift the way that I think about and present things. As a student I was constantly learning, and was surrounded by experienced counselors and professionals who I looked to as the "experts." But now everyone looks to me as the expert, and while I enjoy that role, it takes some mental adjustment. So I'm trying to remind myself to speak up more, and present myself with confidence. But I'm also reminding myself that I don't have to know everything, that no one will hold it against me if I say that I have to do some research before answering a question.

—Quote from recent graduate

The NSGC Code of Ethics guides the conduct of the profession. Each genetic counseling training program sets its own guidelines for student conduct, and all use the NSGC Code of Ethics as a foundation. The relationship of the student to his/her clinical supervisors and teaching faculty facilitates the acquisition of knowledge, skills, and *values* that will endure throughout the student's genetic counseling career.

Both students and practicing genetic counselors must abide by the agreed-upon set of principles found in the Code of Ethics. These principles include obligations for how genetic counselors should conduct themselves and keep abreast of current standards of practice and how they should interact with their clients, colleagues, and society. In all interactions, genetic counselors should maintain professional boundaries, be mindful of conflicts of interest and dual relationships, and make sure that they are acting ethically, professionally, and responsibly. The Code of Ethics is discussed in Chapter 12. In addition, genetic counselors need to abide by the profession's Scope of

Practice, which can be accessed at the NSGC website and is appended to Chapter 1. The Scope of Practice outlines the responsibilities of genetic counselors who provide patient care and covers the components of genetic counseling, professional ethics, and values. Genetic counselors working in clinical care should also be cognizant of the profession's position statements and practice guidelines, accessible at the NSGC website, in addition to guidelines for geneticists and genetics guidelines in their medical specialty. All genetic counselors, regardless of work setting, also need to conduct themselves professionally in accordance with their institution's employee policies.

CERTIFICATION AND LICENSURE OF GENETIC COUNSELORS

Certification

Certification is considered the "gold standard" in our profession. *Diplomates* is the term used to describe genetic counselors who are certified, and CGC® after one's name is the designation for certified genetic counselor. Certification for genetic counselors has existed since 1982 [originally through the American Board of Medical Genetics (ABMG); since 1993, through the ABGC] and has had an impact on other health professionals' and the public's awareness of this professional group. Current candidates for certification must have graduated from an accredited graduate program in genetic counseling and must submit letters of recommendation. Once these credentials have been approved, the candidate must pass a national certification examination.

Genetic counselors certified by the ABGC in or after 1996 are required to recertify on a regular basis in order to remain a certified genetic counselor (CGC®). Genetic counselors certified before 1996 are encouraged to voluntarily recertify. Maintaining certification status is becoming increasingly important as states pass licensure laws for genetic counselors and, based on current licensure laws, will probably be a requirement to practice in any state offering licenses to genetic counselors. The pathways for ABGC recertification in genetic counseling are (1) re-examination or (2) continuing education. Only one pathway can be attempted during any given recertification cycle. All requirements concerning certification and recertification may be found at the ABGC website.

In Canada, the Canadian Association of Genetic Counsellors (Association Canadienne des Conseillers en Génétique) administers the certification examination. Currently, the certification is valid for 10 years and recertification is achieved by (1) re-examination or (2) continuing education. Individuals may choose to recertify by using a combination of Continuing Practice Credits (CPC) and Continuing Education Credits (CEC). Counsellors are required to accrue a total of 150 credits from a combination of these activities during a 10-year period. (CAGC, 2008)

As more genetic counseling programs emerge internationally, requirements for certification of genetic counselors and accreditation of genetic counseling programs will continue to evolve.

Licensure

Licensure is the mark of a professional. Licensure sets a professional standard and provides at least a baseline expectation for the quality of services rendered. Licensure serves to protect not only the professionals who hold the license, but also members of the public who interact with the licensed individual. Licensure serves as one means of protecting public health, safety, and welfare by ensuring a standard of practice, education, and qualification. Physicians, nurses, and most allied healthcare professionals are licensed by each state.

In the case of genetic counseling, licensure would safeguard the public from the harms of substandard service that can lead to misinformation and misguided decision-making. Licensure creates clear education, certification, and continuing education standards for a field and allows consumers to better identify who is an adequately trained practitioner. Licensure laws may define the practice of genetic counseling; set forth licensure requirements; provide for the confidentiality of patient information in the practice of genetic counseling; and establish penalties for violations of the law. Licensure demonstrates a commitment to the high standards of professionalism to which the genetic counseling profession subscribes.

Over the past two decades, advances in our understanding of human genetics have expanded out of the research laboratory and into the clinical practice of mainstream medicine. The Human Genome Project has led to major breakthroughs in the diagnosis, prevention, and treatment of a wide array of conditions, from cancer and heart disease to developmental disabilities and psychiatric illness. Across the country, there is a growing need for qualified professionals who can help patients to translate complex genetics concepts and technology into practical information that has relevance to their own lives and medical decisions. Most healthcare professionals are not experts in genetics, and they do not always know how to counsel concerned patients about these important issues. Physicians, nurses, and other professionals often refer their patients to genetic counselors for the accurate, understandable, and patient-focused information and support we can provide.

Despite the growing need for competent, qualified genetic counselors, our numbers are still small. Most states have not yet enacted legislation to ensure that individuals claiming to be genetic counselors are truly qualified to provide such services. Professional licensure can ensure that patients and consumers feel confident that they are receiving quality genetic counseling services from reliable professionals. State licensure efforts have a direct impact on practice. Once enacted, legislation will ensure that only licensed professionals can use the title "Genetic Counselor". By recognizing the special skills and training of licensed genetic counselors, patients and consumers will be protected from unqualified providers. Licensure may also have a positive impact on reimbursement and billing for genetic counseling services. Our profession has worked hard to achieve a level of expertise and competence in genetic counseling. Licensure formally recognizes our expertise and protects the patients and families we serve.

Until recently there were simply not enough master's-level genetic counselors in individual states to warrant a serious discussion of licensure. As the profession has grown and with increasing pressures from health systems regarding billing and reimbursement practices, licensure discussions have increased. California was the first state to pass genetic counselor licensure legislation in 2000, but Utah was the first state to issue licenses in 2002. As of March 2009, fewer than ten states have enacted licensure laws for genetic counselors; however, many other states are working on licensure legislation. Information about licensure of genetic counselors is available at the NSGC website.

LIFELONG LEARNING PRACTICES

The goal of graduate training in genetic counseling is to help students develop the knowledge and skills necessary to approach any genetic counseling case or situation with accurate information, appropriate counseling skills, and confidence. Since no student can come into contact with patients or families with every known genetic condition, program directors and instructors prepare students to know where to access the information and resources necessary to serve a broad spectrum of clients. As new areas of practice emerge, genetic counselors must develop pertinent skills. A commitment to lifelong learning has always been valued by genetic counselors. A primary goal of the NSGC has been to support continuing education for its members (Rollnick, 1984). Practices and policies of the NSGC highlight this value. The mission statement of the NSGC states: "The National Society of Genetic Counselors advances the various roles of genetic counselors in healthcare by fostering education, research, and public policy to ensure the availability of quality genetic services" (NSGC website, accessed 8 December 2008). This is reinforced by the NSGC Code of Ethics, which states that "genetic counselors strive to seek out and acquire sufficient and relevant information required for any given situation; [to] continue their education and training; [and] to keep abreast of current standards of practice" (NSGC website, accessed 8 December 2008). Therefore, continuing education is a necessary element and an *obligation* of being a professional genetic counselor.

The commitment to professional development is illustrated in the following ABGC practice-based competency: "[The student] can demonstrate initiative for continued professional growth. The student *displays a knowledge of current standards of practice and shows independent knowledge-seeking behavior and lifelong learning*" (Fine et al., 1996). The requirement embodied by this competency for an entry-level genetic counselor again highlights the value the profession places on professional development.

Whether you are in a clinical or non-clinical position, clearly lifelong learning is valuable and in fact essential for genetic counselors from a personal and professional point of view. Genetic counselors are obliged to remain current regarding advances in genetics, medical genetics, and other relevant areas and to be aware of changes in pertinent clinical standards. Professional development depends on accessing educational opportunities, many of which are available through genetics, medical, and scientific professional organizations and in individual work settings. Some of these resources are discussed in the subsections that follow.

Continuing Education

"Continuing education" is a general term used to connote formalized learning after graduation. Many employers and professional organizations require documentation of continuing education activities. The number of continuing education units (CEUs) awarded is determined by the amount of time spent participating in a continuing education program.

Continuing education and related activities enable practicing genetic counselors to remain current about new technologies and testing modalities and about relevant psychosocial, ethical, and legal implications. In essence, genetic counselors must practice at a level consistent with the standard of care even as they help to define guidelines for appropriate practice. Maintaining the status quo is not a viable alternative in a field as rapidly changing as this one!

In 1981, the NSGC developed a continuing education model to ensure quality education programs (Rollnick, 1983). Since 1996, all courses and conferences sponsored by the NSGC have had to meet established criteria for offering CEUs. This means that genetic counselors can accrue CEUs by attending NSGC-sponsored education programs and other health professionals can attend NSGC meetings to help fulfill their own CEU requirements. Genetic counselors can also accrue CEUs by attending other genetics and medical conferences with NSGC approval.

CEUs are classified as category 1 or category 2. *Category 1 CEUs* are granted for programs with content targeted to genetic counselors and preapproved by the NSGC. *Category 2 CEUs* are available for programs approved by organizations other than NSGC for CEUs or Continuing Medical Education (CME) credits. Even though these programs are targeted to other healthcare providers, their content may be considered by NSGC to be relevant to a genetic counselor's continuing education. In addition to conferences, other options for obtaining CEUs include online courses, quizzes on *Journal of Genetic Counseling* articles, and PACs (Professional Activity Credits) (Table 15-1). PACs are awarded for participation in a variety of activities determined by ABGC to promote professional development. These activities include authorship, clinical supervision, leadership and teaching (Table 15-1). For a detailed list of approved PAC activities, please see the ABGC website. The ABGC has set specific CEU and PAC requirements for recertification. It is important to keep aware of these ABGC guidelines. While continuing education should in principle be standard practice for genetic counselors adhering to the Code of Ethics, documentation of such activities is necessary for recertification and licensure.

Conferences

Conferences and professional meetings are a major forum for acquiring continuing education. The NSGC holds a national education conference each year. The format and content of the NSGC conference are designed to meet the broad range of educational needs of the membership. More than half of NSGC members attend this annual conference. Lectures, workshops, practice-based symposia, and contributed paper and poster sessions address issues in clinical genetics and genetic

TABLE 15-1. Pathways for Obtaining Continuing Education Units (CEUs)*

Conferences (Need to be approved by NSGC)	
NSGC conferences and short courses	Other genetics conferences
Other medical conferences	State genetic counselor meetings/workshops

Online Opportunities (Need to be approved by NSGC)	
Online courses	*Journal of Genetic Counseling*

Professional Activity Credits (PACs) (Need to be approved by ABGC)	
Clinical supervision	Presentations given to professional groups
Publications	Teaching
Genetics education outreach	Patient education publications
Leadership activities	Undergraduate or graduate coursework
Volunteer service to ABGC	

*CEUs available in 2008. Check ABGC website for current listing of activities.

counseling, as well as the psychological, cultural, ethical, legal, and professional implications of our work. Conference speakers include NSGC members and guest faculty from a variety of disciplines. Informal networking and sharing of ideas make this conference an extremely important forum for professional development. Usually, an orientation is held for first-time meeting attendees and genetic counseling programs typically hold reunions. Short courses on genetic counseling specialties, such as cancer genetics and neurogenetics, and courses on skill development, such as research skills, often are held in conjunction with the NSGC meeting. NSGC also sponsors regional meetings and online conferences.

The American Society of Human Genetics (ASHG) hosts an annual scientific meeting in the fall, attended by several thousand researchers and clinicians in genetics from around the world. This conference focuses on genetics research and includes presentations relevant to clinicians including concurrent sessions on genetic counseling and genetic testing, clinical genetics, cancer genetics, and reproductive genetics and sessions on education, policy, and ethical issues. The American College of Medical Genetics (ACMG), primarily comprised of genetics clinicians, holds an annual conference in early spring that focuses on clinical genetics and the medical issues raised by genetics research. Both ASHG and ACMG offer educational workshops on topics of special interest in conjunction with their conferences. Usually at the meetings, there are programs specifically for students/trainees. A key benefit of attending ACMG and ASHG meetings is the ability to network and the opportunity to be with our physician and research colleagues. In addition to conferences hosted by genetics professional organizations, counselors are increasingly attending and presenting at conferences focusing on their specialty area of practice.

Finally, many local and national meetings address specific issues in genetics. For example, the various genetic disease support groups sponsor medical and scientific conferences that genetic counselors are welcome to attend; often genetic counselors are asked to give presentations at these meetings. Online meetings, webinars, pod casts, and other distance education services also offer important opportunities for education and networking.

Genetic counselors can learn about meetings from announcements in genetics and other journals, direct mailings, the NSGC Listserv, websites maintained by specific institutions or organizations, and colleagues.

Journals in Genetics and Related Fields

Literature review is probably the best method of day-to-day continuing education. Medical journals relevant to the practice of genetic counseling are available in medical libraries or by subscription, and many journals can be accessed via the Internet. It is prudent to at least review the tables of contents of the major genetics journals each month. Of course, most members of the profession carefully read the *Journal of Genetic Counseling* (official journal of the NSGC). Other journals include *Genetics in Medicine* (official journal of the ACMG), the *American Journal of Medical Genetics,* the *American Journal of Human Genetics* (official journal of the ASHG), the *Journal of Medical Genetics, Public Health Genomics, Genetic Testing*, and *Prenatal Diagnosis.* Genetic counselors residing outside the U.S. may have genetics journals published in their own countries. Most pediatric and obstetrics and gynecology journals contain several pertinent articles per issue. The *New England Journal of Medicine,* the *Journal of the American Medical Association, Science, Nature,* and *Nature Genetics* are broader in focus and often contain articles of interest. In addition, journals devoted to specific medical specialties such as oncology or neurology, or to public health or biomedical ethics, are important to read if your work is focused in a subspecialty area. Because there is so much to read and often so little time to do it, a journal club in your own institution can help everyone to keep up to date. Set one up if none exists!

Advanced Education and Training

The multidisciplinary nature of genetic counseling provides many avenues for professional development. Some genetic counselors find that their graduate training sufficiently equips them to learn new material through self-study or other means, while others may take courses or obtain a second master's degree or a more advanced degree. Genetic counselors can choose to pursue advanced education in bioethics, public health, policy, psychology, sociology, molecular genetics, and other pertinent disciplines. For example, some genetic counselors have enrolled in certificate programs in family and marital therapy as a means of expanding their practices to include long-term psychotherapy for individuals and families dealing with genetic disorders. Genetic counselors also may choose to expand their research capabilities through additional training, workshops, online resources, collaborations, or finding mentors. Additional training in epidemiology, health policy, and research design are pos-sibilities for genetic counselors working in public health settings. The involvement of genetic counselors in newborn and other screening programs and in administrative positions in state health departments has grown; formal training or self-study in this area may be required. Genetic counselors moving into specialty areas such as cancer genetics may learn by doing or may be able to create "apprenticeships," learning from genetic counselors with significant experience and expertise. For some, employers have covered the expenses associated with this sort of additional training; others have taken advantage of sabbatical or fellowship funds. For example, the Jane Engelberg Memorial Fellowship awarded through the NSGC was created to provide an opportunity for genetic counselors to enhance skills, develop new areas of expertise, and conduct research.

For over twenty years, debate has occurred regarding the development of a Ph.D. degree for genetic counselors (Atzinger et al., 2007; Bedard et al., 2007; Biesecker, 1998; Biesecker and Marteau, 1999; Clark et al., 2006; Gaupman et al., 1991; NSGC, 2007; Jolley, 2007; Parrott, 2004; Parrott and Clark, 2007; Resta, 2006; Scott et al., 1988; Trent, 1993; USNEI, 2004; Walker et al., 1990; Wallace et al., 2008; Warren et al., 2005). The development of a Ph.D. is a natural progression for professionals and academic institutions. The critical issues in this debate have been in regard to employability and the practicality of having an advanced degree for genetic counselors. A study by Wallace et al. (2008) surveyed potential employers; the results suggested that there is an employment niche for individuals who have a Ph.D. in genetic counseling that complements, and does not compete with, master's-prepared genetic counselors. The role of the Ph.D. genetic counselor would be to perform research. The employers surveyed expected individuals with a Ph.D. in genetic counseling to perform different roles than genetic counselors with a master's degree.

In essence, advanced education and training enhance the genetic counselor's practice and help to redefine the boundaries of genetic counseling. The genetic counselor with advanced training can share his or her expertise with others in the profession through consultations, presentations, and publications and can act as a role model for colleagues with similar interests.

PROFESSIONAL OPPORTUNITIES IN ONE'S OWN INSTITUTION

Professional development is important within the individual genetic counselor's place of employment, both for personal fulfillment and to augment professional status. It is important to keep in mind that creating a new clinical service, organizing case conferences, serving on a hospital committee, or educating students and health professionals may do as much to positively affect institutional perceptions of a genetic counselor's "worth" as an increased caseload. The skills genetic counselors possess can be applied in contexts outside the traditional genetic counseling sphere.

Professional development within one's institution can be pursued in two ways. First, one can identify opportunities for professional growth through educational offerings in the workplace. For example, one can attend grand rounds, seminars, and journal clubs. Many institutions offer skill enhancement programs in areas such as computer proficiency, grant writing, and public speaking.

Second, one can pursue opportunities for professional growth by participating in educational, clinical, and administrative activities. For example, a genetic counselor interested in ethical issues could volunteer to serve on a hospital ethics committee; these multidisciplinary groups provide guidance to healthcare providers facing difficult dilemmas in patient care. In many medical schools, genetic counselors teach medical students in didactic genetics courses. Medical students and residents on clinical service in genetics units are often taught through more informal interactions with genetic counselors. Genetic counselors may hone their administrative skills by coordinating a multidisciplinary clinic, such as a craniofacial, hemophilia, or muscular dystrophy clinic. The genetic counselor coordinator generally oversees patient referrals to appropriate specialists, provides genetic counseling, and leads the case conference discussion on each patient, ensuring that appropriate follow-up is in place.

Genetic counselors can also serve on Institutional Review Boards (IRBs), service delivery committees, and other committees at their institution. Counselors often author articles for their institution's magazines, websites, or newsletters. Many employers also view active relationships with area support groups as service. Generally, genetic counselors provide exposure to the profession by service to their institutions and communities.

Faculty Appointments

According to the 2008 NSGC Professional Status Survey (Smith et al., 2008) 16% of respondents (246/1508) hold a faculty appointment. Among those with faculty appointments, 66% are at their institution of employment and the rest are at an institution other than where they are employed. Over half of those with faculty appointments (65%) work at a school of medicine, and another 21% work in a genetics graduate program. In 2008, the faculty appointments were: Instructor/Lecturer (57%), Assistant Professor (26%), Associate Professor (12%), Professor (3%), and Research Assistant or Associate Professor (2%).

Faculty appointments can be tenure-track or non-tenure-track, primary or adjunct. At your institution, faculty appointments may not be offered, but if you regularly teach students at another institution, you may qualify there for an adjunct appointment. Generally, academic institutions can appoint faculty on the instructional, clinical or research track (these may be identified by other names at your institution). Faculty appointments may be granted at the time of hire or later in your career. Faculty appointments are based on your professional track record and can take into consideration clinical work, teaching, scholarship, service (organizational and institutional committees, administrative and leadership positions), and publications. Associate-and professor-level faculty appointments generally require a regional or national reputation and depend on evaluations from impartial external sources. There will be set expectations for faculty appointments, reappointments, and promotion that will vary depending on the faculty track and the institution. You can access information about faculty appointments from your institution's website and Office of Faculty Affairs. You should keep accurate records of your academic activities and an up-to-date CV in the specified institutional format starting from day one of your job.

Faculty status comes with advantages and disadvantages. Whether it is the best option for a particular genetic counselor depends on that counselor's preferences and goals. On the one hand, counselors who are interested in scholarship and service or want to improve the teaching quality of their institution may find that faculty status helps them reach these goals. Faculty status is also desirable because it brings opportunities for participation in campus governance, continuous appointment usually in a non-tenure stream, sabbaticals, and higher salaries.

On the other hand, counselors who want to support the research productivity of other faculty at their institution or to maintain a primary clinical focus (i.e., seeing patients) may find that faculty status diverts energy from these goals. Faculty status may not be the best choice for a counselor who does not enjoy the research and publication process or who prefers to spend more time on more "traditional" genetic counseling activities. In addition, faculty status often requires a counselor to spend personal time on professional pursuits, which may affect lifestyle and outside interests.

Some institutions grant faculty status to genetic counselors. At other institutions, genetic counselors may have to advocate for their academic appointments. The choice to pursue a faculty appointment at an academic institution is often a personal one that a counselor can make only after carefully considering the advantages and disadvantages of such a position and his/her own values and goals.

PARTICIPATION IN PROFESSIONAL ORGANIZATIONS

Opportunities for professional development through participation in genetics organizations exist at local, state, regional and national levels. The Appendix to this chapter provides contact information and an overview of the structure and function of the major professional and research-oriented genetics organizations. Visiting the websites of these organizations, reading their publications, and attending the business meetings held at annual conferences (and accessing business meetings/board reports) are the most effective avenues for learning about their activities, resources, and opportunities for participation. The NSGC, ACMG, and ASHG all offer student memberships. At a minimum, as a genetic counselor you should join the NSGC (or the genetic counselor organization in your country) as a student member or as a full member after graduation. NSGC student members are welcome to join one of the SIGs (Special Interest Groups), help plan an Annual Education Conference, and submit an abstract for presentation at a meeting. As a full member of NSGC, you are eligible for appointment to different committees. There are many ways to get involved, and you should consider your own background, talents, and special interests when making this decision. The benefits include the satisfaction associated with contributing to the profession, opportunities for networking and research collaboration, and professional and personal relationships with colleagues. Information about ways to become involved in NSGC is available at the website.

Some genetic counselors have chosen to channel their energies through the ABGC, ASHG, or ACMG. NSGC members have also worked together with ACMG to develop joint practice guidelines and policies. Genetic counselors have contributed their expertise and become involved in other medical organizations, such as the American Society of Clinical Oncologists.

Some states have established state chapters of NSGC, and many states have their own genetics organizations, which include practicing clinical geneticists and genetic counselors. Ask colleagues in your own or neighboring institutions how to become involved. Other cities and states have either formal or informal meetings where genetic counselors can obtain continuing education, discuss challenging cases, provide and receive support, and work together to influence policy-making at local and state levels.

INVOLVEMENT IN POLICY-MAKING

Some genetic counselors have chosen to become involved in policy-making activities on an institutional, statewide, regional, or national level. For instance, some genetic counselors have been involved in activities to further the goals of individuals and families working in a specific advocacy group such as the Huntington's Disease Society of America or Facing Our Risk of Cancer Empowered. Genetic counselors have also contacted senators and representatives to provide input on genetics policy issues and legislation. Other genetic counselors have submitted written comments and provided oral testimony to the Secretary's Advisory Committee on Genetics, Health and Society and other advisory committees. Genetic counselors have worked with colleagues to reach out to legislators to lobby for licensure. Before getting involved with such policy activities, make sure to clarify whether you are acting as an individual or representing your institution or professional society, and be aware that you may need to participate in such activities on your own time. The NSGC website has helpful resources on policy and advocacy, including how a bill becomes a law and how to contact and communicate with congressional representatives.

A FINAL THOUGHT ON PROFESSIONAL DEVELOPMENT

Genetic counseling is a field that requires continued growth as a professional to remain current in the field, to provide optimal care to our clients, and to contribute to the development of expanding roles in the workplace and at state, regional, and national levels. Taking on new responsibilities can lead to new learning and new challenges. Participation in continuing education programs, on committees, and in professional societies will ultimately enhance job satisfaction and the professional status of the individual genetic counselor, while furthering the goals of the profession. In response to recent and rapid changes in technology and healthcare delivery systems, genetic counselors have pushed the boundaries of the profession to meet the needs of patients and the society at large. As a consequence, personal and professional satisfaction among genetic counselors has been enhanced and the original conception of the genetic counselor has not proven large enough to encompass all facets of the current genetic counseling professional's "being." Although it's impossible to predict the future, the authors would not be surprised if the chapter on "professional development" written for the next edition of this book describes a new set of possibilities available to the next generation of genetic counseling professionals.

ACKNOWLEDGMENTS

The authors acknowledge Beth Fine, initial co-author, for her contributions to this text and for all her valuable and considerable contributions to the profession of genetic counseling.

APPENDIX: CLINICAL GENETICS PROFESSIONAL SOCIETIES

American Board of Genetic Counseling (ABGC)

Year founded/incorporated: 1993

Focus: Accrediting body for graduate programs in genetic counseling and certifying body for master's-level genetic counselors

Membership: Certified genetic counselors (designated by the acronym CGC®) are diplomates of ABGC.

Board of directors: 10 elected members; Board elects officers

Standing committees: Committees include the Accreditation Committee, Credentials Committee, Operations Committee, Communications Committee and Executive Committee. Subcommittees of the Credentials Committee include the Certification Examination Committee and the Practice Analysis Committee. Subcommittees of the Accreditation Committee include Accreditation Review and Site Visitors. Subcommittees of the Operations Committee include the Nominating Committee, the Finance Committee, and the Grievance Review Committee. Members can be appointed as site visitors, item writers and to ad hoc committees.

Publications/Resources: *Bulletin of Information for the American Board of Genetic Counseling Certification Examination; Required Criteria for Graduate Programs in Genetic Counseling Seeking Accreditation by the American Board of Genetic Counseling*; Practice-based Competencies (Fine BA et al., *Journal of Genetic Counseling* 1996), Practice Analysis (Hampel H et al., *Journal of Genetic Counseling* 2009); list of accredited graduate programs; brochures, fact sheets, consumer information about genetic counseling and genetic counselors; directory of certified genetic counselors.

Annual meeting: Business meeting and program directors' meeting held each fall during the NSGC Annual Education Conference

Student activities: Guidance with completing an application to become an Active Candidate. An Active Candidate is eligible to take the ABGC certification examination.

American Board of Medical Genetics (ABMG)

Year founded/incorporated: 1981

Focus: Accrediting body for doctoral training programs in human genetics; certifying body for doctoral level providers; genetic counselors were also certified through 1990.

Membership: Certified doctoral level geneticists; certified genetic counselors (1981–1990)

Board of directors: 14 elected members; Board elects officers.

Standing committees: Committees are composed of elected board members (Accreditation Committee, Credentials Committee, Maintenance of Certification Committee, and Finance Committee); members of the ABMG are appointed to the Nominating Committee, which also includes one member of the board of directors.

Publications/Resources: ABMG Certification Exam Information; "Learning Guides" to define competencies for geneticists; list of accredited training programs; website also has information on specialists in genetics, number of certified specialists, job postings and search function "Find a Certified Geneticist."

Annual meeting: Business meeting and program directors meeting held in conjunction with annual ASHG meeting

Student activities: Not applicable

American College of Medical Genetics (ACMG)

Year founded/incorporated: 1991

Focus: Continuing education and professional issues of medical genetics professionals

Membership: Medical genetics professionals at all educational levels (clinicians, genetic counselors, researchers) fit into one of several membership categories: Fellow (doctoral level), Associate (certified genetic counselors), Junior (in postdoctoral training program in medical genetics), Student (in graduate training program in genetics), Corresponding (resides outside U.S. and Canada), Emeritus (in retirement), Affiliate (demonstrated interest in medical genetics, but does not fit another category).

Board of directors: 19 members

Standing committees (appointed members): Economics of Genetic Services; Education and CME; Finance; Genetics Review Course; Governance; Intellectual Property; Laboratory Quality Assurance; Maintenance of Certification; Membership; Nominating; Professional Practice and Guidelines; Program Committee for Annual Meeting; Social, Ethical, and Legal Issues; Therapeutics; Website

Special Interest Groups: Adult Genetics, Public Health Genetics, Quality Improvement

Publications/Resources: *Genetics in Medicine*; *The Medical Geneticist* (quarterly newsletter for members only); ACMG Online Library of presented abstracts; genetics frequently asked questions; genetics resources for healthcare professionals; job board (for members); website has search function "Find a Geneticist."

Annual meeting: Held each March in a U.S. or Canadian city

Student activities: Not applicable

American Society of Human Genetics (ASHG)

Year founded/incorporated: 1948

Focus: Human genetics research (basic and clinical) and education

Membership: Human genetics professionals at all educational levels (clinicians, genetic counselors, clinical and laboratory researchers) and other interested professionals

Board of directors: 17 members; president and general board members are elected; editor of *American Journal of Human Genetics,* secretary, and treasurer are appointed.

Standing committees (appointed members): Program Committee; Information and Education Committee; Social Issues Committee; Awards Committee; Nominating Committee; Professional Development (Ad hoc)

Publications/Resources: *American Journal of Human Genetics* (monthly); *SNP-IT Newsletter* (4 times/year); presented abstracts from previous meetings; Conversations in Genetics (interviews with scientists who made major contributions to genetics); educational tools, activities and resources for K-12 and college students; consumer genetics resources; policy and advocacy resources; job postings; member search available at website.

Annual meeting: Held each fall in a U.S. or Canadian city

Student activities: Student-mentor breakfast held at annual meeting; job search opportunities

Canadian Association of Genetic Counsellors (CAGC-ACCG) (Association Canadienne des Conseillers en Génétique)

Year founded/incorporated: 1990

Focus: To promote high standards of practice, encourage professional growth and increase public awareness of the genetic counselling profession in Canada. The CAGC's Certification Board oversees the certification process for Master's-level genetic counsellors.

Membership: Majority of members are genetic counsellors by training. There are four classes of CAGC membership: Full, Associate, Student, Emeritus.

Board of directors: 9 elected members (President-elect, President, Past-president I, Past-president II, Secretary, Treasurer, Central, Eastern and Western Regional Representatives)

Standing committees: Education, Professional Issues, Liaison, Finance, Membership, Communications, Scientific Program, Nominating and Certification Board

Publications/Resources: *Crossover* (published quarterly); Certification Board Examination Information; website has directory of Canadian Medical Genetics Clinics and searchable Directory of Genetic Support Groups.

Annual meeting: Annual conference and annual general meeting each fall. A short course is held biennially before the conference.

Student activities: Regional representatives are encouraged to make contact with students in their respective regions annually. Meet and greet session specifically for students at the annual conference.

International Society of Nurses in Genetics (ISONG)

Year founded/incorporated: 1988

Focus: Continuing education and professional issues of nurses working in genetics

Membership: Nurses at all educational levels (doctoral, master's, baccalaureate) who are professionally involved with or interested in genetics, and other interested genetics professionals, fit into one of several membership categories.

Board of directors: 7 elected members

Standing committees (members volunteer): Bylaws/Awards, Communications Committee; Education; Ethical Issues and Public Policy; Global Membership; Nominating; Professional Practice; Research; Annual Educational Program Committee

Special Interest Groups: Metabolic, Pediatric, Oncology

Publications/Resources: *ISONG Member Newsletter* (quarterly); *What is a Genetic Nurse* brochure; Buddy Program (for members); Job Board.

Annual meeting: Held each fall in a U.S., Canadian, or European city

Student activities: Preconference seminar/workshop held in conjunction with Annual Education Conference; educational lectures and mentor arrangements through individual ISONG members

National Society of Genetic Counselors (NSGC)

Year founded/incorporated: 1979

Focus: Continuing education and professional issues of master's-level genetic counselors

Membership: Full members (master's-level genetic counselors), associate members (clinical geneticists, researchers, interested others), student members (genetic counseling students)

Board of directors: 12 elected members; President, President-Elect, Immediate Past President, Secretary/Treasurer, Secretary-Treasurer-Elect, 7 directors at-large

Standing committees: Communications; Education; Finance; Genetic Counseling Access and Service Delivery; Membership; Nominating; Public Policy Committee. Recruitment to these committees is via the Leadership/Volunteer Development Program. Members can be appointed to the Ethics Advisory Group, Jane Engelberg Memorial Fellowship Advisory Group and Audrey Heimler Special Projects Award Committee.

Special Interest Groups (SIGs): ART/Infertility, Cancer, Cardiovascular Genetics, Disabilities, Fetal Intervention and Therapy, Hematology, Industry, International, Metabolism/Lysosomal Storage Diseases, Neurogenetics, Pediatrics, Prenatal, Psychiatric Disorders, Public Health, Telegenetics, Students/New Genetic Counselors

Publications/Resources: *Journal of Genetic Counseling* (six issues/year); *Perspectives in Genetic Counseling* newsletter (quarterly); website has wealth of resources for genetic counselors, consumers and healthcare professionals, including search function for "Find a Genetic Counselor."

Annual meeting: Held each fall in a U.S. or Canadian city

Student activities: Student Listserv; mentor program; student workshops at regional and national meetings; job connection service

Transnational Alliance for Genetic Counseling (TAGC)

Year founded/incorporated: 2006, incorporated 2008

Focus: Promoting international communication and collaboration

Membership: Open network of genetics professionals interested in genetic counselor education and international exchange.

Board of directors: 15 participating countries; each has an appointed representative to the Board of Directors. Board elects officers.

Standing committees: Executive Committee, Conference Planning Committee

Publications/Resources: Website has several resources including links to international genetic counseling education programs and professional societies. Searchable database with master of science thesis research abstracts. TAGC supports a Listserv for TAGC Partners and Wiki for collaborative projects.

Annual meeting: Biannual meeting, location varies.

Student activities: Students are encouraged to access resources on the website and participate in TAGC activities and conferences. International clinical rotations are promoted.

REFERENCES

American Board of Genetic Counseling. www.abgc.net. Accessed September 2008.

Atzinger CL, Blough-Pfau R, Kretschmer L, Huether CA, Johnson JA, Warren NS (2007) Characterization of the practice and attitudes of genetic counselors with doctoral degrees. *J Genet Couns* 16(2):223–239.

Bedard AC, Huether CA, Shooner K, Buncher CR, Warren NS (2007) Career research interests and training of genetic counseling students. *J Genet Couns* 16(5):645–653.

Bell EL, Nkomo S (2001) *Our Separate Ways: Black and White Women and the Struggle for Professional Identity.* Boston, MA: Harvard Business School Press.

Benveniste G (1987) *Professionalizing the Organization: Reducing Bureaucracy to Enhance Effectiveness.* San Francisco, CA: Jossey-Bass Inc, Publishers.

Biesecker BB (1998) Future directions in genetic counseling: Practical and ethical considerations. *Kennedy Inst Ethics J* 8:145–160.

Biesecker BB, Marteau TM (1999) The future of genetic counseling: An international perspective. *Nat Genet* 22:133–137.

Canadian Association of Genetic Counsellors (2008) Recertification Protocol. http://www.cagc-accg.ca/. Accessed September 2008.

Clark HM, Gamm J, Huether CA, Buncher CR, Blough-Pfau R, Warren NS (2006) Genetic counselors and research: Current practices and future directions. *Am J Med Genet* 142C:276–283.

Cox T (1993) *Cultural Diversity in Organizations: Theory, Research, and Practice.* San Francisco: Berrett-Koehler Publishers, Inc.

Cystic Fibrosis Foundation (2007) http://www.cff.org/AboutCF/. Accessed September 2008.

Fine BA, Baker DL, Fiddler MB, ABGC Consensus Development Consortium (1996) Practice-based competencies for accreditation of and training in graduate programs in genetic counseling. *J Genet Couns* 5(3):113–122.

Gaupman KM, Edwards JG, Brooks KA, Young SR (1991) The doctoral degree in genetic counseling: Attitudes of genetic counselors. *Am J Hum Genet* 49:488–493.

Hogg MA (2003) Social identity. In M. R. Leary & J. P. Tangney (eds.), *Handbook of Self and Identity.* New York: Guilford Press, pp. 462–479.

Jolley J (2007) Choose your doctorate. *J Clin Nurs* 16:225–233.

Kenen R (1997) Opportunities and impediments for a consolidating and expanding profession: Genetic counseling in the United States. *Soc Sci Med* 45(9):1377–1386.

Lavin DE, Hyllegard D (1996) *Changing the Odds: Open Admissions and the Life Chances of the Disadvantaged.* New Haven: Yale University Press.

Maister D (1997) *True Professionalism: The Courage to Care About Your People, Your Clients and Your Career.* New York: Free Press.

Morrow PC, Goetz J (1988) Professionalism as a form of work commitment. *J Vocat Beha* 32(1):92–111.

National Society of Genetic Counselors. National Society of Genetic Counselors' Code of Ethics. Accessible at NSGC website.

National Society of Genetic Counselors (2007) Genetic Counselors in "Nontraditional Roles". www.nsgc.org/nontraditional. Accessed September 2008.

Olesen HS (2000) Professional Identity as Learning Processes in Life Histories, Roskilde: Papers from the Life History Project 12. Reprinted in Weber K (ed.) (2001) *Experience and Discourse. Theorizing Professionals and Subjectivity.* Roskilde: Roskilde University Press.

Parrott S, Clark C (2004) National Society of Genetic Counselors, Inc. Membership Trends 1980–2002. Boston Information Solutions. Accessible at NSGC website.

Parrott S, Vecchio MD (2007) National Society of Genetic Counselors, Inc. Professional Status Survey 2006. Boston Information Solutions. Accessible at NSGC website.

Ragins BR, Cotton JL, Miller JS (2000) Marginal mentoring: the effects of type of mentor, quality of relationship, and program design on work and career attitudes. *Acad Management J* 43:1177–1194.

Resta RG (2006) Defining and redefining the scope and goals of genetic counseling. *Am J Med Genet* 142C:269–275.

Rollnick BR (1983) Continuing education criteria and continuing education units: Policy issues. *Perspect Genet Couns* 5(1):1.

Rollnick BR (1984) The National Society of Genetic Counselors: An historical perspective. *Birth Defects Orig Artic Ser* 29(6):3–7.

Scott JA, Walker AP, Eunpu DL, Djurdjinovic L (1988) Genetic counselor training: A review and considerations for the future. *Am J Hum Genet* 42:191–209.

Smith M, Freivogel ME, Parrott S (2008) National Society of Genetic Counselors, Inc. Professional Status Survey 2008. Boston Information Systems. Accessible at NSGC website.

Strausbaugh SD, Davis PB (2007) Cystic fibrosis: A review of epidemiology and pathobiology. *Clin Chest Med.* 28(2):279–288.

Trent JT (1993) Issues and concerns in master's-level training and employment. *J Clin Psychol* 49(4):586–592.

U.S. Network for Education Information (USNEI) (2004) Structure of U.S. Education-Graduate/Post Education Levels. http://www.ed.gov/about/offices/list/ous/international/usnei/us/edlite-research-doctorate.html. Accessed September 2008.

Walker AP, Scott JA, Biesecker BB, Conover B, Blake W, Djurdjinovic L (1990) Report of the 1989 Asilomar meeting on education in genetic counseling. *Am J Hum Genet* 46:1223–1230.

Wallace JP, Myers MF, Huether CA, Bedard AC, Warren NS (2008) Employability of genetic counselors with a PhD in genetic counseling. *J Genet Couns* 17(3):209–219.

Warren NS, Callahan N, Leroy B (2005) "Nontraditional" is the new "mainstream" genetic counseling. *Perspect Genet Couns* 27(4):4.

16

Genetic Counselors as Educators

Debra L. Collins, M.S., C.G.C. and Joseph D. McInerney, M.S., M.A.

I was asked to give a talk next month to audiologists on genetics—can anyone share their experience?

I have to give a talk for 5th graders on genetics—does anyone have materials appropriate for this age?

—Inquiries posted to NSGC listserv

INTRODUCTION

Genetic counselors have unique perspectives and knowledge to contribute to the education of other healthcare professionals, teachers, students, and the general public. Throughout your career, you will be asked to speak about genetic topics to professional and lay audiences because of this expertise. Healthcare providers seek genetic experts to update their knowledge of genetic conditions, new genetic tests, management, and treatments, while science teachers value real-world experiences to enhance their classes. Requests for talks, workshops, or interviews also stem from interest generated by current genetic news stories. You can also proactively promote your availability to give presentations through mentor networks and speakers bureaus of the National Society of Genetic Counselors (NSGC), the American Society of Human Genetics (ASHG), the March of Dimes, and other genetic and medical professional societies.

There are many resources to help you prepare a presentation, including teaching tools and activities that can be used with different audiences. Several national

A Guide to Genetic Counseling, Second Edition, Edited by Wendy Uhlmann, Jane Schuette, and Beverly Yashar
Copyright © 2009 by John Wiley & Sons, Inc.

organizations have established genetic education guidelines and science standards for students, elementary grades through high school. There are also guidelines that recommend content to improve healthcare providers' genetics knowledge and skills. Other guidelines help you develop your personal education style through awareness of different learning styles and teaching strategies. The guidelines and learning tools in this chapter will help you develop presentations appropriate for audiences of different ages and backgrounds, as well as help you effectively speak with the media.

EDUCATION FOR HEALTHCARE PROFESSIONALS

Healthcare professionals are the most common audience for genetic counselors. Presentations may vary from a one-hour lecture to longer workshops, short courses, or a semester-long course. Additional curriculum materials may be required, such as written course competencies (objectives) and outcomes (evaluations). The National Coalition for Heath Professional Education in Genetics (NCHPEG) has developed a helpful set of core competencies for healthcare professionals and produced a set of core principles in genetics for health professionals, as well as a framework for teaching about genetics and common diseases. These core principles also provide guidance on the development of genetic courses and curricula.

Integrating genetics into mainstream healthcare is limited by the current nature and extent of genetics education for healthcare professionals (Baars, 2007; Guttmacher et al., 2007; Harvey et al., 2007a; Harvey et al., 2007b; Hayflick and Eiff, 2002; Suther and Goodson, 2003). Increasingly, genetic counselors will likely serve as educators of health professionals because of their training in genetics and in the interpretation of complex information for non-geneticists. However, there are challenges as Hayflick and Eiff 2002 captured in a *Genetics in Medicine* editorial: "Primary care providers are asking for instruction on specific content, and there is no debate about this need. However, with the rapid pace of change in genetic medicine, specific content will fall short of what PCPs really need . . . a thoughtful, deliberate, and informed refinement of the 'usual' cognitive strategies will have the greatest impact on integrating genetics into all of healthcare." Non-geneticist providers need practical examples of how genetics relates to practice, but they also need conceptual education that helps them think genetically. The former will meet immediate needs while the latter will prepare providers for the future of genetic medicine. The following recommendations will help you address these objectives as you plan genetics education programs.

- **Appropriate content.** Experience indicates that healthcare providers do not respond well to genetics instruction designed to train geneticists. Instead, providers need practical information relevant to patient care that holds the prospect of improving patient outcomes. Do not overload practitioner courses with content that covers the structure of DNA, patterns of inheritance, the arcana of DNA sequencing, or other content that generally is important only to geneticists. Before you develop your instruction, work with representatives of the intended audience to determine their needs and to identify the clinical issues that are most important to them. Structure your genetics content around that information. When possible, organize your instruction around real or hypothetical cases that are familiar to the audience and illustrate the genetics concepts you have identified as central to your program. Make the instruction as interactive as possible.

o Choose instructional examples that address common diseases, such as cancer or heart disease, and the related issues clinicians encounter daily. Many healthcare providers hold the misconception that genetic medicine is defined by rare, Mendelian disorders and circumscribed by two disciplines, obstetrics/gynecology and pediatrics. You can broaden their knowledge of the increasingly important role of genetics in common, chronic diseases that are the major causes of mortality and morbidity worldwide.

o Use examples specific to your audience or particular medical subspecialty, such as cystic fibrosis with pulmonologists, or Waardenburg syndrome, connexin 26, and velocardiofacial syndrome with audiologists.

o Define all terms; do not assume all healthcare professionals understand key genetics terms, since genetics may be a small, or little-used, aspect of their training curricula or professional interests.

- **Recognition of differences between genetic evaluations and routine healthcare visits.** Offer primary care providers tools and content to incorporate into their evaluations and provide examples of appropriate referrals for genetic services. Typical healthcare visits involve one individual, usually with a single focused problem (sore throat, rash, ear infection, headache, and so on) (Groopman, 2007). In contrast, genetic evaluations involve a greater depth and breadth, and may involve inquiries about a person's prenatal exposures, birth weight, length, head circumference, and extensive past medical history. In addition, the genetic health history involves inquiries about the health/chronic conditions of first- second-, and third-degree relatives. Family planning goals, vocation, and other long-term issues may be discussed. In your talk, suggest medical information needed for referrals to a genetics center. For example, if a pediatrician refers a child with developmental delay, a growth curve and pregnancy history records are helpful. If an internist refers an adult with colon cancer, information about biopsy tissue availability and numbers of polyps are helpful. If a teenager is referred for evaluation of possible Marfan syndrome, a recent eye exam and echocardiology report are helpful.

- **Behaviors and attitudes.** A central objective of education for healthcare professions is to change the way the learner thinks and acts in the clinical setting. As you develop educational interventions, define clearly what you would like the learners to do differently or how you would like them to think differently after completing your program. For example, you may want the provider to be able to take a more complete family history, refer to genetic services more frequently and appropriately, or order the correct genetic tests. On the cognitive side, you may want the provider to recognize that virtually all disease has a genetic basis, or that genetic data are family data and have implications for privacy and confidentiality. Encourage people-first language, by referring to people first, then their condition. For example, refer to "a boy with diabetes" rather than "a diabetic."

- **Level of detail.** Accurate and complete are different concepts. **You are not trying to turn your audience into geneticists,** and you should resist the temptation to overload your instruction with content that has no immediate relevance for the practitioner.

- **Defining and measuring success.** How will you know your intervention has succeeded? This will require you to define your objectives carefully at the outset. To measure changes in knowledge, pre-tests and post-tests can be administered. If your objective is to increase genetics referrals from a given practice, or improve the ability to take a family history, you can assess those objectives by direct, concrete pre- and post-intervention measures. If, however, your objective is to improve patient outcome as a result of genetics education, the approach to evaluation will be considerably more complex and nuanced. Whether you are preparing an individual lecture or developing a longer course, if you plan to do an evaluation, this should be developed at the outset, not after it is already underway. For more involved assessment, you may consider consulting with an outside evaluator to help define your objectives clearly and design the appropriate evaluation scheme and instruments.

- **Resources.** Before you embark on the development of new educational materials, explore the wealth of existing resources. The development of good instructional materials is time consuming and expensive, and you can use the time and money you save on such development instead for implementation and evaluation of your program.

EXAMPLES OF TRAINING AND CONTINUING EDUCATION OF HEALTHCARE PROFESSIONALS

There are many ways to be involved in healthcare professional education; you can:

- Plan or participate in genetics course offerings for CME (Continuing Medical Education) credit. Present at local, regional, and national medical conferences.

- Work with others in healthcare training programs—for example, schools of nursing and medicine, residency programs, and schools of allied health—to determine where genetics fits most appropriately. Provide concrete examples for the integration of genetics across the curriculum, as most programs will not have room in their crowded curricula for a separate course. For instance, you may be able to provide a seminar on taking a family history, patterns of inheritance, pedigree analysis, the process of genetic evaluations, and how to screen families appropriate for genetic referrals. NCHPEG, for example, has educational programs for speech-language pathologists/audiologists that are well-suited for graduate students.

- Teach or help train faculty in genetics from other disciplines, such as medicine, nursing, and dietetics. Many healthcare training programs do not have sufficient faculty to teach basic genetics or its applications to patient care, and they may welcome your input.
- Work with faculty in charge of student clinical rotations to include genetic aspects of patient care. This will help connect their basic sciences training with clinical experiences, since those responsible for clinical training may lack substantive education in genetics.
- Establish a formal clinical genetics rotation for students, residents, fellows, and other healthcare professionals.
- Work through local and state professional societies, as well as providers, to raise awareness of genetic counseling, including ways to access services. Help make local providers aware of genetic education opportunities. This is a way for the relatively small number of formally trained genetic counselors and medical geneticists to provide genetics expertise to primary care providers, who may lack basic knowledge and confidence to deal with genetics-related issues that arise in clinical settings.
- Conduct educational programs on the importance of family history and the availability of reliable tools that patients can use to collect family history data. Highlight genetic red flags that might appear in family histories taken by healthcare providers. Present the family history as an effective, and relatively inexpensive, genetic test. Instill confidence in the provider's ability to take an informative family history and to recognize symptoms and signs that indicate genetic contributions to disease. They can then provide better patient management through the use of genetic perspectives.
- Plan programs which recognize that a primary physician needs to have enough knowledge to recognize a problem as genetic and enough familiarity with genetic principles to be able to use the literature wisely, or to consult with a geneticist intelligently (Hsia et al., 1979).
- Work with professional societies and certifying agencies to lobby for genetics-related questions on certifying exams, and help write and review questions. This can help increase training in genetics, since testing often drives topics taught in the curriculum.

Recommended* Genetic Concepts for Healthcare Professionals and Medical Students

1. Gene organization, control, and segregation
2. Mutations and premutations

---

*Abstracted from

1. Curricula Recommendations, Medical School Core Curriculum in Genetics, Association of Professors of Human and Medical Genetics/American Society of Human Genetics, *December 2001*.
2. NCHPEG Core Competencies in Genetics for Health Professionals, September 2007

3. Mendelian patterns of inheritance (autosomal v. X-linked, dominant v. recessive)

4. Phenotype and clinical manifestations (variable expression, incomplete penetrance, anticipation)

5. Mitochondrial inheritance and diseases

6. Organization of genes into chromosomes, mitosis and meiosis

7. Chromosomal anomalies (numeric, structural, and mosaic)

8. Genetic imprinting and uniparental disomy

9. Inborn errors of metabolism

10. Complex/multifactorial inheritance and traits

11. Teratogenesis, effects of major human teratogens

12. Genetics and pathogenesis of neoplasms, and in predisposition to malignancies/cancer

13. Ethnic group variability in disease frequency and population genetics

14. Prenatal genetic diagnostic procedures and diseases detected prenatally

15. Genetic counseling methods

16. Predictive testing for genetic disease (advantages, limitations, and concerns)

17. Elicit a comprehensive medical genetic family history and construct a pedigree

18. Carry out a comprehensive physical examination for major and minor anomalies

19. Formulate differential diagnoses, including use of specialized tests

20. Understand cytogenetic, biochemical, and molecular laboratory reports

21. Diagnostic and predictive tests for the condition in family—advise patients of benefits, limitations, and risks of tests

22. Treatments available (dietary, pharmacological, enzyme-replacement, transplantation, gene therapy, other)

23. Pharmacogenetic variations

24. Resources (support groups, services, and agencies)

25. Options available for family decision-making

26. Cultural/religious/ethnic issues in communication of genetic information

27. Confidentiality and the difficulties when relatives are found to be at risk for a serious and potentially preventable disease

NCHPEG has developed a series of targeted educational programs and teaching tools for a broad range of health professionals, such as audiologists, psychologists, and physician assistants. You can find continuing educational resources for interdisciplinary collaboration through ASHG, American College of Medical Genetics (ACMG), NSGC, the Association of Professors of Human and Medical Genetics (APHMG), and other resources at the end of the chapter.

EDUCATION FOR THE LAY PUBLIC

Genetic counselors often receive invitations to speak to the general public or lay advocacy groups. Community groups, such as women's clubs, business groups, and churches, may ask you to speak at a meeting, serve on a panel, participate in a book discussion, or take part in another informal gathering. Lay advocacy groups may ask you to talk to families about a new genetic test or discovery, or psychosocial issues such as sibling issues, coping, or advocacy. Presentations to the general public and lay advocacy groups are wonderful opportunities to share your knowledge and expertise in genetic counseling and to promote awareness of genetic services.

You can "get the word out" proactively through presentations annually each November for National Family History Day, declared by the Office of the U.S. Surgeon General. This day, initially focused on Thanksgiving and extended to the winter holiday season, is promoted through public service announcements and other activities to emphasize the importance and value of a genetic family history and genetic counseling. National Family History Day and DNA Day (discussed below) help health professionals and the public understand the work we do, and are occasions to dispel myths and misconceptions about genetic counseling.

Members of lay audiences generally differ widely in their knowledge of biological processes and genetics, but you can bridge these gaps by including brief definitions of terms and conceptual explanations throughout your talk and using clear diagrams. With these groups, it is particularly important to anticipate and prepare for audience questions. Their questions may distract from your intended topic, including personal health issue questions or questions requiring complex explanations. Lay audience questions may inadvertently divert you to issues in the news such as stem cells, cloning, genetic engineering, eugenics, or non-paternity. Be ready to bring the discussion back to your planned topics. For questions of a personal nature, invite the questioner to speak with you after the presentation.

Many of the educational materials and ideas for high school or college students, presented later in this chapter, can be adapted for lay audiences. Prepare a lay audience talk as you would for a media interview. Helpful hints for this are in the NSGC media kit, "A Primer for Communicating Effectively through the Media" (2002), in the members-only section of the NSGC website. The kit has tips for speaking clearly and giving effective presentations, including how to present a professional image and how to deal with potentially controversial issues.

SCIENCE EDUCATION STANDARDS

Genetics education activities often fit within the framework of national and state science education standards and guidelines. Biotechnology teaching standards exist for high school biology classes, particularly for Advanced Placement, Honors Biology, and Biotechnology classes. These standards are also helpful in preparing presentations for two-year and community colleges as well as four-year colleges and universities (see Resources). Most K–12 science teachers utilize the content standards specified by the ***National Science Education Standards*** (***NSES***) and state-level science standards. Many teachers link their curricula to these science standards, so it can be helpful to identify the standards that fit with your talk.

The National Science Education Standards help guide selection of appropriate content for different grade levels. Standards differ at the state level, however, and change often, so it is wise to consult with teachers to ensure that you are familiar with the most recent iterations and that you are preparing your lessons to address current requirements.

The following concepts and principles are recommended for K-8 students:

- Cellular organization of life
- Cellular differentiation
- Chromosomes
- Disease processes
- Genes
- Heritable traits
- Interactions with environment
- Systemic organization of the human body

Most states ask high school teachers to provide students with basic information about

- Reproduction
- Cellular organization, genes, and chromosomes
- Genetic material (DNA) that carries information for heredity
- Mitosis and meiosis

Science for All Americans, Benchmarks for Science Literacy by the American Association for the Advancement of Science (AAAS, 1993) describes the project developed by many interested professional organizations to establish science literacy goals for all Americans by the year 2061 (the year Halley's comet is to return). The science literacy goals related to genetics include detailed recommendations for each of these categories:

- Science as Inquiry
- Life Sciences
- Science and Technology
- Science in Personal and Social Perspectives
- Biology/Life Science
- Investigation and Experimentation

Other national science organizations also promote U.S. science education for kindergarten through 12th grade, including curriculum standards and guidelines. The

National Academy of Sciences and the National Science Teachers Association (NSTA) publish national guidelines that individual states often use to establish standards for grade-level groups (K–4, 5–8, and 9–12). Familiarity with these grade-level standards helps you choose appropriate genetics activities. These standards (1995) are available online, as well as through ASHG and NCHPEG. The Resources section provides more detailed current national standards related to genetic education in the life sciences as well as important concepts to convey.

Tips Before You Go into the Classroom

1. Talk directly with the teacher to obtain explicit information about your topic and how it fits within the unit.
2. Get a sense of the genetic or biology knowledge of the students in the session you are teaching.
3. Check the national, state, and district guidelines for science teaching at the class grade level. Relevant national and state science guidelines are at the education section of the ASHG website.
4. Do not try to cover everything there is to know about your topic; focus instead on two or three major concepts and illustrate those concepts. Think about what you want the students to be able to do with the information after you leave the classroom.
5. Rather than just planning a lecture, think about ways to engage the students directly in the lesson through hands-on activities.
6. Look for existing resources developed and vetted by reliable sources. The reference section lists ideas from the ASHG, the Biological Curricula Study (BSCS), the National Human Genome Research Institute (NHGRI), the Department of Energy, Eccles Institute at University of Utah, Access Excellence, the Community of Genetics Education at NHGRI, the University of Kansas Genetics Education Center, and others.
7. Once you have planned your presentation, if possible, discuss it with the teacher in advance to determine its appropriateness and whether it can be done in the allotted time with your available resources.

Tips for You in the Classroom

1. Minimize the amount of time you spend lecturing to the students. Instead, engage students directly in the lesson.
2. Minimize the amount of specialized vocabulary you use; choose only the vocabulary you need to convey the major concepts.
3. Consider starting with a question or a discrepant event to get the students' attention. For example, "Identical twins share all of their genes, but when one twin has bipolar disorder, the other twin is affected only about 40 percent of the time. What does that tell you about the causes of bipolar disorder?" This serves as an introduction to genetic and environmental contributions to common disease.

Another, non-clinical, example is: "Antibodies are proteins, which are gene products. Immunologists tell us that the human body can produce hundreds of thousands of different antibodies. But we only have about 20,000 genes. Does that make sense?" This might serve as an introduction to the cell's ability to increase the information content of the genetic material, in this case to produce antibodies.

4. Do not give the students information or an answer that they might be able to produce themselves if given the time to think about it. For example, provide some data and ask, "What might explain these observations?"

5. When you ask a question, wait for an answer. Research shows that most teachers wait about one second after asking a question before providing the answer if no student offers one. That simply is not enough time for anyone to process complex information and formulate an answer. Don't be afraid of silence. Count to three, slowly, after you ask a question—wait for someone to respond. If there is no response, try asking the question differently.

6. Be aware that some students will always be more aggressive than others in providing answers to questions. Research shows, for example, that girls often are more reticent than boys to ask or answer questions in science and math classes. Be sensitive to such differences and call on students who might not be volunteering. Or, if one student asks most of the questions, say, "Let's hear from someone who hasn't had a chance to participate in the discussion yet."

7. Be sensitive to misconceptions about genetics and biology in students' questions or in their answers. If you hear what you think might be a misconception, ask for more information from the student. You might say, "Let's talk about that a bit, because the science tells us something different."

8. Tie your lesson to other areas of biology. Remember that genetics informs our thinking about other areas of life science such as evolution, development, behavior, systematics and taxonomy, and ecology. This will help the teacher make the cross-disciplinary connections that are important to an integrated understanding of biology.

9. Although you may be teaching about genetic counseling, avoid leaving the impression that all of genetics concerns disease and developmental disabilities. Remind the students that this is just one area of genetics, the broad discipline that is concerned with inherited biological variation.

10. Any classroom is a virtual living laboratory of human variation; don't lose the teaching opportunity that laboratory presents. Remember as well to emphasize the overwhelming likeness of all human beings. This is one of the most important lessons of biology and genetics: unity in diversity.

EDUCATION FOR STUDENTS AND SCIENCE TEACHERS

At some point in your career, a colleague, friend, relative, or your own child's teacher may ask you to speak to students. If you are a parent, this is a legitimate way to visit your child's classroom! At back-to-school night or conferences, let the science teacher know that you are a genetic counselor and are willing to talk to the class. Presenting to students can be a great opportunity for early genetics education, and can leave a lasting impression that could influence their choice of study and career. There are also opportunities for genetic counselors to provide continuing education for teachers in training (pre-service teachers) and for those already teaching in the classroom. It is very rewarding to work with teachers, as well as students to provide up-to-date and relevant information. Once you've done a few talks, your name is likely to be passed around!

You can proactively contact schools in your area, or teachers may find you through a colleague who has already become involved in local teacher education and mentor programs. You can promote your availability through genetic societies' speakers' bureaus and explore your institution or state health department speakers' resource list. You can volunteer at community events, judge a science fair or a genetic essay contest, participate in an interscholastic science competition, or provide a talk at a museum special exhibit. You can participate in DNA Day celebrations, an annual event to promote genetics awareness. It celebrates the sequencing of the human genome (as well as the anniversary of Watson and Crick's discovery of the structure of DNA), and is sponsored by major genetic research organizations and professional societies including the National Human Genome Research Institute (NHGRI), ASHG, NSGC, the Genetic Alliance, the Centers for Disease Control and Prevention (CDC), and others.

Collaborative learning and inquiry-based strategies, such as the 5E Instructional Model, are well-suited for student and professional education. This instructional model was developed by the Biological Sciences Curriculum Study (BSCS) [Bybee, R. W. 1996]. This guided-inquiry approach involves students actively in developing their understanding of concepts or skills with the teacher acting as the instructional director. It involves five elements (each beginning with the letter "E"): engage, explore, explain, elaborate, and evaluate. Most teaching models encourage active learning, rather than a lecture where the student is generally a passive participant.

The Resources section includes modules, teaching tools, activities, exercises, and resources. For single lectures as well as for longer genetics units, teaching should focus on active learning, whenever possible. Presentations/classroom activities should challenge students to apply their scientific understanding, analyze and interpret data to solve problems, and use models to illustrate scientific concepts. In genetic modules, students can work in small discussion groups to collect and analyze data, propose hypotheses to explain observations, suggest strategies to test hypotheses, and develop presentations. Challenge students to use higher-order thinking skills while balancing group work with individual learning.

EDUCATION FOR OLDER STUDENTS (HIGH SCHOOL, COLLEGE, AND ADULTS)

Most U.S. high school students complete at least one biology course by graduation. The genetics content in this course may constitute their only formal exposure to genetics concepts. Genetic counselors can enhance this education by classroom presentations that demonstrate "real-world" applications of these genetic concepts. Teachers from science or other disciplines (family development/life skills) may invite genetic counselors to participate in school programs, student shadowing (following institutional and Health Insurance Portability and Accountability Act [HIPAA] requirements), student assignments (i.e., career interviews), and teacher workshops. Schools hold career programs and welcome the addition of a new career and speaker. These programs provide opportunities to meet science educators and develop a network to improve genetics science education.

Many professional organizations websites provide vetted ideas for genetics education. Some address basic, general genetics content, while others focus on genetic counseling, genetic research, or social and legal issues. Some activities for elementary school students, listed later in this chapter, can be adapted for high school students and adults. For instance, the jelly bean activity called Generations from BSCS works with many age groups. Many teaching ideas and developed curricula are available on the Internet and are updated regularly, such as those at NHGRI, ASHG, Cold Spring Harbor, and the Eccles Institute. Table 16-1 has some successful ideas for teaching high school-age students and beyond, and there are additional tools and activities in the chapter resources.

TABLE 16-1. Teaching Ideas for High School Students, College Students, and Adults

Genetic condition assignment	Ask students to prepare a report, or compile a pamphlet, on a genetic condition. Provide students with a list of conditions, or pre-approve topics. Give them instructions on information to include in the report or pamphlet, as well as a grading rubric, so they know what is expected.
Simulated genetic counseling session	Students are assigned "cases" for a genetic counseling role play utilizing a list of provided conditions. Students prepare a family history; then you arrive for "clinic" and simulate an abbreviated counseling session. Provide the audience with pre-clinic preparation information and insight into the directed discussion during the role play; discuss issues that could be addressed after the "clinic," and articulate psychosocial issues you "observed." This simulation is a particularly rewarding way to show the process of genetic counseling.
Family panel	Moderate a panel of individuals with genetic conditions. Ask each panelist to describe his or her condition for 15–20 minutes, including how he or she first learned about the diagnosis and misconceptions about the condition, based on personal experience. Encourage audience questions. If the moderator notices that one panelist is disproportionally asked questions, balance the discussion to involve all panelists, by generalizing questions, or globalizing questions on topics like health insurance or dealing with new healthcare providers.

TABLE 16-1. (*Continued*)

Demonstrate genetic concepts	Use pop-it beads (from Ward's, or Carolina Biological Supply Company—see Resources) to demonstrate a gene, DNA replication, gene alterations, chromosomes, and other concepts. These beads, used by many biology teachers, provide opportunities to involve students in active learning.
Game show	Reinforce genetic concepts and information through competitions or activities based on a game or game show (Jeopardy, 20 questions, other). Ideas for these can be found through the ASHG website, Education section, and other online genetics education sites.
Simulated genetic testing ethics exercise	Provide an audience with a little information about a "research project" and give them the opportunity to "participate." Then, ask students to role play the family, provide them with the genetic "test" results in sealed envelopes, and discuss ethical issues in genetic testing, informed consent, privacy issues, insurance issues, and changes in family relationships. Opening the envelopes is optional. Discussion is the focus of this exercise.
Ethical discussions	Provide a case example from a current topic in the news, or use a prepared curricula such as the Nathanial Wu lesson plan on testing for Huntington Disease from the BSCS curricula (1992). This case deals with possible discrimination at work, privacy, and employer genetic testing. This lesson plan can be supplemented with information on state or national genetic privacy legislation.
Genetic art models	Assign groups of students genetics concepts (for example, a gene with exons and introns, crossing-over, gene-to-protein, chromosomes) to make with recycled materials. Allow preparation time to gather appropriate materials, and have reference books on hand. Each group can show their model and explain their concepts.
Interscholastic competitions between schools	School teams can compete against each other, using multiple choice or open-ended genetics questions appropriate for the levels of student knowledge and abilities. When possible, have a plaque or certificate for the winning team, and try to get information to the media about the competition award winners.

EDUCATION FOR YOUNG STUDENTS (ELEMENTARY TO MIDDLE SCHOOL)

You may be asked to teach young children about genetics in an elementary school, not infrequently by your own child's teacher or a friend's child. It can be challenging to simplify genetics concepts for young students with virtually no science background, but the effort will be well worth your time. Young children are eager to learn and fun to teach because everything is interesting to them. The late Paul de Hart Hurd, a leading authority in science education, once observed that all children are "curious naturalists." Your approach to teaching young children should trade on that inherent curiosity by providing interesting observations, specimens, or objects to engage their interest.

Young children have little to "unlearn" and are receptive to new experiences. Focus on a few fun facts that you and the students can elaborate in an interactive manner. They will enjoy, for example, learning the science behind the human variation they have already observed—why people are different or alike—and how science works. They will be interested in twins and why siblings look alike. They may have a heightened interested in genetics from a current movie or TV show. Group activities and hands-on activities work well with this age, for example, using a beach ball or a deck of cards to illustrate probability (Table 16-2).

TABLE 16-2. Teaching Ideas and Elementary/Middle School Activities

Concept	Teaching Idea
Careers	Provide overview of genetic careers, including those requiring a bachelor's or master's degree as well as a Ph.D. or M.D.
Cell	Create a cell with a small plastic ball (from a craft store) inside another ball (nucleus inside cell); use yarn for chromosomes in the inner ball.
Chromosomes	Create chromosomes with beads, yarn, or other material to show sizes, crossovers, other concepts.
Difference and variability	Identify normal "traits" (earlobes—attached or unattached, widow's peak, tongue rolling, ability to taste PTC paper, other).
DNA	Use pop-it beads to demonstrate base pairing; one section of beads represents a gene.
Family history	Draw a simple family tree *(Note: Keep adoption, and other potentially sensitive issues in mind)*.
Genetic conditions	Describe conditions familiar to students, such as Down syndrome, dwarfism, albinism, other.
Genetic conditions	Ask an individual with a condition to speak or use a video.
Genetic counseling	Role play a simulated genetic counseling session to demonstrate a clinic visit.
General genetics	Utilize videos targeting young viewers developed by NHGRI (Spanish version available) or others.
Inheritance	*Family Trees and Characteristics,* BSCS Genes and Surroundings, Activity 6, shows inheritance of traits over 3 generations using jelly beans.
Inheritance of traits	*From One Generation to Another,* BSCS Genes and Surroundings, Activity 12, shows inheritance of traits using a fantasy character
Probability	Beach ball with 4 different colors, discuss random chance of touching colors each time *(Note: creates fun chaos that neighboring classrooms may not appreciate)*.
Probability	Deck of cards to demonstrate $1/4$ chance, or toss coin to demonstrate $1/2$ chance.
Variability	Make fingerprints by rubbing students' hands across paper with a thick graphic pencil rubbing, "lift" print with clear tape, observe prints, discuss variability (whorls, loops, arches), family traits.
XX vs. XY	Toss a coin to demonstrate 50/50 ratio.

Children can also be empowered to help make a difference in the lives of children with genetic conditions. They obviously cannot cure a condition; however, they can make a big difference in the day-to-day experiences of a classmate with a difference or disability. You can discuss ways they can help make another child's limitations easier, such as sticking up for the classmate if there is teasing, inviting the classmate to sit at their lunch table, and including the classmate in birthday parties. Sometimes, with parental permission, you can ask a child with a genetic condition to give a short presentation. The other students are usually very respectful and interactive. The student can be asked to talk about when he or his parents first learned he had this condition, and discuss some of the misconceptions about it to get the discussion started. The student can explain how any specialized equipment works and helps maintain health. You can read a book involving a central character with a disability. Choose books in which the problem does not just disappear. The main characters should not be treated with too much pity, or have to possess superhuman/heroic capabilities to overcome their limitations. Select a book for which you can later discuss how the main character (person or animal with a difference) and/or others around them learn to accept their short stature, wheelchair, slow progress, or other differences. You could also use a book like *People* (Spier, 1988) that describes many types of differences and acceptance.

Table 16-2 includes ideas for activities for K–8 students that stimulate young students' interest in genetics; some of these activities are also appropriate for older students. There are more activities in the chapter resources section "Teaching Ideas for Education in Medical Genetics."

TEACHING ABOUT ETHICS AND PUBLIC POLICY

Most audiences have questions about ethical issues and public policy. These questions provide opportunities for formal and informal discussions that can be used to clarify issues, heighten awareness, and engage the audience in thoughtful analysis of current media topics, or of topics they have not yet encountered. Critical thinking always has been an important aspect of science education. Ethical analysis is increasingly important because the rapid progress in science and technology often challenges long-standing societal values and policy positions and outstrips the ability of our social and political institutions to accommodate to those challenges. In educational discussions:

- Ensure that students understand the underlying science and technology.
- Address the principles of technology as well as the principles of science that relate to the issues at hand.
- Provide a clear framework for ethical analysis.
- Make sure your instruction emphasizes and demonstrates that ethical analysis is a form of rational inquiry.
- Recognize that controversy often is inherent in such dialogue.

Students should understand that sound ethical analysis is impossible in the absence of sound understanding of the relevant science and technology.

Introduce genetics content by presenting an ethical dilemma, and then asking the students what they need to know about the underlying science and technology before they can discuss the ethical issues knowledgeably. For example:

Josh is a college junior. He was identified as a carrier of sickle cell trait in a screening program at his university. During the follow-up counseling, he tells the counselor that he is engaged and that he has two teenage sisters. The counselor encourages Josh to share his test results with his fiancée, his parents, and his siblings. Josh refuses and tells the counselor that she should not reveal that information either. What should the counselor do?

Before beginning a discussion of this case, ask, "What do we have to know about the underlying scientific and clinical issues before we can discuss this case in an informed manner?" With your help, the students should come to recognize that they must first understand facts and concepts such as:

- The pattern of transmission of the disorder
- The frequency of the sickle cell (HbS) allele in various populations
- Josh's geographic ancestry, and his fiancée's
- The difference between sickle cell trait (AS) and sickle cell disease (SS)
- Availability of prenatal diagnosis for sickle cell disease (SS)
- The severity of the disease
- Prospects for treatment, and the cost of treatment
- Insurance coverage for related services

Work with the students to clarify this information, and emphasize that in the absence of such understanding one might make inaccurate assumptions about the case. Some of the topics that can be part of the case discussion include controversy, principles of technology, and ethical analysis.

Controversy

- Be clear about the underlying sources of controversy in the ethical issues you are addressing, and ask the students to help identify those sources. For example, in ethical dilemmas involving privacy and duty to warn, the underlying source of the controversy may be that genetic data are family data; that is, once you know something about your patient's genotype, you automatically know something about the genotypes of certain family members. With respect to issues such as stem cells, cloning, and recombinant DNA, the ultimate source of the related controversies is our ability to analyze and manipulate the genetic material.
- It helps to call attention to two different types of controversy rooted in science and technology:
  o ***Controversies within the scientific community***. Scientists disagree, for example, about whether there is a substantial biological basis for our

traditional conceptions of race, and about the unit of selection in the course of evolution.

o *Controversies about the use of science and technology that extend into society as a whole.* Should we, for example, use race as a variable in the clinical encounter or in biomedical research, or should we teach intelligent-design creationism in the biology classroom as coequal with evolution theory?

- Check with the teacher in advance if you suspect that some of the information you will cover is controversial. Determine whether the school or district has policies about the teaching of controversial issues, and be certain you understand who needs to know *in advance* if your lesson will address controversial topics (for example, ask if you need to check with the principal, department chairman, or even in some cases, parents).

In Josh's case, the underlying sources of controversy involve the ethical issues of privacy and duty to warn. Is Josh's sickle cell genotype family data? Identifying Josh as a carrier of sickle cell trait means that his sisters each have a 50% carrier risk and he and his fiancée could have a 25% risk to have a child with sickle cell anemia, if his fiancée is also a carrier of sickle cell trait.

Principles of Technology

Most people never encounter the underlying science of a particular controversial issue in genetics; they generally encounter its technological manifestations such as prenatal diagnosis or genetic testing for late-onset disease. The American Association for the Advancement of Science (*Science for All Americans*, 1989) recommends that educational activities highlight basic principles of technology such as:

- All technologies have unintended consequences.
- All technologies are fallible.
- All technologies serve the interests of particular individuals, groups, or agencies.

In Josh's case, you might discuss the accuracy of screening and prenatal diagnosis for sickle cell disease, and the sources of any potential inaccuracies.

A Clear Framework for Ethical Analysis

Discussions of ethical issues in science classes run the risk of becoming unstructured and unfocused exchanges of information that have no clear goal or end point. It helps to provide a mechanism that structures the analysis and the attendant discussions. Consider using frameworks such as the following to structure discussions of ethical issues and dilemmas:

- Competing interests of the parties involved in the case
- Conflicting goals, rights, and duties of the parties
- Ethical principles (autonomy, beneficence, nonmaleficence, justice)

In this case, there are competing interests and conflicting rights that the genetic counselor must consider between Josh and his family members, including his fiancée. Should Josh's autonomy-based position trump the counselor's commitment to nonmaleficence? The genetic counselor has to weigh Josh's right to privacy versus the duty to warn his sisters of their 50% carrier risk for sickle cell trait and his fiancée of the 25% risk to have a child with sickle cell anemia, if she is a carrier of sickle cell trait.

It also is important that students understand the types and relative quality of the information they are using and hearing. Consider these distinctions, for example:

- **Facts:** It is a fact that others in the family might be at risk for disease if an individual tests positive for a genetic variant associated with that disorder.
- **Values:** It is a value position to state that the patient's right to privacy—the right to control that information—is more important than the duty to warn other members of the family.
- **Opinions:** It is an opinion that healthcare providers should not be permitted to violate a patient's right to privacy.

Ethical Analysis is a form of Rational Inquiry

In the discussion of ethical issues, one often hears that "there is no single, correct answer to this (or any) ethical dilemma." That often is true, but the statement does not go far enough. In ethics, as in science, there are well-reasoned and badly reasoned answers. One should expect the same level of intellectual rigor in ethical discourse that one expects in discussions of scientific issues.

One of the most important aspects of introducing ethical analysis in the classroom is that it helps students engage in and practice civil discourse. It is possible to become quite passionate about one's views, but ethical analysis requires civility. One can disagree with another's views and can be quite critical of them, but one cannot resort to personal attacks. Aside from being inappropriate, such attacks used as a form of argument are logical fallacies.

EFFECTIVE PRESENTATIONS: HOW TO PREPARE

Whether your audience is students, healthcare professionals, or the general public, it is valuable to know the context of your presentation, so you can effectively provide relevant information in the time allocated. Whenever possible, you should:

- Clarify the title and content for your talk and how your program fits into the curricula/program
- Know the scheduled time frame, and allow time for discussion
- Discuss and practice audiovisual technology in advance
- Consider different learning styles and educational standards for your audience

Every audience will be a mixed group of learners with different learning styles, such as a spatial-visual style (seeing or creating images, illustrations or diagrams), a kinetic style (moving or touching), a language-oriented style (verbalizing, reading, hearing), or a logical style (thinking, questioning, pondering ideas). Adult-learner styles often are described broadly as visual (images), kinesthetic (tactile), or auditory (verbal) styles. It is important to keep in mind different learning styles as you put together your presentation. The chapter resources include more information on learning styles.

As a new graduate, you may be confident in your knowledge of genetics, and teaching individuals and small groups; however, you may need more preparation to teach to a large audience. Preparation will help you avoid unpleasant surprises during your presentation. Prepare visual aids that can be accommodated by the technology available on the site of your presentation. Microsoft PowerPoint™ is currently used universally. Your talk can be enhanced or diminished by the use of visual aids and handouts. Visual aids and handouts are useful to reinforce information, provide summaries and reading lists, and supply supporting data that would otherwise be difficult to present within your talk. A hard copy of your lecture may encourage your audience to become actively engaged in the lecture and provides an effective way to review lecture content. However, you may want to just provide key slides with to avoid the possibility that your audience will "tune out" and just read the handout. Consider the proprietary issue of your content, as well.

Tips for Using Handouts

- Handouts are simple, need no power supply, and serve as back-up if the technology fails. Determine the size of the audience in advance so everyone has a copy. Remember to refer to the handouts during your talk.
- Handouts can be distributed before, during or after your talk, with an advantage to each:
  - *Before your talk*—if handouts contain important material and you want your audience to follow along while you speak, place the handouts near the entrance to the room.
  - *During your talk*—if you want the audience to view some information right as you are speaking about it, you should distribute the handouts quickly to avoid losing momentum.
  - *After your talk*—if you plan to distribute handouts at the conclusion, tell your audience members so that they will be encouraged to listen rather than divide their attention taking notes.

Tips for Creating and Using Visual Aids

- Visual aids should enhance understanding of your spoken words. People retain best what they see and hear simultaneously, so good visual material can provide insights that would otherwise require lengthy explanations.

- All visual aids should clarify and support your talk; anything on a screen will draw an audience's attention.
- Visual aids must be legible and clearly visible to the entire audience. Use font sizes visible from the back row.
- Be careful not to include too much information on any given slide. Keep the slides simple, with clear data, graphs, figures, and acronyms (define verbally).
- Some concepts can be explained, and then illustrated visually with animations and recordings. However, use dazzling electronic visuals in moderation. You want your audience to absorb and retain the substance of your talk rather than be mesmerized by your special effects.
- Many online textbooks have supplementary animations to aid in explaining concepts.
- Do not read content on your slides that audience members can read for themselves. Your spoken comments should extend or clarify the information on slides.

Graphics, Quotes and Analogies

You can add interest and emphasis to your talk through well-placed illustrations, analogies, and quotes. Cartoons and quotes can be used as transitions between topics and can also provide a humorous break during a talk. Be sure to properly credit/provide the website or source of these graphics, quotes, and analogies.

- Many genetics professionals use cartoons to emphasize a point, particularly those of Gary Larson (Universal Press Syndicated). You also can do an Internet search for "genetics cartoons."
- University libraries subscribe to databases with medical illustrations and graphics for your use. The American Medical Association has a publicly available atlas of the human body.
- Pictures and graphics can be obtained from an Internet search such as Google Images.
- Analogies help convey complex concepts to an audience through familiar associations. Use age-appropriate examples (remember that some very young children may not have seen a toaster, and in contrast, the intricacies of computer software such as spell-checkers may not be familiar to an older lay audience). However, an everyday analogy can make an abstract concept crystal clear. Use them as a strategy for making concepts in genomics easily understandable. The resource section lists several analogies that we have heard or collected, many from colleagues.
- Well-placed quotes may also help emphasize your points.

Judicious use of quotes, cartoons, and other illustrations can support your points. Use them sparingly, however; if overused, they can lose their effect.

Effective Slide Presentations

ASHG and NSGC both provide suggestions for slide preparation through their annual meeting websites, to optimize viewer visibility and readability. Suggestions from these and other sources include the following.

For slides, use:

- No more than 36 words per slide (maximum of 6 lines with 6 words each)
- Two or three facts or information points per image (maximum of six)
- A simple standard Microsoft® PowerPoint™ design. Historically, a diazo blue background with yellow titles and white text is used at professional meetings.
- Black text on white slides for presentations 1) distributed as handouts, or 2) if the audience is provided the slides digitally in order to write notes using a notebook computer.
- Approximately 10% of the male population is color blind, usually red-green. So, if possible, avoid those colors for important points (i.e., do not emphasize the main point in red).
- For complicated images, build the image layer by layer, using a succession of slides, instead of presenting the audience with a complex visual all at once.

When presenting data, consider:

- Pie charts for percentages
- Column charts (vertical) or bar graphs (horizontal) for comparisons and rankings
- Column or line charts for changes over time and frequency
- Bar graphs and dot charts for correlation

For the presentation:

- Rehearse your talk with the visual aids. Practice talking while changing visual materials to avoid losing momentum, your own train of thought, and the audience's attention. Utilize the "speaker ready room" frequently available at large national meetings.
- Check that the correct visual piece is on the screen each time, before you continue.
- Explicitly point to information on the screen you are discussing, and tell your audience why it is important. However, do not annoy or distract the audience by continuing to circle your point.
- Know how long you are scheduled to speak, and do not go over the allotted time. Allow time for questions and comments for the last 5 minutes.
- Do not be diverted by a member of the audience, so that you go over your time or get off track. Let the audience know when you will answer questions.
- Respect your audience and plan to cut information if needed. End the presentation on time.

Logistics:

- Learn what audiovisual equipment will be available and request needed equipment.
- Check whether special requests are needed, such as for a video player (check compatibility, especially sound) or Internet access.
- Ask about the screen size and location and whether your presentation will be projected on more than one screen.
- Minimize text on the lower part of the slides, if the lower part of the screen is difficult to see from the back of a room.
- Know the room size and arrangement, including the lectern's placement and light.
- Determine the type of microphones you will be using (e.g., podium, clip-on) and what type of pointer will be provided (wear clothes with a belt, pocket, or waist band if the microphone transmitter clips on).
- Verify whether an audiovisual technician will be on hand during your presentation, and, if not, who will handle problems such as extra projector bulbs.
- Determine who will monitor and adjust the lights. A dark room may invite some to sleep, so be cautious about low lights.

Bring your presentation on a back-up jump drive and/or compatible CD (not rewriteable) and print out a hard copy. You can also e-mail yourself a copy of your presentation if you will have Internet access. Never assume that all the equipment you plan to use will be waiting and will run smoothly; have back-up plans. Even if your requirements have been confirmed in writing, check that everything is actually there when you arrive at the site.

Challenges and Tips for Effective Presentations

- *Be knowledgeable of current hot topics about genetics in the news and other media.* The mass media tends to focus on stories involving conflict and change, which catch the attention of the public. While you are versed in many topics, some may require more in-depth expertise, such as cloning, stem cell research, genetic engineering, eugenics, direct-to-consumer tests, newborn screening, adoption, or a topic related to a recent movie, crime show, or news event. It can be challenging to respond to your audience's interests on these if your planned focus was for a general genetics overview or genetics careers talk. Current topics can provide teaching opportunities, however, and humor, patience, and anticipating the unexpected will get you through these questions.
- *Be clear about the limits of your knowledge.* Be honest: No one can know everything, and no audience will expect you to be omniscient. When you don't know the answer to a question, some possible responses include:
  o "I don't know, but my best estimate is. . ..." (if you feel you can make an informed judgment).

    o "I don't know. That area is outside of my expertise, but I think I can find the answer and get back to you."

    o "I don't know, and I think that's one of those questions for which no one has an answer at the moment. There is still a lot we don't know about . . .."

- *Set the stage for your talk.* Prepare a brief introduction about yourself and your expertise so the audience knows why you are the one presenting the information. If you are not introduced formally, introduce yourself briefly, using the opportunity to promote the genetic counseling profession's credentials (ABGC certification, etc.) and your experience. The audience will benefit from knowing who you are, how you gained your expertise, where you work, and what you do. You can use this opportunity to interact with your audience, exploring what they know, their exposure to genetics, and what they are interested in learning.

- *Know the audience and the purpose for your being there.* You may be providing required course content on which the students will be tested. For this audience, you may need to provide handouts and more in-depth materials including several multiple-choice exam questions. On the other hand, you may be there because genetics is an ancillary topic, of interest but unfamiliar to your audience. In this case, keep the content simple and informative, without providing overwhelming details.

- *Technology can always fail.* PowerPoint™ slides are currently in favor. However, you should also have a back-up plan, including handouts, notes, stories, or anecdotes; these will be handy if technical issues disrupt your talk.

- *Non-technical programs are very successful.* A simple discussion of what you do, what genetic discoveries you are excited about right now, and some of your current cases can be fascinating. Keep HIPAA privacy issues in mind, however, and consider changing age, sex, location or other identifying information in case anecdotes. Never use real patients' names.

- *Privacy.* Audience members may have a burning genetic question or personal issue. They may share intimate details with the entire audience. You can offer to stay for questions at the session's conclusion for individual questions or give out your contact information, so you can address complex or personal questions in a more appropriate format.

- *Consider whether you are the right spokesperson for a topic.* Determine why you were asked to talk. Is the topic one that you feel qualified to address? Perhaps you are up for the challenge of learning something new to present to an audience and have enough time to develop a presentation. If not, consider referring the talk to another genetic counselor or professional.

- *Consider who you represent and who requested your talk.* Do you represent your institution, your profession, a support group, or yourself? Review appropriate policy statements or positions of relevant organizations, as needed. If the subject of the program is controversial, inquire about the position of the host organization beforehand. If you do not support their position, consider declining.

- *New communication and electronic technology provides challenges for teaching.* New technical devices to access information changes rapidly and will affect future teaching methods. Take advantages of opportunities to learn new educational skills, about distance learning and remote instruction, developing rubrics, online testing, and interdisciplinary and multicultural teaching. Keep abreast of developing technology such as webinars, podcasting, social networking, virtual worlds, collaborative editing and shared work space, Wikis, YouTube, blogs, Twitter and other developments. Attend faculty development seminars offered at your institute, nearby university or community college, or online. There is an exciting growth of methods for future education.

There are additional presentation tips in the chapter resources.

TIPS FOR SPEAKING WITH THE MEDIA

In addition to giving talks and presentations to various audiences, you may be asked to reach an even wider audience through a media interview. A journalist may contact you from a newspaper, magazine, news program, or other media outlet, and this can provide you with another opportunity to provide accurate genetic information to a broad audience. Through this, you can educate the public about a genetic condition, clarify the significance of new research, therapies, or tests for inherited disorders, or explain the value of genetic counseling in helping families with heritable conditions. However, you should explore your institution's policy about media interviews. Some institutions require all interviews to be vetted through their media office, and may have a representative present during interviews to ensure that the reporter sticks to the agreed-upon topic. They may also be familiar with particular reporters, talk show hosts or radio program formats to help you judge the appropriateness of the media request.

An interview may seem like a simple conversation between two individuals, especially if you are discussing a topic in which you are well versed. Yet much of your interview is often edited out. *Ask questions and be prepared.* Ask about the subject of the interview, who the audience is and who else the reporter has interviewed, as well as when the story will run. Ask how long the interview will take; be careful with interviews, especially those on controversial topics, which are scheduled to last longer than 20 minutes. Keep your answers short; a 30-minute interview for TV may result in a 10 to 20-second sound bite. Print reporters are usually looking for quotes. Try to use familiar terms rather than medical jargon. In advance, consider the message you wish to communicate, and prepare key "take-home" points on the topic.

Effective communication through the media requires preparation. Be sensitive to the possibility that the reporter may edit your interview to forward his or her own biases about the subject rather than the message you hope to convey. If you are being interviewed for an article, you can request to review the content before it is printed. However, a publication review is not standard practice. "Dealing with Media: A Primer for Communicating Effectively through the Media" (NSGC 2002) prepares genetic counselors to communicate effectively with the media and is available at the Members section of the NSGC website and summarized in the chapter resources.

DEVELOPING EDUCATION MATERIALS

This chapter is focused on giving oral presentations. Your educational efforts may also extend to development of printed materials or web-based resources, which is beyond the scope of this chapter. Some of the same considerations regarding giving oral presentations, such as type of content to present and appreciating different learning styles, all apply to the development of printed and web-based materials. Helpful resources for developing educational materials are included in the resources section.

CONCLUSION

Educational activities will be a very rewarding part of your professional career. When you give a talk on a genetic topic, not only are you providing genetics content, but your presentation is part of a bigger picture. You are contributing to genetic literacy at every level, a goal of most professional genetic societies. You are providing information that will make a healthcare provider better able to recognize genetic conditions, integrate genetics into his or her practice, and recommend appropriate genetics referrals. You are providing some students with their first (or only) exposure to genetic concepts. Members of your audiences may think about information you presented as they make healthcare decisions and may later consider accessing genetic services. The students may become scientists, healthcare providers, legislators, journalists, ministers, or other professionals with careers in which accurate genetic knowledge will be valuable. You are laying the foundation for this knowledge, not only by the content of your presentation, but also by the resources you recommend. Your audience will gain an appreciation and a better understanding of genetics. You will inspire some to pursue a genetic career. All will be better consumers of genetic healthcare, regardless of their career or profession.

> *A teacher affects eternity; he can never tell where his influence stops.*
> —Henry Brooks Adams

REFERENCES

Reference materials have a limited shelf life and Internet resources are dynamic by nature. The following references may change, but similar new resources are likely to become available.

Curriculum Standards for Health Professionals

Baars M (ed.) (2007) *Genetic Knowledge, Opinions, and Self-Perceived Competence of Non-Genetic Heathcare Providers.* Amsterdam: EMGO Institute.

Clinical Objectives in Medical Genetics for Undergraduate Medical Students, Association of Professors of Human Genetics, *Gen Med* 1(1):54–55, Nov/Dec 1998. Clinical training and competencies for medical students to apply genetic principles in diagnosis, management, and prevention of human disease.

Core Curriculum Recommendations for Medical Schools, American Society of Human Genetics. Knowledge, skills, and attitudes related to medical genetics needed by medical students during their careers as physicians, *Am J Hum Genet* 1995 (56):535–537.

Core Competencies in Genetics for Health Professionals, (3rd edition), 2007, National Coalition for Health Professional Education in Genetics (NCHPEG) Accessible at NCHPEG website.

"Development of New Curriculum" National Standards and the Science Curriculum: Challenges, Opportunities, and Recommendations, Rodger Bybee, (ed.) Biological Sciences Curriculum Study, Kendall Hunt Publishing Company, 1996.

Groopman J (2007) *How Doctors Think*, Houghton Mifflin Company.

Guttmacher AE, Porteus ME, McInerney JD (2007) Educating healthcare professionals about genetics and genomics. *Nat Rev Genet* 8: 151–157.

Harvey EK, Fogel CE, Christenson K, Peyrot M, Terry SF, McInerney JD (2007a) Providers' Knowledge of Genetics: A Survey of 5,915 Individuals and Families with Genetic Conditions. *Genet Med* 9 (5): 259–267.

Harvey EK, Stanton S, Garrett J, Neils-Strunjas J, Warren NS (2007b) A case for genetics education: Collaborating with speech-language pathologists and audiologists. *Am J Med Genet A* 143A: 1554–1559.

Hayflick S, Eiff MP (2002) Will the learners be learned? *Genet Med.* 4 (2): 43–44.

Suther S, Goodson P. 2003. Barriers to the provision of genetic services by primary care physicians: A systematic review of the literature. *Gent Med* 5 (2): 70–76.

Hsia YE et al. (1979), *Service and Education in Medical Genetics.* Academic Press.

Principles of Genetics for Health Professionals (2004) *National Coalition for Health Professional Education in Genetics* (NCHPEG). Accessible at NCHPEG website.

Recommended Curriculum Guidelines for Family Practice Residents: Medical Genetics, 1999, *American Academy of Family Practice*

Spier P (1988) *People*, Random House Children's Books, ISBN-13: 9780385244695.

RESOURCES

Note: All of the following resources are easily found online through a search of the Internet using the article title, or the name of organization (or acronym).

I. Curricula Standards, Guidelines and Ideas, K–12

II. Teaching Ideas

III. Dealing with the Media: NSGC Tips

IV. Analogies

Genetic Societies and Organizations (Mentor Networks, Speakers Bureau, DNA Day, Family History Day)

- American Society of Human Genetics (ASHG), mentor network
- National Society of Genetic Counselors (NSGC), mentor network
- National Human Genome Research Institute (NHGRI), NIH, DNA Day
- U.S. Surgeon General's Family History Initiative and Family Health Portrait

I. Curricula Standards, Guidelines and Ideas, K–12

National Science Education Standards state genetics/biology concepts that all students should know and be able to do. These come from *Science for All Americans* and *Benchmarks for Science Literacy*, the National Research Council of the National Academy of Sciences, and the American Association for the Advancement of Science's Project 2061. State, school, and school district curriculum committees and those who develop instructional and assessment materials strive to meet these content standards. All are online through a variety of web portals.

- National education standards/guidelines—Project 2061, AAAS
- *Benchmarks for Science Literacy*, American Association for the Advancement of Science (AAAS). New York: Oxford University Press, 1993.
- *Science for All Americans: A Project 2061 Report on Literacy Goals in Science, Mathematics and Technology*. Washington, DC: AAAS, 1989.
- *Developing Biological Literacy: A Guide to Developing Secondary and Post-Secondary Biology Curricula*. Biological Sciences Curriculum Study (BSCS). Colorado Springs, CO: BSCS, 1993.
- *National Standards and the Science Curriculum: Challenges, Opportunities, and Recommendations,* Biological Sciences Curriculum Study (BSCS), Bybee, R. W. (ed.). Dubuque, Iowa: Kendall-Hunt Publishers, 1966.
- *Fulfilling the Promise: Biology Education in our Nation's Schools*, National Research Council (NRC) Washington, DC: National Academy Press, 1990.
- *Scope, Sequence and Coordination of Secondary School Science*, The Content Core: A Guide for Curriculum Developers, National Science Teachers Association (NSTA). Vol.1. Washington, DC: NSTA, 1992.
- National and state science guidelines at the education section of the ASHG website.

Curricula Education Ideas

Look for online teaching ideas, activities, CD-ROM, videos, glossaries, and workshops provided by these long-standing organizations with an interest in genetics education:

- *Access Excellence @ the National Health Museum*: Lesson plans for biology, health and life science teachers and students.

- *BSCS (Biological Science Curriculum Service)*: Curricula supplements for grades K-12. Four Human Genome modules for high school students on inheritance, bioinformatics and the Human Genome Project, *Genes and Surroundings* for younger students, other curricula for high school students.
- *CDC Genomics Home*: National Office of Public Health Genomics, integration of advances in human genetics into public health research, policy and programs
- *Cold Spring Harbor*: DNA Lab. DNA resources, workshops, field trips, courses, and products (make your own slide presentation within their web site). DNA from the Beginning, information, pictures, animated primers on Classical Genetics, Molecules of Genetics, and Genetic Organization and Control.
- *DOE, Department of Energy*: Human Genome Project description, progress, history, goals; issues associated with the project.
- *Exploring Genes and Genetic Disorders*: Images of all 24 human chromosomes and different genes mapped to them.
- *GeneTests* (professional audiences): Expert-authored peer-reviewed medical genetics descriptions of inherited disorders. Genetic testing, diagnosis and management, genetics clinic directory, genetics modules and teaching cases. Links for "Educational Materials" and "Genetic Tools."
- *Genetic Alliance*: Educational resource repository for patient advocacy groups including basic genetic concepts and policy issues.
- *Genetic Education Center*: University of Kansas Medical Center. Gateway to education resources on human genetics, curricula ideas, lesson plans, activities, genetic conditions, professional genetic organizations, and other topics.
- *Genetic Science Learning Center*: Eccles Institute, University of Utah. Genetic resources: our lives and society. Grades 5–7 activities, puzzle based activity "Find the gene for Whirling disorder," "Traits bingo," and "tree of genetic traits." Printable karyotypes, chromosome matching activity, instructions on extracting DNA from anything living, and a mystery to solve.
- *Genetics Home Reference (GHR)*: Information on medical genetics and basic genetic concepts for patients and their family members, others.
- *Greenwood Genetics Center, Education Division*: Useful teaching tools and ideas.
- *NCHPEG, National Coalition for Health Professional Education in Genetics*: Health professional education and access to information about advances in human genetics, curricula guidelines and competencies. Teaching tools, family history exercises, matching pedigree exercise, pedigree red flags, and curricula for healthcare professionals.
- *March of Dimes. Birth Defects and Genetics*: Fact sheets, brochures, resources on birth defects, pregnancy complications.
- *NHGRI, National Human Genome Research Institute*: Genetics education materials including an easy-to-use talking glossary of genetic terms.

Learning Styles and Teaching Models

- Index of Learning Styles, BA Soloman, North Carolina State University, Raleigh (includes a self test)
- Learning styles. Includes chart to help you determine your learning style, Charminade School
- Genetic Variation, using 5E Model, Science Education, NIH
- 5E Model, Biological Sciences Curriculum Study (BSCS), Bybee, R. W. (Ed.). *National Standards and the Science Curriculum: Challenges, Opportunities, and Recommendations.* Dubuque, Iowa: Kendall-Hunt Publishers, 1966.
- Fogarty, Robin. "Ten Ways to Integrate Curriculum," *Educational Leadership* 49:2, Palatine, IL: Skylight Publishing, Inc., 1991.Fogarty's 10 curriculum integration models (fragmented, connected, nested, sequenced, shared, webbed, threaded, integrated, immersed, and networked).
- Gardner, Howard. (1993) Multiple Intelligences: The Theory Into Practice. New York: Basic Books.

Slides and medical images

- Google.com—search images, video, or Scholar
- Atlas of the human body, American Medical Association, publicly available: ImageMD—over 50,000 images from Current Medicine's series of illustrated atlases. Each image is accompanied by detailed text (institutional subscriptions),
- HEAL (Health Education Assets Library)—a digital library with digital teaching resources for health sciences educators
- WebPath: The Internet Pathology Laboratory, images, text, and tutorials for pathology education, University of Utah
- NSGC slide swap, NSGC (members only)

Emerging Technology

- 7 things you should know about series, EDUCAUSE Learning Initiative, eLearning, virtual worlds and meetings, social networking, collaborative editing, wikis, podcasting, clickers, digital storytelling, e-books, YouTube, more!
- WikiGenetics, an open source, user-generated encyclopedia on human genetics for the public, information on human genetics.

National and State Science Education Standards (related to genetics)

Examples of the National Science Education Standards (NSE) Standards for curricula involving genetics. Other state standards are linked off the National Coalition for Professional Health Education in Genetics (NCHPEG) web site.

Grades K–4 Standards: establish the foundation of scientific knowledge, including understanding the characteristics and life cycles of organisms. For example:

- plants and animals resemble their parents
- many characteristics are inherited, while others are the result of interactions with the environment

Grades 5–8 Standards introduce the concepts of human biology, to investigate living systems, including cells, and to understand reproduction and heredity. For example:

- observable traits (focus for younger children)
- genetic material carries information

Grades 9-12 Standards:

Science as Inquiry (Content Standard A): Students should develop the ability necessary for science inquiry, for example, they should learn to:
- identify questions and concepts that guide scientific investigations
- design and conduct scientific investigations
- formulate and revise scientific explanations and models, using logic and evidence
- communicate and defend a scientific argument

Life Science (Content Standard C): Students should develop an understanding of these concepts:

- cells store and use information to guide their functions
- genetic information stored in DNA is used to direct synthesis of the thousands of proteins each cell requires.
- in all organisms, the instructions for specifying the characteristics of the organism are carried in the DNA, a large polymer formed of subunits of four kinds (A, G, C, and T).
- the chemical and structural properties of DNA explain how the genetic information that underlies heredity is encoded in genes (as a string of molecular "letters").
- the human body is formed from cells that contain two copies of each chromosome – and therefore two copies of each gene (this explains many features of human heredity).
- changes in DNA (mutations) occur spontaneously at low rates.
- some DNA changes make no difference to the organisms; others can change cells and organisms.

Science and Technology (Content Standard E): Students should develop an understanding of science and technology. They should learn to communicate the problem, process, and solution and understand that:

- science often advances with new technologies.
- new technologies often extend scientific understanding and introduce new areas of research.

- technological solutions may create new problems.
- sometimes scientific advances challenge people's beliefs and practical explanations concerning aspects of the world.

Science in Personal and Social Perspectives (Content Standard F): Students should develop an understanding of science in local, national, and global challenges, since science and technology involve human decisions about the use of knowledge. They should:

- understand basic concepts and principles of science and technology, then engage in active debate about economics, policies, politics, and ethics of various science-and technology-related challenges.
- understand that decisions about new research involve assessment of alternatives, risks, costs, and benefits.

II. Teaching Ideas for Education in Medical Genetics

Sample ideas used successfully by teachers or recommended by genetic counselors. Online content may change, and similar activities will be available. This is a list of the types of materials and activities available; updates can be found at the Genetics Education Center at the University of Kansas Medical Center

Complexity of Genetic Counseling/Testing

- Simulated Genetic Counseling Session, Genetics Education Center, Lesson Plans
- Genetic Condition Fact Sheets, March of Dimes
- *Chance Choices*, Foundation for Blood Research, by Paula K. Haddow, a curriculum designed to demonstrate the practical applications of human genetics
- Family panel—contact local chapters of support groups, ask them to come speak to a class as part of specific curriculum. See Genetic Alliance for local chapters of national patient advocacy groups.

Developing Educational Materials

- Access to Credible Genetics Resource Network, the Genetic Alliance
- Simply Put, Centers for Disease Control (CDC)
- How to Write Easy to Read Health Materials, Medline Plus (National Library of Medicine)
- An Author's Guide, University of Utah
- Writing Reader-Friendly Documents, Federal Plain Language Guidelines
- Principles for Clear Health Communication, Pfizer
- Developing Easy-to-Read Educational Materials: Breast Health
- Genetic and Rare Conditions examples, the Genetics Education Center, University of Kansas Medical Center

Ethical Issues in Genetic Testing and Debate/Genetics

- Nathanial Wu Lesson Plan, Mapping and Sequencing the Human Genome: Science, Ethics, and Public Policy, Activity 3, 1992 BSCS and the American Medical Association. In this activity, students take different positions on an employer's requirement for a genetic test (for Huntington Disease) of an employee.
- Current Genetic ELSI topics—ethical, social, legal, public policy—numerous sources
- An Ethics Casebook for Genetic Counselors, NSGC, 2006 (2nd ed.)
- Spiritual Discernment: A Guide for Genetic and Reproductive Technologies, United Methodist General Board of Church and Society, 2008

Chromosomes/Karyotyping

- Karyotype Activity, the Biology Project, University of Arizona
- Making a Karyotype, Genetic Science Learning Center, University of Utah
- Karyotype Activities, eduMedia-sciences.com, search for interactive karyotype
- Problem sets and tutorials, the Biology Project, University of Arizona

Inheritance of Genetic Characteristics

- Genes And Surroundings (2nd ed.) 2000, BSCS (Biological Science Curriculum Study), Kendall/Hunt, Dubuque, IA, ISBN: ISBN: 0-7872-3024-3 (student guide), ISBN: 0-7872-3026-X (teacher guide)
  - *Generations*, Activity 5 and Family Trees (p. 21–28), All people have the same number of legs, ears, noses and so on. But people are different in size, shape, color and other characteristics. What causes the similarities? What causes the differences?
  - *Family Trees and Characteristics*, Activity 6 (pp. 29–33) This activity uses jelly beans in small paper cups to convey concepts about inheriting characteristics through three generations.
  - *From One Generation to Another*, Activity 12 (p 64–68). This lesson shows inheritance of traits, and variety, using a fantasy character, and compares differences and similarities.
- Pop-it Beads, DNA simulation, Carolina Biological Supply Company, or Ward's Natural Science

Testing Knowledge/Review Genetic Concepts

- Genetic Games, Sargent-Welch
- Genetic Jeopardy, Modern Genetics, DNA & RNA, Quia Corporation
- Human Genetics Matching Game or Concentration Game, Quia Corporation
- Genetic Disorders [Create a] Pamphlet - Teacher Guide, ProQuest

Art and Genetics

- Use scrap materials to create 3-dimensional models of genetic concepts (chromosomes, genes with exons and introns, other)
- Genetic Conditions Activity/BSCS (elementary activity with fantasy characters and various characteristics and traits in parents & offspring)
- Genes And Surroundings, Kendall/Hunt, Dubuque, IA 52004-0539, ISBN: 0-8403-3066-9, ISBN: 0-8403-3065-0 (teacher guide)
- Reebops, small characters (imaginary organisms) made of marshmallows and inexpensive materials, illustrating meiosis and variation, developed by Patti Soderberg, University of Wisconsin
- Use full-size self-portraits illustrating the sameness and differences in traits discussed in previous classes (young students). Discuss observed differences, such as hair, straight or curly, dark or light colored, to teach about individual uniqueness.

Genetics and Current Events, History, and Media Stories

- Lessons utilizing classic or new movies, events, or books such as *Jurassic Park*, OJ Simpson case, *GATTACA*, *Harry Potter*, Middlesex, other
- Science in the Cinema, National Institutes of Health (NIH), science-education. nih.gov/cinema, current films, scientist comments.
- Argentina's "disappeared" and efforts to match grandmothers and children of the Argentine citizens who "disappeared" from 1976–1983, using mitochondrial DNA, can be used to link science and real-world events
- Genetic Themes in Fiction Films: Genetics meets Hollywood, by Michael Clark, Wellcome, UK, 2006.
- Screening DNA: Exploring the Cinema-Genetics Interface, DNA Books, Stephen Nottingham, 2000, ISBN 1-903421-00-4
- Teach with Movies, movie lesson plans and learning guides
- Genetics take starring role on silver screen, USA Today, D Vergano and S Wloszczyna, 06/17/2002, superheroes and others discussed.
- Telling Stories, Understanding Real Life Genetics, genetics education for health professionals, 2007, Cardiff, UK. Stories illustrate the impact and utility of genetics on healthcare.
- YouTube—search for genetic examples

Probability/Chance

- Beach ball to teach probability/math—Throw a 4-colored beach ball around the room to demonstrate the chance of each student hitting a particular color (may create noise for adjoining rooms).

Elementary Curriculum

Use the simplest words possible and only technical terms you define.

Variability and Traits

- Demonstrate objects that are the same and different. Group objects according to colors or other criteria, or use articles of clothing to observe student differences. For example, some students wear sneakers, and can be asked to stand up. Students can also observe their own clothing and sort themselves, or observe other traits such as hair color, hair type, eye color, eye glasses, skin color, and gender).

- Observe characteristics that are similar or different from each other. Graph the number of individuals in their class with specific trait differences to use visual kinesthetic learning.

- Discuss identical twins; each twin is still unique because he or she has his or her own personality.

- Discuss a children's book; several provide an introduction to heredity, while others deal with a disability the main character(s) and those around them learn to accept, or value (short stature, birth defects or differences, mobility, visual or auditory limitations). These books are more appropriate for genetics than those in which the problem goes away, as in an ugly duckling, bed-ridden boy in a secret garden, or frog that becomes a prince.

- Draw family trees—children can draw simple family histories, but be sensitive to issues of adoption and blended families. Try to avoid emphasizing blue/brown eyes or traits that are not that different in some ethnic groups such as Asian, African American, Hispanic/Latino, and others.

- Observe photographs of a child and other family members, and discuss similarities and differences between family members.

- Use Attribute Blocks by MacMillan Early Skills Manipulatives. Students sort objects by a single attribute. Then the teacher increases the difficulty by including more traits. Students are given blocks for two to three attributes in a single pile without naming the attributes, and make piles of things that are the same, then verbalize or point to the similarities and differences.

III. Dealing with Media, a Primer for Communicating Effectively through the Media

Abstracted from the Press/Media Subcommittee of the NSGC Education Committee Subcommittee: Meagan Krasner and Angela Trepanier, 2002

Overview

A media interview is an opportunity to inform the public about your cause. Through it, you can educate the public about a genetic condition, clarify the significance of new research into therapies or tests for inherited disorders, or explain the purpose of genetic counseling in helping families with heritable conditions. However, effective communication through the media requires preparation. An interview may seem like a simple conversation between two individuals, especially if you are discussing a topic with which you are well versed. Yet, much of what you communicate during an interview is often edited out. In the absence of adequate preparation, the reporter may be able to use editing to forward his or her own biases about the subject versus the message you hope to relay. The NSGC media primer helps teach genetic counselors how to communicate effectively with the media.

Tips

- Prepare for an interview. Ask the purpose of the interview. Determine why the topic is in the news now, if it is associated with controversy. Ask the reporter about the focus of the story, and the expected length of the article/program. If there is controversy, try to anticipate questions and prepare statements. Find proposed solutions to the controversy. If you are involved in a television or radio interview, preview the interviewer's work, if possible, to determine his/her style.
- Identify the target audience: is it professionals or the lay public?
- Communicate and develop your message effectively, have one to three major message points, and prepare short, concise statements for each. Short answers (10–15 seconds) are easier to quote and less likely to be taken out of context.
- Use language that will be readily understood by the target audience, and minimize the use of medical or technical jargon for lay audiences.
- Limit the number of statistics used to avoid confusing the audience, and present statistics in laymen's terms, for example "nearly 9 in 10" rather than "85%".
- Prepare and rehearse for questions pertaining to hot buttons or controversial topics.

References Dealing with the Media/Speaking and Writing Tips

- Media Reporting in the Genetic Age: Points to Consider. Alliance of Genetic Support Groups, 1993.
- Effective Media Interview Techniques. American College of Emergency Physicians, 2008.
- Practical Tips on How to Speak Effectively to Reporters. NSGC Annual Educational Conference, Oct 3, 1993, Beth Balkite & Mary Ahrens.
- NSGC Dealing with Media, A Primer for Communicating Effectively through the Media, Members only Section, NSGC, Prepared by the Press/Media Subcommittee of the NSGC Education Committee Subcommittee: Meagan Krasner and Angela Trepanier, 2002.
- Deborah St. James, Stephanie Barnard, Kirk Hughes, Writing, speaking, and communication skills for health professionals, Healthcare Communication Group, 2001, (ISBN: 0300088612) p. 158.
- Hindle, Tim. Making Presentations, DK Publishing, 1998.

IV. Analogies

An analogy can sometimes help convey complex concepts to an audience through familiar associations, showing the similarities between two different things. However analogies are never examples of a concept. Example: lightning is not *like* an electrical spark because lightening *is* an electrical spark. Analogy: Lightning is *like* a bright light turned on and off in a dark room. Analogies can serve as a learning aid. This list, compiled from a number of sources, may be helpful. However, a word of caution: Analogies can be overused. Use them sparingly in your talk, or to help clarify your responses to questions. They can lose their effect if they are overdone.

Concept	Analogy [concept] is like the relationship between [this] and [that], OR [concept] can be compared to [something]
Alleles (of a gene)	**Sodas.** In a soda machine, you could choose between a variety of name-brand sodas (regular, diet, etc.), "Soda" can represents the gene, the specific types of drinks represent various "alleles" of the "soda gene."
Autosomal recessive	**Two lamps on,** in a dark room (if one doesn't work, there is still some light, if both aren't working, there is no light).
Autosomal recessive	**Toaster** (if one side doesn't work, some toast is still produced, but reduced product [rate], if both sides aren't working, no toast).
Autosomal dominant	**Bicycle tires** (both need to function, if one tire is flat, the bicycle doesn't go).
Autosomal dominant inheritance	**Mixing chocolate cake batter and vanilla cake batter.** When the two batters are combined, observe the chocolate batter "taking over" the vanilla batter. The chocolate batter is the stronger or "dominant" batter.
Cell [regulation]	**Car factory:** product is made (such as wheels, steering wheel, or axel). When manufactured normally, a car runs smoothly. If one particular part is not working, the car does not move. The brake and accelerator serve to regulate the speed.
Cell structure	Compare to seeds; They increase in number to form various life forms. All information needed to create a life form is locked within the seed (like a cell).
Chromosome	Like a computer, it contains all the instructions for all the other cells and processes.
Chromosomes	**File cabinets that store information.** The information that chromosomes store is called DNA.
DNA code	"Secret" protein message in a two step coding system—the genetic "code" has 20 amino acids.
DNA replication/base pairing	**A zipper:** Teeth align [or pair up] when zipped.
DNA replication/ transcription	**Xerox copies:** identical copies of the original

Exons & introns	**A poem** (i.e., William Blake, Kipling) where words run together, or are split into words [exons/introns], random italicized words [exons] can represent a gene.
Genes	Like managers, they tell the different cells what jobs or work that they have to complete. Direct the cells to perform various tasks within the body.
Genetic control	**Computer program** [like a set of instructions to do something)]
Genetic material, organization and size	**An encyclopedia set** [genome] is a group of books [chromosomes] with words [genes], made up of letters [DNA base pairs]
Genotype/phenotype and variation	**Cookie recipe** [genetic makeup]: small variations in the ingredients [genotype] can lead to a cookie [phenotype] with different results [variation]
Genetic variation, phenotype/genotype	**Black bear and panda:** In appearance [phenotype], both look similar. However, each has a very different DNA makeup [genotype]. One is a bear, the other is not.
Genetic repair	**Spellchecking software:** can be set to automatic correct as you type
Genome project	**Roadmap:** Searching for genes first involved a large map, then exploring a smaller area, a city, then a specific block, and finally a house.
Heredity: Autosomal recessive inheritance	Harry Potter books by J.K. Rowlings: Muggles are normal folks with no magical power. Wizards have the power to do magic. Wizarding appears to be hereditary, but occasionally a muggle child will appear with natural magical ability, such as Harry's friend Hermione Granger. This can be explained by recessive genes. The gene for magical ability has two alleles, M creates muggles (MM or MW), and W is needed for wizardry (WW) and magical ability. If two MW muggles have a child, there is a one in four chance that the child will be WW. (i.e., Hermione, a wizard born of muggle parents, and Harry Potter's mother whose parents were muggles). Pure-blooded wizards are WW children of WW parents (i.e., Draco Malfoy).
Linkage map	**Road map** [gene map] identified the correct location [gene].
mRNA	**Music:** mRNA is like a long piece of magnetic recording tape, and the ribosome is like a tape recorder. As the tape passes through the recorder playing head, it is "read" and converted into music or other sounds. When a "tape" of mRNA passes through the "playing head" of a ribosome, the "notes" produced are amino acids and the resulting musical pieces are proteins.
Mutations	Various typographical errors in a sentence (insertions, deletions, duplications, etc.)
Mutations	**Sentence:** shift a letter [nonsense], change letter or word, change meaning of sentence [substitution], etc.
Multifactorial inheritance	**Glass of water:** each unaffected parent with a glass partially full, poured together [child] could overflow, resulting in an affected child
Probability of 50%	**Flipping a coin** (50% heads, 50% tails)
Probability of 25%	**Deck of cards:** drawing one card of the 4 suits (25% chance)

Protein synthesis	**Construction process:** Finished product is a protein (i.e., enzyme) assembled according to directions from the "master plans" [DNA] in the nucleus. First, blueprint copies of the building plans are made from the Master Plans [DNA] in the nucleus, and sent out to the construction site [ribosomes in the cytoplasm]. The construction supervisor [ribosome] reads the blueprints [mRNA] for the building [protein], and directs the assembly of all the building parts [amino acids] into their proper places to make the finished building [protein]. Ribosome is like supervisors' blueprint table [makes it easier to read the blueprints].
Recombination length	Compare to highway miles between particular fast food restaurants
Ribosomes	Factories churning out products
Same and different	**A flower seed:** Many cells or seeds of the same species can develop different end-products. Each marigold seed results in a flower with different characteristics [large or small flowers, tall or short, variety of colors]. The flowers are all different, but belong to the same marigold family. There are similarities and differences among family members.
Similarities and differences	**Fingerprints:** Everyone has fingerprints; however, no one has the same fingerprints, not even identical twins.
Triple repeat	Holding down a set of 3 keyboard letters too long: abcabcabc…
Variability of genes	**Single note in a song:** You can play variations on the theme by playing the song in a different key or changing the harmony, but the overall tune is still the same.

17

Evolving Roles, Expanding Opportunities

Elizabeth A. Balkite, M.S., C.G.C. and Maureen E. Smith, M.S., C.G.C.

Do not go where the path may lead. Go instead where there is no path and leave a trail.
—Ralph Waldo Emerson

INTRODUCTION

From the first introduction of the phrase by Sheldon Reed (Reed, 1955), genetic counseling has been a flexible, evolving, and maturing profession in which genetic counselors themselves have shaped the roles and opportunities available to them. In 1971, when the first class of genetic counselors graduated from Sarah Lawrence College, they defined the profession by creating jobs where none had existed before that time. The first genetic counselors filled a need that physicians were not able to fulfill. Mainly, this was by helping pediatric geneticists take family and medical histories, researching genetic conditions and medical records, explaining genetic concepts to patients and families, and assisting families through emotional support. Expansion to the obstetric setting quickly ensued as the technology to provide prenatal testing and screening became available. Over the past 30+ years, the roles of genetic counselors have expanded with the evolution of genetics knowledge and the gradual integration of genetics into healthcare.

Genetic counselors now serve their clients in an ever-increasing number of areas—both clinical and non-clinical. Clinical counselors work in medical subspecialties such as oncology, infertility, mental health, neurogenetics, and cardiovascular disease. They

A Guide to Genetic Counseling, Second Edition, Edited by Wendy Uhlmann, Jane Schuette, and Beverly Yashar
Copyright © 2009 by John Wiley & Sons, Inc.

practice not only in medical centers but in community hospitals, research centers, public health clinics and physicians' offices—closer to the point of care. Bridging the gap, with roles that are both clinical and non-clinical, are genetic counselors working in commercial and academic genetic testing laboratories, health maintenance organizations (HMOs), and research settings. These counselors are coordinating clinical research studies, managing laboratory-based cases, and/or providing genetics education and care coordination. Non-clinical genetic counselors can be found in pharmaceutical and biotech companies, non-profit organizations, and governmental agencies, where they are acting as intellectual support for sales and marketing teams, managing people and organizations, or developing public policy. All are evolving roles and expanding opportunities for graduates of genetic counseling programs to apply their knowledge and skills for the benefit of their clients.

This chapter explores the expanding clinical and non-clinical roles genetic counselors have developed over the past decades. It also describes how they have transitioned their genetics knowledge and professional skills in communication, critical thinking, counseling, and ethics into roles in new clinical and non-clinical settings, gained new skills, and obtained advanced degrees. Finally, it considers potential new areas for genetic counselors as the profession continues to develop and mature. The chapter presents these topics broadly but not in depth. The authors wish to acknowledge the limitation of the language that defines our profession and recognize the graying of the lines between clinical and non-clinical roles.. We hope to expand the definition of our profession here without excluding the very competencies that make the profession unique.

EVOLUTION OF THE PROFESSION

The profession of genetic counseling has evolved over time from a core group of individuals in New York, trained at Sarah Lawrence College (where the first genetic counseling training program was established in 1969), to several thousand individuals practicing in the field worldwide. As of 2008, over 2500 genetic counselors are located in North America, but genetic counselors are also members of healthcare teams in the United Kingdom, Australia, New Zealand, South Africa, Europe, China, Japan, the Middle East, and other countries. There are also training programs for genetic counselors in many of these countries, often initiated by genetic counselors trained in the U.S.

Numerous internal and external forces have helped shape the evolution of the profession. Most significantly, genetic counselors have driven the profession from within. They diligently applied their knowledge, skills, and abilities, and their value was recognized by other healthcare professionals. This recognition led to increased job opportunities. Some job opportunities were offered by a greater number of clinicians (i.e., perinatologists and neurologists) in medical specialties that increasingly relied on genetic test options and genetic counseling. Other opportunities were generated by genetic counselors with the vision to create jobs to meet the need for genetic information in new clinical areas, such as cancer, and in new settings, such as community hospitals. Their vision allowed them to see needs that were not being met and to respond to these needs—to develop new roles not previously considered for a genetic counselor. Another internal factor affecting the profession was an increased number of genetic counseling training programs, resulting in a greater number of genetic counselors. As the numbers of counselors grew, the profession matured as well. The forming of the National Society of Genetic Counselors in 1979 was a significant force driving recognition of the role of genetic counselors and becoming a unified voice for genetic counselors. Later, the forming of our own credentialing organization, the American Board of Genetic Counseling, in 1993 encouraged greater autonomy and increased levels of professionalism. In addition, the recognition of the profession as a healthcare provider has led to the realization of a need to protect patients from inadequately trained, non-credentialed persons through state licensure.

Externally, an increase in genetics knowledge and awareness of the genetic contribution to disease by healthcare professionals has created opportunities for genetic counselors in medicine. The information that has come out of, and is still being mined from, the Human Genome Project has led to an ever-increasing knowledge base, many new technologies, and the "industrialization" of genetics: automation of tests, high throughput testing, faster transfer of technology to the clinic and the marketplace, and an increased need for accurate genetic information. This has resulted in greater industry interest and employment opportunities in genetics as well as new arenas for exploration in public policy and ethics. Industrialization of genetics and the use of new technologies have also led to research into different models of genetic counseling and the delivery of genetic services to meet the needs of healthcare providers, organizations, and consumers.

While there have been a number of factors, both internal and external, that have helped to change the profession and allow its progression, genetic counselors themselves have played the most vital role in increasing the scope, professionalism, and opportunities in the field.

EXPANSION OF THE PROFESSION

Genetic counselors have often sought out new areas in which to exercise their skills, including new clinical realms as well as in business, government, and the not-for-profit sector. As documented by early NSGC Professional Status Surveys, the majority of genetic counselors worked within university medical systems, outreach clinics, publicly funded health clinics and hospitals, and private hospitals. In 1981, when the first survey of genetic counselors was published, most genetic counselors worked in university medical centers (60%) and provided general genetic counseling services (78%) (Begleiter et al., 1981). Since that time, each subsequent survey has documented steady professional growth in other practice areas. In 1987, 1.7% of genetic counselors listed a diagnostic laboratory as their primary work setting (Collins, 1987), and in just five years' time this number had more than doubled to 4.8% in 1992 (Uhlmann, 1992). In 2008, 9.0% of genetic counselors listed diagnostic laboratories as their primary employment setting (Smith et al., 2008).

TABLE 17-1. General and Selected Specialty Areas of Practice in Clinical Genetics

General Areas of Practice
Prenatal Genetics
Pediatric Genetics
Adult Genetics
General Genetics
Selected Specialty Areas of Practice
Assisted Reproductive Technologies/Infertility
Cancer Genetics
Cardiovascular Genetics
Metabolic disorders
Neurogenetics
Ophthalmologic Genetics
Psychiatric Genetics
Specialty Diseases/Single Gene Disorders

New roles emerged in the 1990s; genetic counselors began working in business and marketing and as customer liaisons in genetic testing laboratories. The employers of genetic counselors also began to change during this time period to more private medical centers and clinics (27.5%), diagnostic laboratories (4.8%), and private practice (3.6%) (Schneider and Kalkbrenner, 1998). New employment settings since 2000 have included health advocacy and professional organizations and Internet, pharmaceutical, bioinformatics, research development, and biotechnology companies (Smith et al., 2008). In 2008, genetic counselors were still working predominantly in university medical centers (37%) and private hospitals (19%) (Smith et al., 2008). However, this trend appears to be decreasing as other employers are increasing (Parrott and Clark, 2004). In 2008, two biotechnology companies and one health maintenance organization were the three largest single employers of genetic counselors (personal communication). Looking within the biotechnology companies that have hired genetic counselors, the roles have expanded from clinically oriented roles into marketing, sales, and product development. Changes in healthcare delivery and advances in science and technology related to genetic services have increased the demand for genetic counselors in many clinical and non-clinical sectors. Genetic counselors have moved into new areas of practice (Table 17-1), roles, and work environments (Table 17-2) in response to the marketplace.

DEVELOPMENT OF CLINICAL SPECIALTY AREAS IN GENETIC COUNSELING

Genetic counselors have had an increasing impact on genetic healthcare while becoming more specialized in the clinical setting. One example is the development of the cancer genetics specialty. Genetics counselors played a primary role in the establishment of cancer genetics clinics by collaborating with other professionals working in cancer and using their knowledge about genetics and genetic testing.

Counselors who established this specialty combined their skills as genetic counselors and their interest in applying genetics in a new area with a desire to help patients.

Genetic counseling in oncology grew out of research and increased knowledge about the genetic contributions to cancer. Other clinical specialties, such as assisted reproductive technologies (ART) and infertility, emerged along with increased reproductive technology capabilities. Still other specialties have arisen because of the discovery of genes and genetic risk factors associated with diseases, such as in cardiology, neurology, and ophthalmology. New specialties will continue to develop out of research discoveries as technological advances in testing and risk analysis become more sophisticated.

As genetic counselors have brought their competencies into new clinical areas, they have often narrowed their focus and truly become subject matter experts in a clinical area. For example, some prenatal counselors have developed such a depth of knowledge in genetic counseling for abnormal ultrasound findings that it has become their specialty area of practice. Approximately 10–20% of cancer counselors counsel for only one form of cancer (e.g., breast or colon) (H Hampel, personal communication, 2007). Cardiovascular genetic counselors specialize in areas such as cardiomyopathies, cardiac arrhythmias, and coronary artery disease. As genetic counselors move further into different areas of clinical medicine, specialization within a clinical area is expected to increase along with the increase in knowledge in the area, and the needs of patients, professionals, and payers.

PULLING IT ALL TOGETHER: THE EMERGENCE OF A SPECIALIZATION IN CANCER GENETIC COUNSELING

Cancer genetic counseling provides an excellent example of how the skills of genetic counselors can be applied to a specialty. In the 2008 Professional Status Survey (Smith et al., 2008), cancer was the second highest specialty listed by genetic counselors seeing patients (25%) after prenatal (38%). In 1994, when cancer was first added to the list of specialty areas, only 10% of genetic counselors were working in that specialty (Boldt, 1994). Why the enormous transition over the years? Did the training of genetic counselors change drastically to support this new specialty? With only 10% of genetic counselors working in oncology in 1994, how could new counselors be receiving training in cancer genetics? In fact, there were very few formal training opportunities at the time, and most of these were outside of the graduate school curricula.

In the early 1990s, a small group of genetic counselors decided to pass on their burgeoning experience in cancer genetic counseling by developing the first NSGC short course in cancer genetics. At that time, these genetic counselors were the only ones working in cancer or spending time with cancer genetic questions. By bringing their unique experiences back to the profession via an educational course, they were able to enrich the collective professional knowledge of their colleagues and thereby begin to prepare them for a new specialty in cancer. NSGC held the ABCs of Cancer Genetics short course in 1992; the first scientific paper on BRCA1, the first hereditary breast cancer gene, was published in 1992 (Hall et al., 1992); and Dr. Henry Lynch, an expert in cancer genetics, organized a training program for genetic counselors in 1994. Also in 1994, genetic counselor, Katherine Schneider, MPH, through funding from NSGC's Jane Engelberg Memorial Fellowship, published her book, *Counseling About Cancer: Strategies for Genetic Counselors.* In 1998, the American Society of Clinical Oncology, with genetic counselors on their curriculum committee, held their first educational program in cancer genetics for healthcare providers. Genetic counselors were leaders in the education of other medical specialists in this specialty and were instrumental in shaping this field and the care of patients with hereditary cancers. The need to focus on cancer as their primary interest and to meet the educational needs of this group of counselors resulted in the development of the Cancer Special Interest Group of the NSGC, which was the first Special Interest Group NSGC established.

Genetic counselors have repeatedly responded to emerging healthcare needs by working in new clinical specialties and bringing their experiences back to teach other genetic counselors, thereby encouraging the growth of new specialties. There are numerous examples of genetic counselors who have moved into unique settings, such as laboratory liaison, or new specialties such as cardiology and have brought these experiences and knowledge back to their colleagues by giving lectures, holding workshops, organizing courses, mentoring, and starting Special Interests Groups in NSGC. These activities encourage an environment that promotes constant learning, growth, and improvement.

TRANSLATABLE SKILLS

If you think you can, you can. Instead of talking yourself out of something because you didn't have special training, talk yourself into why you could do it as well as anyone else. We are all very smart with a set of skills different from the person next to you. Believe in your skills and take advantage of what you have to offer. You may have to sell yourself to others to get the opportunity, but you should have the confidence to give a try.
—a genetic counselor in a commercial laboratory

Genetic counselors have multiple skills that enable them to transition into new and exciting roles. Some of these new roles are closely related to traditional roles in the field of genetic counseling, while others are more distant. A non-clinical role for a genetic counselor usually relies on applying clinical experience, knowledge and skills in new ways. For instance, a genetic counselor managing a research study may use the experience gained with consenting patients for genetic tests as well as knowledge of patients' understanding of genetics to write consent forms or develop protocols for a study. A genetic counselor in a marketing role may draw upon his/her experiences counseling patients and the knowledge of what information was key for a patient's decision-making in developing marketing materials for a testing company or when talking with the company's clients. Genetic counselors working in non-clinical roles use their clinical experience everyday, just not for counseling patients.

What the new roles have in common is dependence on the skill base acquired during training, which prepares genetic counselors for the transition into new knowledge areas. The ability to take on new roles demands that you use your knowledge and experience as well as build on existing skills. The knowledge and skill base that helps genetic counselors to transition into other areas of healthcare or other professions are grounded in the practice-based competencies, which form the foundation for managing a genetic counseling case (Fine et al., 1996) and are a central part of training. The four domains of genetic counseling skills are an appendix to Chapter 1 and are described below as a foundation for translatable skills.

Domain I: Communication Skills

Genetic counselors develop unique skills in verbal and written communication, which translate well into different clinical and non-clinical areas requiring the communication of complex, emotionally laden, and technical information. Strong communication skills are the basis for many business interactions; including sales and marketing activities and management. Genetic counselors may be particularly adept at any career that requires strength in teaching medical or technical information, such as trainers or teachers, and developing written materials for both public and professional audiences, such as medical writing. Their communication and knowledge base are also ideal for working with support organizations, or in organizations in which the genetic counselor provides expertise in genetics and clinical care, such as in a pharmaceutical company. Persons with strong skills in this domain are able to manage complex discussions, negotiations, and meetings in a culturally sensitive and skillful manner.

Domain II: Critical Thinking skills

The skills that genetic counselors use to present and evaluate risks for patients are also useful in weighing risks and making decisions in a variety of clinical roles and non-clinical situations as well. A major role of many genetic counselors is sifting through large amounts of information and resources and analyzing what information is most critical to the case. The skills and knowledge required to manage a genetic counseling case, including gathering appropriate information and resources, analyzing and synthesizing data, and presenting information in a logical manner, are pertinent to many positions in research, product management, and marketing. These skills are also useful in demonstrating to clinicians the value of genetic counseling services. Weighing risks and making critical decisions, as well as expertise in privacy and confidentiality gained through clinical practice, can be useful for many managers, in policy creation, and in business development.

Domain III: Interpersonal, Counseling, and Psychosocial Assessment Skills

While these are the skills central to interviewing, counseling, and supporting clients, they are also very useful in interactions with others, outside the clinical genetic counseling arena. For instance, using these skills in a meeting will enable one to have a better understanding of both verbal and nonverbal cues that may impede communication or reaching an agreement. Persons using these skills may work as hiring managers, in situations requiring an understanding of people's motivations, in sales, and in coaching roles. Genetic counselors demonstrating these skills are flexible in working with different types of people and are able to put people at ease. Just as genetic counselors must be able to assess a patient's needs and concerns quickly, they may use these same skills to assess business and other professionals they interact with to put them at ease and focus a discussion or meeting. Roles fitting these areas may include supervisor of other genetic counselors, research coordinator, sales, management, consultant, and discussion leader.

Domain IV: Professional Ethics and Values

Skills in this area are needed in healthcare businesses, insurance companies, technology industries and in research, where decisions about patients, genetic, and health information and the intersection with science and technology are critical. Often business is not aware of or sensitized to the issues genetic testing raises for consumers as well as businesses. Laboratories and testing companies performing genetic tests and developing new methods for reaching out to clients require individuals who possess an understanding of the needs of patients and can balance this with ethical decisions around the uses of technology. Companies need to think about balancing the need to satisfy shareholders with an ethical approach to marketing a test or service. Utilizing their understanding of ethical decision making, genetic counselors can be involved in these decisions in the company or institution. They can also alert the company and/or researcher to cultural differences and sensitivities in the marketplace as they expand their products/research globally.

Thus the training of genetic counselors, with a focus on the practice-based competencies, provides preparation for transition into a variety of roles and related professions. Focusing on their skills, along with their knowledge and experience, enables genetic counselors not only to expand their current responsibilities but to be promoted into positions of increasing value to employers as well. Acquiring the knowledge for a new position may allow a genetic counselor with the right interests and desires to move outside of genetic counseling into other roles in industry, healthcare, not-for-profits, and government.

In 2001, the Industry Special Interest Group (SIG) of the NSGC compiled a list of the specific skills, knowledge, and attitudes possessed by genetic counselors that can be useful in looking for positions outside of clinical genetics. The document is titled *Tools for Working Outside the Box* (Appendix). This document can also be found under the member benefits section of the NSGC website.

ROLE EXPANSION: FROM THE TRADITIONAL GENETICS CLINIC SETTING AND BEYOND

Since all three of my industry jobs had some connection to genetics, the fact that I had a degree in genetics really was a plus as well as the fact that I had seen patients with genetic conditions.

—a genetic counselor in a biotech company

The experience of being one of the first genetic counselors in a new specialty or role can be both invigorating and daunting. It is invigorating because of the opportunity to work with new populations, with new colleagues, and with new knowledge, issues, and ideas. It is daunting because there is so much to learn, new people to work with, and no guidelines for how to proceed. With increasing ease and often in advance of tests and firm risks, genetic counselors are finding their services are needed and well utilized in many different clinical specialties and in non-clinical roles as well. Often, it is the genetic counselor's own interest and curiosity that motivates her/him to seek out other roles and new specialties. However, genetic counselors would not have moved into some of the new specialties and roles if it were not for their individual vision and creativity, and the collective efforts of all genetic counselors to increase knowledge, provide optimal care, and respond to the healthcare needs of the marketplace.

Continuing advances in genetics and genomics have added to the growing understanding of human variation and its contribution to disease. These discoveries impact not only medicine but individuals, communities, and societies as well. Seventeen percent of genetic counselors have taken their subject matter expertise and applied it successfully in non-clinical roles (Smith et al., 2008). These individuals address healthcare needs, provide clinical and educational expertise, participate in policy making and research, and contribute in a variety of ways that translate genetic advances into benefits for the public. The percentage of individuals moving into non-clinical roles is expected to continue to rise to meet the ever-growing needs of the marketplace.

Genetic counselors have moved into the roles of managers, salespersons, marketers, communication specialists, educators, policy makers, research coordinators, health advocates, healthcare administrators, and faculty/program directors. These positions are found in a wide variety of settings such as universities, commercial genetic testing laboratories, as well as biotech, pharmaceutical, and Internet companies. Counselors have also chosen to move into government and non-government organizations, advocacy groups, and new roles within universities. Many have the word "clinical" in their title because their clinical experience is important for their job and their employer organization wants to recognize their genetic counseling experience and professional certification. A sample of genetic counselors' work settings, roles, and responsibilities is provided in Table 17-2.

ACQUIRING NEW SKILLS AND KNOWLEDGE

Genetic counselors have many opportunities to gain new skills and learn new information that can be used to enhance their current positions as well as help them transition into new areas of both clinical and non-clinical work. These new skills may be gained by (1) a commitment to learning—a lifelong journey to grow and improve; (2) networking opportunities—meeting and working with others to enhance one's own experiences; and (3) through work, internships, and other experiences, where a vision can be developed for one's career and professional development. These topics are discussed below, and Chapter 15 is devoted to professional development.

TABLE 17-2. A Sample of Titles, Work Settings, and Responsibilities of Genetic Counselors*

GENETIC SERVICES POSITIONS

Clinical Genetic Counselor
University medical center, private hospital, public hospital, health maintenance organization (HMO), physician's private practice, diagnostic labs, outreach clinics

- Provide genetic counseling services to patients and their families
- May also be involved in supervision, education, and clinical rotations of genetic counseling students, medical students, residents, fellows, and other healthcare professionals
- Senior genetic counselor: supervise genetic counselors

Manager of Clinical Services
Biotech, HMO, university clinics

- Coordinate delivery of genetic services and research projects
- Manage budgets, personnel
- Develop guidelines for provision of clinical care
- May have limited or no involvement in direct patient care

Genetics Specialist
Laboratory, biotech company

- Genetics case management; coordination of samples/special studies; assistance with patient assessment and interpretation of test results
- Collaborate with local genetic counseling centers/private practices to encourage appropriate referrals
- Genetics education of physician clients and/or consumers about a product or services via phone or in person through seminars, workshops, community events

POLICY POSITIONS

Ethics and Policy Advisor
Biotech company

- Advise company on corporate issues related to genetics
- Promote corporate genetics/genomics policy initiatives
- Liaison with genetics community and advocacy groups

Policy Specialist
Professional/medical organizations
Non-profit organizations
Policy organizations

- Work on genetics policy issues
- Develop policy statements on genetics issues
- Develop white papers
- Educate/work with lawmakers at local and national level

RESEARCH POSITIONS

Researcher

- Initiate and contribute to research studies (clinical and non-clinical)
- Obtain funding for genetic research

Research Study Coordinator
Non-governmental organizations, pharmaceutical companies, contract research organizations, universities, and medical centers

- Design, implementation and management of clinical trials/research projects with a genetic component
- Act as liaison with clinical research organizations, physicians and study personnel
- Write/assist in writing IRB protocols/applications
- Recruit patients, provide education of study personnel, co-author consent forms for study, coordinate family studies

COMMERCIAL POSITIONS

Regional Genetics Specialist
Biotech, pharmaceutical, genetic testing companies

- Liaison with sales and or marketing staff
- Provide medical genetics support for sales personnel
- Develop client and/or consumer educational materials
- Provide consultation, as needed, to company policy group

Sales/Marketer
Biotech company, pharmaceutical company

- Responsible for the promotion of a company's services to physicians and study staff
- Develop materials for physicians, staff, consumers

Consultant
Genetic testing companies, government/non-government organizations

- Market expertise and services
- Develop contracts, outline responsibilities
- Provide content and management services as agreed upon

Project Manager
Biotech company, genetics professional organization, non-governmental research organization, community education project

- Development of enhancements to a product (i.e., a genetic test, service, or therapy)
- Develop product materials: brochures, educational pieces, website, advertisements, technical advisories, conferences
- Network and form alliances with professional/advocacy groups

Director /Vice President
Commercial company, policy center, non-governmental research organization, biorepository for a commercial/health plan, and own company

- Assume major leadership responsibilities for program development, hiring of personnel, and management of budget for organization
- Direct marketing of organization
- Oversee all aspects of company directly or by delegating to staff as appropriate

PUBLIC HEALTH, ADVOCACY AND EDUCATION OUTREACH POSITIONS

State Genetics Coordinator
Public health departments

- Oversee genetic programs (i.e., screening programs)
- Manage funding, education, legislative issues
- Network with public sector
- Principal investigator for local and multistate research projects
- Participate in policy development activities on federal and state levels

(continued)

TABLE 17-2. (Continued)

Medical Director
Education department of a contract research organization

- Manage education department
- Develop and manage educational materials (print and media) for healthcare professionals, regulatory authorities, and consumers

Education Director/Advisor
Community education projects, pharmaceutical, biotech companies, HMOs

- Development of materials and coordination of educational programs (lectures, websites, pamphlets)
- Outreach to health professionals and consumers
- Represent organization at conferences, community events
- Deliver targeted education in genetics and applied research ethics via conferences, workshops, and online learning

Executive Director
Genetic disease advocacy groups
Genetics professional organizations

- Lead and implement initiatives according to the strategic direction set by the group/organization
- Represent the group/organization at community activities to enhance the organization's community profile, to build relationships, and to market the group/organization

Director/Coordinator of Genetic Resources and Services
Genetics advocacy group

- Provide accurate genetic disease information and resources for consumers
- Develop relevant educational materials, write funding grants, liaise with professional and consumer groups

ACADEMIC POSITIONS

Director/Associate Director, Genetic Counseling Program
Medical schools, colleges, and universities

- Direct genetic counseling graduate program (teaching, administration, faculty liaison, admissions) in accordance with American Board of Genetic Counseling standards
- Provide administration and faculty expertise needed for successful management of academic program

Faculty
Medical schools, schools of public health, schools of allied health professionals, colleges, universities

- Professors, associate professors, assistant professors, instructors, adjunct faculty
- Teaching medical genetics and genetic counseling at all levels

*It should be noted that there is overlap between these categories. For example, administrative positions could have been grouped together but instead are listed in the different position categories. Education and academic roles also occur in different types of positions.

Commit to Learning

In addition to the skills and knowledge that genetic counselors acquire during their formal training, other opportunities for continued training and learning of new skills and knowledge are available. Many medical and genetic conferences, for example, will have programs useful for the genetic counselor wanting to gain new knowledge or specialize in a particular area of medicine or genetics. Short courses or other topical programs can provide in-depth learning in a particular subject area. This special training can ease the transition into a new clinical area or new role. While many genetic counselors learn new skills on the job, such as writing a business plan or marketing a program to the public, other skills can be learned by more formal methods. Among the formal methods are training opportunities at their institution, certificate programs, and special courses both in person and web-based. For example, many large medical centers offer leadership and management training programs, organization development, business writing skills, project management, and a variety of other courses for employees and faculty. Additionally, useful new skills can be gained through leadership roles in professional organizations or by serving on boards for foundations or support organizations. Many of these activities and courses can also be used to satisfy CEU requirements of the American Board of Genetic Counseling (ABGC). Having a commitment to lifelong learning, through formal and informal methods, enables a process for continued growth and development throughout one's career.

Network, Network, Network

Networking is how I got my first job in industry. I cannot stress enough how important this is. You never know who knows who or what discussion will lead to another lead that will lead to a job—so leave no stone unturned!
                    —a genetic counselor in a biotech company

Genetic counselors can also use their well-developed interpersonal skills to network with colleagues to learn about positions both within and external to clinical genetics. You are networking when you attend professional or trade association conferences; attend meetings, lectures, and case conferences at work; talk to others when attending a social event; join a virtual social and/or professional network; post messages in chat rooms or on mailing lists; talk to sales persons who visit your office; or join a professional special interest group (SIG) or online forum. Networking has a purpose. You are developing relationships that will be beneficial to your work and professional goals. Very often, it is mutually beneficial in that you often have knowledge and a clinical perspective to impart that is useful for the other individual as well. Networking is also done over time; developing a relationship doesn't happen in just one meeting. Sharing information and ideas also occurs over a period of months to years; as you gain experience and a knowledge that is unique, you become more helpful and valuable to others as well.

Networking can also help you identify new job opportunities; it is consistently cited as the #1 way to get a new job. Approximately 80% of new jobs available never get advertised (Crispin and Mehler, 2008). The authors' own experiences in job hunting have been through extensive networking and rarely through an advertised position. Former clinical supervisors, instructors, program directors, co-workers, friends, and colleagues are often the best resource for job seekers. Studies have shown that approximately 34% of new hires brought in from outside an organization were due to employee referrals because the people who do the hiring would much rather hire someone who's been recommended by a person they already employ. Also, they have your first reference and it saves them considerable effort in advertising the position and sorting through all the resumes and phone calls (Crispin and Mehler, 2008).

Through genetic counseling colleagues or other contacts cultivated during career and training experiences, one may begin to form a network of people who can assist in the transition to a new role. The Industry SIG of the National Society of Genetic Counselors provides an ideal opportunity to meet and learn from genetic counselors who have branched out into positions that are generally outside of clinical genetic counseling. Other SIGs, such as Neurogenetics or Cardiology, provide opportunities to meet counselors who have become specialists in one content area. Non-genetics meetings are also an excellent opportunity to meet people from new areas and to research information key to non-traditional roles. In addition, consider setting up informational interviews, meeting with key stakeholders and human resource professionals.

Use technology to network *virtually*. Connecting with people who you know, or even casually have met, via one of the Internet social networks continues to gain momentum. Done properly, it can serve as a way to cultivate relationships with a variety of people with similar professional interests and career aspirations (Brock, 2008). People will always want and need the human, in-person experience. However, technologies provide the ability to get close to a specific group of people with a shared special interest. Also, more and more jobs are being found through social networking. There are probably some who still get hired by traditional newspaper classified ads. However, that market is fading fast. Social networking and blogs are used by many employers today. More and more jobs are offered and accepted through social networks like Twitter, MySpace, Facebook, LinkedIn, Plaxo, and others.

Mentoring Matters

A mentor is an individual, usually older, often more experienced, who helps and guides another individual's development. This guidance is not done for personal gain. Finding mentors both inside and outside the genetic counseling profession can be invaluable. Many experienced genetic counselors consider mentoring as a key step in their own professional development and are willing mentors when asked. They have first-hand experience in the problems genetic counselors face and know how we can translate our skills. Mentors outside of the genetic counseling profession can provide insight into the skill sets needed in a different type of role and the culture of the business or organization. One can find mentors through NSGC's Mentor Program and SIGs and by asking people who they have networked with or through E-mentoring networks, which group mentors and mentees by knowledge areas such as biological sciences, engineering (MentorNet), or business (www.novations.com). Other networks offer mentoring more broadly to a variety of mentees (www.mentoringgroup.com).

A mentor should know you and care about your progress as a professional; a mentee needs to initiate the relationship and be an active participant. Don't assume that a person is too busy or uninterested to want to talk to you about their professional experiences. Most people enjoy talking about their experiences and sharing their mistakes and successes. Realize, too, that mentors may come and go as your needs change. This doesn't mean one should discard previous mentors and never recontact them; it does mean that you may have several mentors over the course of your career to meet the changing needs of your life.

As a mentee, be clear about what you need mentoring in and set aside time to regularly meet with your mentor. This can be face to face, but may often be by phone, email, Internet chat room, blog, or message board. Mentoring matters, and the way you find a mentor or are mentored may vary.

POSITIONING ONESELF FOR A NEW ROLE

My advice is to talk to as many people as possible before and while (and after!) you are making the change. Ask them as many questions as possible about what they do, what they like and don't like about it, what skills are necessary to be successful in the roles, etc. And don't limit these interviews to people in the roles you are most actively considering— branch out to less appealing roles so you don't look back later and wonder. And finally— listen to the advice they give you! Too often we seek advice and then ignore it.
            —a genetic counselor in the Industry SIG

What skills are useful to genetic counselors transitioning into new roles and settings? As a start, when you build relationships with other healthcare providers and answer their questions about genetics, you are networking and showing your value. Providing presentations about genetic services, testing, and counseling in ways that are fundamental and easily translatable to other specialties invites other healthcare providers to think about how they could use the same services. By attending and commenting during case conferences in other departments, you can demonstrate ways in which genetic counselors' knowledge and critical thinking skills can be useful in other areas. Attending business or technology conferences where genetic topics will be discussed and in which you can contribute will highlight your interest in other areas outside of clinical care. Being flexible in your work style and working well as a team member can open opportunities to work in other clinical areas.

There are many reasons one decides to branch out into a new clinical area or to expand into a non-clinical role. A new path, regardless of the ultimate destination, has self assessment, exploration, and implementation phases.

Self-Assessment Phase (Choosing an Itinerary)

Starting down a new path begins with self reflection and evaluation. One needs to thoughtfully and honestly answer several key questions:

1. What do I want? What interests me? Why do I want a new position/role?

The reasons for moving into a new position/role may depend on where one is in their personal and professional life and will vary over time.

- Professional: You want a new challenge or to develop expertise in a new area; your position is eliminated; new opportunities present themselves; you have developed a passion for a new area in genetics or a new way to contribute to quality healthcare

- Personal: You decide to move to a new location or a spouse/partner gets a new job and you have to relocate and make the best of limited opportunities in a specific geographical region; you find yourself burning out in your current role; to balance work and parenting you may need a part-time position or more flexible hours

- Financial: funding resources may not be available, or you need to increase your earning power

2. Am I a pathfinder?

Being the first genetic counselor in an area, whether clinical or non-clinical, means you will be breaking new ground, establishing yourself once again, taking on new responsibilities, acquiring new knowledge/content, applying your skills and experience in a new way. You will also be marketing the profession, and yourself, in this new role. You may need to prove to your colleagues what a genetic counselor does, what your skills are, and what you bring to the organization. You may also be moving into a new culture that calls for using newly acquired skills, language, and information technology and that has a steep learning curve. You have to be honest about whether you have the personality and persistence to be a pioneer in a new area.

3. What is the risk?

Moving into a new role has an element of risk associated with it regardless of whether you are a new graduate of a genetic counseling program or an experienced genetic counselor. You must honestly evaluate the level of risk you are comfortable with before moving into a new role. If you are risk aversive, it may be best to consider moving into a role that is new for you, but is in a setting that has previously employed genetic counselors. If you are able to tolerate a higher level of risk, the more entrepreneurial path of being the first genetic counselor in a setting may be a wonderful opportunity for growth and professional development.

4. What path is right for Me?

Genetic counselors measure success and satisfaction at work in a variety of ways, depending on personal values and strengths. However, some factors seem to be common themes for persons in different roles and may be useful in determining future satisfaction in a given clinical area (Sogol, 1999). A workshop at an NSGC annual education conference addressed some key factors for genetic counselor job satisfaction including:

- Autonomy

- Direct patient care

- Continuity of care (long or short term)
- Diversity of responsibilities
- Focus of expertise
- Innovative thinking
- Intellectual content
- Interaction with healthcare professionals (HCP)
- Psychosocial counseling
- Schedule (regular or varied).

In general, a genetic counselor for whom **caring for patients** and **autonomy** are critical factors for satisfaction in his/her role may consider prenatal counseling and/or working in a specialty/disease clinic such as cancer or neurology in order to achieve greatest job satisfaction. He or she would be less likely to find satisfaction in industry or research. If **diversity of the position** is critical, having a role in pediatrics, adult, industry, or research where one can apply one's knowledge and expertise in medical genetics in a variety of different ways may be preferred to a position in prenatal, which can be less diverse. A role in industry or research may bring satisfaction to genetic counselors for whom **innovative thinking** is important. **Intellectual content** is a critical factor for genetic counselors in pediatrics, adult, and laboratory roles, which are broad in their scope of medical genetics. It is less critical in prenatal and specialty disease counseling because these positions require a depth of knowledge in an area rather than a broad base. If frequent **interaction with other healthcare professionals** is a critical factor, then a role in a clinic or as a laboratory genetic counselor may be preferred to a research role. **Autonomy** or working independently is an important factor for most professionals, but it seems to be a critical factor for counselors in industry, prenatal, and specialty disease areas. Thinking through one's personal preferences and professional needs may help to better define the role best suited to oneself. Self-assessment and input from colleagues or supervisors can help one identify the path most likely to provide the greatest satisfaction. By documenting what your successes are and what factors contribute to your success, you will be able to identify the one or two factors critical to you for job satisfaction. By identifying those factors and exploring the roles where they are key, other factors will support or disallow the choice of one role versus another. Only you can determine whether personal, professional, or financial factors outweigh the factors critical to job satisfaction to choose the path that is right for you.

5. What are my strengths?

We all acquire knowledge and develop skills via education and work experience. However, our strengths are innate to us, are part of our basic makeup and personality; they are our natural abilities or aptitudes. Examples of strengths include empathy, competitiveness, communication, strategic thinking, and creativity (Buckingham and Clifton, 2001). Identifying one's strengths/talents, and building knowledge and skills around them, can assist in finding the path forward. Some standardized tests can be useful to help one identify strengths and personality type suited for one or more genetic counseling roles (Myers-Briggs Type Indicator® or StrengthsFinder®).

6. Do I want to see patients?

Because both clinical and non-clinical roles are open to genetic counselors, one has to assess whether one is ready to move into another clinical role and continue to see patients, or whether a very different role, not involving direct patient care, is the next step in one's career. It is important to remember that one can go back to patient care if the experience of not seeing patients is not fulfilling. However, it is also possible to affect patient's lives and their care indirectly in non-clinical roles in science and healthcare.

Exploration Phase (Mapping It Out)

Once you have an understanding of the role you want, you need to focus your efforts and energy on moving forward with your decision.

There are a number of ways to prepare for either a clinical or a non-clinical role. One is to find a genetic counselor who has a similar position and learn as much as you can about why s/he decided on this career path, what s/he did in preparation, and ask him/her to help/mentor you. Others not in the genetic counseling profession can be very instrumental in helping one enter a different job market, particularly if they understand the genetic counseling training and skill set.

Utilize "People," Print, and Intenet Resources

I started working with a career counselor, this helped me to focus as well as realize my skills and what I wanted out of a job. I decided I could combine my previous work skills in clinical research with my skills as a genetic counselor. I also talked to people in the industry SIG to find out about the jobs they had, the skills needed, and how they used their genetic counseling skills and sold them. I started contacting biotech, pharma, and personalized medicine companies.

—a genetic counselor in a biotech company

"People" Resources

- Network—discuss what you are looking for in a career with your peers, your mentors, basically everyone you know. Use your past and present network of contacts and discuss your goals. See if they can help you reach your goal. What else do they suggest?
- Talk to counselors and company representatives (at NSGC, ASHG, ACMG meetings) that offer genetic services and products to learn what sorts of skills and knowledge they are looking for in employees and what types of positions are available.
- Hire a "career coach" or advisor as your guide into new territory.

Print and Internet Resources

- Use the NSGC job postings to review different positions advertised, become familiar with the responsibilities associated with different positions.
- Read journals, magazines, other literature, and Internet resources associated with the area/role you are considering, for background information and learning about the culture and the vocabulary/terms used by those already working in the area. Read *Business Week* and *Fortune* along with genetics and medical journals.
- Use search engines to research the field in which you are interested.
- Search for genetics educational sites and genetic testing laboratories. Look into genetics Internet companies, as many offer genetic tests and information via the web.
- Visit the website of any company, organization or institution that you are interested in—be familiar with the website wherever you apply.

Job Postings

- Search the websites of genetics and medical professional organizations for job postings.
- Search online, using resources such as www.monster.com and www.medzilla.com for positions.
- Visit websites of universities, academic medical centers, not-for-profit organizations, and individual companies, as many post available jobs with descriptions of positions. As you look at what positions already exist, think of new positions that could exist and consider approaching the appropriate organization about establishing such a position.

Just as genetic counselors have been trained to thoroughly research the information related to a case, determine the most appropriate courses of action, and present all options, these same skills can be of incredible use when moving into a new role. Some questions to seek answers to include: Who is working in this role? What training and experience do they have? What services do they offer? Can you speak with them directly or contact them with questions? What are companies looking for in an employee? What are their needs? Are they willing to consider someone who does not have the standard background for the position? Find out about their culture and values by looking at their website and by talking to people who work in the industry, that is, people that work for the company as well as their competitors.

Take on New Professional Roles Take on roles within NSGC or other professional organizations to expand your skills. Join a SIG, plan a meeting, help with a project, assist with educational sessions at the annual education conference. These experiences help develop skills in management and organization and will broaden your network of contacts. Move outside your role wherever you are currently working. Become involved in such activities as research, teaching, lecturing, creating patient education materials, and/or publishing interesting cases. Serve on a hospital committee or ask to be appointed to one. Consider networking with representatives from foundations, not-for-profits, and businesses who are interested in genetic issues. Can you develop relationships that might help you learn about how these organizations function and the roles within the organizations? Serving on a board, whether volunteer or paid, is an excellent opportunity to develop relationships with leaders, experts and persons with business and research connections, learn about organizational behavior, gain confidence in decision-making, and develop leadership skills. These experiences, gained in developing professionally, can provide valuable skills and information that you might not otherwise acquire in a clinical position.

Obtain an Additional Degree   Some genetic counselors find they need to go back to school to earn additional degrees in order to prepare for a specific role. The desire may be formed shortly after graduation or more gradually, over the course of working as a genetic counselor. Of those who do get additional degrees, some remain in fields related to genetic counseling such as medicine, public health, social work, or psychology, for example. Other degrees may take the genetic counselor further out from the genetic counseling profession, such as an MBA, a law degree, or teaching.

Develop new skills that will expand your opportunities either through courses or on your own. Useful skills to add to your repertoire would include bioinformatics, strategic planning, experience with different databases, management/supervision of others, and familiarity with global medicine and/or policy. Wherever desires and interests may lead, genetic counselor training provides a foundation for multiple valued roles.

Implementation Phase (Going For It!)

Prepare a CV or Resume   Once you have an idea of the area you wish to work in, you will need to prepare your curriculum vitae (CV) or resume to market yourself. A CV or resume needs to be appropriate for whatever position you are interested in applying for. This may be a particular challenge for genetic counselors moving into a role that is outside the clinical setting. As one counselor writes about her experience:

> *I often had difficulty communicating what my skills were and what I could do outside of genetic counseling. My CV didn't fit many of the jobs I was applying for and I didn't have many connections. I wasn't focused because I didn't know what to focus on. It was a long learning process.*
>
> —a genetic counselor in research

This comment stresses the importance of knowing the position you are applying for and tailoring your CV or resume to fit the job. It is also critical to your success to have others, particularly those with experience in the position or business in which you are applying, to read and critique your CV or resume.

The primary differences between a resume and a CV are the length, what is included, and what each is used for. In the United States, the CV is used primarily when applying for academic, education, scientific, or research positions. It is also applicable when applying for fellowships or grants. When seeking a job in Europe, the Middle East, Africa, or Asia, expect to submit a CV rather than a resume. Also, overseas employers often expect to read the type of personal information on CVs that would never be included on an American resume, such as date of birth, nationality, and place of birth. United States laws on what information job applicants can be asked to provide do not apply outside the country.

A resume is more concise than a CV. It is usually a one-, or possibly two-, page summary of your background, education, and work experience. It is preferred by business and/or industry employers. It highlights skills and experience from your background that is most relevant to a potential employer's needs and focuses on your specific achievements in these areas.

CVs and resumes have many purposes. Often they are both the first impression you will make on a prospective employer and demonstrate for them that you meet the minimum requirements for a position. Hopefully, after reviewing your resume, the employer will grant you the opportunity to make a second impression. CVs and resumes also facilitate an interview and discussion. They present your education and/ or work history in detail as well as highlighting your skills. They are a tool to assist you in organizing and analyzing experience, skills, and competency in different areas. They are useful in a job search as well as for networking contacts. Most importantly they are a positive and factual picture of YOU.

As more and more companies rely on online applications, you may need to compose individual paragraphs that describe your knowledge, skills, abilities, and accomplishments. These paragraphs can then be inserted into online applications, which often will not request either a CV or a resume but provide a template of targeted questions for applicants.

Interviewing The type of interview you will have depends on who conducts it as well as their goals. For example, a person from the human resources office may have a different goal in conducting the interview than the hiring manager (Martin and Tulgan, 2007).

Typically there are four types of interviews you may encounter since organizations approach interviewing differently: human resources, supervisor or manager, co-worker, and group. However, regardless of the kind of interview, be thoughtful and concise with your answers. A useful technique to organize your thoughts and answer questions about your accomplishments is the **STAR** (situation, task, action, results) technique: **Situation**: first describe or give a little background about the situation. **Task**: outline the task that needed to be done. Next describe the **Action** taken. Finally, give the **Results** of your action. (Hansen, 2007). Conclude with a summary of your skills and abilities that match the job requirements and a statement of your interest in the job.

Human resource interview Because human resource representatives are trained interviewers, their role is to evaluate your overall potential and decide how well you would fit within the organization. They focus more on how you present yourself than on your technical expertise. They tend to ask questions about your goals and attitudes. Your preparation, how you dress, how effectively you answer questions and your general motivation are all areas they evaluate.

Supervisor/manager interview   When talking to supervisors/hiring managers, the interview questions are more technical. Since these people are directly responsible for getting the work done, they want to be sure you can handle the job for which you have applied. They will want to know, "Can you do the job?" and/or "Will you fit into my existing team?" Therefore, expect to talk about the basics of the job, to show that you are flexible and are a team player. Researching the position in advance is key to helping you answer and ask specific job-related questions.

Co-worker interview   Often your future co-workers may also interview you to see if they like you and can work with you. Usually these people are busy working when you are introduced to them. Be courteous of their time, give short statements about your background, and show your willingness to be a member of the team.

Group interview   Occasionally, you will find yourself facing more than one interviewer at the same time. Use your introduction and answers to steer the interview in the direction you want.

It is especially important to realize that those interviewing you may not have a medical or genetics background and may need additional information about the skills and experiences of a genetic counselor—what a genetic counselor can/cannot do. Be prepared to describe your experiences and skills succinctly and to describe how they translate to the position in which you are interested, how you can meet a need they have. Ultimately, the goal of any interview is for the interviewer to get to know you well enough to determine whether you are a right fit for their organization. This is your chance to shine—and your chance to also determine whether the organization is a right fit for you.

LOOKING AHEAD: VISIONING

I guess you could say I have been able to see the next opportunity for a genetic counselor to apply their skills—and have not been afraid to go for it.
> —a genetic counselor in a pharmaceutical company

Vision for the genetic counseling profession and one's own professional development may grow out of continuous learning, experience, and networking. For some genetic counselors, visioning, the ability to see new opportunities and/or "think outside the box," is an innate talent. For others, it is an acquired skill that is developed through experience. Developing vision is more a matter of discovery than design. It may be developed by associating with visionaries internal and external to the genetic counseling profession, working on strategic planning projects, and/or taking on new challenges. One must be alert to changes in the healthcare system, medicine and genetics, and be willing to question the adequacy of current models to meet future needs. Working on an organization's strategic planning team or having a visionary as a mentor is one way to develop "visioning" skills. Others develop this skill over time as their experience grows in depth and breadth. Some areas where one can envision role expansion for genetic counselors include the following.

Primary Care

Primary care is one of the areas of medicine in which genetic counselors have not yet expanded into a formal role. However, it is well known that most patients rely on the advice of their primary care physician when thinking through healthcare decisions (Harvey et al., 2007) making this a natural place for one to think about family history, genetic risks, and testing. In 1998, the American Medical Association sponsored "Genetic Medicine and the Practicing Physician," a conference for educating primary care physicians about basic medical genetics. There have been a number of other programs and initiatives, most notably the National Coalition for Health Professional Education in Genetics (NCHPEG), aimed at educating the same audience. While there have been a number of studies citing the inability of primary care healthcare professionals to understand and explain genetic tests or their lack of education in this area (Aalf et al., 2003; Howlett et al., 2002; Suther and Goodson, 2003; Yong et al., 2003), there has been a slow, but increasing effort to change the education and practice around genetics. This will increasingly become an issue as medicine becomes more "personalized."

At its most basic, **personalized medicine** refers to using information about a person's genetic makeup to tailor strategies for the detection, treatment, or prevention of disease. Michael Leavitt, past Secretary of the United States Department of Health and Human Services, gave it credence when he stated that healthcare in the United States needed to emphasize "prediction, prevention and personalization" (www.hhs.gov/myhealthcare/goals/index.html#Goal1). Since many healthcare professionals have not been trained sufficiently in genetics and thus may not be able to interpret and use the results of genetic tests, genetic counselors have the expertise to contribute to this evolving approach to patient care. Much remains to be done to enhance the knowledge of genetics and genomics among doctors, nurse practitioners, pharmacists, physician assistants, and allied health professionals, as well as to facilitate the availability of referral networks of medical geneticists and genetic counselors.

As medicine continues to move closer to the point of care, genetic counselors may find themselves in a new clinical role, as a valued member of a new team. They will be the genetics/genomics subject matter expert on the primary care team committed to delivering greater personalized medicine/care to patients. Knowledge of pharmacogenetics (individual response to medicine) will be key in all disease areas—and is already applied in oncology. Expertise in risk assessment, counseling, and knowledge of appropriate testing for complex diseases will be essential for members of this team. Personalized medicine will also need counselors working in non-clinical areas to address policy and ethical, legal, and social issues.

Policy

As not-for-profit organizations and for-profit companies become more invested in genetic medicine and technology, there will be opportunities for subject matter experts in genetics, clinical medicine, and ethics to help guide organizations in supporting policies, sponsoring legislation, and developing policy statements, as well as influencing policy and policy makers. Licensure is anticipated to open new political opportunities at the national and local levels, and genetic counselors may become lobbyists or policy makers in an increasing number of settings.

Research

The NIH roadmap has created opportunities in clinical and basic science that will enable the rapid translation of research into clinical medicine (www.nihroadmap.nih. gov). The emphasis on translation creates many opportunities for genetic counselors to expand research, clinical, ethical, and patient care experiences into many areas of the research enterprise within both public and private institutions. Genetic counselors may broaden their expertise into areas involving data sharing, community engaged research, regulatory oversight, best practices for educating and consenting patients, new models for genetic counseling and the delivery of genetic services, and the translation of technologies directly to the bedside.

Private Practice

It is anticipated that another growth area will be private practice. Future growth is going to depend on gains in state licensure as well as billing and reimbursement. Another contributor to genetic counselors working in private practice will be the increased ability of genetic counselors to bill directly for their services. There have always been a small percentage of genetic counselors who have maintained a private practice counseling patients referred through private, mostly physician, referrals. Some genetic counselors have developed creative ways of working around the lack of ability to collect payment from insurance through charging a fee to the physician, who in turn adds the additional cost to patients (www.bayareagc.com). Genetic counselors who have been able to align themselves with physician groups or a network of physicians, clinics, or smaller hospitals are more likely to sustain a practice over a longer term. Maintaining this type of relationship with physicians and groups of healthcare providers could be enhanced by the counselor's ability to bill directly to insurance as a provider.

Consultants to Healthcare Payers/Providers

The role of consultant is anticipated to grow as genetics is more fully integrated into medicine. Personalized medicine may present opportunities for more genetic counselors to move into the insurance/payer industry as case managers, educators or consultants. Their subject matter expertise will be invaluable to public and private payers considering whether a test is appropriate for a patient and whether they should provide a level of compensation for it. Genetic counselors may also consult/advise case managers when genetic testing is involved to ensure testing is performed appropriately.

Virtual Roles

In 2009, there are several Internet genetics companies that have combined different technologies (phone, web, and algorithms) to deliver genetic risk assessment and counseling. These innovative companies have recognized the benefit of having genetic counselors' expertise and advice in the development of their company as well as their products and delivery of services. If successful, genetics and genomics Internet companies will be a growth area for genetic counselors. Also, healthcare blogs are one of the fastest-growing areas on the Internet and offer additional *virtual* roles for genetic counselors as educators and advisors.

Public Health

As health is increasingly framed by the genetic contribution to disease and technology allows for increased testing and screening, health professionals with knowledge of public health systems and genetics/genomics will be needed to bring genetics and public health together to benefit the public and society. Genetic counselors' knowledge of genetic services delivery and patients' perspectives on illness will be of great value when translated from individuals to populations. Genetic counselors in public health are already state coordinators of genetic services and program managers in maternal and child health, newborn screening programs, and chronic diseases. They will play a larger role as educators, policy makers, and developers of patient and consumer materials as well as work in public health research.

CONCLUSION

The genetic counseling profession has made many inroads into a variety of clinical and non-clinical roles, and there are still many new areas for genetic counselors to explore and expand their careers. Does thinking about some of these challenges or new roles speak to you? Don't be afraid to push the limits of your training and experience—genetic counselors are trained in a manner that provides them with a foundation of skills and knowledge to take on the challenges of a variety of professional roles.

What keeps genetic counselors from pursuing these roles? Many genetic counselors are fearful of losing the respect of their colleagues when they move into a new, expanded role—often a non-clinical role. As a profession, we must be open to the changing roles and diversity within our profession and accept that we are no longer solely a profession of clinicians, but one of clinical professionals, business people, policy makers, educators, investigators, administrators, and managers to name a few. These additional roles will enrich who we are as professionals and expand our experiences so that we are better prepared for what the future offers us.

Where do genetic counselors of today find the resources to shape our field for the future? Many genetic counselors have gained inspiration into new career paths from genetic counseling colleagues with similar interests, by meeting others outside our profession with an interest in genetic healthcare but different approaches to providing care, by listening to new directions of research at meetings, and by being a keen observer of the business, policy, and regulatory arenas relating to genetic healthcare.

New roles will continue to be carefully planned as well as serendipitous. One must be resourceful in shaping one's own professional life. As in the past, genetic counselors must continue to expand into clinical arenas, respond to healthcare needs, promote safe and ethical use of genetic technologies, and be an active voice in the ever-changing healthcare environment and global integration of genetics into medicine.

APPENDIX: TOOLS FOR WORKING OUTSIDE THE BOX: WHAT GENETIC COUNSELORS CAN BRING TO A NON-TRADITIONAL ROLE

As genetic counselors, we have skills that are marketable to a wide variety of organizations. However, sometimes, we fail to see how our experiences and training in genetic counseling can be applied to other avenues. This document is a "brainstorm" of ideas regarding how our talents can complement more non-traditional positions in various industries.

Please check those that apply to the field you are exploring. When using these attributes in an interview situation, it is ideal to be prepared to support them with a "story" that illustrates a time when you demonstrated this quality.

1. **Knowledge**
   - ☐ Expertise in genetics
   - ☐ Medical knowledge and experience (prenatal/pediatrics/adult medicine, daily workings of a hospital/clinic/medical office/laboratory)
   - ☐ Experience with consumers, professionals, and the genetics community
   - ☐ Knowledge of healthcare industry/billing/insurance
   - ☐ Understanding of basic business principles/concepts
   - ☐ Knowledge of biotechnology or other genetics-related industries
   - ☐ Familiarity with access to genetics services and referrals
   - ☐ Understanding of and sensitivity to ELSI issues in genetics
   - ☐ Knowledge of educational methods
   - ☐ Direct patient care experience; understanding of people's response to genetics information
   - ☐ Familiarity with available resources and research
   - ☐ Understanding of research principles and technical writing
   - ☐ Experience with grant writing
2. **Skills**
   - ☐ Genetic counseling
   - ☐ Leadership abilities

- ☐ Reliability
- ☐ Explaining complex information in simple language
- ☐ Responsiveness
- ☐ High-quality work
- ☐ Flexibility
- ☐ Research abilities and ability to access information
- ☐ Being a liaison
- ☐ Being an advocate
- ☐ Attention to details
- ☐ Project/case management
- ☐ Facilitation
- ☐ Listening
- ☐ Decision-making skills
- ☐ Problem solving/conflict resolution
- ☐ Interpersonal skills
- ☐ Working independently and as a part of a team
- ☐ Multitasking
- ☐ Ability to get things accomplished within a system
- ☐ Ability to manage expectations
- ☐ Ability to weigh benefits and limitations of situations
- ☐ Ability to assume varying roles, depending on the situation at-hand
- ☐ Communication (written and verbal)
- ☐ Ability to prioritize
- ☐ Ability to identify appropriate resources
- ☐ Creativity, innovativeness and forward thinking
- ☐ Business skills (i.e. marketing, presentations, proposals)
- ☐ Ability to organize a meeting
- ☐ Ability to grasp business concepts
- ☐ Ability to think "outside the box"
- ☐ Ability to see the big picture
- ☐ Computer skills: Word, PowerPoint, Excel, internet/intranet information searches, email, etc.

3. Attitudes

- ☐ Passionate
- ☐ Committed to personal growth
- ☐ Dedicated to learning
- ☐ Willing to assume responsibility
- ☐ Educated risk-taker
- ☐ Assertive, but sensitive

☐ Perseverant

☐ Committed to educating others

☐ Altruistic

☐ Objective/non-directive

☐ Outgoing and personable

☐ Open and approachable

☐ Enthusiastic

Strategies for Transitioning into a Non-Traditional Role

Sometimes, it's hard to know where to start when "branching out" from a position that is comfortable to you. Here are some tips for making a transition in your career. Please check those that would apply to you and then begin to use them.

- **Exploration and Preparation**
  - ☐ Take on roles within NSGC or other professional organizations: join a SIG, plan a meeting, help with a project, assist with a PBS or workshop at the national meeting. These experiences can help you land that non-traditional position.
  - ☐ Become involved with "extra-curricular" activities such as research, teaching, lecturing, creating patient education materials, publishing your interesting cases. These provide valuable skills that you would not otherwise get in your clinical position.
  - ☐ Find a mentor within NSGC that has made similar transition.
  - ☐ Hire a "career coach" or advisor as your guide into new territory.
  - ☐ Read industry magazines to become familiar with the field in which you are interested. Some examples are Wired.com, Theindustrystandard.com, Red-herring.com
  - ☐ Read Business Week/Fortune along with the New England Journal and JGC.
  - ☐ Use search engines to research the field in which you are interested (Google, Copernic, AOL, Yahoo, etc.).
  - ☐ If you are interested in an organization, visit their corporate website.
  - ☐ Revamp your CV to be appropriate for a non-clinical position by reframing your genetic counseling skills into more general attributes.
  - ☐ Draft more than one CV and highlight different skills in each one—customize them to the specific job for which you are applying.
  - ☐ Use a title that reflects your skills; you may need to avoid calling yourself a "Genetic Counselor." Use "Clinical Genetic Specialist," "Genetic Educator," or some other term that sells your skills but does not pigeon hole you into a traditional genetic counselor salary.
- **Prospecting**
  - ☐ Discuss what you are looking for in a career with everyone you meet.

☐ Use your network and contacts. Who do you know and how can they help you to reach your goal?

☐ Utilize your resources: make use of NSGC Listserv, Perspectives, Industry SIG, and other SIGs.

☐ Don't just look at what positions already exist—think of new positions that should exist and sell the organization on hiring you for that position (convince them that they need this position and write a job description for it).

☐ Search online for jobs (Monster.com, etc.).

☐ Approach companies that offer genetic services and products.

☐ Approach recruiters or "head hunters" in the applicable field.

- **Interviewing**
  ☐ Research the organization at which you are interviewing.

  ☐ Learn about your interviewer. Who are they? What is their background?

  ☐ Practice interviewing skills for the business world—there are plenty of web sites that give practice interview questions and tips.

  ☐ Use the STAR technique when interviewing: describe the **S**ituation/**T**ask, **A**ction, **R**esult.

  ☐ Cite examples of your skills during the interview process and give examples when you have used those skills.

  ☐ Talk to other individuals already in the new position/organization to gain insight.

  ☐ Always "close" the interview by asking if they have enough information from you in order to make a decision on who the best candidate for the job is and find out if they have any concerns about you before you leave—get a timeline for the hiring process.

  ☐ Send a thank you note or email and follow-up with a call if you haven't heard from the organization by the deadline they promised.

REFERENCES

Aalf CM, Smets EM, de Haes HC, Leschot NJ (2003) Referral for genetic counseling during pregnancy: limited alertness and awareness about genetic risk factors among GPs. *Fam Prac* 20(2):135–141.

Begleiter M, Collins DL, Greendale K (1981) NSGC Professional Status Survey. *Perspect Genet Couns*, Vol 3, No 4. Available from: National Society of Genetic Counselors, Inc., Chicago, IL.

Boldt AH (1994) Professional Status Survey, 1994. Available from National Society of Genetic Counselors, Inc., Chicago, IL.

Brock, T (2008) Social networking and bottom line business. www.bizjournals.com/extraedge/consultants/succeeding_today/2008/06/16/column518.html?market=portland, accessed December 8, 2008.

Buckingham M, Clifton D (2001) Now, Discover Your Strengths. The Free Press, New York, NY.

Collins DL (1987) Results of the NSGC professional status survey. *Perspect Genet Couns* Vol 9, No 2. Available from National Society of Genetic Counselors, Inc., Chicago, IL.

Crispin G, Mehler M (2007) Career X Roads 7th Annual Source of Hire Study: What 2007 Plans Mean for Your 2008 Plans. www.careerxroads.com/news/SourcesOfHire08.pdf, accessed December 8, 2008.

Fine BA, Baker DL, Fiddler MB, ABGC Consensus Development Consortium (1996) Practice-based competencies for accreditation of and training in graduate programs in genetic counseling. *J Genet Counsel* 5:105–112.

Hall JM, Friedman L, Guenther C, Lee MK, Weber JL, Black DM, King MC (1992) Closing in on a breast cancer gene on chromosome 17q. *AJHG* 50(6):1235–1242.

Hansen R (2007) Quintessential Careers www.quintcareers.com/STAR_interviewing.html, accessed December 8, 2008.

Harvey EK, Fogel CE, Peyrot M, Christensen KD, Terry SF, McInerney JD (2007) Provider's knowledge of genetics: A survey of 5915 individuals and families with genetic conditions. *Genet Med* 9(5):259–267.

Howlett MJ, Avard D, Knoppers BM (2002) Physicians and genetic malpractice. *Med Law* 21(4):661–680.

Leavitt M. www.hhs.gov/myhealthcare/goals/index.html#Goal1, accessed December 8, 2008.

Martin C, Tulgan B (2007) Managing the Generation Mix 2007. RainmakerThinking, Inc. www.rainmakerthinking.com/rschrpts.htm, accessed December 8, 2008.

Parrott S, Clark C (2004). Membership Trends 1980–2002. Available from National Society of Genetic Counselors, Inc., Chicago, IL.

Reed S (1955) *Counseling in Medical Genetics*. Philadelphia: W.B. Saunders.

Sogol E (1999). Pathway Evaluation Program. Glaxo Wellcome, Inc.

Schneider KA, Kalkbrenner KJ (1998). Professional Status Survey 1998. *Perspect Genet Couns*. Vol 20, No 3. Available from National Society of Genetic Counselors, Inc., Chicago, IL.

Smith M, Freivogel ME, Parrott S (2008) Professional Status Survey 2008. Available from National Society of Genetic Counselors, Inc., Chicago, IL.

Suther S, Goodson P (2003) Barriers to the provision of genetic services by primary care physicians: A systematic review of the literature. *Genet Med* 5(2):70–76.

Uhlmann WR (1992) Professional Status Survey Results. *Perspect Genet Couns*. Supplement to Vol 14, No 2, Summer 1992. Available from National Society of Genetic Counselors, Inc., Chicago, IL.

Yong MC, Zhou XJ, Lee SC (2003) The importance of family history in hereditary breast cancer is underappreciated by healthcare professionals. *Oncology* 64(3):220–226.

18

Putting It All Together: Three Case Examples

Jane L. Schuette, M.S., C.G.C., Donna F. Blumenthal, M.S., C.G.C., Monica L. Marvin, M.S., C.G.C., and Cheryl Shuman, M.S., C.G.C.

INTRODUCTION (Jane L. Schuette)

The best way to capture the nature of the genetic counseling process is in the presentation or recounting of an actual "case." As the reader reviews the unfolding of the interaction, it is then that he begins to understand the intricacy of balancing information, education, the exploring of options, decision-making, and support for choice. The following cases each exemplify this process in three different realms: the pediatric genetics clinic, the reproductive genetics clinic, and the cancer genetics clinic. Readers who are unfamiliar with the conditions in each of the cases (fragile X, Lynch syndrome, and Klinefelter syndrome) should consult a medical genetics textbook or other resource for background information.

In the pediatric case the counselor encounters issues related to the competing needs of individual family members and the importance of supporting the family dynamic. In this particular case, the counselor's cultural awareness and sensitivity are key in creating a relationship of mutual trust and respect with the family.

In the reproductive genetics case, the counselor facilitates decision-making for a couple confronting an especially problematic dilemma. They are faced with unexpected results that involve a range of potential outcomes in their pregnancy from "normal" to infertility and speech and language delay. As the couple sorts through

A Guide to Genetic Counseling, Second Edition, Edited by Wendy Uhlmann, Jane Schuette, and Beverly Yashar
Copyright © 2009 by John Wiley & Sons, Inc.

their individual tolerances for risk and uncertainty, the counselor must remain aware of her own feelings and perspectives in order to present balanced information. Such cases are difficult; they are not "neat and tidy" with satisfying outcomes. There are often heartbreaking choices to be made and lingering questions for the patient. It is a challenge for the counselor to support the couple as they process the "information" while they attempt to incorporate its meaning into their lives.

The cancer genetics case illustrates the complex process of cancer genetics evaluation and counseling. The author guides the reader through the various components of patient medical history, family history, risk assessment, informed consent, testing, provision of test results, and management. Throughout all the steps, the counselor is confronted with issues related to the patient's own mortality, her concern for family members, and the complex process of decision-making.

Case presentation facilitates discussion and exploration, thereby enhancing learning. This process should be considered essential to student skill acquisition and development, as well as for the continued growth of the more experienced genetic counselor. It is our hope that these cases will stimulate discussion and serve to demonstrate the value of analyzing our work.

PEDIATRIC CASE (Cheryl Shuman)

This case involved a referral for a pediatric genetic assessment, testing, and genetic counseling, and it demonstrates some of the complexities involved in defining who the patient is within the context of a nuclear family. In this case, all of the family members ultimately pursued genetic testing, and it was important to help each individual explore the unique issues relevant for his/her decision-making. Competing needs can arise within some families, and consideration should be given to the potential impact of test results on other family members. In addition, the child (often the proband in a pediatric setting) should be evaluated within the context of the family and the family dynamic preserved unless there is concern that the child may be at risk for abuse. In this specific case, the family presented as a cohesive and caring family unit. This case also demonstrates that while pediatric issues may incorporate a wide age range, the approaches and relevant issues shift with different cognitive and emotional maturation stages. As well, the parents had immigrated to North America from New Delhi and were practicing Muslims. Therefore, cultural awareness and sensitivity were essential to appreciating their concerns and supporting a respectful dialogue; however, assuming that all family members would incorporate their religious convictions or cultural identity in a similar manner could have undermined the professional relationship and potentially inhibited their willingness to engage in an open dialogue.

Background

Maya's family doctor initiated a referral to the Genetics Clinic when Maya's mother, Inaya, told him that her great nephew (i.e., Maya's maternal first cousin once removed), Adam, was recently diagnosed with fragile X syndrome. (Fig 18-1). Maya

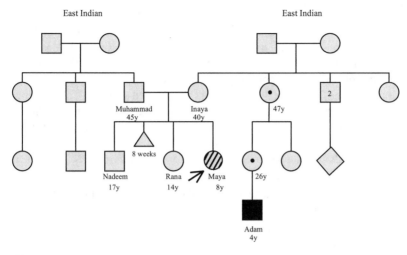

East Indian   East Indian

Key

⦸ learning difficulties

■ fragile X syndrome

▣ ⊙ heterozygous for fragile X premutation

Historians; Inaya & Muhammad
Taken by: Cheryl Shuman, MS, CGC
Consanguinity denied

FIGURE 18-1

was 8 years of age at the time of referral and was reported to be having some learning difficulties. Her parents had become more concerned about Maya's educational issues upon learning of the fragile X diagnosis in Inaya's family. Inaya's sister, who lives in London, England, forwarded a letter to her at-risk family members that provided confirmation that Adam had a molecular test result of 657 CGG repeats in the FMR1 (fragile X mental retardation 1) gene. As well, Adam's mother and maternal grandmother (Inaya's sister) were confirmed to be heterozygous for premutation range repeats. This information was provided before the initial appointment along with preliminary information regarding the pedigree obtained via a family history questionnaire.

Goals and Preparation

As a component of case preparation, a review of updated references on fragile X syndrome was undertaken, especially given the rate at which new information is generated regarding the clinical findings (e.g., current considerations regarding potential psychiatric and/or behavioral findings in premutation carriers) and the molecular underpinnings. A reference list compiled for the appointment is provided here: Hagerman, 2001; Hagerman and Cronister, 2002; McConkie-Rosell et al., 2005; Sherman et al., 2005; Saul and Tarleton, 2007; McConkie-Rosell et al., 2007. To facilitate review of this case, classification of CGG repeat sizes will be included as follows: normal alleles: approximately 5–40 repeats, intermediate alleles: 41–59 repeats, premutation alleles: 59–200 repeats, full mutation: >200 repeats (Saul and Tarleton, 2007).

An agenda for this appointment was developed before the consultation. Note that, as for any genetic counseling situation, this agenda was flexible and developed for preparation purposes only, since family members can present with unanticipated issues or concerns that may become apparent at the outset of the appointment. Contracting provides an opportunity for the family to become fully engaged by contributing to the framing of the session and being asked to dialogue about issues that are personally relevant. The detailed agenda for this session included the following components but would not necessarily be presented in the following order:

- Learning about the specific questions and concerns from each of the family members present, including Maya
- Learning what the parents understood about fragile X syndrome in general and specifically about Adam
- Reviewing the family history obtained via the questionnaire and collecting further information
- Obtaining Maya's medical, developmental, and social histories
- A physical examination to be undertaken by the medical geneticist to ensure that there were no clinical features suggestive of a different underlying etiology for Maya's learning difficulties

This would be followed by a discussion of the genetic testing available, possible approaches to testing (i.e., who could have testing first), and the potential implications of both positive and negative test results for those present at this appointment as well as other family members—primarily Maya's sibs. While many genetics clinic appointments are limited to a single interaction or consultation, the discussion with the family would include a plan to organize additional appointment(s) if the family chose to pursue testing and a positive result(s) was obtained. The intention would be to present this in a positive manner so that the family would not feel that they had only one opportunity to raise all of their concerns and that they would not feel abandoned to cope with the test results and to navigate through the clinical and social waters on their own.

It is important to involve any child attending an appointment in the discussion to whatever degree they are comfortable as noted by Reich in the previous edition of this text (p. 409). That is to say that the child should not be pressured into responding to numerous questions, but by being asked several simple, age-appropriate questions about school, after-school activities, friends, birthday parties, etc., the child may feel more comfortable in this setting. During the session, some children may appear to be engaged in play but may still be listening to fragments of the discussion or glancing at their parents, especially during any expressions of stress or distress (Weil, 2000). This can lead to increased anxiety in the child and a need for additional reassurance, and if the parents are not attentive the genetic counselor may redirect their focus to their child. This requires a heightened awareness on the part of the genetic counselor. It can also be quite distressing for children to be the focus of a discussion but not be included or even to be talked about in the third person, and disturbing misconceptions may develop. For children who have a number of issues meriting ongoing medical attention, a sense of being 'medicalized' can result in feeling as though any sense of autonomy over their own body has been lost (Weil, 2000). Throughout the genetic counseling appointment, depending on the cognitive level and other issues, the genetic counselor should continue to check in with the child and, with either tacit or overt agreement from the parents, to frame portions of the discussion toward the child. The simple act of involving the child/children in the session demonstrates a respect for their autonomy and that they are regarded as integral members of the session. Certainly, with older children/adolescents, the counselor should consider contracting with the child as well as the parents, directing the counseling to the child, checking in and soliciting questions from both the child and parents, and providing the child with contact information for any questions/issues arising (e.g., business card). As adolescents are encouraged to assume responsibility for their own health and well-being, such measures may be viewed as nurturing this transition.

Session 1

The initial appointment was attended by Maya and her parents, Inaya and Muhammad. During the contracting, certain information and cues came to light that merited integration into the session. Muhammad informed the genetic counselor that he worked as a civil engineer and Inaya worked as a data architect. Both were observant Muslims. This was learned during the family history acquisition, when they stated that while their own brothers and sisters lived in distant cities for the most part, they derived a sense of belonging and community from attending mosque each week. At that point, the genetic counselor was able to ask them to recount a few of their experiences immigrating to North America and how they had adjusted to the cultural and lifestyle differences. This provided an opportunity for the family to talk about an area of familiarity, allowing them to become more comfortable in this setting, and for the genetic counselor to gauge their acculturation. Throughout this brief discussion, the questions were asked in a sincere and interested manner and with the understanding that they need not answer. Had the couple given very short, terse answers indicating that they viewed this as either too personal or a distraction from the focus of the session, the genetic counselor would have followed their cues and shifted the dialogue to the referral indication. Inaya and Muhammad told the genetic counselor that they had maintained a very strong commitment to their cultural values and traditions and viewed themselves as being religiously observant. Later in the session, the couple noted that while their marriage had not been arranged and they met during their university education, that it was very important to them that their children wed within their community. All of this information was helpful in guiding the genetic counselor in her approach.

Before the appointment, the parents had searched the Internet for information about fragile X syndrome and had some familiarity with the overall features in addition to having talked with Inaya's sister about her grandson. They appreciated that Inaya and their children were at increased risk but were not clear what this risk actually implied. As such, there remained a palpable level of tension in the room, some of which was manifested by their body language—Inaya sat quite rigidly with her feet crossed and her hands clenched in her lap. Muhammad sat in the chair just next to Inaya, but his posture was tipped just slightly away from her. Both cast nervous glances at each other and at Maya, who sat quietly holding on to but not yet playing with an electronic toy. They had not been able to independently synthesize the specific information regarding repeat sizes and variability in expression. They agreed that they would like the genetic counselor to include a general description of fragile X syndrome in the discussion.

The family history (Fig. 18-1) revealed that Inaya and Muhammad had three children, all of whom were generally healthy. The eldest, a son, Nadeem, was 17 years of age and a senior in high school; there were no concerns about Nadeem's academic or social skills. Inaya had a first trimester miscarriage before having two daughters, Rana and Maya. Rana was 14 years of age and was noted to be having some difficulty focusing on schoolwork; as well, she had a tendency toward being emotionally labile. Rana had not undergone any formal psychoeducational evaluation, and her parents attributed some of her issues to hormonal fluctuations associated with puberty. As noted above, at the age of 8 years, Maya was having problems processing information at school. This had first come to light during a parent-teacher meeting the prior year when Maya was in grade 2. Maya was described by her parents as being a socially shy child, but she did provide answers to the genetic counselor when directly questioned. She told the genetic counselor that she had one 'best' friend and liked her teacher. As the appointment continued, she became more comfortable and began to play with her computerized virtual pet. Pregnancy, medical, and developmental histories were obtained and did not yield any new information of significance. Other than the index case with fragile X syndrome, the remainder of the family history was non-contributory, and Inaya and Muhammad denied consanguinity.

Although the reason for referral was straightforward and there had not been any concern raised by the referring pediatrician regarding dysmorphism or other clinical issues, a physical examination by the clinical geneticist was indicated to rule out other potential clinical diagnoses for Maya. While it was important to have this take place relatively early in the session as clinical suspicion of another disorder could have redirected the session significantly, the parents were asked if they would prefer to have a general discussion of fragile X syndrome first or to proceed to the physical examination. This provided the parents with some control of the appointment and demonstrated that this was a negotiable session. They preferred to proceed with the examination. The genetic counselor explained to Maya and her parents that these examinations are typically somewhat different from more traditional physical exams with respect to the features examined and the measurements taken. Maya was asked whom she wanted to be present for the examination (i.e., just one or both of her parents), and she had no preference as long as her mother was there. The physical examination did not note any additional clinical findings suggestive of another syndromic diagnosis. In addition to offering molecular testing for fragile X syndrome, the clinical geneticist suggested that a karyotype be initiated at the same time.

The family returned to the counseling room, and the genetic counselor asked if any of the family members had thought of any additional questions or concerns, but nothing further was raised. A brief discussion of fragile X syndrome ensued. Since the family did not have first-hand experience with this disorder, key issues about fragile X syndrome were contextualized so that Inaya and her husband could make an informed decision about testing. As with any testing, it is critical to consider the potential impact of both positive and negative results.

In their situation, Inaya and Muhammad could have chosen to stage the testing beginning with Inaya and then, depending on test results, to pursue testing for Maya. Although this approach would not have provided definitive reassurance with respect to Maya's learning difficulties, it might have allowed the parents more time to adjust to their newly learned family information. For some families, this provides a welcome relief from focusing on pathology, while for others, the delay may exacerbate any underlying anxiety. Nonetheless, having this option and being involved in decision-making provides families with some degree of control. Given that Inaya's sister was heterozygous for a premutation, Inaya's a priori risk to also carry a premutation was 50%; the potential implications for all of her children, including Maya, were explored in anticipation that Inaya's test results might indicate heterozygosity for a premutation. This would mean that each of her children would be at increased risk for inheriting a premutation or a full mutation. Some time was devoted to discussing the transmission of genes and the sense of guilt felt by many parents when they learn that they had indeed transmitted a genetic alteration. The genetic counselor asked Inaya how she thought she might feel were such a situation to unfold. She said that she was already feeling exceedingly worried about Maya, but since her learning difficulties were not severe in comparison to what she had come to understand about fragile X syndrome, she said that she didn't really know what to think. She was apprehensive about exploring her feelings in depth both because Maya was present and because she said that she was afraid to do so. The genetic counselor suggested an opportunity to speak with Inaya privately but Inaya declined, preferring to wait until the results became available.

An alternative approach to testing involved initiating testing for both Inaya and Maya at the same time because of Maya's learning difficulties. Had Maya not had any reported difficulties, the genetic counselor would have undertaken a discussion about the implications of initiating genetic testing on a minor when there were no clear cut health-related benefits (Clarke, 1994; ASHG/ACMG Report, 1995; Bioethics Committee, Canadian Paediatric Society, 2003). However, given her learning difficulties the testing was considered diagnostic, and establishing a genetic etiology would likely allow this family to access additional supports through the educational system than would otherwise be available to them. Inaya and Muhammad chose to initiate testing on both Maya and Inaya at the same time.

Test Results and Follow-Up

Inaya's molecular result revealed 30 and 62 CGG repeats. Maya's result was surprising; the test revealed that Maya was a compound heterozygote for the FMR1 premutation with 70 and 81 CGG repeats. The laboratory coordinator asked whether the parents were consanguineous, and a review of the chart indicated that they had denied consanguinity.

The genetic counselor sought out published data and expert guidance regarding the clinical implications of this test result before contacting the family (Mazzocco and Holden, 1996; McConkie Rosell, personal communication). This represented a rare occurrence and the one published family with 3 sisters who were compound heterozygotes for the FMR-1 premutation suggested no deficits or difficulties. However, the implications for reproductive risk were significant. The genetic counselor also consulted with colleagues within her work setting, including clinical geneticists, genetic counselors, social workers, and bioethicists as she planned how to communicate this information.

Different approaches may be considered for providing test result information. Some genetic counselors may prefer to have an appointment scheduled without providing information via telephone, but others feel that once initial genetic counseling is provided that individuals are appropriately prepared to receive the results by telephone and delaying information transfer serves to increase anxiety. The latter was felt to be true for this family. The genetic counselor telephoned Inaya to provide some preliminary information regarding the available test results. During the telephone conversation, Inaya's carrier status was disclosed and she was told that Maya's results were available and that she had, as well, inherited the premutation but that there was a finding that was difficult to interpret given the information provided.

Given that Inaya and Muhammad had denied consanguinity in the first appointment, the genetic counselor considered other possible explanations for Maya's result, including a laboratory technical issue, unacknowledged consanguinity, or misattributed paternity. Individuals may not always be forthcoming about their family information, either by intent or otherwise. Although the genetic counselor asked to schedule another appointment to discuss the results, she began with the most parsimonious explanation for the molecular findings and told Inaya that she wanted to check the family history she had taken during the first appointment. She then asked Inaya again if she and Muhammad were related by blood. To this question, Inaya expressed some surprise and said that, in fact, they were second cousins; during the first appointment, they hadn't really focused on this question and in retrospect thought that being second cousins would not be relevant for a disorder that was being passed through her family. The genetic counselor indicated that this information was very helpful and that she would explain everything during the follow-up appointment. Inaya did not ask for additional information at that time but asked if she could come in with only her husband for the next appointment so that they could speak more openly and to seek advice about how to proceed. Although Inaya's affirmation of consanguinity provided resolution to the unexpected molecular result in Maya, it also led to mixed emotions in the genetic counselor, somewhat easier to mask given that the conversation was via telephone. This entire outcome clearly merited deeper reflection, but the initial feelings involved both relief at having an explanation and embarrassment that the issue of consanguinity hadn't been confirmed during the appointment, the latter emotion potentially arising from a lack of due diligence in soliciting the family history and/or that the question may have been presented in such a manner as to have inhibited the truthful response from the family, although certainly other explanations, including Inaya's, were also plausible.

Session 2: Follow-Up Appointment—Results Disclosure

Although the original referral criteria pertained to Maya, there were now two other individuals in this family with testing results that required further discussion (an adult female carrier of a premutation and an adult male carrier of a premutation), hence three patients. At this follow-up appointment, the genetic counselor chose to begin by reviewing Inaya's results, as this seemed the most logical approach. Inaya said that she had tried to mentally prepare herself for a positive (premutation) testing result; nonetheless, her reaction to reviewing the test results was clearly one of distress and she had been crying on and off since the telephone call several days earlier. Inaya admitted that she had been hoping for a normal result and that her worry about the well-being of her children was almost overwhelming. During this time, Muhammad sat quietly beside his wife; they had chosen seats on a couch for this appointment rather than in separate chairs; this allowed them to sit physically closer to one another. The genetic counselor asked Muhammad about his feelings regarding Inaya's test results. He said that although he was upset he really wanted to focus on helping Maya and was apprehensive about her test results.

The genetic counselor quietly talked about the emotional sequelae experienced by other carriers of X-linked disorders in transmitting an alteration to their children. Inaya calmed during this discussion and was no longer looking down into her lap, but rather she maintained eye contact with the genetic counselor. Had Inaya's result been the only available data for this appointment, the genetic counselor would have spent additional time exploring Inaya's feelings; however given Maya's molecular test result, the focus was then shifted to discussing this issue.

The genetic counselor then explained Maya's test result, drawing a diagram to assist with the explanation. Given the paucity of information available on females who are compound heterozygotes for FMR1 premutations, information was drawn from the data available on heterozygous premutation carriers. Although much of the available literature indicates normal intelligence and appearance for premutation carriers, there exists some concern regarding potential influences on areas of emotional well-being and learning; as well, clinical findings in adults include premature ovarian failure and FXTAS–tremor/ataxia syndrome in older premutation carriers, the latter more frequently diagnosed in males but also reported in some female carriers (Hagerman and Hagerman, 2004; Lachiewicz et al., 2006; Saul and Tarleton, 2007; Wittenberger et al., 2007, McConkie-Rosell et al., 2007). Therefore, Maya's learning problems may have been due to her molecular status or may have been coincidental. Inaya and Muhammad indicated that they were distressed by her test result but were also somewhat relieved to know that she did not have fragile X syndrome. These conflicting emotions led them to feel confused and somewhat helpless as they did not know how to proceed in order to help her. In fact, this situation is not uncommon in the clinical genetics arena, when testing may not clarify a diagnosis or one's risk to develop a disorder (e.g., ambiguous test results, relatively low sensitivity of specific genetic testing, etc.), although certainly this represented a unique situation for all those involved in this case.

The genetic counselor offered to make a referral for a full educational assessment for Maya with the hospital-based team of developmental experts. In the local school system, such assessments are important to access publicly funded remedial interventions and are reviewed and updated at appropriate points in time. This assessment was meant to identify Maya's strengths as well as issues that could benefit from targeted intervention. Her parents were relieved to learn that the assessment would also note areas of strength and not just focus on Maya's deficits. The genetic counselor informed Inaya and Muhammad that if she were to make the referral, then disclosure of Maya's DNA results would be included both because these results could be relevant to her assessment and because this information could be found in her hospital chart. However, because of Maya's unique test result (i.e., compound heterozygote), it was important for her parents to be aware that these results might be misinterpreted by healthcare providers or educators and that Maya could be inappropriately "labeled" as having fragile X syndrome. The intent of raising this issue was not to frighten Maya's parents but rather to allow them to appropriately advocate for their daughter. Alternatively, Inaya and Muhammad could themselves organize a referral with the school psychoeducational team based upon the concerns raised by her teachers or a private referral and choose whether or not to disclose the molecular results. They admitted that they were very private individuals and, in the past, had only shared personal issues with a very select group of family and friends. In this situation, however, they felt conflicted as to what might be the best approach for supporting Maya's development, and they wanted to consider this further. Long-term issues regarding reproductive risks and potentially altered ovarian function had been briefly reviewed in the pretest session, and further discussion of these issues was left to a future appointment given the volume and significance of information left to be covered. Information about fragile X-associated tremor/ataxia syndrome in premutation carriers was raised later in this session.

Inaya began to consider her other two children, and she again became distressed thinking about their future and whether they would be marked in some manner or deemed less desirable for marriage in their community. She didn't know how and when and with whom to share this information without causing harm. But throughout, she and her husband both agreed that they wanted to begin by talking with Maya at an appropriate time. They felt that given Maya's age, they would likely focus their discussion on information about their family history and carrier status. They also felt that it was important to introduce to her the notion of fragile X syndrome, as this term might be used inappropriately by some of the educational or health care providers. The genetic counselor presented the notion of normalizing the educational assessment by indicating that many children have strengths and weaknesses at school or in other activities.

Once a plan for Maya had been established, Inaya and Muhammad wanted to talk specifically about testing for their other children. They felt that after talking alone with Maya, they would follow the same plan with Nadeem and Rana together, that is, talking about their family history and about their own test results and the implications for each of them. If Maya were present and wanted to talk about her results, or what she understood of them, they would be supportive. The genetic counselor suggested that Nadeem and Rana be given the opportunity to consider this information for as long as they needed and that they should not be made to feel under pressure to make a decision regarding testing especially as neither was encountering any significant problem. Even though their children were at very different stages in emotional and intellectual development, Inaya and Muhammad felt that it was important to process this as a family unit. They would schedule a follow-up appointment at an appropriate time in the future depending on the concerns raised by their children. The counselor informed them that the appointment could include any or all of their children and that Rana and Nadeem would be given the opportunity to talk with the genetic counselor independent of their parents and sibs. The parents were not totally comfortable with this last approach but understood its merit (see section on: Considerations: genetic counseling and adolescents).

Finally, the discussion turned to the origin of the second triplet repeat expansion, although Inaya and Muhammad had already begun to anticipate this from the question regarding consanguinity. Testing was offered to Muhammad to confirm his molecular status and to provide information for other family members. As well, Muhammad was aware of information from the initial discussion and his Internet searches regarding fragile X-associated tremor/ataxia syndrome. This information was reviewed with both Muhammad and Inaya along with the recommendation to disclose this to their family physician for appropriate monitoring and neurological assessment if clinically indicated.

The genetic counselor told them that she would telephone Muhammad's results to him (which she did several weeks later) and left it to them to contact her for follow-up as needed. They appreciated that they could schedule a follow-up appointment either together or individually, and the genetic counselor again told them that she would be available to talk via telephone, if they so preferred. While she was concerned about providing them with additional opportunities to work through their new situation, she also respected that they felt that they needed a break from the intensity of coping with so much information about each family member. The genetic counselor also felt that they had displayed appropriate emotional responses and were moving forward in the adaptation process.

Recontact from Family

Approximately 6 months later, Inaya telephoned to provide an update. She said that she and her husband had first spoken with Maya to tell her that they were going to try to obtain help for her in school and that she should not feel embarrassed because many children had extra help. They chose to organize this assessment privately in order to avoid confounding the situation with faulty assumptions that she had fragile X syndrome. Maya remembered having a blood test, and Inaya told her that she and Maya shared similar results and that they would talk with her in the future about her specific test results. They said that Maya accepted this without any apparent distress and seemed reassured that she was like her mother. Inaya and Muhammad then met with all of their children together to discuss their family history and their own test results. She said that their children listened intently and asked several questions about what testing they should or could pursue. They were informed about the availability of blood testing and an opportunity for genetic counseling before any decision they might make. After some time, Nadeem told his mother that he wanted to book an appointment, and when his mother said that she would want to attend, he did not disagree. Rana said that she wasn't really interested, at least not at the present time.

Considerations: Genetic Counseling and Adolescents

Considerations regarding genetic testing offered to children in the institution in which this family was seen generally adhere to the guidelines provided by the Canadian Paediatric Society, the American College of Medical Genetics, the American Society of Human Genetics, and the British Working Party (Clarke, 1994; ASHG/ACMG Report, 1995; Bioethics Committee, Canadian Paediatric Society, 2003). Furthermore, there is no defined chronological age at which medical decision-making automatically transitions to the adolescent. Rather, the health care provider assesses the maturity and the capacity of the adolescent to be able to comprehend the information provided and to make an informed decision. This approach may vary somewhat between different institutions and may be further guided by relevant social and clinical parameters and by local or federal statutes.

Regardless of who would ultimately make the decision about testing (i.e., parent or child), given their chronological ages, genetic counseling was organized for Nadeem and Rana. As such, consideration was given to the emotional and cognitive stages of adolescent development (Weil p. 2000) and this would be explored during the session(s) along with potential psychosocial issues. As well, the genetic counselor considered the language to be incorporated and planned to listen for their verbal cues so as to better tailor the approach. Engaging adolescents in a meaningful dialogue also requires recognition that their thought processes are often concrete rather than abstract and their decisions may involve consideration of issues only relevant to their lives at present; they are unlikely to fully consider the future impact of their decisions and actions. Finally, recent research underscores the importance of first assessing what the adolescents wish to learn before embarking on the planned agenda (Szybowska et al., 2007). However, if there is a significant gap between what the genetic counselor feels is important for decision-making and what knowledge the adolescent wishes to learn, this will require some negotiation and a framing of why the information may be important. This may ultimately involve a delicate balancing act in order for the genetic counselor to provide due diligence and for the adolescent to feel that he or she has exerted some autonomy in the session.

Many have raised concern about subsequent negative sequelae when genetic testing is undertaken during adolescence (Fanos, 1997). Such concerns have included the potential for stigmatization, negative impact on self-esteem and social relationship development, and even a negative self-fulfilling prophecy for those adolescents found to have genetic mutations or alterations. However, a number of studies have demonstrated little basis for long-lasting impact (Clow and Scriver, 1977; Zeesman et al., 1984; Jarvinen et al. 1999; Jarvinen et al., 2000), and, in fact, there appears to be a preference for learning about carrier status in early adolescence (McConkie-Rosell et al., 1997; Fanos and Gatti, 1999; McConkie-Rosell et al., 1999; McConkie-Rosell et al., 2002).

Considerations: Family Systems and Cultural Competence

Constructs of family systems such as Rolland's integrated family systems illness model may not be directly applicable for families dealing with certain genetic disorders that do not present as life-threatening, although there are many highly relevant concepts. This model describes the multifaceted, dynamic interactions between the patient, the family, and the physical disorder (Rolland, 1987). Family systems theories may incorporate a number of life aspects including the role of beliefs systems, cultural, social and historic contexts, ongoing influences of family members on one another, the transgenerational nature of genetic disorders, and the uncertainties of chronic health issues and anticipatory loss (Rolland, 1987; Germain, 1994; Street and Soldan, 1998; Weil, 2000). Frameworks such as those developed by Street and Soldan (1998), which outline typical life-cycle phases (e.g., adolescent to adult), psychosocial issues, and possible transitions (e.g., identification of carrier status), can serve to guide genetic counselors in their practice. Moreover, in combination with the genetic counselor's knowledge about the disorder and the family story, such paradigms can enhance genetic counseling approaches regarding decision-making, coping, and anticipatory management; as well, family systems theories may be used to further support the family in incorporating the genetic issue into their life story without allowing it to define any one family member or the family as a whole (Germain, 1994; Street and Soldan, 1998; Weil, 2000).

Competency in cross-cultural genetic counseling relies upon a commitment from the genetic counselor to actively reflect on personal assumptions, biases, knowledge (or lack thereof), and behaviors. As well, it involves appropriate preparation for genetic counseling through ongoing development of skills, strategies, and knowledge. However, information gleaned should serve only as a jumping off point for genetic counselors to engage individuals from culturally different backgrounds in a sincere and nonjudgmental manner in order to learn about their worldview, acculturation, and assimilation (Ibrahim, 1991; Sue et al., 1995; Weil, 2001; Lewis, 2002).

Session 3

Nadeem attended the appointment with both of his parents. The genetic counselor invited him into the counseling room on his own, and his parents had been prepared for this approach. The genetic counselor spent a short period of time talking with Nadeem about his family history and eliciting information. It became apparent that Nadeem had a good understanding of his personal situation and that he was at risk to have inherited the premutation; he also understood that by virtue of his abilities that he was not at increased risk to have fragile X syndrome. The genetic counselor asked why he had requested this appointment, and he felt that in the following year he would be away at university and the logistics would then become complicated. When asked if he would like his parents to join him in the appointment, he gave a positive response. The genetic counselor also asked him to consider if he did pursue testing after the appointment, how he would want the results disclosed to him. Would he want to schedule a follow-up appointment now, have the results telephoned to him personally, or telephoned to one of his parents to communicate to him? He would need to select an option by the end of the appointment, although certainly this could be altered at his direction.

Inaya and Muhammad joined Nadeem and information was reviewed pertaining to fragile X syndrome, the inheritance, the molecular etiology, and the risks for transmitting males including the increased risk for tremors/ataxia later in life. Nadeem accepted the information with few questions but maintained eye contact and appeared fully engaged. He seemed to appreciate having the session focused on his needs, with his parents being there primarily for his support. Inaya and Muhammad were very respectful of his autonomy, letting him know that they were there to support him and help with his decision-making. Nadeem chose to pursue testing and asked if the result could be telephoned to him at home and to have one of his parents on the extension. His molecular result indicated that he had 95 CGG repeats and he accepted the information, saying that he "kind of expected it." Marriage and the possibility of adult-onset tremors seemed a long way off to him, and he felt that he would deal with it when the appropriate time came. He declined a follow-up appointment but said that he would call if he had any concerns or wished to schedule an appointment either alone or with a potential life partner in the future.

Session 4

Several months later, Inaya again called and said that Rana was asking many questions and she and her husband felt that it would be best to schedule an appointment for all three of them. She felt that Rana would not want to meet on her own but understood that the option would be presented. Indeed, when the genetic counselor asked Rana if she preferred to proceed on her own for a portion of the session or meet with her parents, she emphatically stated that she wanted her parents present. Upon questioning, Rana summarized what she understood about fragile X and said that she had been thinking about this a lot. She indicated that she had selected this topic for a project in her Health Education class and now she really wanted to know what her status was. Rana had achieved excellent grades in school and presented at the appointment as a quiet, but relatively mature adolescent. She said that she knew she was a carrier because of her father's carrier status but that she still wanted to know her repeat size. This seemed to be of significant importance to her and when asked what this information might mean to her, she took some time to reply but eventually said that perhaps she would stop thinking about it so much. She said that she was curious but it really wasn't that important to her. This contradicted somewhat her comments about it occupying so much of her thinking and perhaps was an attempt to reassure herself. Inaya and Muhammad agreed to support her decision to pursue testing.

The genetic counselor explored (somewhat) Rana's psychological status and her ability to cope with the test results. Her parents felt that she was emotionally stable and that her shyness was in keeping with their family's emotive/behavioral gestalt. They were concerned about her future, as well as Maya's, including marriageability, but felt that fortunately this was still a long way off for both of their daughters. They held out hope that research would provide them with additional options that would be culturally and morally acceptable. They wanted to disclose the test result to Rana themselves, and Rana told the genetic counselor that this would be fine with her. The family knew that ongoing support and guidance would be available by telephone, email, and/or appointment.

Final Reflections

This complex case presented numerous learning opportunities for the genetic counselor. The eventual uncovering of consanguinity was humbling in that the family history acquisition had seemed to be a straightforward and an easily completed component. As noted above, further reflection was merited regarding the approach to interviewing (including verbal cues and body language) and whether this may have inhibited a more forthcoming response. Moreover, perhaps along with the family, the X-linked basis of inheritance may have limited this line of questioning. In addition to personal reflection, much input was sought and subsequently incorporated from colleagues during small group discussions and case presentation. Maya's molecular result also presented an unanticipated challenge for communication, especially because of the limited correlative data. Trying to meet the needs of each family member as autonomous individuals and within their family construct required a thoughtful, measured approach as well as review of appropriate developmental literature. Finally, the generosity of the family in sharing their experiences, feelings, and perceptions was enriching for the genetic counselor. This case seemed to unfold, and with each layer, subtle nuances were revealed about the family dynamic and life story. Ongoing reflection throughout this case and afterwards provided opportunities for the genetic counselor to grow professionally and to consider approaches to better serve the needs of each family member and the family unit as a whole—approaches that would then be transferable to other families.

REPRODUCTIVE GENETICS CASE (Donna F. Blumenthal)

Introduction

The following case illustrates the decision-making process of one couple in response to their amniocentesis result. This case was specifically selected because it demonstrates that the counselor can serve as facilitator of that process, regardless of the patient's final decision. It is incumbent upon the counselor to help the patient see the factors that are relevant to him or her. Since there is no one right decision for all patients, the same set of circumstances can result in a very different decision for another couple. The same genetic counseling principles and interviewing techniques apply. As counselors, it is our responsibility to help patients articulate their circumstances, values, beliefs, and priorities so that they can base their decision on all the factors that are relevant to them. If that can be accomplished, then the counselor has done her job.

Background

Cathy C., a 38-year-old woman of Irish Catholic descent, was referred at 19 weeks of gestation because her amniocentesis, performed for advanced maternal age, revealed a karyotype of 46XY/47XXY (mosaic Klinefelter syndrome). When asked their understanding of why they came for genetic counseling, the couple said that they had come because of Cathy's Ehlers–Danlos syndrome (EDS) and the amniocentesis result. The counselor had been unaware of any history of EDS, but it was apparent that the patient wanted to address it. The first 10 minutes of the session was spent discussing Cathy's chronic condition. Asking open-ended specific questions such as "What was it like to grow up with this condition?" and more focused questions such as "How were you diagnosed?" helped the counselor to get a sense of who Cathy was and how her condition had impacted her. The counselor learned that Cathy was a physician in the Department of Pediatrics. She had a history of mitral and tricuspid valve insufficiency and chronic orthopedic problems. She recalled spending much of her public school career in crutches because of recurrent joint dislocations and ankle sprains. She had always had "cigarette-paper scars," as she now referred to them, which were never biopsied. No one realized the connection between the scars and her knee and ankle problems until she entered medical school, where she was finally diagnosed with Ehlers–Danlos syndrome. Her 36-year-old Ashkenazi Jewish husband, Mark L., is also a physician and has an orthopedic practice at another location. They have one healthy three-year-old son. They had no genetic counseling before their amniocentesis.

Commentary

The couple's impression was that they were referred for two reasons, EDS and their amniocentesis results. The counselor assumed that the primary purpose of the visit was to interpret the amniocentesis result. Their expectations of the session were quite different from the counselor's in that they focused on the patient's condition for a significant amount of time. Perhaps their medical backgrounds led them to approach the session from a clinical standpoint. The difference between the couple's and the counselor's agendas illustrates the importance of asking and not just assuming. As the session progressed it became apparent that EDS was such a big part of the patient's identity that her narrative would have been necessary to explore eventually, if not initially. There is no one right order for facts to be revealed.

Equally curious was the omission of any mention of the risk to their offspring for EDS. Recognizing a potential gap in the patient's narrative, the counselor asked the couple if they had concerns about having a child with EDS, and if they knew their options for molecular studies and prenatal diagnosis. They said that they were not interested in prenatal diagnosis for EDS because it would not influence their plans for this child or pregnancy. This questioning served to close the gap and redirect the focus of the conversation to the amniocentesis result.

Before their amniocentesis, the couple had not been prepared for the possibility of any abnormal result other than Down syndrome. When their obstetrician told them that the result was mosaic Klinefelter syndrome, they researched the condition on the Internet. The information they obtained paralleled the description that the counselor provided: Klinefelter syndrome is characterized by tall stature, infertility, and an increased risk for speech and language delays. Other features are highly variable and include female distribution of body fat, shy personality, delays in motor skills, learning problems, and poor school performance. (Pai, 2003; Linden et al., 2002; Ratcliffe and Paul, 1986). IQ averages 10–15 points below that of their siblings. Testosterone therapy improves body habitus, self-esteem, ability to concentrate, and libido, but not fertility. Fifty percent of individuals develop gynecomastia, which may be treated surgically if it does not resolve on its own. Klinefelter syndrome is not associated with mental retardation, major physical anomalies, or shortened life expectancy. Some individuals are only mildly affected and may never come to medical attention. It is not possible to predict the severity based on the karyotype. The fact that a normal cell line was identified further increases the likelihood of a normal phenotype, but the prognosis for any one individual can still fall anywhere in the spectrum (Gardner and Sutherland, 2004; Christian, 2000).

I asked what it would mean to them to have a child that met this description. They were more or less in agreement that it would be difficult to raise a child with Klinefelter syndrome and, more importantly, to *be* a child with Klinefelter syndrome. However, they could not come to grips with the fact that there was also a normal cell line present and the possibility that this could be a perfectly normal child. Cathy could not see terminating a pregnancy that might result in a perfectly normal or mildly affected child, while Mark could not see his way to continuing a pregnancy with the risk of a child with the full-blown syndrome. I asked each of them what they felt were the pros and cons of each decision and if they could describe the worst- and best-case scenarios. To Mark, the worst case would be a son with academic and psychosocial problems who would drain their financial and emotional resources to the detriment of their older child. To Cathy, the worst case would be to terminate the pregnancy, and to wonder for the rest of her life what this child would have been like, believing that she did the wrong thing, and that she in some way would ultimately have to answer for her wrongdoing. They went over the symptoms of Klinefelter syndrome again and again.

Commentary

The earlier conversation about Cathy's EDS was quite relevant after all. Did she see this child as no more or less perfect than herself? What if her mother had terminated for EDS of unknown severity? Now she was carrying a pregnancy that would result in a child with mosaic Klinefelter of unknown severity.

The counselor's perspectives impact the genetic counseling session, and therefore it is important for the counselor to ask herself how she feels about a particular circumstance and decision. There may be little correlation between what the counselor thinks she would do in a hypothetical situation and what she actually does if faced with that situation. However, if she is not aware of her feelings and opinions, she may mistakenly believe that her feelings are also what the patient is feeling. If the counselor is self-aware, she might be better able to keep her statements and questions unbiased. It is possible, perhaps even probable, that Cathy and Mark had made some assumptions about the geneticist's and genetic counselor's opinion of their case. "Patients may scrutinize the genetic counselor for an eyeblink or a shrug of the shoulders that, at a crucial point in the discussion, might indicate to them the counselor's own feelings" (Tishler, 1981). Patients can be very sensitive to what they imagine the counselor's opinion to be, and may be reluctant to divulge feelings that they think are contrary to hers.

Cathy then focused on the termination procedure itself, wanting to know exactly how it was performed. Mark kept asking her to think instead about the big picture, that this decision would have a lifelong impact and needs to be viewed in that larger context. He explained to her that the procedure would consume just a few short days, while the child would present lifelong challenges.

Commentary

There is a trap in describing phenotypes to prenatal patients that is very easy for students and new counselors to fall into. It stems from a natural inclination to answer a question when it is asked, as you might in normal conversation, instead of wondering about the reason for the question. Consider the following dialogue:

> *Patient: "Will my baby be mentally retarded?"*
>
> *Counselor: "No. He may have delayed speech and learning problems, but most boys with Klinefelter syndrome attend regular high school and may even go further in their education."*
>
> *Patient: "Will he be infertile?"*
>
> *Counselor: "There is a chance he will, but he may not be; the presence of the normal cell line makes fertility a possibility. Besides, 10% of couples today are infertile for a variety of reasons and there are many options available for reproduction."*
>
> *Patient: "Will he be handicapped?"*
>
> *Counselor: "No, he won't."*
>
> *Patient: "You want me to continue this pregnancy!"*

In truth, the counselor may have had no preference one way or the other for how the couple should proceed, but it is easy to see how the patient may have reached the conclusion that she did. It may be helpful, instead of answering her questions, to ask what each of the symptoms means to her. For example: "How do you feel about the possibility of learning disabilities?" "How do you feel about the chance for infertility?" and "What about the chance for social problems, the chance that he won't fit in with his peers?" (Kessler, 1992, and personal communication). The couple may never have consciously considered the weight of each of these issues before. In hearing themselves state how important or unimportant academics, fertility, and independence are, they will be better able to make the best decision for themselves and less reliant on their perceptions of others' opinions and perspectives.

As difficult as it is for some patients to decide what to do when the diagnosis is clear, this couple had the added burden of having to make a decision without knowing as much about the outcome of the pregnancy as they would like. I explained to Cathy and Mark that ultimately their decision would be based on their tolerance for risk, because prenatal confirmation of the severity of Klinefelter syndrome would not be possible. They said that they needed a few days to mull it over and left that session undecided.

Tolerance for risk is related to one's comfort with uncertainty. Uncertainty is a major motivating factor in the decision to undergo prenatal as well as other types of genetic analysis, such as presymptomatic testing. For couples faced with prenatal results that present a range of risk, a great deal of uncertainty remains. The decision-making process often involves a sorting through of worst- and best-case scenarios while weighing the likelihood of those types of outcomes. For some the persistence of uncertainty for an indefinite period of time, for example, throughout childhood, is envisioned to be difficult. Some couples would expect to be watching and waiting for any sign of developmental delay and problem behavior. Would Mark and Cathy be scrutinizing their child for any sign of Klinefelter syndrome, and if so, for how long?

Decisions are made within an individual's frame of reference or context. Having a genetic diagnosis in Cathy played a role not only in this husband's and wife's perception of the potential for problems in their pregnancy but also in their perception of their severity. Having a child or children, whether healthy or not, also contributes toward an individual's frame of reference. Furthermore, this couple's experiences as physicians may have increased their sensitivities to possible medical problems. Marteau (2002) observed that patients counseled by geneticists were less likely to terminate than those counseled by other medical specialists, presumably because of their more accurate understanding of the diagnoses as relatively benign conditions. It is possible that geneticists have a different bias than their patients. The patient, by contrast, isn't comparing her future child to the patients that routinely present to a genetics clinic. The patient may be comparing her potential child to the children of her friends and relatives and to the child she hopes to have. As a result, the patient may perceive mosaic Klinefelter syndrome to be a greater burden than a medical geneticist would perceive it to be.

Christian et al. (2000) studied 169 couples from 1971 to 1997 whose prenatal diagnosis revealed a sex chromosome abnormality including mosaicism. The authors observed that the rate of termination decreased over the 26 years of the survey (from 100% termination rate at the beginning to 54% by 1997). They attributed the decrease in termination to the long-term prospective outcome studies that proposed a more optimistic prognosis than originally provided. Mezei et al. (2004), who also noted a decrease in termination rate over time (1990–2001), found that the most common reasons for which parents in their study were likely to terminate for a

diagnosis of a sex chromosome aneuploidy were fear of abnormal sexual develop-
ment or infertility. Sagi et al. (2001) interviewed 60 parents whose amniocenteses
revealed sex chromosome aneuploidy with or without mosaicism from 1989–1998. In
his study, 80% terminated. The most common reasons given were "fear of a
nonspecific abnormality" and "concerns about abnormal sexual development."

I called Cathy and Mark three days later to find out how they were doing. Cathy
answered. She told me that they had decided to terminate. In fact, she had just gotten
home from the laminaria placement. She said that "One of us had to compromise to
save our marriage, and I couldn't see him compromising." She was expressing her
priorities, and they were that her marriage was more important to her than continuing
this pregnancy, despite her belief that she would ultimately have to answer for her
decision.

Commentary

Kenen (2000) examined the role of the male in the decision-making process. He might
*categorize this couple's decision-making style as one of **saliency**. Kenen hypothesized*
that the male partner's impact seems to depend in part on the couple's decision-
*making style. In the **domain** style of decision-making, the couple has divided up their*
responsibilities and concedes to the partner who has the brunt of the responsibility in
*that area. The **joint-delegated** style involves lengthy discussion between the partners*
*and compromise. In the **saliency** style, "if there is still disagreement, it is decided in*
favor of the partner who feels the strongest about the matter." In Cathy and Mark's
case, it appears that Mark's need to terminate was stronger than Cathy's need to
continue. It would have been interesting to explore how other decisions of theirs were
resolved and whether they adhered to a specific style.

Cathy expressed concern about what to say to her son. He was very much expecting
a younger brother or sister. I asked her what she was thinking of saying. She said that
she was going to say "the baby went to heaven." Her son was familiar with heaven
because his friend's grandmother had died and that's where she went. Her other
thought was to say that "the seed that was planted was not growing." She had used a
seed analogy to explain how the pregnancy came to be, and felt this seed-not-growing
metaphor logically followed from that. I commented that, in spite of everything, she
was still able to think of her son's best interests. I recommended additional resources
for her such as *A Time To Decide, A Time To Heal* (Minnick and Delp, eds.) as well as
psychological counseling. I relayed to her some suggestions about how to approach
her son, recommending not to draw a connection between the hospital and the loss, to
remind him that this is something that can only happen to babies before they are born,
that is, not him (his seed "grew") and not his parents, and that he did not cause this loss
by anything he may have said, felt, or thought. I told her I would call again after the
procedure.

I called three days later and Mark answered. The following is my transcript of that
phone conversation: I asked how it went and he said, "It went." Then he added, "It was
pretty tough. It wasn't easy. The day before was difficult. The day of was torturous for
both of us, more for her, because she was in pain, and concept-wise. The procedure

went well. There was minimal bleeding. The doctor said there should be no problem conceiving in the future." I noticed how he quickly changed the subject from her pain to the procedure. I said that I was glad that the procedure went smoothly, and that she was lucky to have someone like him who recognized how difficult it was for her, physically and emotionally.

I asked him when he planned to return to work. He said that he was returning to work tomorrow, but that she planned to take off an indeterminate amount of time. I asked what he planned to tell his co-workers. He said he was going to say his "wife had some cramping and bleeding and when they went to the doctor there was no heart beat." He added that he hoped that no one would push for further details. He tried to imagine if he would put someone in the awkward position of having to divulge details, and decided that he would not. They decided to tell everyone that they had had a miscarriage. In fact, he was in the process of devising a list of people to call. "Only our families know the truth," he said. "We did not tell her sisters the truth because they would judge her, and no one really knows what they would do faced with the same situation."

Commentary

Apparently, when Mark said that their families know, he did not include Cathy's sisters. By the nature of our jobs, genetic counselors are privy to information about our patients' diagnoses and decisions that they might not even share with their closest friends and relatives. In their book, Men Don't Cry... Women Do, Martin and Doka (2000) explain that social support varies for given losses. They define **disenfranchised loss** *as a loss that is not openly acknowledged, socially sanctioned, or publicly shared such as divorce, prenatal loss, or relationship loss, respectively. Therefore patients experiencing disenfranchised loss can't avail themselves of their usual support networks. Although the genetic counselor can't replace friends and family, she can provide a sympathetic ear.*

Mark continued that he had observed a pregnancy termination in medical school and that it was very upsetting. At that point Cathy got on the phone and cut Mark off. She was anxious to relate her ordeal. She said that during the procedure, "no one talked to me, only to my husband." I asked, "Why do you think that was?" and she said, "They didn't want to talk to me because of what I did." I said, "You felt they were judging you." She went on to elaborate about how very upset she was that no one talked to her. She mentioned that she had antiabortion literature at home that exacerbated her distress. She couldn't come to grips with the details of the procedure. Cathy was also upset because people kept telling her "not to think about it." All the doctors avoided answering her "questions about how they stop the baby's heart." I asked why that was. She said, "I think it's because it's too horrible to say." She continued, "As I was leaving, one nurse said 'I hope to see you soon on the third floor'." I asked what that was, and she said 'L&D' (the Labor & Delivery floor). I asked her what she thought the nurse meant by that. She said, "She hopes that next time I'll continue the pregnancy."

Commentary

The counselor had interpreted the nurse's comment to mean that she hoped that Cathy had better luck in the future. Cathy was feeling so guilty, though, that she interpreted the nurse's comment as judgmental and accusatory.

I referred Cathy to our social worker, Shelly, who sees patients privately and also facilitates a group for parents who have terminated a pregnancy because of prenatal test results. She was reluctant to call Shelly at first since she and the social worker know many people in common. However, after a very upsetting interview with an outside therapist, she relented.

Cathy has since spoken with Shelly in person and by phone, but declined the group. Cathy had told her that she felt like a murderer. She also said that she would have been able to deal with a son with Klinefelter since she treats children with medical problems every day. Over time, the social worker helped her deal with her feelings of guilt and regret.

The counselor never had the opportunity to continue her conversation with Mark. He seemed very distressed by the termination procedure, but he conceded the phone immediately once his wife picked up the receiver. He may have felt less deserving of a counselor's time and sympathy since the option he wanted was the one that was chosen. He might have benefited from the chance to express his feelings to a neutral party, and it is possible that he pursued this course on his own at a later time.

Commentary

Counselors don't often obtain long-term follow-up information on their patients, so it is hard to learn what was helpful and what was not, or even harmful. Exploring some of the variables that mitigate or complicate the recovery period after a termination might help the couple down the road. Korenromp et al. (2005a) surveyed 196 women in the Netherlands two to seven years after they terminated a pregnancy for abnormal prenatal diagnosis. The majority of women had adjusted well. However, the authors found a significant risk of posttraumatic stress syndrome, especially if the women terminated after 14 weeks' gestation, for a condition that was compatible with life, and if the women were less well-educated and lacked the support of their partners, compared to women who terminated before 14 weeks' gestation, for lethal conditions, who were better educated, and had the support of their partners. Lack of partner support at the time of the termination procedure was a significant predictor of posttraumatic stress, grief, anxiety, and depression (Korenromp, 2005b). In this study, both men and women viewed termination as more of a traumatic event than a loss. In fact, 17% of women had pathological levels of posttraumatic stress and were more likely to express doubt and regret about their decision, compared to 2.5% of women ten months after a normal pregnancy and delivery. An area for future investigation might be to compare the extent of these same variables, posttraumatic stress, loss, grief, doubt, regret, anxiety, and depression, with parents who choose to continue their pregnancies after receiving abnormal prenatal test results.

A couple may appreciate some anticipatory guidance relating to the grieving process. Martin and Doka (2000) suggest that there are differences in the way in which men and women grieve. Women are more likely to need to express their sadness and seek the company of others. They tend to their feelings of grief. Men, although not exclusively, tend to address their thoughts about grief. They tend to express their grief through actions such as directing their energy in creative or constructive ways, for example, in maintaining a garden or building a car. Korenromp (2005b), in his survey of Dutch couples who terminated for abnormal prenatal diagnosis, found that women had higher levels of grief, stress, and anxiety than men but men had higher levels of avoidance, where avoidance is defined as "an intrapsychic process in which the implications of the event are denied or avoided." Korenromp may have stumbled upon one of the differences between the way men and women grieve. Consequently, they misinterpreted a more cognitive style of grieving as avoidance. A patient himself or herself may wonder whether something is wrong with him or her because he or she is not grieving in the conventional way.

Summary

It is not hard to see that another couple in the same position could have chosen a different path. Cathy could just as easily have said, "In order to save our marriage, Mark decided that we should *continue* the pregnancy." We really don't know enough about the strength of their marriage to predict which stresses would be too great for it to withstand. The point is that the role of the counselor would be the same either way. The principle of genetic counseling to facilitate the decision-making process is the same regardless of the decision that patients make. What is critical is that patients are supported in making what they believe is the best choice at a particular point in time while confronted with a particular set of circumstances. Support should not only include full access to resources and information, but an exploration of beliefs, values, and priorities.

Some issues illustrated by this case were (1) the decision to terminate or continue was extraordinarily difficult, (2) the husband and wife took opposite positions, which can put a stress on the marriage, (3) accurate anticipatory information could have restored some sense of control, (4) shame and guilt may have deprived them of their usual support system, (5) the path not chosen may become idealized since we do not have to endure its consequences, and (6) we are all shaped by the experiences that we encounter in our lives. In this case, Cathy's orthopedic problems may have made her more accepting of the less-than-perfect child. Their decision-making styles and degree of psychological support, their occupations, and the reasons that they became physicians may have all played a role in what the diagnosis meant to them and in what they decided to do.

CANCER GENETICS CASE (Monica L. Marvin)

This case is discussed to illustrate common principles and considerations related to the provision of cancer genetic counseling. The case involves a 39-year-old woman,

Anne, referred to our Cancer Genetics Clinic by her oncologist because of her personal history of early-onset ovarian cancer and her family history of colorectal cancer. The structure of our clinic was such that the patient was seen by both a genetic counselor and a physician during her visit.

Medical History

We were able to review Anne's medical history by obtaining records from the referring physician and by eliciting information via a questionnaire the patient completed before her appointment.

Through the review of Anne's questionnaire and medical records, we learned that Anne was recently diagnosed with ovarian cancer at age 39. Her cancer was a stage IIC ovarian cancer, meaning that the cancer had spread to pelvic organs and that washings from the abdomen found evidence of cancer cells. The pathology report described this as an endometriod ovarian carcinoma with focal clear cell ovarian carcinoma. Anne's cancer treatment included a total abdominal hysterectomy with bilateral salpingooo-phorectomy (removal of the uterus, both ovaries, and Fallopian tubes) and chemotherapy. Imaging studies performed two months before her scheduled appointment in cancer genetics revealed no residual disease. In terms of screening for other cancers, the patient had undergone a number of normal screening colonoscopies in the past because of a family history of colorectal cancer. Her most recent colonoscopy was performed six months before her cancer genetics appointment. Anne had also undergone a baseline screening mammogram at age 35.

Commentary

The personal medical history collected from patients being seen for cancer risk assessment should include age, personal history of benign or malignant tumors, major illnesses, hospitalizations, surgeries, biopsy history, reproductive history, cancer screening and surveillance, and environmental exposures. For patients who have had a cancer, additional information collected should include the organ in which the tumor developed, age at diagnosis, number of tumors, pathology, stage and grade of malignant tumors, pathology of benign tumors, and treatment regimen (surgery, chemotherapy, and radiation). This information can be collected prior to the session through a questionnaire or at the time of the session (Trepanier et al., 2004).

Review of the patient's medical records is important for a number of reasons. First, documentation of the specific type of cancer (including both the site of the primary cancer and the pathology findings) is critical in an accurate assessment of a possible inherited risk for cancer. In addition to knowing the primary site of a cancer, review of the pathology report may reveal findings characteristic of cancers that arise in the setting of specific hereditary cancer syndromes. Second, it is important to document what the patient's treatment entailed, as it may impact the future cancer risk and/or management. For example, it was important to document that the patient had both ovaries and uterus removed. It is also important to note what previous cancer screening the patient has undergone. In this case, the fact that Anne had undergone screening colonoscopies in the past because of her family history of colorectal cancer suggested that she had some awareness of the importance of her family history. It also provided some reassurance regarding the possibility of a current colorectal cancer in Anne.

From a counseling standpoint, an understanding of the patient's personal experience with cancer, including the time since diagnosis, the status of her treatment, and her prognosis are also important in anticipating the needs and concerns that may arise in a session. In this particular case, the patient was diagnosed with a moderately advanced ovarian cancer, completed her treatment, and recently received reassuring news from her imaging studies and pelvic exams. At the time of her visit, her cancer appeared to be in remission. One would anticipate her needs, expectations, and frame of reference to be quite different if, for example, she had recently been diagnosed with a recurrence of her cancer or if we were seeing her just after the original diagnosis.

Finally, the fact that Anne completed her questionnaire and returned it before her appointment suggested that she intended to attend the counseling session and that she was at least minimally motivated to facilitate the process.

Family History

Family history information was also collected from Anne before her appointment through the questionnaire. In the setting of cancer genetics counseling, the information typically collected regarding family members includes at least a three-generation pedigree with attention to cancer diagnoses, ages of onset, the presence of multiple primary cancers, the presence of precancerous lesions, the presence of possible shared environmental factors, consanguinity, and ancestry/ethnicity. Both maternal and paternal histories should be collected, including both affected and unaffected relatives. Anne reported a striking family history of cancer, as shown in Figure 18-2.

Commentary

In reviewing the family history, it was worth noting that not only did Anne have an extremely strong family history of cancer, but nearly all of her relatives who had cancer died within just a few years of their cancer diagnoses. She had not witnessed any relatives survive their cancers. In a family such as Anne's, the genetic counselor might anticipate the patient equating a cancer diagnosis with a death sentence.

When reviewing a reported family history, it is also important to recognize that erroneous cancer reporting may occur (Love et al., 1985; Theis et al., 1994). Because the accuracy of the reported family history can have a profound impact on the counselor's assessment, it can be helpful to confirm cancer diagnoses reported in relatives. Studies suggest that the accuracy of reporting depends on the site of cancer and the degree of the relationship to the affected individual. The reporting of cancers in first-degree relatives is more accurate than reporting in second-or third-degree relatives. Furthermore, reporting of abdominal malignancies is particularly prone to inaccuracies, while reporting of breast cancers tends to be highly accurate (Douglas et al., 1999). When possible, family histories should be documented with medical

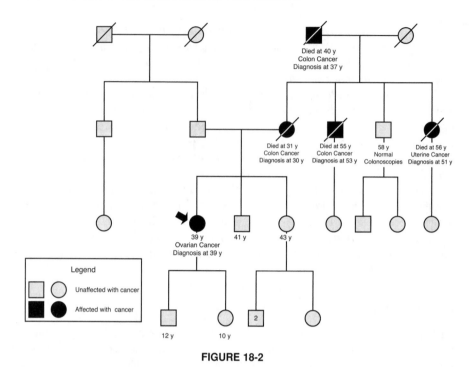

FIGURE 18-2

records. *This can be a time-consuming process, and engaging the patient in the process is essential. In some cases, documentation of the family history will not be possible or practical. Lack of documentation of the history should not serve as a barrier to services, but should be noted.*

Risk Assessment

Anne's personal history of ovarian cancer and family history of colorectal cancer were consistent with an autosomal dominant hereditary cancer predisposition. The findings of multiple generations affected with cancer, early ages of onset, and multiple primary cancers are hallmarks of a strong hereditary cancer risk in a family.

Approximately 10% of epithelial ovarian cancers are believed to be associated with a strong hereditary risk (Boyd, 2003). Patients with a strong hereditary risk for ovarian cancer typically come from three different types of families: (1) site-specific ovarian cancer, (2) hereditary breast and ovarian cancer syndrome, and (3) Lynch syndrome (also known as hereditary nonpolyposis colorectal cancer syndrome or HNPCC) (Lynch, 1997; Boyd, 2001). Families with site-specific ovarian cancer or hereditary breast and ovarian cancer syndrome most often harbor mutations of the BRCA1 or BRCA2 tumor suppressor genes (Ford et al., 1998). Families with Lynch typically harbor mutations of mismatch repair genes, including MLH1, MSH2, MSH6, and PMS2 (Lynch and de la Chapelle, 2003).

Review of the patient's striking family history of colorectal cancer made Lynch syndrome the obvious diagnosis in this family. Colorectal cancer is the main feature of Lynch syndrome. Other cancers including uterine, ovarian, biliary tract, stomach, and urinary tract cancers can also be found in families with Lynch syndrome (Marra and Boland, 1995; de la Chapelle, 2004; Hampel et al., 2005). The risk of developing cancer in Lynch syndrome is age dependent, with higher risks at increasing ages. The lifetime risk (by age 80) of developing colorectal cancer is estimated to be 69–82% in men and 52–82% in women (Aarnio et al., 1999; Hampel et al., 2005). The second most common cancer in Lynch syndrome is uterine cancer, with a lifetime risk estimated to be 40–70% (Dunlop et al., 1997; Aarnio et al., 1999; Cederquist et al., 2005). The lifetime risk for ovarian cancer is approximately 10–12% (Aarnio et al., 1999; Vasen et al., 2001).

Lynch syndrome generally results from a germline mutation in one of at least four mismatch repair genes. The two genes most commonly implicated are MLH1 and MSH2, accounting for 34% and 42% of families, respectively (Casey et al., 2005). Defects in the genes involved with mismatch repair lead to an accumulation of somatic mutations in a cell, which may result in a cancer. Colorectal cancers that arise in individuals with Lynch syndrome due to defective mismatch repair gene function exhibit a "molecular fingerprint" known as microsatellite instability (Lynch and de la Chapelle, 2003; Umar, 2004). Microsatellites are stretches of DNA with a repetitive sequence of nucleotides that are particularly susceptible to acquiring errors when mismatch repair gene function is impaired. Microsatellite instable tumors exhibit inconsistent numbers of microsatellite nucleotide repeats compared with normal tissue. The finding of microsatellite instability in a tumor is a highly sensitive indicator of defective mismatch repair (Jass, 1995).

A diagnosis of Lynch syndrome can be made based on clinical findings or through genetic testing. The criteria for a clinical diagnosis are known as the Amsterdam Criteria. These criteria were initially established in 1991, before the availability of genetic testing, and were revised in 1999 (Vasen et al., 1991; Vasen et al., 1999). The original and revised criteria for a clinical diagnosis of HNPCC are described in Table 18.1.

Anne's family history met the Amsterdam I criteria for a clinical diagnosis of Lynch syndrome.

Commentary

Reviewing Anne's medical records and family history questionnaire before her appointment allowed the genetics team to establish well-defined goals for the initial counseling session. These goals included eliciting and addressing the patient's concerns, discussing our assessment of her history, establishing and discussing her clinical diagnosis of Lynch syndrome, discussing the implications of a diagnosis of Lynch syndrome for Anne's risk for future cancers and related management issues, discussing the availability of genetic testing, and discussing implications for her family members.

TABLE 18.1   Original and Revised Amsterdam Criteria for Hereditary Nonpolyposis Colorectal Cancer (Vasen, 1991;Vasen, 1999)

Amsterdam I Criteria (Families must fulfill all criteria); "3-2-1-0" criteria
At least 3 relatives should have a histologically verified colorectal cancer; 1 of them should be a first degree relative of the other 2.
At least 2 successive generations should be affected.
In 1 of the relatives, colorectal cancer should be diagnosed under 50 years of age
Familial adenomatous polyposis should be excluded (0).

Amsterdam II Criteria (Families must fulfill all criteria)
There should be at least 3 relatives with an HNPCC-associated cancer (colorectal cancer, cancer of the endometrium, small bowel, ureter, or renal pelvis).
One should be a first degree relative of the other 2.
At least 2 successive generations should be affected.
At least 1 should be diagnosed before the age of 50.
Familial adenomatous polyposis should be excluded in the colorectal cancer cases, if any.
Tumors should be verified by pathological examination.

Genetic Counseling Visit I

Anne was accompanied to each visit by her husband, John. In contracting with Anne and John, we learned that they had been told that Anne was referred to discuss a possible inherited cause for the cancer in her family. Anne stated that she knew that "cancer ran in her family" and was uncertain what she might learn from us. She seemed skeptical of the utility of the visit, but appeared willing to participate in the process. When questioned further about her own concerns, she shared that she was most anxious about her children developing cancer and truly hoped that we could provide some guidance for their care. We validated the concern Anne had for her children and commended her for taking time to fill out the questionnaires and to come to the appointment. We informed Anne and John that after reviewing Anne's information, we were confident that we could provide valuable information for both Anne and her family, including her children. We explained the general structure of the visit:

- We would briefly review her medical and family histories,
- Discuss our impressions of why there was so much cancer in her family,
- Discuss the possibility of genetic testing,
- And discuss plans for managing cancer risks in the family.

Given the stated concern for their children, we assured Anne and John that we would discuss the children explicitly. Although Anne had not expressed any concerns or questions related to her own care, we discussed that we would also be making some recommendations for Anne's care. The patient and her husband agreed with this plan and denied any additional concerns.

Commentary

Anne's stated concern for her children is quite typical of cancer survivors seen in cancer genetics clinics. Studies suggest that the main reasons to undergo genetic testing for cancer susceptibility, and presumably to seek genetic counseling, are to assess the risk to one's children, to make decisions related to one's own management, and to reduce uncertainty about being a carrier (Esplen et al., 2001; Brandt et al., 2002; Foster et al., 2002; Hadley et al., 2003). Our patient did not initially seem to recognize that a diagnosis of a hereditary cancer syndrome in her would have implications not just for her relatives, but also for her own health management. Specifically, Anne did not voice concerns related to her risk for another cancer or for recurrence of her previous cancer. A diagnosis of a hereditary cancer syndrome in Anne would, in fact, place her at increased risk for a second primary cancer. Therefore, we introduced this topic as part of the agenda for the counseling session.

The review of her medical history during the session included confirmation of Anne's cancer history and treatment, as well as confirmation of her current surveillance and screening practices, including the dates and findings of previous colonoscopies. Her medical and screening histories were consistent with what we had ascertained from the medical records. Anne reported no other significant medical history. We also commended Anne for her vigilant colorectal cancer screening.

We next reviewed the pedigree that we had constructed from Anne's questionnaire, highlighting the hallmarks of a hereditary cancer syndrome found in her family history. In doing so, we validated Anne's assumption that "cancer ran in her family." We also acknowledged the devastating toll that cancer had taken in her family. While some patients may use the family history as a chance to recount their family's experience with cancer, Anne provided little personal or emotional information about her family's cancer history. This initial reluctance to share her personal reaction to cancer changed later in the session as she became more engaged in the conversation, especially as it related to the management of her children.

Anne was informed that we recognized the pattern of cancers in her family as consistent with a clinical diagnosis of Lynch syndrome. We described that Lynch syndrome was the most common inherited colorectal cancer syndrome and that her family contained many of the hallmarks of the condition. Her family tree was used as a visual aid as we described how this diagnosis could be made with the Amsterdam criteria. Anne indicated that she had never heard of Lynch syndrome or HNPCC before and stated, "You mean there are other families like mine out there?" We assured her that not only were there other families like hers, but that we had experience taking care of many families with Lynch syndrome. Anne and John did not seem shocked or upset at the "label" of Lynch syndrome we had given her family. Rather, their body language (moving to the end of their seat and leaning in closer) suggested that their interest in the discussion was increasing. Anne and John were informed that given a diagnosis of Lynch syndrome, it was our hope that by making specific recommendations related to management of the risk for cancer in her family, we could change what cancer meant in the family. Specifically, we hoped that the information we could provide would mean that fewer family members would die from cancer.

Commentary

Anne stated early in the session that she believed that "cancer ran in her family." She had watched many relatives, including her mother, die of cancer at young ages. Telling her that there was an inherited risk for cancer in her family appeared to be stating the blatantly obvious to her. As we proceeded to provide an actual name for the condition, promised to offer a plan for managing the cancer risk in the family, and informed Anne that her family was not alone in having Lynch syndrome, her interest and attention increased.

In general, the identification of a specific inherited cancer syndrome within a family often allows for the provision of information regarding the spectrum of cancers that individuals are at risk for, quantitative risk estimates for the different associated cancers, and a defined management plan. The degree of reassurance that can be provided to patients regarding the medical benefit of recognizing an inherited cancer syndrome varies based in part on differences in the efficacy of screening and preventative methods available for the stated cancers. As described further below, there is evidence supporting the benefit of cancer screening in individuals at risk for Lynch syndrome (Jarvinen et al., 2000; Renkonen-Sinisalo et al., 2000). Therefore, our approach to counseling families with Lynch syndrome tends to stress that knowledge of the condition can be empowering.

We discussed Lynch syndrome with Anne and John and described that the condition was associated with a higher than average risk for certain cancers, especially colorectal cancers and uterine cancers, as well as ovarian and other cancers. We discussed that Lynch syndrome provided an explanation for Anne's early-onset ovarian cancer and for the striking family history of cancer. Given her stated concerns about her children, we told Anne and John that not everyone in the family necessarily inherited the risk for cancer and that not everyone in the family who inherited the risk would necessarily develop a cancer. We promised Anne that we would discuss risks and management issues related to her children later in the session, but that we first wanted to discuss the implications of the diagnosis of Lynch syndrome for her own health and management. Anne and John agreed to this approach.

In considering implications of the diagnosis of Lynch syndrome for Anne, we discussed that she was at increased risk for additional primary cancers, most notably colorectal cancer. We were able to provide some reassurance regarding the chance of Anne having a current colorectal cancer given that she had very recently had a normal colonoscopy. We discussed that unlike the less than optimal screening options for ovarian cancer, screening for colorectal cancer with colonoscopies was highly effective in detecting colorectal cancers at an early stage and also provided the potential to prevent colorectal cancers by identifying and removing precancerous polyps. Anne was also informed of the increased risk for uterine cancer in Lynch syndrome, but was reassured that given her hysterectomy, she was not at risk for that cancer. We also discussed screening options for other Lynch syndrome-related cancers.

Anne was also informed that, in general, a diagnosis of Lynch syndrome did NOT make it more likely for ovarian cancer to recur. Preliminary data suggest that survival rates are similar for gynecologic cancers occurring in patients with Lynch syndrome and for those occurring in the general population (Boks et al., 2002; Crijnen et al., 2005). Furthermore, there is evidence that colorectal cancers occurring in the setting of Lynch syndrome have a better prognosis than those in the general population (Watson et al., 1998).

Commentary

A choice was made early in the counseling to discuss implications for Anne first, rather than initially discussing implications to her children. When such a choice is made, it is critical to let the patient know you have heard her concern and that you plan to address it. In retrospect, it may have been useful to first more fully address the couple's stated concern for their children before discussing implications for Anne. As described below, the couple asked very few questions about Anne's health until we moved on to the discussion of their children.

As one might expect, telling a cancer survivor that she has an increased risk of developing yet another cancer can be distressing and anxiety provoking. When discussing increased risks for cancer, it is important to include information about how that risk can be managed. In general, options include screening, chemoprevention, and prophylactic surgery. The availability and utility of each of these options varies based on the cancer. For Anne, it was important to discuss the proven utility of colorectal cancer screening in families with Lynch syndrome. Importantly, the risk for colorectal cancer can be decreased by at least 50% in families with Lynch syndrome with appropriate screening, including frequent colonoscopies beginning at a young age, typically between ages 20–25 years or 10 years before to the earliest diagnosis in the family (Jarvinen et al., 2000).

Throughout the discussion of Anne's risk for additional cancers and management, Anne and her husband asked few questions about Anne's own medical care. Rather, they remained focused on implications for family members and began asking related questions. Anne and John were able to anticipate some of the issues we had planned to discuss, including the chances their children inherited the risk for cancer and what could be done to prevent cancer in them.

In discussing implications for relatives, we described autosomal dominant inheritance, using the pedigree to demonstrate which relatives appeared to be at risk for having inherited Lynch syndrome. Close relatives at risk (children and siblings) were discussed explicitly, with a plan to review risks to extended family members in more detail at a later visit. We discussed that each of Anne's two children were at 50% risk for having inherited Lynch syndrome, stressing that not everyone who inherits HNPCC develops cancer and sound management could be initiated for her children, as appropriate, based on results of genetic testing. Anne and John were assured that Lynch syndrome was not generally associated with childhood-onset cancers, so that from a medical standpoint, there was no urgency in having her children screened. Anne and John did not appear surprised by the 50% chance of passing the inherited cancer risk on to their children. Again, they had already recognized that cancer "ran in the family" and were likely expecting a significant risk to the children.

A discussion of the inheritance of Lynch syndrome led us directly into a discussion of the value of genetic testing. We discussed that the most informative approach to genetic testing for inherited cancer susceptibility was typically to begin the genetic testing in a family member who was most likely to carry a gene mutation, such as a family member who had an early cancer. This approach is especially important for a condition like Lynch syndrome, in which there are multiple genes involved and limitations in mutation detection. In Anne's family, she was the only cancer survivor, making her the ideal candidate for genetic testing in her family. Given that a clinical diagnosis of Lynch syndrome had already been made in Anne based on the Amsterdam I criteria, identification of the specific gene mutation responsible for the condition in Anne would not alter our recommendations for her care. Therefore, we told Anne that regardless of the results of her genetic testing, she should be screened as per current screening guidelines for families with Lynch syndrome approved by the National Comprehensive Cancer Network (www.nccn.org).

We discussed with Anne and John that the real utility in genetic testing was for her family members. Specifically, the identification of the gene mutation responsible for Lynch syndrome in the family would allow for genetic testing of unaffected at-risk individuals. Those identified as carriers of the putative gene mutation could then use this knowledge to make informed decisions related to management, including screening, chemoprevention, and surgical options. Those who tested negative for the familial mutation could be spared the increased screening and follow general population screening guidelines.

Commentary

Genetic testing for HNPCC and subsequent management of those at increased risk with regular colonoscopies is cost effective and greatly reduces the rate of colorectal cancer development and overall mortality (Syngal et al., 1998; Jarvinen et al., 2000; de Vos tot Nederveen Cappel et al., 2002). For inherited cancer syndromes in which knowledge of one's genetic status will have implications for screening or preventative strategies, particularly when those screening or preventative strategies are of proven efficacy, the traditional nondirective approach to genetic counseling is not appropriate. A narrow definition of nondirective counseling implies that a genetic counselor should refrain from encouraging a particular course of action (Baker et al., 1998, Chapter 1). In cancer genetic counseling, the genetic counselor may, in fact, encourage a particular course of action (i.e., "Genetic testing for Lynch syndrome is recommended to confirm your diagnosis as well to provide a means for identifying at risk family members. This would help determine who needs increased screening." or "We strongly encourage you to share information about your genetic test results with your family members as it will help them receive the most appropriate risk assessment and management.") Perhaps a more appropriate definition of nondirective counseling in this context is supporting client autonomy and promoting active, self-confident decision-making (Kessler, 1997; White, 1997). Such a definition has more relevance in a setting where evidence exists that a particular course of action is advantageous.

As we expected given Anne's stated desire to help her family, she was eager to pursue genetic testing. We discussed our typical approach to genetic testing for Lynch syndrome, which in our center included microsatellite instability testing (MSI) and immunohistochemistry (IHC) on archived tumor tissue, followed by germline testing from a blood sample to identify the specific gene mutation. For Anne, performing MSI and IHC before germline testing would potentially identify the gene responsible for the condition in her family and would allow a more focused approach to germline testing. We proposed performing the testing in a stepwise manner (MSI/IHC first followed by germline testing), but offered to collect samples for both the tumor testing and germline testing at this visit in an effort to minimize the number of visits Anne would need to make to our clinic.

Informed consent is a necessary precursor to genetic testing for hereditary cancer syndromes. The basic elements of informed consent are described below, including details related to the discussion with Anne (Geller et al., 1997, 2003; Trepanier et al., 2004):

- **Purpose of the test and who to test**: A diagnosis of Lynch syndrome was already made in Anne's family. The purpose of the test was to identify the specific gene mutation responsible for the condition in the family. Anne was the most appropriate person in whom to initiate testing given that she was the only cancer survivor in the family.

- **General information about the gene(s) being tested**: Anne was informed that MSI and IHC would be performed on her archived tumor tissue first and that based on those results, her blood sample would be tested for mutations in one of the mismatch repairs genes, as appropriate.

- **Possible test results**: Ultimately, a mutation in a mismatch repair gene could be identified. This would allow other family members to undergo genetic testing. Alternatively, a mutation in a mismatch repair gene might not be identified. In this case, the clinical diagnosis of Lynch syndrome would remain and all at-risk relatives would need to be followed according to management guidelines for Lynch syndrome. A gene variant of uncertain significance could also be identified. In this case, all at-risk relatives would need to be followed according to management guidelines for Lynch syndrome until the significance of the gene variant could be determined.

- **Likelihood of a positive result**: The probability of identifying the specific gene mutation responsible for Lynch syndrome in the family was estimated with two models, MMRPRO and PREMM (Balmana et al., 2006; Chen et al., 2006). These models suggested a 46% and 44% likelihood of identifying the mutation, respectively.

- **Technical aspects and accuracy of the test**: Anne was informed of the multistep process involved in genetic testing for Lynch syndrome. She was informed that because of limitations in current technologies, genetic testing was not able to identify the specific gene mutation responsible for Lynch syndrome in all families. The spectrum of mutations responsible for Lynch syndrome can include nonsense, missense, and frameshift mutations, as well as mutations that alter splicing, and larger genomic mutations such as deletions, duplications, rearrangements, or other chromosomal abnormalities.

- **Economic considerations**: The patient was informed of the cost of her tests and that the genetic testing would likely be covered by her insurance. Anne stated she wanted to proceed with testing regardless of insurance coverage and did not want to verify insurance coverage before ordering the test.

- **Risks of genetic discrimination**: Anne voiced concern about the potential for genetic discrimination. She stated that she knew her own personal cancer history alone was likely to cause difficulties should she need to purchase new medical insurance or life insurance for herself. She was concerned about the risk for her children to experience genetic discrimination based on her own genetic testing. We addressed these concerns based on current federal and state legislation. Specifically, the patient was informed that at the federal level, the Health Insurance Portability and Accountability Act (HIPAA) of 1996 provided some protection against discrimination with regard to health insurance for individuals with group policies (www.hhs.gov/ocr/hipaa/) (Fleisher and Cole, 2001). We discussed that our state also had legislation to prevent health corporations from requiring members or applicants to undergo genetic testing or disclose genetic test results or information before issuing, renewing, or continuing insurance (www.migeneticsconnection.org). We shared our professional opinion that the proven benefits of genetic testing for Lynch syndrome outweighed the theoretical risks for insurance discrimination. We discussed that similar protections were not in place for life or disability insurance. These are common concerns for patients seeking genetic testing for cancer predisposition and for other adult-onset conditions, making it critical for genetic counselors to have knowledge of current federal and state legislation.

- **Psychosocial considerations**: We discussed Anne's readiness to undergo genetic testing. She was highly motivated and expressed that she felt that genetic testing was a gift she could provide her family. While some patients may fear receiving a positive test result from genetic testing, given that Anne had already been diagnosed with cancer, had been given a clinical diagnosis of Lynch syndrome, and desired to help her family, she expressed that she was not worried about receiving a positive test result. Her minimal concerns related to coping with genetic test results are consistent with data in the literature that suggest that individuals who accept genetic testing for hereditary cancer syndromes may represent a self-selected group who have confidence in their ability to cope with results (Vernon et al., 1999; Aktan-Collan et al., 2000; Hadley et al., 2003).

- **Confidentiality issues**: We discussed that Anne's results would be part of her medical record and would be subject to the same confidentiality requirements as the rest of her medical record. Her results would not be released to family members without her written consent.

- **Utilization of test results for medical surveillance and preventative measures**: We discussed that her management would be impacted by her clinical diagnosis of Lynch syndrome, but NOT by the proposed genetic test results.

- **Alternatives to genetic testing**: Anne was aware that genetic testing was optional. If she declined genetic testing, DNA banking could be helpful by allowing a sample of her DNA to be available to her family members in the future.
- **Storage and potential reuse of genetic material**: Anne's DNA would not be stored by the testing laboratory upon completion of the genetic testing.

After discussing these elements of informed consent with Anne and her husband, Anne signed informed consent documents for genetic testing. We scheduled a return visit for the purpose of reviewing the test results. Anne was provided with patient education materials related to Lynch syndrome and also sent a letter summarizing the visit.

Commentary

We had reviewed a large amount of new information with the family at this initial visit and had accomplished our initial goals. These goals included eliciting and addressing the patient's concerns, discussing our assessment of her history, establishing and discussing her clinical diagnosis of Lynch syndrome, discussing the implications of a diagnosis of Lynch syndrome for Anne's risk for future cancers and related management issues, discussing the availability of genetic testing, and discussing implications for her family members. We also explicitly addressed Anne's stated concerns regarding her children. Specifically, she was informed that her children were at risk for Lynch syndrome and that our hope was that genetic testing would allow us to determine who inherited the condition. Appropriate screening recommendations could be made for her children pending the results of genetic testing. Given that Anne and John had repeatedly discussed their children, we also previewed for them that genetic testing for cancer susceptibility was not generally performed in children unless medical intervention was warranted in childhood (MacDonald, 2000; Prenatal and Childhood Testing for Adult-onset Disorders, NSGC Position Statement 1995). Given that screening for colorectal cancer typically begins at age 20 to 25 or ten years younger than the earliest cancer diagnosis in the family, Anne was told that genetic testing for her children was not recommended before the age of 18.

Genetic Test Results

Genetic screening of Anne's tumor showed high levels of microsatellite instability and negative staining for the MSH2 and MSH6 proteins. These results were entirely consistent with the clinical diagnosis of Lynch syndrome and also suggested that MSH2 was the most likely gene responsible for cancer in the family. MSH2 and MSH6 form a heterodimer, so it was not unexpected to see loss of both proteins.

Germline testing of the MSH2 gene revealed a mutation. This mutation was a two-base pair insertion in exon 6 that, while not previously described, was predicted to result in premature truncation of the protein.

Genetic Counseling Visit II

Results from the germline testing were communicated with Anne and John at a follow-up appointment. This session was started with very brief contracting in which we reviewed that at her previous visit a diagnosis of Lynch syndrome had been made. We confirmed that Anne had returned to receive results of genetic testing for the condition and informed her that she was found to carry a mutation of the MSH2 gene. We told her that the genetic test result provided further confirmation of her diagnosis of Lynch syndrome and allowed at risk relatives to undergo genetic testing. Given that we had repeatedly discussed that Anne had a clinical diagnosis of Lynch syndrome and that knowledge of the specific gene mutation would be helpful for her family, these results were presented to the patient as "good news." Anne stated she was happy that the gene mutation had been identified.

Before moving on with the session, we felt it was important to review some of the "take-home messages" from the last visit and address any of Anne and John's questions. As we reviewed the features and inheritance of Lynch syndrome, Anne and John appeared to have a clear understanding of the natural history and of the inheritance of the condition. It became apparent that they had done a lot of thinking about Lynch syndrome since their last visit. Anne told us that she knew she would need yearly colonoscopies and that removing polyps could prevent cancer, but questioned what we could do to prevent the polyps and colon cancer risk altogether. Was there a pill she could take? Would changing her diet or exercising more lower her risk for colon cancer? Was there a way to fix the gene mutation? We told Anne that these were excellent questions and that, in fact, these were questions that researchers were currently trying to answer. We told Anne that the only way to eliminate the risk for a colorectal cancer was to entirely remove the colon and rectum. We told Anne that this option was very rarely chosen by patients with Lynch syndrome since colorectal cancer screening with colonoscopies was so effective. Although prophylactic co-lectomy is feasible, when quality of life is considered, colonoscopies provide the greatest benefit in quality-adjusted life years (Lee et al., 2001). Regarding the availability of "a pill" to lower the risk for colon cancer, we discussed that while some cancer risks can be lowered with certain medications, chemoprevention of colorectal cancer in Lynch syndrome was not currently available, although much research was being done in this area. We emphasized that the mainstay of colorectal cancer risk management in Lynch syndrome was screening with colonoscopies.

Commentary

It was interesting that at the initial visit, Anne voiced few questions or concerns related to her own cancer risk or management. She had been primarily focused on her children. At this second visit, the patient's initial questions were related to her own management. This is not to say that she did not still have concerns for her children. Rather, it seemed that Anne and John had a deeper understanding of the many implications of the diagnosis in the family. Furthermore, Anne's questions related to fixing the gene mutation were a reminder to us that although we had shared "good news" about having found the gene mutation, better news would have been that we found the gene mutation and that we had a magic bullet to fix it.

As we had at our previous visit, we once again discussed the implications for family members. Anne told us she was eager to share the news with her brother and sister, who had not yet had any colorectal cancer screening. Anne's pedigree was used to explicitly identify other family members in whom genetic testing would be beneficial, including her siblings, her children (when they were a bit older), her maternal cousins, and her maternal uncle. Anne was also encouraged to reach out to her maternal grandfather's relatives, who also appeared to be at risk. Similar to our counseling regarding the benefits of genetic testing for Anne, we were directive in our approach and encouraged Anne to share the information about Lynch syndrome and her genetic test results with these relatives. Once again, the rationale for this directive approach was that knowledge of one's genetic status in relation to Lynch syndrome would have dramatic implications for their management. Anne told us, "That is why I started all this, to try and help my family." She shared that she had already discussed the importance of knowing about their family history of cancer with her children, ages 12 and 10. She shared that she intended to tell her children that "even if I am not around when you turn 18, you need to get checked out for the cancer gene." Anne also planned to enlist the help of her husband, the children's pediatrician, and her sister to remind her children about Lynch syndrome and genetic testing as they approached the age of 18.

Commentary

Anne's discussion of making sure her children were able to avail themselves of genetic testing when they reached the age of 18 was the first time during our interactions that we had discussed the possibility that Anne might die before her children reached adulthood. As one might expect, this was a very powerful moment as Anne discussed her own mortality and concerns for her children. It proved to be one of those moments that "struck a chord" with me on many levels, as a counselor, a parent, and a woman, requiring me to pause, catch my breath, and recognize her for her bravery and dedication to her family's welfare.

To facilitate the process of informing other family members, we provided Anne with multiple copies of a "family notification letter" and her genetic test results which she could share with relatives. This letter included very basic information including (1) the fact that Lynch syndrome had been diagnosed in the family, (2) information about Lynch syndrome and its inheritance, (3) the specific gene mutation responsible for the condition in the family, (4) recommendations to discuss this information with their physician, and (5) contact information for our clinic.

Anne and her husband shared that they were very appreciative of the information they had learned through the course of genetic counseling and genetic testing. In the year following Anne's appointment, we had the opportunity to test Anne's siblings, both of whom tested negative for the familial gene mutation.

Commentary

Discussion of the cancer risks to relatives is a critical component of cancer genetic counseling. Providing written materials for patients to share with relatives can help patients feel confident in their ability to sharing accurate, relevant details to their relatives. Depending on the cancer risks within a family and the potential harm that could result, if the proband does not wish to share information with at-risk relatives, the genetic counselor may wish to seek an ethics consult (ASHG, 1998).

Summary

This case illustrates common issues in providing cancer genetic counseling. These include the following:

- Cancer risk assessment entails careful review of a patient's medical history and family history. Hallmarks of a strong hereditary risk for cancer include multiple generations affected with cancer, early ages of onset, a tendency for multiple primary, bilateral, or multifocal cancers, and patterns of specific cancers within a family.
- A diagnosis of a hereditary cancer syndrome can be made through clinical criteria and/or through genetic testing. A diagnosis of a hereditary cancer syndrome can have implications both for the proband's health management as well as for relatives.
- Depending on the efficacy of interventions available for individuals found to have a hereditary risk for cancer, genetic counseling related to cancer genetic issues may be more directive than is typical for other arenas of clinical genetics.
- Common issues raised in genetic counseling for cancer susceptibility include, but are not limited to, concerns about the development of additional primary cancers in cancer survivors, the risk for cancer in relatives, and the potential for discrimination.
- The process of providing comprehensive cancer genetic risk assessment and counseling is complex. Patients typically have informational, medical, and psychosocial needs and can benefit from a multidisciplinary approach, including access to genetic counselors, medical geneticists, surgeons, oncologists, social workers, oncology nurses, psychologists, and other health professionals (Trepanier et al., 2004). Genetic counselors working independently, without supervision, should be prepared to make referrals to appropriate medical professionals for long-term medical management as needed.
- The identification of a mutation within a cancer family is often viewed as **good news**, empowering family members with options for testing, surveillance and treatment.

This case was particularly rewarding for me as a genetic counselor given Anne's dedication to her family's welfare, including not just her children, but additional relatives as well. Furthermore, given the proven efficacy of interventions for Lynch, it is gratifying to know that we may be able to make some difference in survival in a family that had been devastated by cancer.

REFERENCES

Aarnio M, Sankila R et al. (1999) Cancer risk in mutation carriers of DNA-mismatch-repair genes. *Int J Cancer* 81(2):214–218.

Aktan-Collan K, Mecklin JP et al. (2000) Predictive genetic testing for hereditary non-polyposis colorectal cancer: uptake and long-term satisfaction. *Int J Cancer* 89(1):44–50.

ASCO (2003) American Society of Clinical Oncology policy statement update: genetic testing for cancer susceptibility. *J Clin Oncol* 21(12):2397–2406.

ASHG (1998) ASHG statement. Professional disclosure of familial genetic information. The American Society of Human Genetics Social Issues Subcommittee on Familial Disclosure. *Am J Hum Genet* 62(2):474–483.

ASHG/ACMG Report (1995) Points to consider: Ethical, legal, and psychosocial implications of genetic testing in children and adolescents, *Am J Hum Genet* 57:1233–124.

Baker DL, Schuette JL et al. (1998) *A Guide to Genetic Counseling*. New York: Wiley-Liss.

Balmana J, Stockwell DH et al. (2006) Prediction of MLH1 and MSH2 mutations in Lynch syndrome. *JAMA* 296(12):1469–1478.

Boks DE, Trujillo AP et al. (2002) Survival analysis of endometrial carcinoma associated with hereditary nonpolyposis colorectal cancer. *Int J Cancer* 102(2):198–200.

Boyd J (2001) BRCA: the breast, ovarian, and other cancer genes. *Gynecol Oncol* 80(3):337–340.

Boyd J (2003) Specific keynote: hereditary ovarian cancer: what we know *Gynecol Oncol* 88(1 Pt 2): S8–S10; discussion S11- S13.

Brandt R, Hartmann E et al. (2002) Motivations and concerns of women considering genetic testing for breast cancer: a comparison between affected and at-risk probands. *Genet Test* 6(3):203–205.

Bioethics Committee, Canadian Paediatric Society (CPS) (2003) Guidelines for genetic testing of healthy children. *Paediatrics Child Health* 8(1):42–45.

Casey G, Lindor NM et al. (2005) Conversion analysis for mutation detection in MLH1 and MSH2 in patients with colorectal cancer. *JAMA* 293(7):799–809.

Cederquist K, Emanuelsson M et al. (2005) Two Swedish founder MSH6 mutations, one nonsense and one missense, conferring high cumulative risk of Lynch syndrome. *Clin Genet* 68(6):533–541.

Chen S, Wang W et al. (2006) Prediction of germline mutations and cancer risk in the Lynch syndrome. *JAMA* 296(12):1479–1487.

Christian SM et al. (2000) Parental decisions following prenatal diagnosis of sex chromosome aneuploidy: a trend over time, *Prenat Diagn* 20:37–40.

Clarke A (1994) The genetic testing of children. Working Party of the Clinical Genetics Society (UK). *J Med Genet* 31(10):785–797

Clow C, Scriver C (1977) Knowledge about and attitudes toward genetic screening among high-school students: The Tay-Sachs experience. *Pediatrics* 59(1):86–90.

Crijnen TE, Janssen-Heijnen ML et al. (2005) Survival of patients with ovarian cancer due to a mismatch repair defect *Fam Cancer* 4(4):301–305.

de la Chapelle A (2004) Genetic predisposition to colorectal cancer. *Nat Rev Cancer* 4(10):769–780.

de Vos tot Nederveen Cappel WH, Nagengast FM et al. (2002) Surveillance for hereditary nonpolyposis colorectal cancer: a long-term study on 114 families. *Dis Colon Rectum* 45(12):1588–1594.

Douglas FS, O'Dair LC et al. (1999) The accuracy of diagnoses as reported in families with cancer: a retrospective study. *J Med Genet* 36(4):309–312.

Dunlop MG, Farrington SM et al. (1997) Cancer risk associated with germline DNA mismatch repair gene mutations. *Hum Mol Genet* 6(1):105–110.

Esplen MJ, Madlensky L et al. (2001) Motivations and psychosocial impact of genetic testing for HNPCC. *Am J Med Genet* 103(1):9–15.

Fanos JH (1997) Developmental tasks of childhood and adolescence: Implications for genetic testing. *Am J Med Genet* 71:2–28.

Fanos JH, Gatti RA, (1999) A mark on the arm: Myths of carrier status in sibs of individuals with ataxia-telangiectasia. *Am J Med Genet* 89:338–346.

Fleisher LD and Cole LJ (2001) Health Insurance Portability and Accountability Act is here: what price privacy? *Genet Med* 3(4):286–289.

Ford D, Easton DF et al. (1998) Genetic heterogeneity and penetrance analysis of the BRCA1 and BRCA2 genes in breast cancer families. The Breast Cancer Linkage Consortium. *Am J Hum Genet* 62(3):676–689.

Foster C, Evans DG et al. (2002) Predictive testing for BRCA1/2: attributes, risk perception and management in a multi-centre clinical cohort. *Br J Cancer* 86(8):1209–1216.

Gardner RJ, Sutherland GR(eds.) (2004) *Chromosome Abnormalities and Genetic Counseling* (3rd ed.). Oxford University Press, Inc., p. 393–400.

Geller G, Botkin JR et al. (1997) Genetic testing for susceptibility to adult-onset cancer. The process and content of informed consent *JAMA* 277(18):1467–1474.

Germain CB (1994) Emerging conceptions of family development over the life course. *Families in Society: J Contemp Hum Serv* 75(5):259–267.

Hadley DW, Jenkins J et al. (2003) Genetic counseling and testing in families with hereditary nonpolyposis colorectal cancer. *Arch Intern Med* 163(5):573–582.

Hagerman RJ (2001) Fragile X syndrome. In: Cassidy, S.B and Allanson, J.E. (eds), *Management of Genetic Syndromes.* Wiley-Liss, Inc.

Hagerman RJ, Cronister A (eds) (2002) *Fragile X Syndrome: Diagnosis, Treatment, and Research.* (3rd ed). Baltimore; Johns Hopkins University Press.

Hagerman PJ, Hagerman RJ (2004) The fragile-X premutation: A maturing perspective. *Am J Hum Genet* 74:805–816.

Hampel H, Stephens JA et al. (2005) Cancer risk in hereditary nonpolyposis colorectal cancer syndrome: later age of onset. *Gastroenterology* 129(2):415–421.

Ibrahim, F. (1991) Contribution of cultural worldview to generic counseling and development. *J Couns Dev* 70:13–19.

Jarvinen O, Lehesjoki AE, Lindlof M, Uutela A, Kaariainen H (1999) Carrier testing of children for two X-linked diseases: a retrospective evaluation of experience and satisfaction of subjects and their mothers. *Genet Test* 3(4):347–355.

Jarvinen O, Hietala M, Aalto AM, Arvio M, Uutela A, Aula P, Kaariainen H (2000) A retrospective study of long-term psychosocial consequences and satisfaction after carrier testing in childhood in an autosomal recessive disease: aspartylglucosaminuria. *Clin Genet* 58(6):447–454.

Jarvinen HJ, Aarnio M et al. (2000) Controlled 15-year trial on screening for colorectal cancer in families with hereditary nonpolyposis colorectal cancer. *Gastroenterology* 118(5): 829–834.

Jass JR (1995) Colorectal adenoma progression and genetic change: is there a link? *Ann Med* 27(3):301–306.

Kenen R, Smith ACM, Watkins C, Zuber-Pitore C (2000) To use or not to use: Male partner's perspectives on decision making about prenatal diagnosis. *J Genet Couns* 9:33–45.

Kessler S (1992) Psychological aspects of genetic counseling. VII. Thoughts on directiveness. *J Genet Couns* 1:9–17 (and personal communication)

Kessler S (1997) Psychological aspects of genetic counseling. XI. Nondirectiveness revisited. *Am J Med Genet* 72(2):164–171.

Korenromp MJ Christiaens GCML, van den Bout J, Mulder EJH et al. (2005a) Long-term psychological consequences of pregnancy termination for fetal abnormality: a cross-sectional study. *Prenat Diagn* 25(3):253–260.

Korenromp MJ, Christiaens GCML, van den Bout J, Mulder EJH et al. (2005b) Psychological consequences of termination of pregnancy for fetal abnormality: similarities and differences between partners. *Prenat Diagn* 25(13):1226–1233.

Lachiewicz AM, Dawson DV, Spiridigliozzi GA, McConkie-Rosell A (2006) Arithmetic difficulties in females with the fragile X permutation. *Am J Med Genet A.* 140(7):665–672.

Lee JS, Petrelli NJ et al. (2001) Rectal cancer in hereditary nonpolyposis colorectal cancer. *Am J Surg* 181(3):207–210.

Lewis LJ (2002) Models of genetic counseling and their effects on multicultural genetic counseling. *J Genet Couns* 3:193–212.

Linden MG, Bender BG (2002) Fifty-one prenatally diagnosed children and adolescents with sex chromosome abnormalities. *Am J Med Genet* 110:11–18.

Linden MG, Bender BG, Robinson A (2002) Genetic counseling for sex chromosome abnormalities. *Am J Med Genet* 110:3–10.

Love RR, Evans AM et al. (1985) The accuracy of patient reports of a family history of cancer. *J Chronic Dis* 38(4):289–293.

Lynch J (1997) The genetics and natural history of hereditary colon cancer. *Semin Oncol Nurs* 13(2):91–98.

Lynch HT de la Chapelle A (2003) Hereditary colorectal cancer. *N Engl J Med* 348(10): 919–932.

MacDonald DJ, Lessick M (2000) Hereditary cancers in children and ethical and psychosocial implications. *J Pediatr Nurs* 15(4):217–25.

Marra G, Boland CR (1995) Hereditary nonpolyposis colorectal cancer: the syndrome, the genes, and historical perspectives. *J Natl Cancer Inst* 87(15):1114–1125.

Marteau TM et al. (2002) Outcomes of pregnancies diagnosed with Klinefelter syndrome: the possible influence of health professionals. *Prenat Diagn* 22:562–566.

Martin TL. Doka KJ (2000) In: Beth Schad and Karin McAndrews (eds.), Men Don't Cry...Women Do: Transcending Gender Stereotypes of Grief, p. 13.

Mazzocco MM, Holden JJ (1996) Neuropsychological profiles of three sisters homozygous for the fragile X permutation. *Am J Med Genet* 64(2):323–328.

McConkie-Rosell A, Spiridigliozzi GA, Iafolla T, Tarleton J, Lachiewicz AM (1997) Carrier testing in the fragile X syndrome: attitudes and opinions of obligate carriers. *Am J Med Genet* 68(1):62–69.

McConkie-Rosell A, Spiridigliozzi GA, Rounds K, Dawson DV, Sullivan JA, Burgess D, Lachiewicz AM (1999) Parental attitudes regarding carrier testing in children at risk for fragile X syndrome. *Am J Med Genet.* 82(3):206–211.

McConkie-Rosell A, Spiridigliozzi GA, Sullivan JA, Dawson DV, Lachiewicz AM (2002) Carrier testing in fragile X syndrome: when to tell and test. *Am J Med Genet.* 110(1):36–44.

McConkie-Rosell A, Finucane B, Cronister A, Abrams L, Bennett RL, Pettersen BJ (2005) Genetic counseling for fragile X syndrome: updated recommendations of the National Society of Genetic Counselors. *J Genet Couns* 14(4):249–270.

McConkie-Rosell A, Abrams L, Finucane B, Cronister A, Gane LW, Coffey SM, Sherman S, Nelson LM, Berry-Kravis E, Hessl D, Chiu S, Street N, Vatave A, Hagerman RJ. (2007) Recommendations from multi-disciplinary focus groups on cascade testing and genetic counseling for fragile X-associated disorders. *J Genet Couns* 16(5):593–606.

Mezei G, Papp C, Toth-Pal E et al. (2004) Factors influencing parental decision making in prenatal diagnosis of sex chromosome aneuploidy. *Obstet Gynecol* 104:94–101.

Minnick, MA and Delp, KJ (eds.) (1992) *A Time To Decide, A Time To Heal*, Pineapple Press, MI

Pai GS, Lewandowski RC, Borgaonkar DS (eds.) (2003) *Handbook of Chromosomal Syndromes*. Hoboken, NJ: John Wiley & Sons, Inc. p. 334–336.

Ratcliffe SG, Paul N (eds.) (1986) Prospective studies on children with sex chromosome aneuploidy. In: Nielsen J et al., *Chromosome examination of 20,222 newborn children: Results from a 7.5 year study in Arhus, Denmark, in Birth Defects Orig Art Ser* 22(3): 209–219.

Renkonen-Sinisalo L, Aarnio M et al. (2000) Surveillance improves survival of colorectal cancer in patients with hereditary nonpolyposis colorectal cancer. *Cancer Detect Prev* 24(2):137–142.

Rolland JS (1987) Chronic illness and the life cycle: A conceptual framework. *Fam Process* 26:203–221

Sagi M et al. (2001) Prenatal diagnosis of sex chromosome aneuploidy: possible reasons for high rates of pregnancy termination. *Prenat Diagn* 21:461–465.

Saul RA, Tarleton JC (updated April 2007) FMR1-Related Disorders In: *GeneReviews at GeneTests: Medical Genetics Information Resource (database online)*. Copyright, University of Washington, Seattle. 1997–2007. Available at http://www.genetests.org.

Sherman S, Pletcher BA, Driscoll DA (2005) Fragile X syndrome: diagnostic and carrier testing *Genet Med.* 7(8):584–587.

Street E, Soldan J (1998) A Conceptual framework for the psychosocial issues faced by families with genetic conditions. *Families Syst Health* 16(3):217–232.

Sue D, Arrendondo P, McDavis R (1995) Multicultural counseling competencies and standards. In: Ponterotto, Casas Suzuki and Alexander,(eds), *Handbook of Multicultural Counseling*, Thousand Oaks, Sage CA: Publications, p. 634–643.

Syngal S, Weeks JC et al. (1998) Benefits of colonoscopic surveillance and prophylactic colectomy in patients with hereditary nonpolyposis colorectal cancer mutations. *Ann Intern Med* 129(10):787–796.

Szybowska M, Hewson S, Antle BJ, Babul-Hirji R (2007) Assessing the informational needs of adolescents with a genetic condition: what do they want to know? *J Genet Couns* 16(2):201–210.

Theis B, Boyd N et al. (1994) Accuracy of family cancer history in breast cancer patients. *Eur J Cancer Prev* 3(4):321–327.

Tishler CI (1981) The psychological aspects of genetic counseling, *Am J Nurs*, 81(04):733–734.

Trepanier A, Ahrens M et al. (2004) Genetic cancer risk assessment and counseling: recommendations of the national society of genetic counselors. *J Genet Couns* 13(2):83–114.

Umar A (2004) Lynch syndrome (HNPCC) and microsatellite instability. *Dis Markers* 20(4–5):179–180.

Vasen HF, Mecklin JP et al. (1991) The International Collaborative Group on Hereditary Non-Polyposis Colorectal Cancer (ICG-HNPCC). *Dis Colon Rectum* 34(5):424–425.

Vasen HF, Watson P et al. (1999) New clinical criteria for hereditary nonpolyposis colorectal cancer (HNPCC, Lynch syndrome) proposed by the International Collaborative group on HNPCC. *Gastroenterology* 116(6):1453–1456.

Vasen HF, Stormorken A et al. (2001) MSH2 mutation carriers are at higher risk of cancer than MLH1 mutation carriers: a study of hereditary nonpolyposis colorectal cancer families. *J Clin Oncol* 19(20):4074–4080.

Vernon SW, Gritz ER et al. (1999) Intention to learn results of genetic testing for hereditary colon cancer. *Cancer Epidemiol Biomarkers Prev* 8(4 Pt 2): 353–360.

Watson P, Lin KM et al. (1998) Colorectal carcinoma survival among hereditary nonpolyposis colorectal carcinoma family members. *Cancer* 83(2):259–266.

Weil J (2000) *Psychosocial Genetic Counseling*. New York. Oxford University Press.

Weil J (2001) Multicultural education and genetic counseling *Clin Genet* 59(3):143–149.

White MT (1997) "Respect for autonomy" in genetic counseling: An analysis and a proposal. *J Genet Couns* 6:297–313.

Wittenberger MD, Hagerman RJ, Sherman SL, McConkie-Rosell A, Welt CK, Rebar RW, Corrigan EC, Simpson JL, Nelson LM (2007) The FMR1 premutation and reproduction *Fertil Steril* 87(3):456–465.

Zeesman S, Clow CL, Cartier L, Scriver CR (1984) A private view of heterozygosity: eight-year follow-up study on carriers of the Tay-Sachs gene detected by high school screening in Montreal. *Am J Med Genet.* 18(4):769–778.

Index

Academic opportunities for genetics counselors, 474–475

Acceptance of responsibility, psychosocial issues in genetic counseling and, 154–155

Accreditation for genetic counseling training programs, 21

Accuracy issues:
ethics in genetics counseling, informed consent and, 370
genetic testing, 287
genetic test results, 122–123
medical genetics evaluation, 256
pedigree construction and, 54
research design and, 451–452

Action decisions:
decision-making models and, 226
ethics of genetic counseling and, 380

Action stage of health behavior, 198

Active listening, in interviewing, 80–83

Adolescents:
decision-making models and, 238, 382–383
genetic counseling guidelines for, 564–565

Adoption data, pedigree construction and, 52

Adult learners:
genetics education programs for, 496–497
patient education practices and, 179–181

Adult-onset diseases, genetic counseling and, 15–16

Adult patients, medical genetics examinations, 275

Advanced counseling students, evaluation of, 422

Advanced education and training for genetics counselors, 472–473

Advocacy groups:
discussion during interviewing of, 89–90
importance of, 104
international resources, 104–106
online directories, 104–105
resources for patients, 104–105
support group literature, evaluation of, 105–106

Affective issues:
assessment during interviewing of, 89–90
ethics of genetic counseling and, 10

A Guide to Genetic Counseling, Second Edition, Edited by Wendy Uhlmann, Jane Schuette, and Beverly Yashar
Copyright © 2009 by John Wiley & Sons, Inc.